OXFORD READING

BIOET

Published in this series

Other volumes are in preparation

BIOETHICS

Edited by
JOHN HARRIS

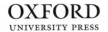

OXFORD
UNIVERSITY PRESS

OXFORD
UNIVERSITY PRESS

Great Clarendon Street, Oxford OX2 6DP

Oxford University Press is a department of the University of Oxford.
It furthers the University's objective of excellence in research,
scholarship, and education by publishing worldwide in

Oxford New York

Auckland Bangkok Buenos Aires Cape Town Chennai
Dar es Salaam Delhi Hong Kong Istanbul Karachi Kolkata
Kuala Lumpur Madrid Melbourne Mexico City Mumbai Nairobi
São Paulo Shanghai Taipei Tokyo Toronto

Oxford is a registered trade mark of Oxford University Press
in the UK and in certain other countries

Published in the United States
by Oxford University Press Inc., New York

Introduction and selection © Oxford University Press 2001

Database right Oxford University Press (maker)

First published 2001

British Library Cataloguing in Publication Data

Data available

Library of Congress Cataloging in Publication Data

Data available

ISBN 0–19–875257–1

3 5 7 9 10 8 6 4

Typeset in Times
by RefineCatch Limited, Bungay, Suffolk
Printed in Great Britain by
Biddles Ltd, *www.biddles.co.uk*

CONTENTS

INTRODUCTION: THE SCOPE AND IMPORTANCE OF BIOETHICS

JOHN HARRIS

The Oxford Readings in Philosophy series aims to collect the outstanding works in a branch of philosophy and present them in a stimulating and an accessible form so that all those interested in the field will have available the best possible introduction to the range, importance, and interest of the area of study in question. The preparation of such a volume inevitably involves serious reflection on the nature of the subject matter itself.

In this introductory essay I will try to say something about the evolution and nature of bioethics and in doing so say something about how bioethics has arrived at the point of being a distinct and important branch of philosophy, and why it is indeed a branch of philosophy and not another thing altogether. We will then look at two different developments in contemporary bioethics which threaten not only to distort the nature of bioethics but to undermine its essential function. In doing so we will have something to say about the distinctive contribution of bioethics in the contemporary world.

THE HISTORY OF BIOETHICS

Bioethics as it is understood today has really two distinct origins. The first is in what might be termed 'traditional medical ethics', which for many years was concerned principally, and at times exclusively, with what we might call matters of 'etiquette', the daily proper conduct of physicians. The second origin is moral philosophy.

Considerations about the ethical implications of medical practice have always been important in the understanding of the Western medical profession and in the education of medical apprentices and later medical students.[1] These concerns were first given expression in the Hippocratic oath, which emerged in early Greek medicine, but which became important because it

---

[1] Here I have been greatly helped by the work of my colleagues Søren Holm, himself both a clinician and a philosopher, and Charles Erin and Rebecca Bennett.

resonated with later Christian values. It is, however, important to note that the Hippocratic tradition has never been the only tradition in medical ethics. There have always been competing traditions.

Certain historical periods have been marked by a distinct lack of reflection on the content of the rules of medical ethics, and in consequence what passed for medical ethics degenerated into the sort of normative system we find in the rules of 'etiquette' or good manners—rules of professional conduct to be learned by rote and which, if followed, assure acceptance by fellow professionals. The Hippocratic oath, often still held up as some sort of guarantee of the ethical bona fides of the medical profession, is in effect the code of conduct of a closed and self-protecting guild, as much if not more concerned with looking after the interests of its fellow members than with the ethics of patient care or duties to society. In other periods medicine has been treated as problematic, and philosophy has been employed in the criticism and reconstruction of medical practice. In the English-speaking world one can date the beginning of modern professional ethics to the 1803 publication of *Medical Ethics* by the Manchester physician Thomas Percival.[2] Percival's ideas formed the basis of the early ethics codes of the American and British Medical Associations, and also influenced the codes of the World Medical Association as late as the 1940s and 1950s. The cornerstone of this conception of ethics was the responsibility of the professional towards the patient, on the one hand, and towards the profession, on the other.

This understanding of ethics has increasingly been challenged in the complex health care systems in the Western world as the users of those systems have become aware of their rights or entitlements as persons, as citizens, and as purchasers (whether directly or indirectly) of the medical services they use. (See Chapters 15, 16, and 17.)

The other foundation of bioethics is moral philosophy. In the tradition dominant in the United Kingdom, North America, and Australasia moral philosophy became increasingly scholastic and removed from the ethical concerns of real people. In this period in the middle of the twentieth century the most prominent academic philosophers turned away from an engagement with real moral problems to discussions of meta-ethics. Moral philosophy thus lost its important role as a critique of, and to some extent a corrective to, the morally problematic aspects of politics and social life. During the 1960s many young philosophers began again to turn to the moral problems of modern society, utilizing the philosophical tools of modern

[2] Thomas Percival, *Medical Ethics; or, A Code of Institutes and Precepts, Adapted to the Professional Conduct of Physicians and Surgeons* (Manchester: S. Russell, 1803).

Anglo-American analytic philosophy. This revival of philosophical attention to real and pressing issues of public concern can be traced to the Campaign for Nuclear Disarmament and the prominent role in that movement played by Bertrand Russell. Although Russell seems not to have thought of his contribution to practical affairs as any sort of distinctly philosophical activity, his populist tract *Has Man a Future*[3] written as a response to what he perceived as a major threat to the continued existence of humankind, formulated a question that is at the heart of bioethics today and which lies at the heart of many of the contributions to this volume. The sharply focused Campaign for Nuclear Disarmament in the United Kingdom, and the equally sharply focused but differently directed civil rights movement in the United States, gave way to a more broadly based 'peace movement' which in turn influenced so-called 'hippie culture'[4] and the rise of protest against the United States prosecution of an aggressive war in Vietnam. All of these issues concerned the (then) young philosophers who have influenced modern bioethics, and some of the philosophical attention that was focused on issues of war and peace, and on the ethics of political dissent and protest, came, via concern with personal and public responsibility for what happens in the world, to be turned towards issues in the field we now call bioethics, and formed the second major foundation of modern bioethics.

THE SCOPE OF BIOETHICS

While medical ethics now makes up a large and central subsection of bioethics, bioethics extends beyond the realms of medicine and health care to encompass areas including environmental ethics, ethical issues of sexuality and reproduction, and for example what is sometimes now called 'genethics', the ethics of genetic choice and manipulation. Central to these concerns are issues around the beginnings of life (see Chapters 1, 2, and 3) and concern with our increasing capacity to determine the sorts of beings that will exist in the future (see Chapters 13 and 14). Bioethics is also concerned with the ethics of scientific research and experimentation and has hence come to be concerned with the ways in which the whole of science is pursued, including of course the activities of the pharmaceutical and other industries that pursue or utilize the products of science, and ultimately with the ways in which science is regulated and controlled.

---

[3] (Harmondsworth: Penguin, 1961).
[4] Whose slogan was 'make love not war', a doctrine still diligently practised by many of today's students.

In short, bioethics investigates ethical issues arising in the life sciences (medicine, health care, genetics, biology, research, etc.) by applying the principles and methods of moral philosophy to these problems. Medical ethics and genethics (ethical issues arising from the discipline of genetics) are subsets of bioethics.

METHODOLOGY

There can be confusion, and indeed there is controversy, about what exactly the methodology of bioethics is. Bioethics is often characterized as a multidisciplinary mode of inquiry. Health care professionals, life scientists, philosophers, theologians, lawyers, economists, psychologists, sociologists, anthropologists, and historians are among those who are typically involved in what might broadly be termed 'bioethical inquiry'. And if we move from the idea of bioethics as disciplined inquiry to the notion of 'bioethical activity' broadly conceived, we must also include journalists, media presenters, and politicians in the list of contributors to contemporary bioethics.

However, while a wide range of disciplines, and some contributions that can only be characterized as ill disciplined, are actively involved in bioethics, the central method of bioethical inquiry is moral philosophy. Bioethics, rather than being a multidisciplinary mode of inquiry, is in fact a branch of applied ethics which is characteristically informed by multidisciplinary expertise and findings. As Ronald Green puts it: 'while ethics and moral philosophy may sometimes represent a relatively small part of the actual work of bioethics, they form in a sense the confluence to which all the larger and smaller tributaries lead, and, more than any other single approach, the methods of ethics and philosophy remain indispensable to this domain of inquiry.'[5] This is one of the reasons why this volume includes only philosophical contributions to bioethics. However, a further word needs to be said about the role of empirical methods in bioethics, because increasingly bioethics is coming under pressure from those who feel the need for an easily recognized and understood methodology which can in turn be quickly evaluated, and from a phenomenon which I have called 'the globalization of bioethics'. These pressures are transforming bioethics as popularly understood, and require some consideration.

[5] Ronald M. Green, 'Method in Bioethics', *Journal of Medicine and Philosophy*, 15/2 (Apr. 1990), 182.

The Globalization of Bioethics

'Globalization' is perhaps the catchphrase of the new millennium. It is a term widely used and misused, and covers everything from the effects of cellular telephones to world peace. Its fashionable connotations have also had their effect on bioethics, and have partly contributed to the pressures to which I have referred. While 'the globalization of ethics' is sometimes a term used to refer to the increasing inclusion of and attention to non-Western voices in the ethical debate, or to the quest for universal and cross-cultural themes in ethics, as I am using the term in connection with bioethics it has a rather different sense.

The globalization of bioethics[6] may be thought of as the phenomenon according to which the ethical agenda is increasingly set, not by religious, cultural, and indeed ethical traditions, nor by competition in the market-place of ideas, nor by community leaders, exceptional sages, or 'saints', nor indeed moral philosophers; but rather in a new and unprecedented way. This agenda is now set by national and international ethics committees, or com-mittees with ethical agendas, and by the conventions, protocols, reports, or conclusions which they produce, and which are disseminated either by the bodies and governments to whom these bodies report or, increasingly, by the press and media interest which they arouse. One feature of this phenomenon is the increasing *institutionalization* of bioethics; but the phenomenon to which I refer owes more, I believe, to the world stage on which bioethical issues are now played out and to the increasing consciousness of a world audience of the ethical pronouncements made by national governments and international organizations. Three features of this phenomenon are particularly important.

The first is that the standard of ethical argument in such reports, where it exists at all, is often poor. Too often indeed argument is excluded from the reports altogether, perhaps because it seems insufficient to support the resonant conclusions and portentous pronouncements they so often contain.

For example, the much trumpeted *Universal Declaration on the Human Genome and Human Rights*[7] of Unesco declares: 'Practices which are con-trary to human dignity, such as reproductive cloning of human beings, shall not be permitted.'[8] The document contains not a scintilla of argument in support of this sweeping pronouncement, nor any indication of just what is

---

[6] See my 'Research on Human Subjects, Exploitation and Global Principles of Ethics', in Andrew D. E. Lewis and Michael Freeman (eds.), *Current Legal Issue, iii: Law and Medicine* (Oxford: Oxford University Press, 2000).

[7] Pub. (as a pamphlet) 3 Dec. 1997.

[8] Ibid., Art. 11.

meant by 'human dignity'.[9] The United Kingdom government is equally intemperate. It states proudly,

The Government has made its position on reproductive cloning absolutely clear on a number of occasions. On 26th June 1997, the then Minister for Public Health stated in response to a Question in Parliament: '*We regard the deliberate cloning of human beings as ethically unacceptable. Under United Kingdom Law, cloning of individual humans cannot take place whatever the origin of the material and whatever the technique is used.*' This remains the Government's position.[10]

The Council of Europe, no more measured than the United Kingdom government, in its *Convention on Human Rights and Biomedicine*,[11] states that 'The human body and its parts shall not, as such, give rise to financial gain.'[12] Again not a breath of argument supports this assertion, and while many see it as an attempt to minimize the unjust exploitation of vulnerable human beings, one might have expected some empirical evidence of the dangers of exploitation, some analysis of the concept of 'exploitation', some guidance on how to distinguish payments for goods and services that are exploitative from those that are not, and, finally, some detailed argument to support a conclusion with very far-reaching effects.

The second feature that should be noticed is that it is these conventions and protocols that are increasingly cited in ethical justification, not only of personal conduct but of national legislation. In other words, it is these reports that are fast becoming the reference-points for ethical decision-making. This is disturbing because, even where the reports are well argued, the argument is necessarily brief and itself pendent upon other sources which, while often referenced, are seldom quoted in any detail and hence do not become part of the debate. We are in danger of seeing an increasing marginalization of serious work in bioethics and an increasing use of, and reliance on, reports and other relatively brief public statements of various sorts. Thus secondary sources of 'authority' for ethical claims are increasingly the ones that enter the debate; and the evidence and argument that might sustain those claims is seldom, if ever, available to the general public or subjected to analysis and critique.

The final telling feature of the globalization of ethics concerns the ways in

[9] For chapter and verse, see my 'Genes, Clones and Human Rights', in Justine C. Burley (ed.), *The Genetic Revolution and Human Rights: The Amnesty Lectures 1998* (Oxford: Oxford University Press, 1999).

[10] *Government Response to the Recommendations Made in the Chief Medical Officer's Expert Group Report*, Cm. 4833 (London: Stationery Office Aug. 2000).

[11] *Convention for the Protection of Human Rights and Dignity of the Human Being with regard to the Application of Biology and Medicine: Convention on Human Rights and Biomedicine* (Oviedo: Council of Europe, 4 Apr. 1997), *http://www.coe.fr/eng/legaltxt/164e.htm*

[12] Ibid., Art. 21.

which these international conventions are arrived at. Classically they are the products of high-level meetings. So they should be, of course, but such meetings are under pressure to achieve consensus and to produce agreed conclusions; and consensus can often only be marshalled around high-minded, resonant, and increasingly abstract and ambiguous principles. Too little attention is paid to the consequences of these principles, when applied to particular circumstances and to the ways in which they are often incongruous with other equally widely held and respected principles that have escaped formal articulation in international conventions. In other words, the sharp, and sharply focused, arguments required to sustain or indeed to challenge conclusions in the field of bioethics are absent from the forums in which conclusions are reached and are unavailable to a general public presented with these conclusions.[13] It is one of the aims of this book to make more available these sharp, and sharply focused, arguments.

Very often, also, the deliberations of public bodies on ethical questions involve so-called 'consultation exercises', through which attempts are made to find out what the public feels about the issues or would wish to see done about them by way of legislation. Of course, no one can object to public consultation: the public should of course be consulted, they have a right to be consulted, democracy requires it. However, there are many different sorts of concern that may prompt public consultation, and many different effects such 'consultation' may have.

What is the Role of Public Consultation in Bioethics?

Many activities fall broadly under the heading of 'public consultation'. Some are structured meetings or events, for example major conferences, focus groups, consensus conferences, public meetings, citizens' juries, and the like. Others are information-gathering or opinion-monitoring exercises, which may include opinion-polling, questionnaires, telephone sampling, structured interviews, selective mail shots, and even referendums.

What is the role and purpose of such activities in bioethics? Almost all publicly funded ethics research of the sort undertaken or commissioned by ethics committees or commissions takes it as axiomatic that some attempt to discover what people think about the issues under consideration is part of the remit. But the point and purpose of obtaining this information is seldom clear.

---

[13] Although the United States National Bioethics Advisory Commission may be an honourable exception.

There are important distinctions between a number of different ideas and activities here. Notably between:

- public consultation
- public participation
- public involvement
- public access
- public accountability
- public control.

Very often so called 'data' about what the public think are gathered without any clear understanding of the purpose(s) such an exercise is supposed to serve, or of the effects it might have. It is simply thought to be 'a good thing', perhaps because it appears to further other, supposedly laudable, obligations of public bodies, namely:

- transparency, and
- openness.

Let us return to the bullets points above that list some of the purposes often thought to be served by activities that come broadly under the heading of 'public consultation'. None of these are clearly defined ideas, and while many of them, like motherhood and apple pie, command fairly universal approbation, it is unclear what point they serve in bioethics research. Worse, while no item on the list implies subsequent items (that is, public consultation does not imply participation, participation does not imply involvement,[14] and so on), the claim that any one of these activities has been undertaken as part of a decision-making process seems designed, and is often somehow taken, to imply all the others.

We need to be clear about the radical differences that obtain between an obligation, for example, to see what people think so that you know what the public reaction might be to the recommendation of something different, and the obligation to see what people think so that you will be sure not to recommend anything different. Equally, there is the idea that it is useful to allow people to *contribute* to the decision-making process and to allow people to *influence* or even to *control* that process.

For a committee or commission that is set up to advise the government of a nation-state, such as the National Bioethics Advisory Commission in the United States, the national ethics committees that operate in many

---

[14] Public participation may, in Wittgenstein's wonderful image, be a cog that is not connected to the machinery, so that while it 'can be turned . . . nothing else moves with it', and so participation in the process may not imply involvement in the subsequent decision-making. See Ludwig Wittgenstein, *Philosophical Investigations* (Oxford: Blackwell, 1963), para. 271.

European countries, or the Human Genetics Commission in the United Kingdom,[15] there is always an acute danger in public consultation or opinion-taking. A government, however independent-minded it might believe itself to be, is unlikely to accept advice that is radically at odds with what are perceived to be the current views of voters. And so there is a danger that to find out those views in advance of an advisory committee or commission forming its own views and presenting them, with supporting evidence and argument for public consideration, that public consultation will simply pre-empt the process that the commission was designed to initiate and result in the bypassing of the advice that it is its responsibility to give.

The Precautionary Principle

The tendency towards conservatism built into processes of public consultation is often thought to be consistent with prudence and with the so-called 'precautionary principle'. This principle, while vague, is generally interpreted as requiring, not unreasonably, that we always proceed responsibly, exposing communities and one another to the least danger. However, the line of 'safety' is not always coextensive with a policy of minimum change. Very often the failure to take radical steps is the policy that costs us most, both in the short and in the long term.[16]

It is often believed that there is some moral imperative to be ultra-cautious in permitting new research, particularly in the biomedical and health fields. However, it is not unusual to find this so-called 'precautionary principle' being invoked in circumstances in which it is far from clear in which direction (if any) caution lies. A similar problem is familiar from the discussions about germ-line gene therapy.[17] Caution was urged to prevent the introduction of germ-line gene therapy on the principal ground that germ-line changes would affect future generations indefinitely and are probably irreversible. Any damage done if germ-line therapy were to go wrong therefore (*a*) would be magnified and (*b*) would continue as long as procreation continued. However, given that the germ-line therapy would likely be

---

[15] I should declare an interest here since I am a member of the United Kingdom Human Genetics Commission and was a member of one of the advisory bodies that preceded it, the United Kingdom Advisory Committee on Genetic Testing.

[16] John Harris and Søren Holm, 'Precautionary Principle Stifles Discovery', *Nature*, 400 (29 July 1999), 398.

[17] *Report of the Committee on the Ethics of Gene Therapy* (London, HMSO: 1992); British Medical Association, *Our Genetic Future* (Oxford: Oxford University Press, 1992); Harris, 'Biotechnology: Friend or Foe', in A. Dyson, and J. Harris, (eds.), *Ethics and Biotechnology* (London: Routledge, 1994).

introduced to correct genetic defects, to fail to carry out the therapy would also adversely affect future generations indefinitely, and thus the harm caused by the genetic defect (*a*) would be magnified and (*b*) would continue as long as procreation continued. We would only know which way lay caution if we could compare the number of times germ-line therapy would go wrong and the magnitude of the damage thereby caused with the number of times a defective gene would be disastrously expressed and the magnitude of the harm that would cause.

Of course, the extent of such risk in any particular case is just what we want committees of the great and the good to assess for us.[18] And their having made this assessment, we need such committees to set out the ethical arguments as to whether, in the light of such assessment, it might be, first, ethical and, secondly, prudent to pursue the research or policies in question.

Judgements about Ethics and Ethical Judgements

Before we leave the question of the role of public values and attitudes in bioethics there is another problem that should be noticed. Discovering what the public thinks about issues of ethical significance is not the same as discovering the ethical values of the public. And finding out what the public thinks it acceptable to do about issues of ethical importance is not the same as finding out what the public finds ethically acceptable. This is because judgements about matters of ethical significance are not necessarily ethical judgements.

This is not the place for any attempt at a complete account (if that were possible) of what makes something an *ethical* judgement. However, some things can and should be said here that bear both on the question of the methodology of bioethical inquiry and on the role of empirical methods in bioethics.

'Morality' is just one of the normative systems that operate within society, albeit the one to which all others are answerable. Other general normative systems include the rules governing religious observance, rules of good manners or etiquette, and, of course, the legal system. Then there are the rules of particular professions, occupations, corporations, or clubs that are often rather misleadingly referred to as codes of professional ethics or corporate ethics. All or any of these normative systems may enjoin or forbid

---

[18] For other examples of this phenomenon and its problematic consequences, see John Harris, 'Goodbye Dolly: The Ethics of Human Cloning', *Journal of Medical Ethics*, 23/6 (Dec. 1997), 353–60; 'Cloning and Human Dignity', *Cambridge Quarterly of Healthcare Ethics*, 7/2 (Spring 1998), 163–8; 'Genes, Clones and Human Rights'.

things in the name of morality, and the operation of these normative systems may generate ethical dilemmas. For example, although it is always wrong (incorrect) to break the law, doing so is not always morally wrong. The law requires us to drive on the left in the United Kingdom. Other countries that regulate road traffic differently are not, for that reason at least, morally inferior to the United Kingdom. There is nothing unethical about driving on the right, even in the United Kingdom, except in so far as it is dangerous (or possibly unfair) to do so where others are conforming to the law. If it is morally wrong to commit murder, it is so not because law forbids it; rather the law forbids it because it is morally wrong.[19]

The terms 'right' and 'wrong' are characteristically used to enforce the rules of all normative systems, so that it is always 'wrong' in some sense to defy the rules of a normative system. For these reasons many people use terms like 'wrong' to describe actions or practices forbidden by a normative system that they happen to accept.[20] But saying that something is morally wrong implies more than the fact that it is forbidden by a normative system that the agent accepts. It implies that it is forbidden by that system because it is morally wrong, or that, in addition to its being forbidden by that system, it is also morally wrong.

Similarly with personal judgements that are not made simply in accordance with the rules of a normative system. When we ask someone whether they think this or that to be 'right' or 'wrong', the answer may reveal their prejudices or personal aversions or likes rather than information about their morality or their moral views or judgements properly so called. Ronald Dworkin has assayed an account of at least some of the factors that make individual judgements moral judgements and that can defeat an individual's claim to be acting from moral conviction.

Dworkin notes that if someone purports to be acting from moral conviction or because his morality requires it, he must at the very least produce reasons in support of such a claim. Moreover, those reasons must meet minimum standards of evidence and argument; they must not, for example, be based on prejudice, or on alleged facts that are both false and manifestly implausible, or on a personal emotional reaction such as 'it makes me sick!' Moreover, such reasons will presuppose a general moral principle or theory. Here the claim to be acting from moral conviction may be undermined by the insincerity of the agent where he clearly does not accept the theory

---

[19] Among other reasons.
[20] So that when opinion-samplers ask whether people believe something is right or wrong, they may be receiving information about what a particular normative system enjoins or forbids, and not information about the moral beliefs of those who accept this system.

presupposed by the stand he has taken, or acts inconsistently with this theory or principle in other areas of his life.

Where individuals consider and evaluate the moral claims of others, such claims command respect precisely because they are *moral* claims, and are thus distinguishable from personal preferences or prejudices. And Dworkin concludes that, when considering my moral claims,

> You will want to consider the reasons I can produce to support my belief and whether my other views and behaviour are consistent with the theories these reasons presuppose. You will have, of course, to apply your own understanding, which may differ in detail from mine, of what a prejudice or a rationalization is, for example, and of when one view is inconsistent with another. You and I may end in disagreement over whether my position is a moral one, partly because of such differences in understanding. And partly because one is less likely to recognise these illegitimate grounds in himself than in others.

Finally, Dworkin insists that

> We must avoid the sceptical fallacy of passing from these facts to the conclusion that there is no such thing as a prejudice or a rationalization or an inconsistency, or that these terms mean merely that the one who uses them strongly dislikes the positions he describes this way. That would be like arguing that because people have different understanding of what jealousy is, and can in good faith disagree about whether one of them is jealous, there is no such thing as jealousy, and one who says another is jealous merely means he dislikes him very much.[21]

While this is by no means a complete account of what it is that makes a judgement a moral judgement, and while any such account would be in some respects controversial, it does establish that there is *something* over and above the fact that it is a judgement about an issue of moral significance that makes a judgement a reflection of the morality of an individual. This gives us some reason to be cautious about claims to the effect that forms of public consultation have revealed the moral attitudes or values of the public, and that these must both be respected and inform public decision-making. If what is informing public decision-making is a collection of recorded prejudices or evidence of a slavish and uncritical adherence to a sectarian normative system, then perhaps the respectability, if not the authenticity, of the voice of the people requires challenge rather than faithful reporting and incorporation into the decision-making process. This challenge cannot come from empirical bioethics, but must come from philosophical bioethics with its long tradition of critical and independent analysis. And we now come to the question of the role of empirical studies in bioethics.

Empirical studies, as I noted earlier, have played an increasingly important role in bioethics, partly because of the felt need to act on evidence of

---

[21] See Ronald Dworkin, *Taking Rights Seriously* (London: Duckworth, 1977), ch. 9, pp. 252–3.

public values and attitudes to the questions and dilemmas of bioethics, and partly because of the nervousness on the part of bodies funding bioethics research about the apparent absence of a clearly recognized and simply evaluated methodology in research applications.

The Role of Empirical Studies

What, then, may we say of the role of empirical studies in the domain of ethical research? Clearly science and empirical research is *relevant* to the study of ethics and to ethics research, but how exactly? Truths in almost any field are established by a combination of evidence and argument. The evidence is primarily empirical in one way or another, but it is the argument about the meaning of the evidence, and the conclusions which it licenses, that make the ethical contribution. If we first think about the role of science, it is clearly essential to ethics in important ways; for example, we need to know what embryo research is and does, or what stem cell research is and what it might be expected to achieve and at what cost. We cannot begin to address the ethics of such research and its applications without knowing the facts in some detail. And, of course, if we don't know the facts, then we have to find them out before we can start to assess the science and its applications from the perspective of ethics. But gathering the facts and *deciding what we ought to think about them* are two different sorts of activity.

In essence this is not a problem about 'methods in ethics'; it is a problem about the *funding* of ethical research. The place of empirical studies in ethics would not be an issue if it did not vitally relate to the funding of ethical research. Ethical research has only relatively recently required funding at all; that is, funding separate from and additional to the public funding that supports most professional academics in their university and research laboratory posts. More recently public bodies have come to see the importance of ethics and the impossibility of rationally proceeding with research programmes in science without paying attention to the ethics of such research. They have accordingly devoted parts of their research budget to ethical issues, most notably the ethical legal and social issues component of the Human Genome Project budget and the ethics strands of the Biomedical and Health Research budget of the European Commission. However, the deployment of research funds requires the peer review of research proposals, and the funding bodies for scientific research do not seem to have greatly altered their peer review process for the inclusion of ethics. Hence, boards of scientists of various sorts have faced the problem of evaluating research proposals in ethics. Scientists look for clear articulation of appropriate methodology. Not understanding or appreciating the methodology of ethics, they have, perhaps understandably, gravitated towards ethical projects with a large empirical component, the methodology of which can be clearly presented and is easily understood by scientists. This phenomenon has had a distorting effect on bioethics and has expanded the scope of bioethics without obviously commensurate gains in ethical understanding.

If one consequence of the publication of this volume is the provision of a series of exemplars of the methodology of philosophical bioethics, one very valuable objective will have been achieved.

Bioethics Today

We have spent some time thinking about what bioethics is not; the remainder of this volume will be concerned with what bioethics is. Bioethics has its roots in medicine and in the ethical issues raised by the practice of medicine. It must therefore have something useful to say to the health professionals who care for patients. It must, among other things, be able to help with decisions to be made about managing the care of 'Mrs Jones in Ward 5 at 4.10 in the afternoon'.

The care of Mrs Jones requires innumerable decisions by many different people, decisions about whether to intervene at all and what sorts of intervention to make or withhold. What are the constraints on those decisions; who should be involved in the making of them; whose consent or authority for them is required; and who may know what is planned and why? We are in philosophically very complex territory, and yet we have not faced anything very dramatic or out of the ordinary. Take the very basic and everyday question whether a drug should be given or withheld. Already this raises issues about what, if anything, the patient should be told, and whether she must consent to the giving or withholding of the drug. If she cannot consent, who may do so on her behalf? Who else may share in the decision and in knowing the reasons for making it and its consequences? We are concerned with issues of privacy and confidentiality, consent and autonomy, truth-telling and information-giving (see Chapters 15, 16, and 17). Since the decision is over whether or not to give or withhold a drug, we need to think about acts and omissions, and about whether doing something has the same consequences, and carries with it the same responsibilities, as omitting to do something (see Chapters 8 and 9).

Now must be added issues about the consequences for the patient, for the health care system, and for society generally. This may sound portentous, but the drug may, for example, be expensive. If this patient has it, she may use up resources that could be 'better' or 'more efficiently' spent elsewhere. What does 'better' mean here? What is meant by 'efficiency'? Another patient may be more deserving—have a better claim to the resource (see Chapters 10, 11, and 12). Mrs Jones is also pregnant. What will be the effect of the drug she needs on her unborn child? How is that child's interests or rights to be balanced against those of Mrs Jones? How, indeed, do the interests or entitlements of future generations figure in our moral agenda (see Chapters 13 and 14)? How are these decisions to be made, and who is to make them? Can general principles be formulated that will help both with Mrs Jones and with all the other patients in this large and busy hospital?

Finally, Mrs Jones will, at some point, have to face death and the prospect of dying,[22] and the professionals who care for her will also have to confront the problems of helping her face death and dying. She may or may not be competent to manage her own affairs, and may have left prior indications about what she would have wanted her care to be like in this final phase of her life (see Chapters 4, 5, and 6).

Fancy has not taken us too far from Mrs Jones in Ward 5 and 4.10 in the afternoon, but thinking about Mrs Jones has made us face most of the main questions and themes of bioethics, with issues about the beginnings of life and the end of life, with scarce resources and future generations, with the value of life and the relative value of different lives (see Chapters 7, 8, and 9) and with the narrower but equally important day-to-day issues of information-giving, consent, respect for patients, and so on.

Ultimate Questions

Bioethics has perhaps attracted some of the best philosophers and produced some of the most important work done in contemporary philosophy precisely because it is concerned with the ultimate questions in their most dramatic form. Questions about the value of life and about the meaning of life are questions that perhaps everyone but professional philosophers believed had always been among the central concerns of philosophy. These were the sorts of question that surely justified the existence of philosophy as a distinct and distinctly important field of study. However, as we have noted, until

---

[22] Although it is conceivable that there will come a time when some will be able indefinitely to postpone this confrontation with death. See John Harris, 'Intimations of Immortality', *Science*, 288/5463 (7 Apr. 2000), 59.

recently these questions, if they were raised at all by philosophers, seemed to lack the specificity and the urgency of real problems. The emergence of nuclear weapons raised the possibility of a war that not only would be unprecedented in its severity, but for the first time raised the real prospect of an end to human life altogether and brought a sense both of reality and of urgency to academic ethics. While the nuclear threat receded, the sense of urgency that it had brought to ethics remained, and philosophers found in the practice of medicine and in the advance of medical and biological science the dramatic and fascinating questions of real importance and seriousness that matched their commitment and concern. Not surprisingly, then, it was the issues of life and death and the hugely consequential choices of medical science that produced some of the most important and demanding ethical responses. Although many of these issues arose in wards and clinics in connection with Mrs Jones and her fellow patients, they were very often addressed in a very general and universal form.

Concern with Mrs Jones is still at the centre of bioethics, but more and more frequently public policy issues are taking centre-stage. These policy issues range from those concerned with health and research policy narrowly conceived to questions of public safety and the future of humankind. Recent controversies in bioethics have, for example, centred on HIV–AIDS and AIDS research, on the introduction of genetically modified plants and organisms and on genetic selection and manipulation.

These debates, like those about 'the fate of Mrs Jones and her unborn child', have become the proving-ground for the central concepts and tenets of our shared morality. Concepts like justice and the sanctity of life, acceptance of imperatives to refrain from killing and to minimize suffering, belief in honesty and truth-telling, and the nature of life itself have all been challenged by scientific and technological developments in the biosphere (see Chapters 7 and 11). It is the better understanding of these central elements of our shared morality that has been the main contribution of bioethics to the end of the second millennium.

Shared Morality

I have talked of the central elements of a 'shared morality'. To what extent is this justified? Moral principles of the sort I have referred to thus far are not just plucked from the air, but neither are they derived from unassailable premisses or immutable absolutes. They articulate central elements of a shared morality. Like the Ten Commandments and other sacred and venerable articulations of central beliefs, they remind us of that morality and our commitment to it; and like the famous Commandments, they require interpretation.[23]

However, they also differ from the Commandments and other theologically derived texts in important ways. Unlike the Commandments, they do not attempt self-justification. They do not purport to explain *why* they ought to be accepted. So, when we articulate a moral principle, we are reminding ourselves of what we believe to be an important part of the morality we already accept. We should follow the principle *because* we accept the morality, but the principle cannot give us *reasons for* accepting the morality. When we encounter a principle, we need first to reflect on our morality to see whether and how the principle fits with it. We then need to explore the consequences of accepting the principle to see whether we can adhere to it consistently with other moral beliefs that we share and wish to retain. If the principle can be applied consistently with our general morality, well and good; if not, we have to choose whether to abandon the principle or abandon the elements of our morality which are not consistent with it.[24]

Ethics-Based Medicine

Before doing so, we must examine another assumption that has been made. I am assuming that bioethics, and so of course medical ethics also, is part of ethics more generally, and that what it is ethical to do to—and for people within a health care system, or 'clinically', or in research settings—and what people are obliged to do for one another are dimensions of our general morality. The assumption, then, is that the delivery of health care, both individually and within a health care system, is part of our more general obligations to one another, and, in particular, that it is entailed by the commitment we have to honour other people's entitlements to concern, respect, and protection. In short, the duties of health care professionals or research scientists, in so far as they are ethical duties, are derived from general morality and are not part of a particular ethics of health care (see Chapters 7, 10, and 11). The ethical *dilemmas* that arise within a health service may be different from those arising within a prison service, for example, but the principles that inform the resolution of those dilemmas are drawn from our general morality. Resistance to this idea often comes from a confusion about

---

[23] Does the proscription on killing include animals and plants? Are some Commandments more important than others? Is the prohibition against coveting one's neighbour's oxen as important as that against coveting one's neighbour's wife?
[24] This does not, of course, purport to be a complete account of either morality or moral reasoning.

the different sorts of normative systems that operate within any society. That we have already noted.

Medical or health care ethics (as opposed to bioethics) may be construed as the ethical code of a particular profession or professions, or of the health care system. So construed, it has limited force and will appeal, at most, only to members of those professions, or perhaps, more pessimistically, to those who wish to become or continue to be members of those professions. As we shall construe it, however, it is the application of our general morality to the dilemmas of research and of health care more generally.[25] Thus construed, research ethics and medical ethics apply as much to research subjects or to patients and their friends and relatives as they do to researchers, doctors, or nurses; and they are as concerned with the general obligations of society to carry out research or to provide health care as they are with the duties of researchers or other professionals to deliver it.

Religious and cultural traditions sometimes claim special status in bioethical debate, suggesting that their approach to the problems of biomedicine must be determined 'from within' and are not therefore vulnerable to the arguments of so-called 'bioethicists'. These traditions contain elements of all the sorts of normative systems that I have noted. They have strands that are more clearly like the rules of a club or a profession (often concerning dress codes and dietary arrangements, for example[26]), and they usually have a body of 'law'. They will also, of course, have important things to say about all the major moral concerns of humankind. However, nothing in any religion or cultural tradition absolves each of us, each member of the religion or cultural tradition, from thinking through moral questions for ourselves. There are three main sorts of reason why this must be true, and it is worth noting these before we continue. I will not have time to develop these points in any great detail or with much sophistication.

Ambiguity
Nothing written in a natural language is unambiguous. As William Empson famously remarked, 'in a sufficiently extended sense any prose statement could be called ambiguous'.[27] Not only are all statements susceptible to interpretation and qualification, but it is scarcely possible to understand any sophisticated statement without interpretation or gloss. Whether the source of our moral guidance is a self-consciously didactic text like the Ten

[25] I have argued this point in greater detail in my *The Value of Life* (London: Routledge & Kegan Paul, 1985), ch. 3.
[26] As Mary Douglas's famous analysis suggests. See Mary Douglas, *Purity and Danger* (London: Routledge & Kegan Paul, 1966).
[27] William Empson, *Seven Types of Ambiguity* (London: Chatto & Windus, 1930; rev. edn. 1970), ch. 1.

Commandments, the Universal Declaration of Human Rights, or, indeed, this volume, it will require at the very least interpretation and qualification, and almost certainly critical evaluation as well.

Moral Relativism

Although a certain degree of moral relativism is now regarded as both polit-ically correct and intellectually required, I do not believe there exists a coher-ent version of moral relativism—if, that is, moral relativism is interpreted as rendering a moral system or set of culturally derived values immune from 'external'[28] critical evaluation. There are many reasons that should be per-suasive in rejecting moral relativism, and I will have time to mention just two. The first is that cultures and religions develop and evolve. There is no major religion that does not have a theological tradition—a tradition of the study and interpretation of religious texts and doctrine. Partly through these trad-itions, religions and cultures, and their values and morality, evolve and develop. At least sometimes religions and cultures change and develop for good reasons; sometimes these changes are even changes for the better. These reasons may be theological; they may sometimes even be logical.

However, whatever counts as a good reason for change or development from within a culture and religion will also count as a good reason when voiced from outside the culture or religion (although, of course, it may seem less appealing when coming from outside). This shows that no religion or culture can be hermetically sealed from outside influence, but it is a relatively weak argument. It only shows that cross-cultural criticism is not *necessarily* imperialistic; it cannot show that it is *never* imperialistic. However, there is one other reason why moral relativism must be false, and it is our third reason for maintaining that ethics is always a rational, not simply a religious or cultural, activity.

Ethics and Theology are Necessarily Independent of One Another

There is an argument familiar to philosophers and indeed to theologians that seems too clever to be true but has never been refuted.[29] It derives from Plato,[30] but I shall use Bertrand Russell's famous formulation of it:

---

[28] This term also requires much interpretation.

[29] See e.g. Anthony Kenny, *A Brief History of Western Philosophy* (Oxford: Blackwell 1998), 25 ff. and his 'Afterword', 346 ff.

[30] Plato *The Dialogues*, trans. B. Jowett, 4th edn. (Oxford: Clarendon Press, 1953), vol. 1: *Euthyphro* 10–11. Socrates is educating Euthyphro about holiness: 'But, friend Euthyphro, if that which is holy were the same with that which is dear to the gods, and were loved because it is holy, then that which is dear to the gods would be loved as being dear to them; but if that which is dear to them were dear to them because loved by them, then that which is holy would be holy because loved by them. But now you see that the reverse is the case, and that the two things are quite different from one another. For one . . . is of a kind to be loved because it is loved, and the other . . . is loved because it is of a kind to be loved.'

... if you are quite sure that there is a difference between right and wrong then you are in this situation: is that difference due to God's fiat or is it not? If it is due to God's fiat, then for God Himself there is no difference between right and wrong, and it is no longer a significant statement to say that God is good. If you are going to say, as theologians do, that God is good, you must then say that right and wrong have some meaning which is independent of God's fiat. Because God's fiat's are good and not bad independently of the mere fact that He made them. If you are going to say that then you will have to say that it is not only through God that right and wrong came into being, but that they are in their essence logically anterior to God.[31]

This argument does not say anything about the existence of God, nor does it deny his or her goodness. It merely points out that the statements 'God is good' and 'God is God' must have different meanings, if 'good' is to have any meaning at all. One of God's great claims to fame is that he wills the good. It is our ability to reason about the nature of the good independently of God's fiat, as Russell calls it, that partially accounts for theology and indeed enables us to say non-vacuously that God is good. For if we believe that God only wills the good, then if we can establish what is good, we have reason to choose between rival interpretations of God's will.

Genetics

Finally, we should look at two areas vital to bioethics in which the philosophical contribution is really just beginning: genetics and global justice. It is genetics that is beginning to create a new generation of acute and subtle dilemmas that will in the new millennium transform the ways in which we think of ourselves and of society. It is genetics, bringing both a new understanding of what we are and almost daily developing new ways of enabling us to influence what we are, that is creating a revolution in thought, and not least in ethics. For the first time in human history we are becoming responsible for the course of human evolution. For the first time we can think about determining not only who will live and who will die, but also what all those who live and die in the future will be like. Not only will phenotypical, and perhaps superficial, traits like hair and eye colour, skin colour, and general body build and degrees of athleticism be susceptible to genetic influence, but also, probably, traits like general intelligence, longevity, susceptibility and resistance to disease,

---

[31] Bertrand Russell, 'Why I am not a Christian', in *Why I am not a Christian and Other Essays* (London: George Allen & Unwin, 1957).

capacity for recovery from infection and tissue damage, and many other features.[32]

Genetics is dramatically reminding us of two features of our existence that are existentially both important and problematic (see Chapters 7, 13, and 14). They are the closeness of our genetic relatedness, not only to one another, but also to other species. 'While a child is 99.95% the same as its genetic mother at the level of genetic information, it is also 99.90% the same as any randomly chosen person on the planet earth.'[33] While we share most of 'our' genes with everyone else, we also share the vast majority of our genetic information with animals and other creatures. We share about 98.5 per cent of our genetic information with chimpanzees, for example, and about 40–50 per cent with cabbages and bananas. It is difficult to know what effect such information will have on us and on our ethical relations with each other and with other species. On the one hand, such knowledge seems to bring all of creation closer together; on the other, it seems to highlight the crucial importance of quite minute differences at the level of genetic information.

Equally important is the change that genetics has reinforced in our understanding of responsibility which involves abandoning one of the most basic and traditional of distinctions, that between what is given and what is done. Traditionally there are those things that seem given, perhaps controlled by fate or by the gods and for which we therefore can neither have nor claim responsibility, and there are those that, because we can affect them, become to some extent our responsibility. Recent advances in genetics have shown us just how much we can actually and potentially do to influence and change the genetic constitution of individuals, and it is philosophy that has reminded us that, once we realize that we have the capacity to change, we are responsible for the consequences of our choices whether or not to exercise that capacity. The idea that 'if we are able to change things, to elect not to do so is also to determine what will happen in the world' is of considerable antiquity—Plutarch, Jesus, and Shakespeare all make prominent use of it— but its revival in contemporary thinking about medical science, and about genetics in particular, has been partly owing to the insistence of contemporary philosophers[34] (see Chapters 8 and 9).

---

[32] As I have discussed elsewhere. See John Harris, *Clones, Genes and Immortality* (Oxford: Oxford University Press, 1998) and Justine Burley and John Harris (eds.), *The Blackwell Companion to Genethics: Ethics and the Genetic Revolution* (Oxford: Blackwell, forthcoming), esp. introd.

[33] Lee Silver, 'The Meaning of Genes and "Genetic Rights"', *Jurimetrics: The Journal of Law, Science, and Policy*, 40/1 (Fall 1999), 77–93.

[34] See e.g. Jonathan Glover, *Causing Death and Saving Lives* (Harmondsworth: Penguin, 1977) and John Harris, *Violence and Responsibility* (London: Routledge & Kegan Paul, 1980), esp. ch. 3.

Global Justice

One thing we do know is that the technology and the investment in scientific research required to implement not only the new genetics, but almost all foreseeable bioscience, will be expensive. Even in technologically advanced countries, therefore, the effects of advances in bioscience are likely to be confined to a minority of the population. In global terms the divide between high-income and low-income countries will be increased. What can be afforded in the United States, for example, will be very different from what can be afforded in countries like Uganda with an annual per capita expenditure on medicine of about $6. This increasing gulf between rich and poor countries, and the injustice, both relative and absolute, that it entails, are perhaps the greatest of the ethical issues facing humankind today. While not principally an issue for or within bioethics, and hence not separately considered in this volume, it is one that requires to be part of any bioethics agenda. This is particularly so when the ethical issues involved in developing and making available new drugs, procedures, or technologies are considered, or when the ethics of biomedical research arise.[35]

---

[35] For the beginnings of philosophical discussion of global justice, see Glover, *Causing Death and Saving Lives*; Harris, *Violence and Responsibility*; and Peter Singer, *Practical Ethics* (Cambridge: Cambridge University Press, 1979), ch. 8.

PART I

BEGINNINGS OF LIFE

1

A DEFENCE OF ABORTION[1]

JUDITH JARVIS THOMSON

Most opposition to abortion relies on the premiss that the foetus is a human being, a person, from the moment of conception. The premiss is argued for, but, as I think, not well. Take, for example, the most common argument. We are asked to notice that the development of a human being from conception through birth into childhood is continuous; then it is said that to draw a line, to choose a point in this development and say 'before this point the thing is not a person, after this point it is a person' is to make an arbitrary choice, a choice for which in the nature of things no good reason can be given. It is concluded that the foetus is, or anyway that we had better say it is, a person from the moment of conception. But this conclusion does not follow. Similar things might be said about the development of an acorn into an oak tree, and it does not follow that acorns are oak trees, or that we had better say they are. Arguments of this form are sometimes called 'slippery slope arguments'—the phrase is perhaps self-explanatory—and it is dismaying that opponents of abortion rely on them so heavily and uncritically.

I am inclined to agree, however, that the prospects for 'drawing a line' in the development of the foetus look dim. I am inclined to think also that we shall probably have to agree that the foetus has already become a human person well before birth. Indeed, it comes as a surprise when one first learns how early in its life it begins to acquire human characteristics. By the tenth week, for example, it already has a face, arms and legs, fingers and toes; it has internal organs, and brain activity is detectable.[2] On the other hand, I think that the premiss is false, that the foetus is not a person from the

From Judith Jarvis Thomson, 'A Defence of Abortion', *Philosophy & Public Affairs*, 1/1 (Fall 1971), 47–66.

[1] I am very much indebted to James Thomson for discussion, criticism, and many helpful suggestions.
[2] Daniel Callahan, *Abortion: Law, Choice and Morality* (New York, 1970), 373. This book gives a fascinating survey of the available information on abortion. The Jewish tradition is surveyed in David M. Feldman, *Birth Control in Jewish Law* (New York, 1968). pt. 5, the Catholic tradition in John T. Noonan Jr., 'An Almost Absolute Value in History', in Noonan (ed.), *The Morality of Abortion* (Cambridge, Mass., 1970).

moment of conception. A newly fertilized ovum, a newly implanted clump of cells, is no more a person than an acorn is an oak tree. But I shall not discuss any of this. For it seems to me to be of great interest to ask what happens if, for the sake of argument, we allow the premiss. How, precisely, are we supposed to get from there to the conclusion that abortion is morally impermissible? Opponents of abortion commonly spend most of their time establishing that the foetus is a person, and hardly any time explaining the step from there to the impermissibility of abortion. Perhaps they think the step too simple and obvious to require much comment. Or perhaps instead they are simply being economical in argument. Many of those who defend abortion rely on the premiss that the foetus is not a person, but only a bit of tissue that will become a person at birth; and why pay out more arguments than you have to? Whatever the explanation, I suggest that the step they take is neither easy nor obvious, that it calls for closer examination than it is commonly given, and that when we do give it this closer examination we shall feel inclined to reject it.

I propose, then, that we grant that the foetus is a person from the moment of conception. How does the argument go from here? Something like this, I take it. Every person has a right to life. So the foetus has a right to life. No doubt the mother has a right to decide what shall happen in and to her body; everyone would grant that. But surely a person's right to life is stronger and more stringent than the mother's right to decide what happens in and to her body, and so outweighs it. So the foetus may not be killed; an abortion may not be performed.

It sounds plausible. But now let me ask you to imagine this. You wake up in the morning and find yourself back to back in bed with an unconscious violinist. A famous unconscious violinist. He has been found to have a fatal kidney ailment, and the Society of Music Lovers has canvassed all the available medical records and found that you alone have the right blood type to help. They have therefore kidnapped you, and last night the violinist's circulatory system was plugged into yours, so that your kidneys can be used to extract poisons from his blood as well as your own. The director of the hospital now tells you, 'Look, we're sorry the Society of Music Lovers did this to you—we would never have permitted it if we had known. But still, they did it, and the violinist now is plugged into you. To unplug you would be to kill him. But never mind, it's only for nine months. By then he will have recovered from his ailment, and can safely be unplugged from you.' Is it morally incumbent on you to accede to this situation? No doubt it would be very nice of you if you did, a great kindness. But do you *have* to accede to it? What if it were not nine months, but nine years? Or longer still? What if the director of the hospital says, 'Tough luck, I agree, but you've now got to stay in bed, with the violinist plugged into you, for the rest of your life. Because remember this. All persons have a right to life, and violinists are persons. Granted you have a right to decide what happens in and to your body, but a person's right to life outweighs your right to decide what happens in and to your body. So you cannot ever be unplugged from him.' I imagine you would regard this as outrageous, which suggests that something really is wrong with that plausible-sounding argument I mentioned a moment ago.

In this case, of course, you were kidnapped; you didn't volunteer for the operation that plugged the violinist into your kidneys. Can those who oppose abortion on the ground I mentioned make an exception for a pregnancy due to rape? Certainly. They can say that persons have a right to life only if they didn't come into existence because of rape; or they can say that all persons have a right to life, but that some have less of a right to life than others, in particular, that those who came into existence because of rape have less. But these statements have a rather unpleasant sound. Surely the question of whether you have a right to life at all, or how much of it you have, shouldn't turn on the question of whether or not you are the product of a rape. And in fact the people who oppose abortion on the ground I mentioned do not make this distinction, and hence do not make an exception in case of rape.

Nor do they make an exception for a case in which the mother has to spend the nine months of her pregnancy in bed. They would agree that would be a great pity, and hard on the mother; but all the same, all persons have a right to life, the foetus is a person, and so on. I suspect, in fact, that they would not make an exception for a case in which, miraculously enough, the pregnancy went on for nine years, or even the rest of the mother's life.

Some won't even make an exception for a case in which continuation of the pregnancy is likely to shorten the mother's life; they regard abortion as impermissible even to save the mother's life. Such cases are nowadays very rare, and many opponents of abortion do not accept this extreme view. All the same, it is a good place to begin: a number of points of interest come out in respect to it.

1. Let us call the view that abortion is impermissible even to save the mother's life 'the extreme view'. I want to suggest first that it does not issue from the argument I mentioned earlier without the addition of some fairly powerful premisses. Suppose a woman has become pregnant, and now learns that she has a cardiac condition such that she will die if she carries the baby to term. What may be done for her? The foetus, being a person, has a right to life, but as the mother is a person too, so has she a right to life. Presumably they have an equal right to life. How is it supposed to come out that an abortion may not be performed? If mother and child have an equal right to

life, shouldn't we perhaps flip a coin? Or should we add to the mother's right to life her right to decide what happens in and to her body, which everybody seems to be ready to grant—the sum of her rights now outweighing the foetus's right to life?

The most familiar argument here is the following. We are told that performing the abortion would be directly killing[3] the child, whereas doing nothing would not be killing the mother, but only letting her die. Moreover, in killing the child, one would be killing an innocent person, for the child has committed no crime, and is not aiming at his mother's death. And then there are a variety of ways in which this might be continued. (1) But as directly killing an innocent person is always and absolutely impermissible, an abortion may not be performed. Or, (2) as directly killing an innocent person is murder, and murder is always and absolutely impermissible, an abortion may not be performed.[4] Or, (3) as one's duty to refrain from directly killing an innocent person is more stringent than one's duty to keep a person from dying, an abortion may not be performed. Or, (4) if one's only options are directly killing an innocent person or letting a person die, one must prefer letting the person die, and thus an abortion may not be performed.[5]

Some people seem to have thought that these are not further premises which must be added if the conclusion is to be reached, but that they follow from the very fact that an innocent person has a right to life.[6] But this seems to me to be a mistake, and perhaps the simplest way to show this is to bring out that while we must certainly grant that innocent persons have a right to life, the theses in (1) to (4) are all false. Take (2), for example. If directly

[3] The term 'direct' in the arguments I refer to is a technical one. Roughly, what is meant by 'direct killing' is either killing as an end in itself, or killing as a means to some end, for example, the end of saving someone else's life. See n. 6, below, for an example of its use.

[4] Cf. *Encyclical Letter of Pope Pius XI on Christian Marriage*, St Paul Editions (Boston, n.d.), 32: 'however much we may pity the mother whose health and even life is gravely imperiled in the performance of the duty allotted to her by nature, nevertheless what could ever be a sufficient reason for excusing in any way the direct murder of the innocent? This is precisely what we are dealing with here.' Noonan (*The Morality of Abortion*, 43) reads this as follows: 'What cause can ever avail to excuse in any way the direct killing of the innocent? For it is a question of that.'

[5] The thesis in (4) is in an interesting way weaker than those in (1), (2), and (3): they rule out abortion even in cases in which both mother *and* child will die if the abortion is not performed. By contrast, one who held the view expressed in (4) could consistently say that one needn't prefer letting two persons die to killing one.

[6] Cf. the following passage from Pius XII, *Address to the Italian Catholic Society of Midwives*: 'The baby in the maternal breast has the right to life immediately from God.—Hence there is no man, no human authority, no science, no medical, eugenic, social, economic or moral "indication" which can establish or grant a valid juridical ground for a direct deliberate disposition of an innocent human life, that is a disposition which looks to its destruction either as an end or as a means to another end perhaps in itself not illicit.—The baby, still not born, is a man in the same degree and for the same reason as the mother' (quoted in Noonan, *The Morality of Abortion*, 45).

killing an innocent person is murder, and thus is impermissible, then the mother's directly killing the innocent person inside her is murder, and thus is impermissible. But it cannot seriously be thought to be murder if the mother performs an abortion on herself to save her life. It cannot seriously be said that she *must* refrain, that she *must* sit passively by and wait for her death. Let us look again at the case of you and the violinist. There you are, in bed with the violinist, and the director of the hospital says to you, 'It's all most distressing, and I deeply sympathize, but you see this is putting an additional strain on your kidneys, and you'll be dead within the month. But you *have* to stay where you are all the same. Because unplugging you would be directly killing an innocent violinist, and that's murder, and that's impermissible.' If anything in the world is true, it is that you do not commit murder, you do not do what is impermissible, if you reach around to your back and unplug yourself from that violinist to save your life.

The main focus of attention in writings on abortion has been on what a third party may or may not do in answer to a request from a woman for an abortion. This is in a way understandable. Things being as they are, there isn't much a woman can safely do to abort herself. So the question asked is what a third party may do, and what the mother may do, if it is mentioned at all, is deduced, almost as an afterthought, from what it is concluded that third parties may do. But it seems to me that to treat the matter in this way is to refuse to grant to the mother that very status of person which is so firmly insisted on for the foetus. For we cannot simply read off what a person may do from what a third party may do. Suppose you find yourself trapped in a tiny house with a growing child. I mean a very tiny house, and a rapidly growing child—you are already up against the wall of the house and in a few minutes you'll be crushed to death. The child on the other hand won't be crushed to death; if nothing is done to stop him from growing he'll be hurt, but in the end he'll simply burst open the house and walk out a free man. Now I could well understand it if a bystander were to say, 'There's nothing we can do for you. We cannot choose between your life and his, we cannot be the ones to decide who is to live, we cannot intervene.' But it cannot be concluded that you too can do nothing, that you cannot attack it to save your life. However innocent the child may be, you do not have to wait passively while it crushes you to death. Perhaps a pregnant woman is vaguely felt to have the status of house, to which we don't allow the right of self-defence. But if the woman houses the child, it should be remembered that she is a person who houses it.

I should perhaps stop to say explicitly that I am not claiming that people have a right to do anything whatever to save their lives. I think, rather, that there are drastic limits to the right of self-defence. If someone threatens you with death unless you torture someone else to death, I think you have not the right, even to save your life, to do so. But the case under consideration here is very different. In our case there are only two people involved, one whose life is threatened, and one who threatens it. Both are innocent: the one who is threatened is not threatened because of any fault, the one who threatens does not threaten because of any fault. For this reason we may feel that we bystanders cannot intervene. But the person threatened can.

In sum, a woman surely can defend her life against the threat to it posed by the unborn child, even if doing so involves its death. And this shows not merely that the theses in (1) to (4) are false; it shows also that the extreme view of abortion is false, and so we need not canvass any other possible ways of arriving at it from the argument I mentioned at the outset.

2. The extreme view could of course be weakened to say that while abortion is permissible to save the mother's life, it may not be performed by a third party, but only by the mother herself. But this cannot be right either. For what we have to keep in mind is that the mother and the unborn child are not like two tenants in a small house which has, by an unfortunate mistake, been rented to both: the mother *owns* the house. The fact that she does adds to the offensiveness of deducing that the mother can do nothing from the supposition that third parties can do nothing. But it does more than this: it casts a bright light on the supposition that third parties can do nothing. Certainly it lets us see that a third party who says 'I cannot choose between you' is fooling himself if he thinks this is impartiality. If Jones has found and fastened on a certain coat, which he needs to keep him from freezing, but which Smith also needs to keep him from freezing, then it is not impartiality that says 'I cannot choose between you' when Smith owns the coat. Women have said again and again 'This body is *my* body!' and they have reason to feel angry, reason to feel that it has been like shouting into the wind. Smith, after all, is hardly likely to bless us if we say to him, 'Of course it's your coat, anybody would grant that it is. But no one may choose between you and Jones who is to have it.'

We should really ask what it is that says 'no one may choose' in the face of the fact that the body that houses the child is the mother's body. It may be simply a failure to appreciate this fact. But it may be something more interesting, namely the sense that one has a right to refuse to lay hands on people, even where it would be just and fair to do so, even where justice seems to require that somebody do so. Thus justice might call for somebody to get Smith's coat back from Jones, and yet you have a right to refuse to be the one to lay hands on Jones, a right to refuse to do physical violence to him. This, I think, must be granted. But then what should be said is not 'no one may choose', but only '*I* cannot choose', and indeed not even this, but '*I* will not *act*', leaving it open that somebody else can or should, and in particular that anyone in a position of authority, with the job of securing people's rights, both can and should. So this is no difficulty. I have not been arguing that any given third party must accede to the mother's request that he perform an abortion to save her life, but only that he may.

I suppose that in some views of human life the mother's body is only on loan to her, the loan not being one which gives her any prior claim to it. One who held this view might well think it impartiality to say 'I cannot choose'. But I shall simply ignore this possibility. My own view is that if a human being has any just, prior claim to anything at all, he has a just, prior claim to his own body. And perhaps this needn't be argued for here anyway, since, as I mentioned, the arguments against abortion we are looking at do grant that the woman has a right to decide what happens in and to her body.

But although they do grant it, I have tried to show that they do not take seriously what is done in granting it. I suggest the same thing will reappear even more clearly when we turn away from cases in which the mother's life is at stake, and attend, as I propose we now do, to the vastly more common cases in which a woman wants an abortion for some less weighty reason than preserving her own life.

3. Where the mother's life is not at stake, the argument I mentioned at the outset seems to have a much stronger pull. 'Everyone has a right to life, so the unborn person has a right to life.' And isn't the child's right to life weightier than anything other than the mother's own right to life, which she might put forward as ground for an abortion?

This argument treats the right to life as if it were unproblematic. It is not, and this seems to me to be precisely the source of the mistake.

For we should now, at long last, ask what it comes to, to have a right to life. In some views having a right to life includes having a right to be given at least the bare minimum one needs for continued life. But suppose that what in fact *is* the bare minimum a man needs for continued life is something he has no right at all to be given? If I am sick unto death, and the only thing that will save my life is the touch of Henry Fonda's cool hand on my fevered brow, then all the same, I have no right to be given the touch of Henry Fonda's cool hand on my fevered brow. It would be frightfully nice of him to fly in from the West Coast to provide it. It would be less nice, though no doubt well meant, if my friends flew out to the West Coast and carried Henry Fonda back with them. But I have no right at all against anybody that he should do this for me. Or again, to return to the story I told earlier, the fact that for continued life that violinist needs the continued use of your kidneys does not establish that he has a right to be given the continued use of your kidneys. He certainly has no right against you that *you* should give him continued use of your kidneys. For nobody has any right to use your kidneys unless you give him such a right; and nobody has the right against you that you shall give him this right—if you do allow him to go on using your kidneys, this is a kindness on your part, and not something he can claim from you as his due. Nor has he any right against anybody else that *they* should give him continued use of your kidneys. Certainly he had no right against the Society of Music Lovers that they should plug him into you in the first place. And if you now start to unplug yourself, having learned that you will otherwise have to spend nine years in bed with him, there is nobody in the world who must try to prevent you, in order to see to it that he is given something he has a right to be given.

Some people are rather stricter about the right to life. In their view, it does not include the right to be given anything, but amounts to, and only to, the right not to be killed by anybody. But here a related difficulty arises. If everybody is to refrain from killing that violinist, then everybody must refrain from doing a great many different sorts of things. Everybody must refrain from slitting his throat, everybody must refrain from shooting him— and everybody must refrain from unplugging you from him. But does he have a right against everybody that they shall refrain from unplugging you from him? To refrain from doing this is to allow him to continue to use your kidneys. It could be argued that he has a right against us that *we* should allow him to continue to use your kidneys. That is, while he had no right against us that we should give him the use of your kidneys, it might be argued that he anyway has a right against us that we shall not now intervene and deprive him of the use of your kidneys. I shall come back to third-party interventions later. But certainly the violinist has no right against you that *you* shall allow him to continue to use your kidneys. As I said, if you do allow him to use them, it is a kindness on your part, and not something you owe him.

The difficulty I point to here is not peculiar to the right to life. It reappears in connection with all the other natural rights; and it is something which an adequate account of rights must deal with. For present purposes it is enough just to draw attention to it. But I would stress that I am not arguing that people do not have a right to life—quite to the contrary, it seems to me that the primary control we must place on the acceptability of an account of rights is that it should turn out in that account to be a truth that all persons have a right to life. I am arguing only that having a right to life does not guarantee having either a right to be given the use of or a right to be allowed continued use of another person's body—even if one needs it for life itself. So the right to life will not serve the opponents of abortion in the very simple and clear way in which they seem to have thought it would.

4. There is another way to bring out the difficulty. In the most ordinary sort of case, to deprive someone of what he has a right to is to treat him unjustly. Suppose a boy and his small brother are jointly given a box of chocolates for Christmas. If the older boy takes the box and refuses to give his brother any of the chocolates, he is unjust to him, for the brother has been given a right to half of them. But suppose that, having learned that otherwise it means nine years in bed with that violinist, you unplug yourself from him. You surely are not being unjust to him, for you gave him no right to use your kidneys, and no one else can have given him any such right. But we have to notice that in unplugging yourself, you are killing him; and violinists, like everybody else, have a right to life, and thus in the view we were considering just now, the right not to be killed. So here you do what he supposedly has a right you shall not do, but you do not act unjustly to him in doing it.

The emendation which may be made at this point is this: the right to life consists not in the right not to be killed, but rather in the right not to be killed unjustly. This runs a risk of circularity, but never mind: it would enable us to square the fact that the violinist has a right to life with the fact that you do not act unjustly toward him in unplugging yourself, thereby killing him. For if you do not kill him unjustly, you do not violate his right to life, and so it is no wonder you do him no injustice.

But if this emendation is accepted, the gap in the argument against abortion stares us plainly in the face: it is by no means enough to show that the foetus is a person, and to remind us that all persons have a right to life—we need to be shown also that killing the foetus violates its right to life, i.e. that abortion is unjust killing. And is it?

I suppose we may take it as a datum that in a case of pregnancy due to rape the mother has not given the unborn person a right to the use of her body for food and shelter. Indeed, in what pregnancy could it be supposed that the mother has given the unborn person such a right? It is not as if there were unborn persons drifting about the world, to whom a woman who wants a child says 'I invite you in'.

But it might be argued that there are other ways one can have acquired a right to the use of another person's body than by having been invited to use it by that person. Suppose a woman voluntarily indulges in intercourse, knowing of the chance it will issue in pregnancy, and then she does become pregnant; is she not in part responsible for the presence, in fact the very existence, of the unborn person inside her? No doubt she did not invite it in. But doesn't her partial responsibility for its being there itself give it a right to the use of her body?[7] If so, then her aborting it would be more like the boy's taking away the chocolates, and less like your unplugging yourself from the violinist—doing so would be depriving it of what what it does have a right to, and thus would be doing it an injustice.

And then, too, it might be asked whether or not she can kill it even to save her own life: If she voluntarily called it into existence, how can she now kill it, even in self-defence?

The first thing to be said about this is that it is something new. Opponents of abortion have been so concerned to make out the independence of the foetus, in order to establish that it has a right to life, just as its mother does, that they have tended to overlook the possible support they might gain from making out that the foetus is *dependent* on the mother, in order to establish that she has a special kind of responsibility for it, a responsibility that gives it rights against her which are not possessed by any independent person— such as an ailing violinist who is a stranger to her.

On the other hand, this argument would give the unborn person a right to its mother's body only if her pregnancy resulted from a voluntary act, undertaken in full knowledge of the chance a pregnancy might result from it. It would leave out entirely the unborn person whose existence is due to rape. Pending the availability of some further argument, then we would be left with the conclusion that unborn persons whose existence is due to rape have no right to the use of their mothers' bodies, and thus that aborting them is not depriving them of anything they have a right to and hence is not unjust killing.

And we should also notice that it is not at all plain that this argument really does go even as far as it purports to. For there are cases and cases, and the details make a difference. If the room is stuffy, and I therefore open a window to air it, and a burglar climbs in, it would be absurd to say, 'Ah, now he can stay, she's given him a right to the use of her house—for she is partially responsible for his presence there, having voluntarily done what enabled him to get in, in full knowledge that there are such things as burglars, and that burglars burgle.' It would be still more absurd to say this if I had had bars installed outside my windows, precisely to prevent burglars from getting in, and a burglar got in only because of a defect in the bars. It remains equally absurd if we imagine it is not a burglar who climbs in, but an innocent person who blunders or falls in. Again, suppose it were like this: people-seeds drift about in the air like pollen, and if you open your windows, one may drift in and take root in your carpets or upholstery. You don't want

---

[7] The need for a discussion of this argument was brought home to me by members of the Society for Ethical and Legal Philosophy, to whom this paper was originally presented.

children, so you fix up your windows with fine mesh screens, the very best you can buy. As can happen, however, and on very, very rare occasions does happen, one of the screens is defective; and a seed drifts in and takes root. Does the person-plant who now develops have a right to the use of your house? Surely not—despite the fact that you voluntarily opened your windows, you knowingly kept carpets and upholstered furniture, and you knew that screens were sometimes defective. Someone may argue that you are responsible for its rooting, that it does have a right to your house, because after all you *could* have lived out your life with bare floors and furniture, or with sealed windows and doors. But this won't do—for by the same token anyone can avoid a pregnancy due to rape by having a hysterectomy, or anyway by never leaving home without a (reliable!) army.

It seems to me that the argument we are looking at can establish at most that there are *some* cases in which the unborn person has a right to the use of its mother's body, and therefore *some* cases in which abortion is unjust killing. There is room for much discussion and argument as to precisely which, if any. But I think we should side-step this issue and leave it open, for at any rate the argument certainly does not establish that all abortion is unjust killing.

5. There is room for yet another argument here, however. We surely must all grant that there may be cases in which it would be morally indecent to detach a person from your body at the cost of his life. Suppose you learn that what the violinist needs is not nine years of your life, but only one hour: all you need do to save his life is to spend one hour in that bed with him. Suppose also that letting him use your kidneys for that one hour would not affect your health in the slightest. Admittedly you were kidnapped. Admittedly you did not give anyone permission to plug him into you. Nevertheless it seems to me plain you *ought* to allow him to use your kidneys for that hour—it would be indecent to refuse.

Again, suppose pregnancy lasted only an hour, and constituted no threat to life or health. And suppose that a woman becomes pregnant as a result of rape. Admittedly she did not voluntarily do anything to bring about the existence of a child. Admittedly she did nothing at all which would give the unborn person a right to the use of her body. All the same it might well be said, as in the newly emended violinist story, that she *ought* to allow it to remain for that hour—that it would be indecent in her to refuse.

Now some people are inclined to use the term 'right' in such a way that it follows from the fact that you ought to allow a person to use your body for the hour he needs, that he has a right to use your body for the hour he needs, even though he has not been given that right by any person or act. They may say that it follows also that if you refuse, you act unjustly toward him. This use of the term is perhaps so common that it cannot be called wrong; nevertheless it seems to me to be an unfortunate loosening of what we would do better to keep a tight rein on. Suppose that box of chocolates I mentioned earlier had not been given to both boys jointly, but was given only to the older boy. There he sits, stolidly eating his way through the box, his small brother watching enviously. Here we are likely to say 'You ought not to be so mean. You ought to give your brother some of those chocolates.' My own view is that it just does not follow from the truth of this that the brother has any right to any of the chocolates. If the boy refuses to give his brother any, he is greedy, stingy, callous—but not unjust. I suppose that the people I have in mind will say it does follow that the brother has a right to some of the chocolates, and thus that the boy does act unjustly if he refuses to give his brother any. But the effect of saying this is to obscure what we should keep distinct, namely the difference between the boy's refusal in this case and the boy's refusal in the earlier case, in which the box was given to both boys jointly, and in which the small brother thus had what was from any point of view clear title to half.

A further objection to so using the term 'right' that from the fact that A ought to do a thing for B, it follows that B has a right against A that A do it for him, is that it is going to make the question of whether or not a man has a right to a thing turn on how easy it is to provide him with it; and this seems not merely unfortunate, but morally unacceptable. Take the case of Henry Fonda again. I said earlier that I had no right to the touch of his cool hand on my fevered brow, even though I needed it to save my life. I said it would be frightfully nice of him to fly in from the West Coast to provide me with it, but that I had no right against him that he should do so. But suppose he isn't on the West Coast. Suppose he has only to walk across the room, place a hand briefly on my brow—and lo, my life is saved. Then surely he ought to do it, it would be indecent to refuse. Is it to be said 'Ah, well, it follows that in this case she has a right to the touch of his hand on her brow, and so it would be an injustice in him to refuse?' So that I have a right to it when it is easy for him to provide it, though no right when it's hard? It's rather a shocking idea that anyone's rights should fade away and disappear as it gets harder and harder to accord them to him.

So my own view is that even though you ought to let the violinist use your kidneys for the one hour he needs, we should not conclude that he has a right to do so—we should say that if you refuse, you are, like the boy who owns all the chocolates and will give none away, self-centred and callous, indecent in fact, but not unjust. And similarly, that even supposing a case in which a woman pregnant due to rape ought to allow the unborn person to use her body for the hour he needs, we should not conclude that he has a right to do so; we should conclude that she is self-centred, callous, indecent, but not unjust, if she refuses. The complaints are no less grave; they are just different. However, there is no need to insist on this point. If anyone does wish to deduce 'he has a right' from 'you ought', then all the same he must surely grant that there are cases in which it is not morally required of you that you allow that violinist to use your kidneys, and in which he does not have a right to use them, and so also for mother and unborn child. Except in such cases as the unborn person has a right to demand it—and we were leaving open the possibility that there may be such cases—nobody is morally *required* to make large sacrifices, of health, of all other interests and concerns, of all other duties and commitments, for nine years, or even for nine months, in order to keep another person alive.

6. We have in fact to distinguish between two kinds of Samaritan: the Good Samaritan and what we might call the Minimally Decent Samaritan. The story of the Good Samaritan, you will remember, goes like this:

A certain man went down from Jerusalem to Jericho, and fell among thieves, which stripped him of his raiment, and wounded him, and departed, leaving him half dead.
And by chance there came down a certain priest that way; and when he saw him, he passed by on the other side.
And likewise a Levite, when he was at the place, came and looked on him, and passed by on the other side.
But a certain Samaritan, as he journeyed, came where he was; and when he saw him he had compassion on him.
And went to him, and bound up his wounds, pouring in oil and wine, and set him on his own beast, and brought him to an inn, and took care of him.
And on the morrow, when he departed, he took out two pence, and gave them to the host, and said unto him, 'Take care of him; and whatsoever thou spendest more, when I come again, I will repay thee.'

(Luke 10: 30–5)

The Good Samaritan went out of his way, at some cost to himself, to help one in need of it. We are not told what the options were, that is, whether or not the priest and the Levite could have helped by doing less than the Good Samaritan did, but assuming they could have, then the fact they did nothing at all shows they were not even Minimally Decent Samaritans, not because they were not Samaritans, but because they were not even minimally decent.

These things are a matter of degree, of course, but there is a difference, and it comes out perhaps most clearly in the story of Kitty Genovese, who, as you will remember, was murdered while thirty-eight people watched or listened, and did nothing at all to help her. A Good Samaritan would have rushed out to give direct assistance against the murderer. Or perhaps we had better allow that it would have been a Splendid Samaritan who did this, on the ground that it would have involved a risk of death for himself. But the thirty-eight not only did not do this, they did not even trouble to pick up a phone to call the police. Minimally Decent Samaritanism would call for doing at least that, and their not having done it was monstrous.

After telling the story of the Good Samaritan, Jesus said 'Go, and do thou likewise.' Perhaps he meant that we are morally required to act as the Good Samaritan did. Perhaps he was urging people to do more than is morally required of them. At all events it seems plain that it was not morally required of any of the thirty-eight that he rush out to give direct assistance at the risk of his own life, and that it is not morally required of anyone that he give long stretches of his life—nine years or nine months—to sustaining the life of a person who has no special right (we were leaving open the possibility of this) to demand it.

Indeed, with one rather striking class of exceptions, no one in any country in the world is *legally* required to do anywhere near as much as this for anyone else. The class of exceptions is obvious. My main concern here is not the state of the law in respect to abortion, but it is worth drawing attention to the fact that in no state in this country is any man compelled by law to be even a Minimally Decent Samaritan to any person; there is no law under which charges could be brought against the thirty-eight who stood by while Kitty Genovese died. By contrast, in most states in this country women are compelled by law to be not merely Minimally Decent Samaritans, but Good Samaritans to unborn persons inside them. This doesn't by itself settle anything one way or the other, because it may well be argued that there should be laws in this country—as there are in many European countries— compelling at least Minimally Decent Samaritanism.[8] But it does show that there is a gross injustice in the existing state of the law. And it shows also that the groups currently working against liberalization of abortion laws, in fact working toward having it declared unconstitutional for a state to permit abortion, had better start working for the adoption of Good Samaritan laws generally, or earn the charge that they are acting in bad faith.

I should think, myself, that Minimally Decent Samaritan laws would be one thing, Good Samaritan laws quite another, and in fact highly improper. But we are not here concerned with the law. What we should ask is not whether anybody should be compelled by law to be a Good Samaritan, but whether we must accede to a situation in which somebody is being compelled—by nature, perhaps—to be a Good Samaritan. We have, in other words, to look now at third-party interventions. I have been arguing that no person is morally required to make large sacrifices to sustain the life of

---

[8] For a discussion of the difficulties involved, and a survey of the European experience with such laws, see James M. Ratcliffe (ed.), *The Good Samaritan and the Law* (New York, 1966).

another who has no right to demand them, and this even where the sacrifices do not include life itself; we are not morally required to be Good Samaritans or anyway Very Good Samaritans to one another. But what if a man cannot extricate himself from such a situation? What if he appeals to us to extricate him? It seems to me plain that there are cases in which we can, cases in which a Good Samaritan would extricate him. There you are, you were kidnapped, and nine years in bed with that violinist lie ahead of you. You have your own life to lead. You are sorry, but you simply cannot see giving up so much of your life to the sustaining of his. You cannot extricate yourself, and ask us to do so. I should have thought that—in light of his having no right to the use of your body—it was obvious that we do not have to accede to your being forced to give up so much. We can do what you ask. There is no injustice to the violinist in our doing so.

7. Following the lead of the opponents of abortion. I have throughout been speaking of the foetus merely as a person, and what I have been asking is whether or not the argument we began with, which proceeds only from the foetus's being a person, really does establish its conclusion. I have argued that it does not.

But of course there are arguments and arguments, and it may be said that I have simply fastened on the wrong one. It may be said that what is important is not merely the fact that the foetus is a person, but that it is a person for whom the woman has a special kind of responsibility issuing from the fact that she is its mother. And it might be argued that all my analogies are therefore irrelevant—for you do not have that special kind of responsibility for that violinist, Henry Fonda does not have that special kind of responsibility for me. And our attention might be drawn to the fact that men and women both *are* compelled by law to provide support for their children.

I have in effect dealt (briefly) with this argument in section 4 above; but a (still briefer) recapitulation now may be in order. Surely we do not have any such 'special responsibility' for a person unless we have assumed it, explicitly or implicitly. If a set of parents do not try to prevent pregnancy, do not obtain an abortion, and then at the time of birth of the child do not put it out for adoption, but rather take it home with them, then they have assumed responsibility for it, they have given it rights, and they cannot *now* withdraw support from it at the cost of its life because they now find it difficult to go on providing for it. But if they have taken all reasonable precautions against having a child, they do not simply by virtue of their biological relationship to the child who comes into existence have a special responsibility for it. They may wish to assume responsibility for it, or they may not wish to. And I am suggesting that if assuming responsibility for it would require large sacrifices, then they may refuse. A Good Samaritan would not refuse—or anyway, a Splendid Samaritan, if the sacrifices that had to be made were enormous. But then so would a Good Samaritan assume responsibility for that violinist; so would Henry Fonda, if he is a Good Samaritan, fly in from the West Coast and assume responsibility for me.

8. My argument will be found unsatisfactory on two counts by many of those who want to regard abortion as morally permissible. First, while I do argue that abortion is not impermissible, I do not argue that it is always permissible. There may well be cases in which carrying the child to term requires only Minimally Decent Samaritanism of the mother, and this is a standard we must not fall below. I am inclined to think it a merit of my account precisely that it does *not* give a general yes or a general no. It allows for and supports our sense that, for example, a sick and desperately frightened fourteen-year-old schoolgirl, pregnant due to rape, may *of course* choose abortion, and that any law which rules this out is an insane law. And it also allows for and supports our sense that in other cases resort to abortion is even positively indecent. It would be indecent in the woman to request an abortion, and indecent in a doctor to perform it, if she is in her seventh month, and wants the abortion just to avoid the nuisance of postponing a trip abroad. The very fact that the arguments I have been drawing attention to treat all cases of abortion, or even all cases of abortion in which the mother's life is not at stake, as morally on a par ought to have made them suspect at the outset.

Secondly, while I am arguing for the permissibility of abortion in some cases, I am not arguing for the right to secure the death of the unborn child. It is easy to confuse these two things in that up to a certain point in the life of the foetus it is not able to survive outside the mother's body; hence removing it from her body guarantees its death. But they are importantly different. I have argued that you are not morally required to spend nine months in bed, sustaining the life of that violinist; but to say this is by no means to say that if, when you unplug yourself, there is a miracle and he survives, you then have a right to turn round and slit his throat. You may detach yourself even if this costs him his life; you have no right to be guaranteed his death, by some other means, if unplugging yourself does not kill him. There are some people who will feel dissatisfied by this feature of my argument. A woman may be utterly devastated by the thought of a child, a bit of herself, put out for adoption and never seen or heard of again. She may therefore want not merely that the child be detached from her, but more, that it die. Some opponents of abortion are inclined to regard this as beneath contempt—thereby showing insensitivity to what is surely a powerful source of despair. All the same, I agree that the desire for the child's death is not one which anybody may gratify, should it turn out to be possible to detach the child alive.

At this place, however, it should be remembered that we have only been pretending throughout that the foetus is a human being from the moment of conception. A very early abortion is surely not the killing of a person, and so is not dealt with by anything I have said here.

2

KILLING AND LETTING DIE

HELGA KUHSE AND PETER SINGER

THE ISSUE

One of the first widely publicized cases of an abnormal infant deliberately being allowed to die is 'The Johns Hopkins Case', so named after the Johns Hopkins Hospital in Baltimore, where the events took place. In many respects the case is similar to that of Baby Doe: the infant had Down's syndrome and a blockage in its digestive system. The blockage could have been removed by surgery, but the mother, who was a nurse, refused to consent to the operation. The father accepted this decision, taking the view that his wife was more knowledgeable about such cases than he was. The baby was therefore left untreated. It could not digest food taken through its mouth, and no attempt was made to feed it by any other method. In contrast to the Baby Doe case, neither the doctors nor the hospital made any attempt to take the parents' decision before a court. A further contrast with the Baby Doe case is that the baby took much longer to die: fifteen days.

A dramatized version of these events was made into a film entitled *Who Should Survive?*, produced by the Joseph P. Kennedy Foundation in Washington, DC. At Monash University, we show the film to students taking an undergraduate philosophy course on 'Contemporary Moral Issues'. The film shows how, after the parents have made their decision, the baby is placed in a side room with a sign on its cot: NOTHING BY MOUTH. Nurses are shown rocking a crying baby, trying to comfort it. The film discusses how difficult it was for the nursing staff to be unable to do anything but watch the baby wither away from dehydration and hunger. The film also shows the doctor talking on the phone to the baby's father, who called daily to find out 'how things were going'. To this the doctor can say nothing, except that everything is happening as one would expect, just a little slowly.

From Helga Kuhse and Peter Singer, 'Killing and Letting Die,' in their *Should the Baby Live?* (Oxford: Oxford University Press, 1985).

Not surprisingly, students find the film disturbing. Most of them believe that what they have seen should not have happened. Less predictably, however, of this large majority who think that these events should not have taken place, by no means all disagree with the parents' decision to refuse permission for the operation. What many of them find objectionable is not the decision that a Down's syndrome baby should not be kept alive; it is to the manner in which that decision was implemented that they object. They are horrified that death should have been a fifteen-day ordeal for the nurses, the doctors, the family, and most important, for the baby. 'If the doctors were not going to challenge the refusal of permission to operate,' a student will often ask, 'why couldn't they do something to end the baby's suffering sooner?'

That is the question we shall examine in this chapter. As in the Johns Hopkins case, the Baby Doe case, and the case of spina bifida infants who have been judged too severely affected to warrant treatment, the question arises only after the crucial decision not to provide life-prolonging treatment has been made. We make no assumption, at this stage, about *when* we are justified in making this crucial decision. In particular, we have said nothing about whether it is a defensible decision in the case of Down's syndrome infants with digestive system blockages. Yet since almost everyone—even, as we saw in Chapter 2, President Reagan's Surgeon General, Dr C. Everett Koop—believes that it is *sometimes* right not to attempt to prolong life, the question arises for almost every doctor treating newborn infants: given that the baby's life will not be prolonged, would it not be kinder—and ethically preferable—to kill it?

In asking this question we are, of course, aware that any doctor administering a lethal injection to an infant would risk a murder charge. This may also be true, however, of a doctor who deliberately allows an infant to die— most legal systems recognize that there can be murder by omission as well as murder by action. The law is, however, too complex for us to discuss here. Nor do we need to discuss it, for we are not asking what any individual doctor, working within a particular legal system, should do. We are asking a more fundamental question: when other things are equal, is there a morally significant difference between allowing a baby to die, and killing that baby? In asking this question we do not need to take account of the law. It is, if anything, the other way round: if we were to discuss what the law in this area ought to be, then we would need to ask whether there is a morally significant difference between killing and allowing to die. The moral issue comes first; only when it has been answered can we assess the law and see if it should be reformed.

THE MEDICAL MAINSTREAM

The feasibility and desirability of treatment of a grossly handicapped infant, especially in the neonatal period, is one of the most difficult decisions in paediatrics ... For centuries the mainstream of medical opinion has abhorred the extremes and has trod the middle path. This was expressed in classical form by the nineteenth-century English poet Arthur Clough (1819–61):

> Thou shalt not kill; but need'st not strive
> Officiously to keep alive.

So wrote G. Keys Smith and E. Durham Smith in their 1973 article in the *British Medical Journal*, reporting on selective treatment for spina bifida at the Royal Children's Hospital in Melbourne. The lines they quote from Clough are often quoted by doctors discussing the difference between killing a patient and allowing that patient to die. In the last chapter we saw that they were referred to with approval by Haas in his contribution to the debate triggered off in *The Lancet* by Zachary's article on the treatment of spina bifida: 'The old dictum we were taught as medical students' is how Haas described them, and this is probably how most doctors think of Clough's couplet. Ironically, it is the very opposite of how Clough himself thought of his most quoted lines. They come from a poem called 'The Latest Decalogue'. Here are the opening lines:

> Thou shalt have one god only; who
> Would be at the expense of two?
> No graven images may be
> Worshipped, except the currency.

As these lines make clear, the poem is a bitingly satirical attack on those who profess to respect the Ten Commandments, but in fact betray their spirit at every point. For Clough the idea that it is all right to allow people to die, as long as one does not actually kill them, is just this sort of betrayal of the spirit of the commandment.

For anyone with an inclination for historical detective work, it would be fascinating to find out just how Clough's satirical lines were transformed into an 'old dictum' taught to medical students, and even into the 'classical form' of the mainstream of medical opinion. We must, however, confine ourselves to more urgent tasks: to show that the author of these oft-quoted lines did not share the views of those who now quote them, is not to refute the view in support of which they are being quoted. Clough, it may now be said, was simply unable to see the valid point behind the attitude he was satirizing. Certainly the attitude is now widely held, especially amongst doctors. In our survey of nearly 200 obstetricians and paediatricians in Victoria, all but two agreed that in some circumstances it was proper to decide against using all available means to keep an infant alive; yet only 31 per cent of obstetricians and 40 per cent of paediatricians were prepared to accept that active euthanasia could ever be justified. In other words 99 per cent of doctors were ready to allow an infant to die, but of these more than 60 per cent were not ready to kill it.

An American survey in 1975 of 457 paediatricians and paediatric surgeons produced even stronger support for the distinction. In this survey, referred to by Dr C. Everett Koop in his testimony before Judge Gerhard Gesell, the doctors were asked to imagine that the parents of a Down's syndrome baby with a blockage had refused consent to surgery, and that they—the doctors—had decided to accept this decision. Would they then stop all supportive treatment, such as tube feedings? Would they terminate the infant's life by an injection of drugs such as morphine? A large majority of the doctors replied that they would stop all supportive treatment, but only six doctors said that they were prepared to give a lethal injection. Admittedly, these results have to be treated with caution. More than a third of those who sent back the questionnaires did not answer this question; it is possible that they were reluctant to put on paper their readiness to break the law. Moreover, a few who said that they were not prepared to kill nevertheless added comments describing this course as 'most humane but illegal' or 'what I would prefer to do but it is illegal under present laws'. These comments make it clear that the doctors were indicating what they would actually do in the present situation, not what they thought ought to be done in an ideal situation. Nevertheless, the survey suggests that in America, as in Australia, most doctors distinguish between allowing to die and killing.

Medical associations support doctors in these views. The American Medical Association, as we have seen, condemns mercy killing as 'contrary to that for which the medical profession stands', but under certain circumstances accepts 'the cessation of the employment of extraordinary means to prolong the life of the body'—in other words, allowing the patient to die. The Australian Medical Association, in a submission to the Law Reform Commission of Western Australia in 1982, has said: 'Surely when it is deemed to be in the best interests of the child that its life should not be prolonged, the ability to refuse to prolong its life should exist.' The submission then went on to admit that on moral or philosophical lines it was extremely difficult to draw a line between actively killing and passively allowing someone to die; nevertheless, the submission said, 'doctors felt the distinction very strongly'.

In the final section of the last chapter, we saw some of the consequences of these attitudes for those spina bifida infants who are not selected for treatment. One consequence already noted is that many babies take a long time to die. Another consequence is that the final outcome—life or death—is often determined not by any rational assessment of the severity of the infant's handicap, but by chance factors, such as whether the infant happens to contract an infection in its first few days of life. This chance element is especially apparent when Down's syndrome infants with simple intestinal blockages are allowed to die, while those without such blockages live. The blockage has nothing to do with the severity of the mental handicap. It ought therefore to be quite irrelevant to the question of whether an infant born with that particular handicap should live or die. Yet because it allows parents the option of refusing consent to an operation, it can be the determining factor in this life or death choice. The accidental presence of the blockage means that parents can choose to let the infant die, whereas if the baby did not need surgery they would not be able to choose to kill it.

An even more striking illustration of the role played by 'accident' comes from the treatment of Andrew Stinson, an extremely premature and marginally viable baby born to Peggy Stinson, a Pennsylvania teacher, in December 1977. Despite a firm statement by Peggy and her husband that they wanted 'no heroics', Andrew was kept alive for nearly six months. Long before the end of that period, it was clear that if he survived at all he would be seriously damaged. Andrew needed a respirator to keep him breathing, but the doctors would not take him off it—to do so they regarded as wrong, presumably because it involved a deliberate human act. As Peggy Stinson put it in her journal:

I shouldn't say they 'took him off'—they couldn't do that, since that would be immoral and illegal. They had to hope for an appropriate accident; once Andrew became accidentally detached from the respirator and had breathed for a couple of minutes, they could declare him 'off' and *omit* to put him back on while they wait for his inadequate breathing to kill him. This is the moral, legal, and 'dignified' way.

Had Andrew not become accidentally detached, he might have gone on being kept alive indefinitely; but such accidental detachings occur routinely. Normally this triggers an alarm, and the re-attachment is equally routine—unless the decision has been made that it is better for the baby to die.

It is striking how far some doctors will go to ensure that infants they are 'allowing to die' actually do die—while still refusing to advocate active euthanasia. Here is a statement from Herbert Eckstein, a London paediatric surgeon, referring to a spina bifida baby that is not to be treated:

It is in my opinion quite impossible to kill off such a baby, but if surgical treatment is withheld then it is only reasonable to withhold other forms of treatment such as antibiotics, oxygen, and tube feeding ... In our experience to date all children with myelomeningocele who were refused surgical treatment have died within a month and if a baby is not to be treated then the surgeons and nursing staff should do nothing to prolong life.

John Lorber takes a similar stance. As we have seen, he has stressed that once the decision not to operate has been reached, 'nothing should be done which might prolong the infant's survival'. Lorber makes no secret of the fact that the object of non-treatment is 'not to avoid treating those who would die early in spite of treatment, but to avoid treating those who would survive with severe handicaps'. In the light of this statement, it is obvious that non-treatment has failed in its object if the patient survives. To say the same thing in positive terms: the object of non-treatment is that the patient should die. Moreover Lorber acknowledges, as any humane person would: 'It is painful to see such infants gradually fading away over a number of weeks or months, when everybody hopes for a speedy end.' Indeed, we have already seen that some doctors think Lorber's use of the sedative chloral hydrate goes a long way towards ensuring that everybody's hopes are fulfilled. Nevertheless Lorber says: 'I strongly disagree with active euthanasia.' We must now examine the reasons why Lorber, Eckstein, and so many other doctors hold this view.

'LETTING NATURE TAKE ITS COURSE'

Apart from the celebrated 'old dictum' of Arthur Clough, the most oft-recurring refrain in this debate is that allowing patients to die is different from killing because the doctor who allows a patient to die is merely 'letting Nature take its course'. We saw Dr Ian Wickes, in his contribution to the debate over Zachary's *Lancet* article, suggest that 'to let Nature take its course' is a middle way between treating all spina bifida infants and killing some of them. In the same debate Dr Haas was thinking along similar lines when he said that 'Nature if left alone will always correct its own mistakes in these cases.' John Lorber has said that selective non-treatment is 'another name for letting nature take its course.' Dr Vincent Collins, writing in the *Journal of the American Medical Association* on 'Limits of Medical Responsibility in Prolonging Life', offered this characterization of the distinction between killing and allowing to die:

In [euthanasia] one directly causes life to end, whereas by discontinuing therapy one permits death to occur by omitting an act and permitting nature to take its course ... When one permits death by not continuing therapy, the harm that is done is done by nature acting.

In his book *The Patient as a Person*, the Protestant theologian Paul Ramsey puts it this way:

In omission no human agent causes the patient's death, directly or indirectly. He dies his own death from causes that it is no longer merciful or reasonable to fight by possible medical intervention.

The thrust of all these comments is that if we kill, we are responsible for the resulting death; if, however, a doctor allows a patient to die, it is nature that is responsible. This is a slightly odd suggestion for medical practitioners to make, since medicine is largely an attempt to prevent nature taking its course. Nevertheless, the suggestion needs closer scrutiny. First we need to distinguish two possible interpretations. Is the suggestion that when death results from an omission the doctor is not *causally* responsible for the death? Or is it that the doctor is not *morally* responsible for the death? To be sure that we have covered the point of the appeal to nature, we must deal with both these possibilities.

The first possibility is that when we allow someone to die, we are not causally responsible for the death. Suppose we are dealing with a severe case of spina bifida, one that we have decided not to treat. The baby develops an infection. We have antibiotics at hand which we know could cure the infection, but because this baby is not being treated, we do not give antibiotics. As we expected, the infection worsens and the baby dies. Can we say that because the baby died of an infection, we did not cause the baby's death? Is this simply 'death from natural causes'?

This approach relies on an intuitive sense of 'cause' which further thought shows is indefensible for two reasons. First, it is unable to tell us which omissions merely permit nature to act, and which go beyond this; for presumably those who take this approach will not describe *all* deaths resulting from omissions in this way. They would not want to say that Dr Leonard Arthur was merely permitting nature to take its course when he wrote 'Parents do not wish baby to survive. Nursing care only' on the medical record of John Pearson—who was, remember, a Down's syndrome baby with no other apparent abnormalities. Obviously, if starving to death were merely allowing nature to take its course, there would be an easy way for the parents of any unwanted infant to ensure that it died without their having caused its death. On the other hand, if death by starvation were not death by 'natural causes', would those who take his approach want to invoke 'natural causes' in a case of death by an infection that is as preventable as starvation?

The second objection to the view we are considering is that there is no satisfactory account of what it is to 'cause' something, according to which deaths by omission are caused by 'nature' rather than by the person who omitted to act. As the Oxford legal philosophers H. L. A. Hart and A. M. Honoré have pointed out in their influential book *Causation and the Law*, we often regard a human omission as the cause of something which, from a different perspective, may seem very much an act of nature:

the cause of a great famine in India may be identified by the Indian peasant as the drought, but the World Food Authority may identify the Indian Government's failure to build up reserves as the cause and the drought as a mere condition.

Here we can see the philosophical naivety of the idea that nature, rather than a deliberate human omission, causes the death of the untreated baby who develops an infection. John Stuart Mill pointed out long ago that the cause of an event is 'philosophically speaking . . . the sum total of the conditions positive and negative taken together'. By 'conditions positive and negative' he means both those that had to exist, and those that had to *not* exist, for the event to occur. Thus the cause of a guest being burnt to death in a hotel fire might be that there was an electrical short circuit *and* that there was inflammable material nearby *and* that there was no sprinkler system *and* that the fire alarm had not been serviced for three years and so did not go off . . . The list could be extended indefinitely, because there would have been no deaths if the hotel had been empty, or if it had never been built in the first place, and so on. There is really no such thing as 'the cause' in the sense of one condition or event which has some objective claim to being the single determining factor. It is only against a background of our particular interest in questions such as how an event could have been prevented that we sometimes single out 'the cause' of an event. In the example just given we are unlikely to refer to the existence of the hotel or the presence of the guest as the cause of the death, since we take hotels and their guests for granted as part of the background. What about the electrical short circuit? Electrical engineers might well single this out as the cause of the death; they might, for instance, use this fire as a case study in electrical hazards, and on this basis suggest improvements in electrical design and safety which would eliminate such occurrences. A public inquiry into the death, on the other hand, would be more likely to focus on who is to blame. From this perspective, the short circuit may not be seen as the cause of the death, since we know that such things do happen from time to time, given the prevailing standards of electrical safety. The inquiry would probably conclude that the death was the result of the management's negligent disregard of standard precautions against fire.

This example shows how the notion of a single event being 'the cause' swiftly breaks down, once we give our attention to a particular consequence and the different reasons why we might be interested in it. Suppose that we are interested in why a baby died. We may be told that the baby contracted pneumonia and died of 'natural causes'. But if we know that many other babies in the same hospital also contracted pneumonia and did not die from it, this answer should not satisfy us. We are interested in why *this* baby died, and a condition which also applies to many other babies who did not die cannot answer our inquiry. So we press the point, and are told that the other babies were given antibiotics which enabled them to overcome the pneumonia; this baby, on the other hand, was a Down's syndrome child, had been rejected by its parents, and so was not given antibiotics. Now we know what differentiates this baby with pneumonia from the other babies with pneumonia: this one was not given antibiotics. Since antibiotics could have cured the pneumonia, the doctor's omission is the causal factor that made the difference between this baby living or dying. Hence we can appropriately describe the doctor's failure to treat the pneumonia as the cause of death.

So it cannot be said that when a doctor refrains from treating a patient, the patient's death is caused by 'nature' rather than by the doctor. Both the illness and the omission are part of 'the sum total of the conditions positive and negative taken together' which is the full causal account of the death. We can properly single out any one of a number of these conditions as *the* cause, depending on our particular interests in the matter.

Let us try the other possible interpretation of the remarks by Vincent Collins, Paul Ramsey, and the other writers we quoted earlier: could it be that when death comes as a result of an omission rather than an action, no one is *morally* responsible for the death, because it is only 'nature taking its course'?

This is even less plausible than the previous claim, especially in the medical setting, where the doctor has a clear moral responsibility for the care of the patient. Of course, we are not morally responsible for all our omissions. If I am standing on the beach while someone drowns in the surf fifty metres away, I will not be morally responsible for the death if, concentrating on a game of beach cricket, I fail to notice the person signalling for help. Even if I did notice the signal, but was unable to help because I cannot swim a stroke and there was no one else who could be summoned in time, I will not be responsible. If, however, I noticed the signal and could easily have carried out the rescue, but refrained from doing so because I didn't wish to interrupt my sunbathing, I bear considerable moral responsibility for the death. If I happen also to be a lifeguard and was on duty at the time, my moral responsibility for refraining from rescuing the drowning person is greater still. Moral responsibility arises only when we have some control over our actions in a situation, and it is strengthened when we have a specific duty that is relevant to what is happening.

When John Lorber and Herbert Eckstein leave infants to die of pneumonia without giving antibiotics, they are not like the person who did not
notice that there was someone drowning nearby. They are well aware of the
condition of the infants and its likely lethal nature. Nor are they like the
person who notices the victim but is unable to help. They have at their
disposal powerful drugs which in almost all cases will effect a cure. They are
not even like the ordinary sunbather; they are more like the lifeguard—not,
of course, in respect of their motives, but in respect of the degree of moral
responsibility they bear. Just as lifeguards have a well-recognized duty
towards swimmers, so doctors have a well-recognized duty towards their
patients. Doctors who deliberately leave a baby to die when they have the
awareness, the ability, and the opportunity to save the baby's life, are just as
morally responsible for the death as they would be if they had brought it
about by a deliberate, positive action. This does not mean, of course, that it
is necessarily wrong for doctors to leave a baby to die: it means only that the
responsibility for doing so cannot be evaded by saying that the harm is done
by 'nature acting'. The responsibility for the baby's death is the doctor's, and
it is one which must be squarely faced.

THE DOCTRINE OF DOUBLE EFFECT

At this point we briefly mention another view, sometimes confused with the
distinction between killing and letting die: the 'doctrine of double effect'.
This doctrine is regarded as important by Roman Catholic theologians and
moralists, and a considerable literature has been built up around it. We shall
not probe the intricacies of this doctrine. We refer to it only in order to show
that, whatever its merits, it is not relevant to the decisions made by doctors
like Lorber and Eckstein.

The doctrine of double effect relies on a distinction between what we
directly intend to do, and what we merely foresee will result from our act.
Thus, in a classic application of the doctrine, Roman Catholic theologians
have permitted doctors to remove a cancerous womb from a pregnant
woman. The doctor foresees, of course, that the foetus will die as a result of
the operation. Nevertheless the doctor does not directly intend the death of
the foetus. The direct intention is to save the woman's life. If there were a
way of doing this which allowed the foetus to live, the doctor would take that
way. Unfortunately there is not. Hence the death of the foetus is an
unwanted side-effect of a laudable intention, and the doctor is not regarded
as killing the foetus.

It is easy to see that this doctrine will give rise to some very fine distinctions, especially when it is coupled—as it is in Roman Catholic moral theology—with the view that the end does not justify the means. For instance, a case which seems very similar to the one just described is that in which the head of the foetus has, during delivery, become lodged in the vaginal passage. If all attempts to dislodge it are unavailing—not likely now-adays, but it did happen when medical techniques were less sophisticated—the only way to save the life of the woman is to insert an instrument which will crush the skull of the foetus. The outcome is then the same as in the case of the cancerous womb. The foetus dies, but the woman lives. Despite the similarity of results, Roman Catholic theologians did not, and still would not, permit doctors to perform this operation. To carry it out, they said, the doctors had to form the direct intention to crush the skull of the foetus, which is of course equivalent to killing it. Even though the motive of the action was the same as in the previous case, the death of the foetus was here not an unwanted side-effect, but the directly intended means to the desired end. As such, it was the direct killing of an innocent human being and absolutely prohibited.

The difficulty of seeing much moral significance in the distinction between these two cases has led many people to reject the doctrine of double effect—and we would, if it were necessary for us to take a stand on the question, reject it for this and other reasons. For our present purposes, however, it is only necessary for us to point out that when, say, John Lorber selects a patient for non-treatment, he does directly intend the death of that patient. To quote him again: 'The main object of selection is . . . to avoid treating those who would survive with handicaps.' Recall, too, Lorber's instruction that the temptation to operate on the hydrocephalus must be resisted 'because progressive hydrocephalus is an important cause of early death'. Clearly Lorber does intend the death of those patients he selects for non-treatment—otherwise selection would not reduce the number who survive with handicaps, and might even—as Freeman's case of the surviving untreated boy suggests—increase the handicaps these patients will have. There is no sense in which these deaths are mere 'unwanted side-effects' of a course of action pursued for some other, more vital goal.

As we can see from Lorber's statements, the fact that a death occurs as a result of an omission rather than as the result of an action has nothing to do with the doctor's intention. One can intend to cause a death by an omission, just as one can intend to cause a death by an action. Whatever its merits, the doctrine of double effect is quite separate from the claim that we are not responsible for the results of our omissions.

THE LORBER–HARRIS DEBATE

We have used John Lorber as a standard example of a doctor who selects some severely handicapped infants for an early death. We have done this not because we believe his practice is unusual, but because he has written so explicitly about what he is doing. We have also mentioned that he is opposed to active euthanasia. Since we have quoted so frequently from his writings, it is only fitting to give his reasons for this opposition.

Lorber raised the question of active euthanasia in his 1975 Milroy Lecture on 'Ethical Problems in the Management of Myelomeningocele and Hydrocephalus'. His objections are worth quoting at length:

It may . . . be inconsistent or hypocritical to oppose active euthanasia, yet support non-treatment, or what is often called passive euthanasia. However, active euthanasia may brutalize the persons who carry it out. It would be wrong for a doctor to order his junior or his nurses to carry out such a task if he cannot bring himself to do it.

I strongly disagree with active euthanasia, especially for babies and children, who cannot possibly ask for it or give their considered consent. It would be impossible to formulate legislation, however humane are the intentions, that could not be abused by the unscrupulous. There have been plenty of horrific examples of this in the past, especially in Hitler's Germany. Few just or compassionate persons would wish to give such a dangerous legal power to any individual or group of people.

Yet for some severely handicapped spina bifida babies or others who are equally severely handicapped it would be the most humane way to deal with a desperate situation. It is painful to see such infants gradually fading away over a number of weeks or months, when everybody hopes for a speedy end. It is this consideration of lingering death that still compels some doctors to treat, reluctantly, all babies, in spite of the suffering such a policy will entail.

Nevertheless, no treatment is not necessarily equivalent to passive euthanasia. No treatment with normal nursing care is a safeguard against wrong diagnosis and against deliberate misdiagnosis for an evil purpose. If an infant's condition is not as grave as was thought, he will live, and he can then be given optimal care if he has any handicaps.

John Harris, an English philosopher whose work has focused on moral responsibility, has published a detailed critique of this passage in the *Journal of Medical Ethics*. He finds four separate arguments in it, and deals with them in turn. Lorber then replies to Harris, in the same journal. This debate gives us an unusual opportunity to see how a practising physician handles a philosopher's critique of his published views on an ethical issue. We shall follow the sequence of arguments set out by Harris, and consider Lorber's reply to each point.

The Argument from Brutalization

Lorber opens his objections to active euthanasia by asserting that active euthanasia may brutalize those who carry it out. Lorber cites no evidence of this, and as Harris points out, evidence would be hard to find. So we are balancing a mere speculative possibility against the real and known pain and distress of patients, family, and medical staff. Anyway, why assume that the more humane approach is the more brutalizing? 'In the absence of any evidence,' Harris says, 'it is plausible to suppose that the responsibility of bringing about a slow and distressing death would be more rather than less brutalizing than would a quick and merciful killing.' Harris might have added that there is plenty of testimony on the harrowing effects of these slow deaths. Writing about the Johns Hopkins case with which we began this chapter, Dr Anthony Shaw has said: 'The baby's lingering death (15 days) severely demoralized the nursing and house staffs. In addition, it prolonged the agony for the parents, who called daily to find out if the baby was still alive.'

In his reply to Harris, Lorber remains unconvinced:

it would be wrong to assume . . . that active euthanasia would be less traumatic, either to parents or to professional staff who may be expected to carry this out. The killing may be quick and painless, but the aftermath of thoughts and guilt complexes in the parents and persons involved is likely to be much worse than caring for the baby in a humane way until it dies. There is no question of self-deception or hypocrisy here. Furthermore, though many parents do express a wish, when their infant is very handicapped, that the doctor should put an end to the life painlessly, this is illegal and I would strongly disagree with any suggestion that we ought to carry out an illegal act however logical it may seem to be to some.

Lorber's reference to the law is indicative of the different perspectives of philosopher and practitioner. Harris is not, as we understand him, advising doctors to flout the law. He would like to see the law changed and he is urging doctors to cease supporting a law which prevents these tragic situations being resolved in the most humane possible manner. It is important to keep these issues separate. The first and more fundamental issue is: what should the law be in this matter? This is the question Harris is discussing. The second issue is: given a law which prohibits active euthanasia, what should doctors do? Harris does not discuss this issue, which would lead us into quite different topics, into political philosophy and the obligation to obey the law. We shall not go into these topics either.

So let us consider the other aspects of Lorber's reply. It may indeed be the case that given the moral attitudes which are widely held in our society, some people would experience greater guilt if they actively killed an infant than if they allowed that infant to die. But is it true that there is no self-deception involved here? The supposition that there would be greater guilt after active killing only makes sense if the people involved believe that deliberately allowing an infant to die is somehow not morally equivalent to killing it. Perhaps they believe that it is only 'letting nature take its course'; perhaps they think there is a commandment against killing, but no commandment to 'strive to keep alive'. Once people come to see that there is no basis for the moral distinction between killing and deliberately withholding treatment so that a severely handicapped infant will die, the psychological burden of guilt and remorse will surely swing the other way: it will be consoling to know that in tragic circumstances one did the very best for all concerned by ensuring that death took place swiftly and painlessly.

Finally, we wonder if Lorber's admission that many parents do ask for active euthanasia does not undercut his assertion that the guilt complexes in the parents are likely to be worse if active euthanasia is performed. Might not the parents be the best judges of their own feelings in this matter?

Lorber adds a separate claim to this argument: 'It would be wrong for a doctor to order his junior or his nurses to carry out such a task if he cannot bring himself to do it.' With this claim Harris has no argument, but he points out that the whole issue is what, in conscience, people ought to do. The implication is that if, on reflection, we can see that active euthanasia is preferable to passive euthanasia, then doctors ought to be able to bring themselves to do it.

Lorber's comment on this follows on immediately from the last passage quoted, in which he pointed out that active euthanasia is illegal. He then said: 'Even if it were legal I should certainly never do it.' Since this statement is made without further explanation, it is presumably to be taken as a personal psychological report. As such, it explains why Lorber stresses the objection to ordering others to do what one cannot bring oneself to do; but it has no bearing on what other doctors, without the same feelings against active euthanasia, might quite properly do. The 1975 survey of American paediatric surgeons and paediatricians revealed that if it were legal at least some doctors would have preferred to carry out active euthanasia, rather than leave a baby to die.

The Argument from Lack of Consent

Lorber said that he strongly disagreed with active euthanasia, 'especially for babies and children, who cannot possibly ask for it or give their considered consent'. This is, however, a peculiar objection for Lorber to make, for it applies equally to selective non-treatment for babies and children. As Harris says: 'selective non-treatment is intended to result in death and it does, and those who die cannot possibly ask for it or give their considered consent'.

This looks a conclusive reply. In his rejoinder Lorber admits, as he must, that 'one cannot get the consent of the baby to non-action' but he adds that equally 'one cannot get their consent for all the major operations and procedures which have been carried out on them'. This is true too, of course, and it would be a valid reply to someone who was arguing that because infants cannot give their consent, one must keep them alive no matter how severe their handicaps will be. It is not, however, a relevant response to Harris, who is arguing that if we are going to allow infants to die by deliberately not treating them, active euthanasia would be preferable. Obviously the consent of the parents is all one could have in either case—and Lorber has admitted that many parents do ask for active euthanasia for their infant. So if active euthanasia were legal, the consent of many parents would be readily forthcoming.

The 'Last Door' Argument

Lorber had said that 'no treatment with normal nursing care' is a safeguard because 'If an infant's condition is not as grave as was thought, he will live and he can then be given optimal care if he has any handicaps.' Harris calls this 'the last door argument' —meaning that a lethal injection would close the last door on the infant's chances, whereas 'no treatment' leaves the door open. It is an argument often made against active euthanasia, for adults as well as for children.

As Harris points out, in the case of the children Lorber selects for non-treatment, the alleged safeguard is a very chancy business: 'If a child selected for non-treatment contracts an infection and dies because it is not given antibiotics, or if it requires resuscitation which is not given and it dies, there will be no opportunity to discover whether the diagnosis was wrong or not.' This is correct. Normal infants can contract infections. Before antibiotics were available, many of them died. Death from this cause is no indication of future handicap. The same can be said of many other causes from which these untreated infants die: while in the rare case of an untreated infant surviving—a very rare case among Lorber's patients—it may be possible to say that a diagnosis was wrong, in most cases of untreated infants dying it will not be possible to say that the diagnosis was right. Moreover, if infants do survive, there will also be some whose condition is every bit as grave as it was thought to be, and now even graver because of non-treatment. In the case of a child dying from an infection without being given antibiotics, the withholding of the drugs was effectively closing the last door on that infant's chance of survival. A lethal injection would have done no more.

Lorber does not respond to this criticism.

The Slippery Slope Argument

Finally we come to Lorber's assertion that no matter how humane our intentions may be, we will find it impossible to formulate legislation that is not open to abuse. Lorber refers to Hitler's Germany as an instance of what can happen when 'such a dangerous legal power' is put in the hands of any individual or group of people. Here Lorber is advancing a 'slippery slope' argument. Once we take the first step on to the slope, so these arguments run, we shall be unable to avoid sliding all the way down the abyss; therefore no matter how innocent that first step may seem, we had better not take it.

Harris makes two points in reply. The first is a point he has made more than once: that what Lorber says of active euthanasia applies equally to Lorber's own practices. Lorber and others already have, Harris reminds us, the power to adopt a course of action that will bring about the deaths of their patients. As Harris says, 'The power is awesome but it is already exercised,' and he adds that if we fear it may be abused, the best safeguard is to bring these life and death decisions out in the open, where there can be the widest possible public debate and scrutiny. To ensure this, Harris suggests, we should legalize non-voluntary euthanasia, restricting it to patients who are clearly incapable of consenting and where death is clearly in the best interests of the patient. We could then build into the legislation whatever safeguards we wished—presumably Harris has in mind procedures like a requirement for a second opinion from a senior physician, or the approval of a hospital ethics committee, or of some other tribunal.

The only reply Lorber makes to this point is that he cannot conceive of any legislation which could draw up a list of criteria as to who should be killed for the sake of mercy and who should carry out such an act. But while it may be politically difficult to get such legislation at present, we can see no ultimate barrier to drawing it up. If there are doctors prepared to consign an infant to death from, say, hydrocephalus, we cannot see why there should not be doctors willing to give a lethal injection. As for the criteria determining who should be killed, there is no reason why legislation would have to spell this out in detail; it could be left to the doctor, acting with the agreement of the parents and in consultation with another senior physician; or it could be left to some other committee or tribunal. It is hard to see why this would be worse than the present informal system of letting infants die. This system effectively gives to one doctor acting alone the power to make the life-or-death decision.

Harris's second point against the slippery slope argument is a brisk rejection of the claim that there is any analogy between Nazism and what he is proposing. Lorber does not respond to this rejection, so perhaps he accepts that the analogy is far-fetched. Nevertheless we see a need for a more thorough discussion, because people persist in raising the spectre of Nazism whenever active euthanasia is mentioned. They frequently cite Dr Leo Alexander, a psychiatrist who worked with the United States Counsel for War Crimes in Nuremberg from 1946–7. In 'Medical Science under Dictatorship', an article published in the *New England Journal of Medicine* in 1949, Alexander asserts that the path to genocide began with the Nazi euthanasia programme which Hitler ordered on 1 September 1939, the day the Second World War began. The gist of Alexander's article, so far as euthanasia is concerned, is to be found in this oft-quoted passage:

Whatever proportions these crimes finally assumed, it became evident to all who investigated them that they had started from small beginnings. The beginnings at first were merely a subtle shift in emphasis in the basic attitudes of the physicians. It started with the acceptance of the attitude, basic in the euthanasia movement, that there is such a thing as a life not worthy to be lived. This attitude in its early stages concerned itself merely with the severely and chronically sick. Gradually the sphere of those to be included in this category was enlarged to encompass the socially unproductive, the ideologically unwanted, the racially unwanted, and finally all non-Germans. But it is important to realize that the infinitely small wedged-in lever from which this entire trend of mind received its impetus was the attitude toward the nonrehabilitable sick.

This passage has evidently persuaded many people that we must resist the idea that there is 'such a thing as a life not worthy to be lived', and that hence we must resist all steps towards euthanasia. Here two important points need to be made. The first we have already argued for, in Chapter 2: everybody accepts that some lives are not worth living. Obviously those who select some spina bifida infants for non-treatment, with the object of reducing the number of infants who survive with severe handicaps, are in no position to deny that they judge some lives as not worth living. It is not, however, only John Lorber and his colleagues who make such judgements. Even C. Everett Koop makes them, for he does not advocate prolonging the life of an infant born without a brain or without an intestine. Unless we are prepared to prolong such lives, we must admit that we judge some lives to be not worth living. As we saw, appeals to such doctrines as the distinction between ordinary and extraordinary means also rely on quality of life judgements, albeit in a camouflaged form. So if the judgement that some lives are not worth living were enough to put us on the slippery slope towards Nazism, we would already be well down that slope; on the other hand, the fact that such judgements are so inescapable, and must have been made in every society, should be sufficient grounds for doubting Alexander's claim that they have anything to do with the uniquely abhorrent Nazi policies.

Our second point is more specifically addressed to the accuracy of Alexander's understanding of Nazism. In 1976 the Hastings Center, the leading American centre for bioethics research, held a conference on 'The Proper Use of the Nazi Analogy in Ethical Debate'. At that meeting Professor Lucy Dawidowicz, an eminent historian and author of *The War against the Jews, 1933–45*, pointed out that we can easily slip into error when we take terms used by the Nazis and translate them literally, without regard for the way the Nazis used them. As Dawidowicz says of terms like 'euthanasia':

when we apply these terms to the Nazi experience, we should see them in quotation marks, for they do not have our meaning. These terms and the programs they stood for were integral aspects of Nazi racism. Nazi racism derived from a theory about the ultimate value of the purity of the *Volk*, a word meaning 'people' or 'nation' which in Nazi usage took on a quasi-mystical sense.

Dawidowicz then considers a Nazi term of obvious relevance to Alexander's contention:

Those persons or groups of persons that were considered harmful to racial health, that is, racial purity, were characterized by the racial ideologists as 'valueless' life, which was slated for destruction. The German term was *Vernichtung lebensunwerten Lebens*, literally, 'the destruction of life unworthy of life,' generally translated as 'valueless' life. The 'valuelessness' of such life was measured in terms of the health of the *Volk*, itself an abstract concept, not a physical reality. This health had no bearing on individual health, on family health, even on public health, or the health of society.

In the light of these comments, it is easy to see that Alexander has badly misunderstood the Nazi terminology. The misunderstanding vitiates his attempt to use the historical experience of Nazism as an argument against euthanasia as we now understand the term. When the Nazis talked of 'a life not worthy to be lived' they meant that the life was unworthy because it did not contribute to the health of that mysterious racial entity, the *Volk*. Since our society does not believe in any such entity, there is no real prospect that allowing active euthanasia of severely handicapped new-born infants would lead to Nazi-style atrocities.

Having dealt with the Nazi analogy, let us return to the slippery slope argument in itself, rather than to its specific application in the claim that euthanasia will lead to Nazi-like atrocities. Perhaps the best answer to such arguments was given by Sam Gorovitz, an American philosopher, when testifying before a United States Ethics Advisory Board inquiring into the ethics of research on *in vitro* fertilization (the 'test-tube baby' technique). A previous witness had suggested that accepting this technique might put us on a slippery slope, with a society like the one portrayed in 'Brave New World' at the end of it. Speaking as an experienced skier, Gorovitz pointed out that we frequently make judgements about which slippery slopes we can handle and which we cannot: 'It is a question of control, and in part, of judgment.' Another American, Clifford Grobstein, developed this point in his book on new reproductive techniques, *From Chance to Purpose*. Grobstein draws attention to the crucial role played by our purposes. As long as our purposes are clearly spelt out, and we know how far we are willing to go, there is no reason to fear slippery slopes. Any new proposal that lies outside our original purposes will have to be considered afresh, and at that point we can always refuse to take the further step.

BEYOND 'LETTING DIE'

In this chapter we have examined several ways in which philosophers, theologians, and doctors have attempted to find moral significance in the distinction between killing and letting die. Some appealed to philosophical doctrines about responsibility and intention, others made pragmatic objections about the finality of killing and its liability to abuse. None of the philosophical doctrines succeeded in showing the distinction to be morally significant. On the pragmatic issues Lorber struggled hard, but in vain, to defend an essentially indefensible position against Harris's criticisms. We therefore conclude that, at least in the medical cases we have been considering, killing an infant is not worse than letting that infant die. Often it will be better, because the swifter death will cause less suffering.

For many of our readers, we suspect, this conclusion will have been plain all along, and the present chapter a philosophically laboured defence of the obvious. These readers will agree with John Freeman who, as we saw at the end of the previous chapter, said that society and medicine should stop 'perpetuating the fiction' that killing and letting die are ethically different. We agree that this view is a fiction, but we have considered it necessary to deal with it at length because it is a fiction that is widely believed, and believed with deep conviction. To give up the fiction is to give up the belief in the sanctity of human life; and this is something that few people are prepared to do.

The thrust of this book so far is that no one really believes that all human life is of equal value, but many people pay lip-service to this belief and adopt disguises which make it difficult to recognize that they are not in fact acting in accordance with what they say. Other people are open in their rejection of the view that all human life is of equal worth, but still are not prepared to admit that it would be right to take the quickest means to end a life that is not worth living. They too are trying to draw a veil over the extent to which their policies and practices are incompatible with the traditional Judaeo-Christian doctrine of the sanctity of human life. Thus all our argument to this stage has been a kind of philosophical undressing. The point has now been reached at which we can gaze on our practices in their naked truth. Many people find nudity shocking, however, and this instance, we can safely predict, will prove no exception. We must therefore ask ourselves: do we dare openly to confront the traditional views about the sanctity of human life that are so deeply embedded in the moral consciousness of our society? Or should we hastily cover ourselves up again with our inadequate, but comforting, fig leaves?

In the next two chapters we shall see whether the traditional views are as solidly based as they appear to be. If not, the fact that our arguments have led us into confrontation with these views is no reason for refusing to follow these arguments where they lead.

3

ABORTION: IDENTITY AND LOSS

WARREN QUINN

Most philosophers who discuss abortion seem to presuppose that during any period of time in which a human fetus is not yet a human being abortion remains a matter of negligible moral consequence.[1] The extreme antiabortionist, of course, denies that there is any such period; but he too seems to accept the presupposition. For he argues as if everything depended on establishing conception as the point at which human life begins. The extreme proabortionist relies on the same presupposition. It enables him to move from the premise that no fetus ever fully qualifies as a human being to the conclusion that abortion at any fetal stage is permissible on demand.[2] Even moderates are generally so classified because they take some intermediate point in pregnancy (for example, viability) to be the beginning of human life, and hence to be the moral watershed at which abortion begins to be objectionable. Thus all parties to the debate as traditionally conducted seem to regard the fetus itself as entering the moral drama in only one of two ways: either as a mere mass of cells which can be excised at the pregnant woman's

From Warren Quinn, 'Abortion: Identity and Loss,' *Philosophy and Public Affairs*, 13/1 (Winter 1984), 24–54, and in his *Morality and Action* (Cambridge: Cambridge University Press, 1993). Copyright © 1984 by Princeton University Press. Reprinted by permission of Princeton University Press.

Many thanks to Philippa Foot, Miles Morgan, Christopher Morris, Gerald Smith, and other Los Angeles philosophers for their encouragement and criticisms. And thanks above all to Rogers Albritton for his patient advice.

[1] The fact that the following discussion will be carried on in terms of 'human being' rather than 'person' requires some comment. This will, of course, make no difference to those who conceive of human beings as essentially persons. But to those who think that human beings *become* persons I would suggest the following defense of my procedure. Whatever new, and undoubtedly more serious, moral aspects come into play when persons are killed, the killing of a genuine human being, especially where this is not done wholly in the name of its own interests, raises serious enough moral issues just on the face of it to be worth considering. In the following I shall try to show that this appearance is correct.

[2] To speak strictly, a fetus is the prenatal organism from about the eighth week on and is preceded by the zygote, conceptus, and embryo. In this paper I allow myself the common philosophical (and perhaps bad) habit of using 'fetus' and 'fetal' as general terms covering the entire series from single-cell zygote to full-term fetus.

discretion or as a human being with a full right to life of the very sort possessed by those who ponder its fate.[3]

But this presupposition may be false. At least it is at odds with two intuitions I have long found persuasive: (1) The first of these is that even a very early abortion stands in need of moral justification in a way that the surgical removal of a mere mass of tissue does not. Abortion is morally problematic not only because of its impact on the pregnant woman but also because of its impact on the organism that is killed and removed. The extreme antiabortionist will, of course, share this intuition, but it is deliberately weaker and vaguer than anything he could endorse as a final position. This is shown by its apparent compatibility with my second intuition: (2) That abortion occurring early enough in pregnancy, at least before all the organ systems of the fetus are complete, is not morally equivalent either to the killing of an adult or the killing of an infant. The early fetus not only fails to be morally protected by the same kind of right to life that mature persons possess, but its moral status also differs in some important way from that of the neonate.

The extreme proabortionist will, of course, endorse (2) but not the idea that it can be conjoined consistently to (1). But it is this conjunction that I find plausible. The early fetus is not, as the conservative thinks it is, under the full moral protections appropriate to a mature human being, but it is also not the morally negligible thing the liberal seems to think it is. To these two intuitions I shall add a third which sometimes strikes me as equally compelling: (3) As pregnancy progresses abortion becomes increasingly problematic from the moral point of view. More, and perhaps considerably more, is required to justify an abortion at six months than at one month. This intuition, which may well be widely shared, almost never finds a secure place in philosophical discussions of the abortion issue.

In this paper I shall discuss, in what will have to be a somewhat rough and schematic way, two alternative metaphysical theories of the status of the fetus and the nature of fetal development in which these moral intuitions could be seen to be satisfied. These theories attempt to articulate, each in its own way, the kind of individual identity that the fetus possesses, especially in relation to the identity of the future human being it will in some sense become. Each of them is offered as plausible quite apart from the question of abortion, for each does considerable justice to intuitions about fetal identity that arise from an attempt to take man seriously as a biological being. But their special relevance to this discussion lies in the way they satisfy

---

[3] Although some proabortionists think like Judith Thomson that even the possession of a full-fledged right to life would be rendered irrelevant by the fact that the fetus locates itself where it has no right to be and makes demands it has no right to make. See 'A Defense of Abortion,' *Philosophy & Public Affairs*, 1 (1971), 47–66.

certain requirements imposed by the first two moral intuitions. (1) will seem to have serious weight only if the fetal being affected by abortion is thought to be capable of receiving morally significant harms and benefits. If the fetus were viewed as a special kind of short-lived individual destined at birth to fade from existence as the human being replaces it, or as the early stage of a complex piece of biological machinery which a human being will only later come to possess, abortion would seem to pose no serious moral problem. It seems then that (1) demands a theory in which the future human being in some sense already exists in the fetus.[4] Intuition (2), on the other hand, with its denial that abortion is strictly comparable to standard cases of murder or even to infanticide, seems to require that there be a sense in which a human being does not yet exist *in utero*, or at least a way in which it does not yet fully exist there.

Any ontology of the fetus suitable for my purposes must thus satisfy both of these superficially conflicting demands. Each of the two theories to be presented in Sections II and III seems to me to do this and to satisfy other independent requirements more plausibly than other theories I have seen discussed or have been able to construct. As indicated, the discussion will be programmatic rather than complete. In particular I shall set aside the obviously important question as to the precise time at which the human creature first exists as a full-fledged human being. My concern here is instead with the clearly identifiable but morally problematic period that comes first. In Section III I shall go on to argue that if either of the theories is true, then there is some way in which we shall be forced to see standard cases of abortion as inflicting on a fetus the loss of a future fully human life. In Section IV I shall reflect on the ethical implications of this result, trying to show that the initial moral intuitions are indeed secured.

I

The theory to be developed in this section starts with an examination of the extreme antiabortionist's premise that conception marks the beginning of

---

[4] That we can refer to a possible but as yet nonexistent human being who, if he comes to exist, will have some significant relation to that which the fetus will become is not, I think, enough to make abortion seriously problematic. For while it seems possible now to harm the interests of an as yet nonexistent human being who will in fact come to exist, I do not believe that one can in any way affect the interests of a merely possible human being who does not now and never will in fact exist—even by the very act that prevents it from ever existing. This is why birth control does not seem to raise a comparably serious moral issue. Richard Hare, it must be noted, does take the interests of merely possible people seriously in 'Abortion and the Golden Rule,' *Philosophy & Public Affairs*, 4 (1975), 201–22, esp. 219–21.

human life. This premise includes at least two distinguishable claims: First, that conception marks the beginning of the individual, for example Socrates; and second, that it marks it as the beginning of a human being. The theory under consideration rejects the second claim, but finds something importantly suggestive in the first. For it does seem plausible to think that some individual entity begins to exist at conception to which the later human being will be intimately related, an individual biological organism of the species *Homo sapiens*. And this organism, while living within its parent, does not have the biological status of an organ. Its development is explained by reference to its own needs; and its emerging parts are assigned functions within *it* rather than within its parent. I shall call this entity, upon which our theory focuses, the *human organism*. This serves not only to give it a name but to distinguish it from the *human being* who will, as we shall see, only enter the picture later.

Now what is absolutely central to this theory is the claim that the human organism persists and continues to develop through fetal, infant, child, and adult forms, remaining numerically one and the same individual organism throughout the entire human life cycle. The theory regards this claim as conceptually unobjectionable and empirically verifiable. Despite its remarkable changes of form, there are no stretches in the life of the human organism, even in the amazing developments of the fetal stage, at which it is plausible on biological grounds to suppose that a previously existing organism ceases to exist.[5] The smooth gradualism of fetal development is, of course, part of the reason.[6] But even more important to the case for organic continuity is the fact that this development proceeds according to a tendency and plan that we believe to have been fully present in even the earliest form of the zygote. (That 'plan' is used in this context metaphorically is not, I think, a problem. The point is that the subsequent development is causally determined by special goal-directed factors present in even the earliest stages.) Throughout its life, the fetus has need of external objects and stimuli, whose absence will retard or even end its development. But we do not,

[5] This may have to be qualified where monozygotic (identical) twins are concerned. If such twinning is genetically determined, then the pretwin zygote may have to be regarded as some special kind of proto-organism that ceases to exist in its own right as the twinning process takes place. If twinning is contingently produced by environmental factors, the pretwin zygote can be regarded as a human organism that might have gone on to develop through a normal human cycle but, as a matter of fact, ceases to exist in the twinning process. Since twinning is a striking discontinuity of normal development there may be nothing objectionably ad hoc in these qualifications. See Lawrence Becker's 'Human Being: The Boundaries of the Concept,' *Philosophy & Public Affairs*, 4 (1975), 334–59, esp. 340.

[6] Continuity from conception onward is also emphasized by Richard Warner in 'Abortion: The Ontological and Moral Status of the Unborn,' *Social Theory and Practice*, 3 (1974), 201–222.

according to the theory, interpret its interaction with them as altering its basic plan of development.

For this reason there is a clear difference between any event in the life of the fetus and the event of fertilization in the life of the ovum. The ovum has a developmental history of its own which is dependent on its own determinate nature and the internally encoded plan that this nature includes. But we do not suppose that this nature and plan by themselves account for the later development of the zygote and conceptus. We rather think of the latter as a new form of life to whose nature both the ovum and the spermatozoon have made significant contributions. Parthenogenesis, should it become possible, will be best conceived as a transformation rather than a development of the ovum—the parthenogenic agent being seen as having the power to change the ovum's essential nature, to make of it a new organism with a quite different teleology. The now purely imaginary possibilities of cloning and wholesale gene splicing should be viewed, according to the theory, in much the same way.

The second central thesis of the theory concerns the nature of the human (or, for that matter, animal) body, that is, the body of a human being. The theory rejects a certain, perhaps philosophically common, idea according to which the human body is a fully real organic *subentity*—one which, while logically incapable of intentional actions (that is, unable to read, converse, perceive), is the *primary agent* of a human being's metabolic and purely reflexive activities. So conceived, it is our body that digests, that converts nourishment to protoplasm, that sweats, that jerks when struck in certain ways, and *we* (human beings) are seen to metabolize, jerk, sweat, or even simply to occupy physical space only because our bodies do. According to this conception, we supervene upon, contain, or bear some other exotic relation to a distinguishable source of activities which then become attributable to us by a kind of logical courtesy. This idea can be seen most clearly in a certain perspective on extreme senility in which it is seen as the emerging or separating off of the body. The higher parts of the human person having, as it were, evaporated, the body is left behind unhappily bereft of its former companions.

The theory being considered rejects the idea of the body as real subentity. It instead takes the body, insofar as it is conceived as something incapable of higher activity, to be a product of *mere* abstraction. So taken, the body of a man is nothing other than the man himself, *just insofar* as he is a subject for physical, chemical, and biological inquiry.[7] This abstraction produces an

---

[7] See Douglas Long's interesting discussion of an abstractionist account of the body as it fits into the issue of other minds in 'The Philosophical Concept of a Human Body,' *Philosophical Review*, 73 (1964), 321–37.

object of thought which, in virtue of the relevant stipulations, is logically capable of movement and biological activity but not thought and volition.[8] But the abstraction of the body from the man, although no doubt culturally and psychologically profound, is seen by the theory as lacking the metaphysical significance often assigned it. Our living bodies are capable of behaving as they do only because *we* are, and senility is the deterioration of what was previously able *both* to metabolize and to think into what is now able only to metabolize.

The importance of the idea of the body to the abortion issue is clear. Given the availability of the conception of the body as subentity, the fetal organism could be dismissed as nothing more than that human subentity in its early stages.[9] On such a view, the fetus is the beginning of the body of an as yet nonexistent human being.[10] But, given the abstractive conception of body, things look very different. When man is seen as a single organism capable of a wide repertoire of behaviors ranging from the metabolic and automatic to the intentional and cerebral, a quite different picture of the relation of the primitive to the mature human organism becomes attractive: The primitive organism is seen as something which in the course of *its* normal development will take on new physical, psychological, and eventually rational powers. It will first acquire a form and capacity that will qualify it as animal; and it will subsequently take on mental, emotional, and volitional powers that will qualify it as a human being. But through all these changes it will remain one and the same biological organism. It must be admitted that only a perfectly amazing kind of organism could have this protean capacity, an organism which, even in its initial stages, would have to contain some kind of representation of all the structures of its maturity. But, according to the theory, that is exactly the kind of organism that modern biology has revealed the human fetus to be.

Is the zygote then nothing other than the human being in its earliest phase of development? Not, I believe, according to the conceptual intuitions of most people nor according to the present theory's interpretation of the grammar of 'human being.' Human organisms qualify as human beings

[8] No doubt there is something appealing in the availability of such an object of thought, considerably more appealing than the availability of (say) the *nonmusical self*, an object of thought that includes everything in the human being other than his musical powers and capacities and is therefore logically incapable of composition and musical performance. Only people bizarrely obsessed with musical activity and ability would find it psychologically possible to think in such terms, while most of us find it convenient and satisfying to think in terms of the body.

[9] Hugh McLaughlin identifies the fetus with part of the future person's body in 'Must we Accept either the Conservative or the Liberal View on Abortion?' *Analysis*, 37 (1977), 197–204.

[10] This is of course not the position that the fetus is a mere mass of cells, and so it might be taken to generate a rather weak kind of antiabortion argument.

only when they have reached a certain developmental completeness. 'Human being' thus brings in reference to a certain (typically very long) noninitial phase in the development of the human organism, just as 'adolescent' brings in reference to a certain developmental phase of the human being. But this reference does *not* establish a distinguishable individual. The adolescent is not distinct from the human being who is adolescent, and the human being is not distinct from the human organism which is a human being. The theory thus denies what in some philosophical circles has come to have the status of an axiom: that being a human being is an essential property.[11] Just as common sense discloses that the individual who is in fact an adolescent might never have been one (for example, might have died in childhood), so biological science shows us that the organism which is in fact a human being might never have been one (for example, might have been spontaneously aborted as a fetus).

It is not surprising that status as a human being should *seem* to be an essential property. The stage of the human organism in which it is a human being takes up, at least in familiar cases, the longest and most conspicuous part of its life. And there may be another, less respectable, reason. In determining whether the sortal 'human being' individuates a substance per se or merely a stage of it, one must distinguish the question, Was there an earlier time at which the individual who is now a human being existed as a mere fetus? from, Did the human being already exist as a mere fetus? There is certainly a way of hearing the second question which requires that it be answered in the negative. But this fact by itself is metaphysically inconclusive, for it leaves us free to answer the first question affirmatively. In fact, something similar occurs for even the most uncontroversial stage sortals. Thus there is a way of hearing the assertion that the adolescent already existed as a mere child which makes it seem just as false. It seems that a certain, possibly deceptive ambiguity arises when such predicates as 'already existed as' or 'still exists as' are applied to subjects individuated by stage sortals such as 'adolescent.' But we can protect ourselves from metaphysical error here by simple linguistic measures. Thus we can see clearly that the child before us is the very same ongoing biological individual as the future adolescent, and, according to the present theory, that the human fetus is the very same ongoing biological individual as the future human being.

'Human being' may seem to have two further peculiarities not shared by

---

[11] I now find that W. R. Carter also advocates the stage-sortal conception of human being in 'Do Zygotes Become People?', *Mind*, 91 (Jan. 1982), 77–95. His basic argument is that there is no 'natural breaking point' between conception and birth at which we could locate the beginning of a new substantial individual, and therefore that we may be forced to say that the fetus becomes, that is, takes on the attributes of, a human being.

other terms that sort out the stages of human organisms. First, it may seem that we give proper names to human begins as such. And second, it may seem that we reserve, again for human beings as such, a special set of pronouns, including the philosophically fascinating 'I'. While both claims are arguable, I doubt that either is quite right. Even a convinced extreme pro-abortionist might be caught off-guard wondering exactly when he or she was conceived and whether he or she occupied a breach position in the womb. And it is difficult to suppose that because the Chinese regard themselves as already one-year-old at birth, their personal names and pronouns must be seen to have a different logic. But even if there were linguistic contexts in which it was off-limits to refer to fetuses by human names and personal pronouns, nothing devastating to the present theory would be entailed. For human names and personal pronouns might be restricted in this way simply because they carry in these contexts an implication that their referents are, at the time indicated by the reference, in the relevant developmental stage. Indeed, if 'human being' were a stage sortal then any names given to human beings *as such* would have to carry some such restriction. The theory is thus inclined to treat the alleged fact of names and pronouns unextensible to the fetus as no more metaphysically telling than the fact that in certain cultures children's nicknames cannot be extended to adults. That we could not in such a culture properly refer to an adult as 'Timmy' or 'Freddie' (or that to do so would be either an insult or a joke) would not in the least entail that the individual before properly referred to as Timmy does not still exist. Without prejudice to the issue of the extensibility of human names, it will be convenient to introduce a convention yielding names that without question apply to biological organisms: Thus if 'Smith' is the name of a human being we may refer to the human organism with whom he is identical as 'Smith°.'

Since the theory holds that the normal fetal human organism is going to become a human being it also asserts that the history of every human being is part of the history of some human organism. Thus whatever happens to Smith at t also happens to Smith° at t, whatever Smith does at t Smith° also does at t, and whatever state Smith happens to be in at t is also a state that Smith° is in at t. So if Smith is bored at t, happy at t, engaged in philosophical reflection at t, so is Smith°. Of course, on the assumption of special reference conditions for human names, it will not follow from the fact that Smith is at t 'just beginning to exist' (that is, is just entering the stage in which it can be referred to as 'Smith') that Smith° is as well. But this is perfectly compatible with the theory. For this alleged fact about Smith does more than characterize the way Smith is at t; it also refers us to the Smithless pre-t world. Facts really confined to reporting the condition of Smith at t will transfer to Smith Smith°.

So much for the outline of the theory as it bears on our present interests. As to the point in the normal life of the human organism when it becomes a human being, I offer only this observation: The biological perspective which we have been adopting tempts one to regard as especially significant the point at which the major organ systems, most especially the central nervous system, are completely formed.[12] This criterion is attractive even insofar as human mentality is concerned. For if we distinguish between the mental faculties that are developed as a normal human infant collects and sorts experiences of himself and the world, that is, the mental faculties that the infant or child comes to have in virtue of the learning he has done, from the underlying mental capacities that make this learning possible, it seems attractive to identify the latter as what is essential. (One also thereby avoids the somewhat awkward necessity of ascribing early learning to something other than a human being.) And it may well be that the underlying mental capacities that support the learning processes of the neonate are already contained within the fully developed nervous system of the very late fetus.

II

The first theory, as we have seen, connects status as a human being to the achievement of a certain advanced developmental *stage* in the life of an underlying organism. (We may therefore call it the 'stage theory.') The theory to be developed in this section, however, returns to the more familiar idea of 'human being' as a substance sortal which applies to an individual throughout its entire career. The central idea is that fetal development is a *process* in which an individual human being gradually comes to exist.[13] (So we may call it the 'process theory.') This conception presupposes a general metaphysics in which it is possible for individual substances to come into (and go out of) existence *gradually*. And because of the problematic nature of this general metaphysics, the strategy of this discussion will have to be somewhat different. With the stage theory, what most needed discussing was

[12] Although the overall morphology is sketched in quite early in pregnancy, the distinctively human convolutions of the brain may still be developing in the eighth month. See Jean Blumenfeld's excellent discussion of fetal brain development in 'Abortion and the Human Brain,' *Philosophical Studies*, 32 (1977), 251–68. Also see Becker, 'Human Being,' 341–5.

[13] Lawrence Becker, ibid., p. 335, also adopts the view that 'entry into the class of human beings is a process.' But, unlike me, he seems to think the partial human reality of what he calls the 'human becoming' to be in itself of no moral interest. For him the whole problem is when the process is finished. Joel Feinberg also discusses a 'gradualist potentiality criterion' which may be compatible with my idea of the becoming process. See 'Abortion,' in *Matters of Life and Death*— Thomas Regan (ed.), *New Introductory Essays in Moral Philosophy* (New York: Random House, 1980), 183–216.

not the perfectly familiar and apparently noncontroversial general metaphysics of underlying substance and developmental stage but rather the somewhat surprising application of that schema to the case of human organism and human being. In the present case, however, the problems are reversed. If one thought that genuine processes in which substantial individuals gradually came to exist were really possible, it would seem immediately plausible to identify fetal development as just such a process. The trouble is that one is likely to think either that there is no plausible general argument in favor of the existence of such processes or that there is some logical incoherency in the very idea of them. I shall therefore have to make some brief remarks in response to both these doubts before applying the general theory to interpret the identity of the fetus.

The central feature of the process theory is that the coming to be of substantial individuals may be a genuine *process* in time in the course of which the prospective individual comes into existence gradually, entering the world by degrees. The ontology in question thus involves the idea of the extent to which an individual has at a given time become fully actual or real—or, as I shall sometimes say, the degree to which it already fully exists. It will be helpful in understanding this conception of coming to be, which we may call *gradualist*, to contrast it with the rival *antigradualist* idea. The antigradualist finds only two kinds of processes involved in the typical way in which artifacts such as houses and biological individuals such as human beings are introduced to the world. First there are preparatory processes: Boards and bricks are assembled together in preparation for the coming to be of the house, and cells are organized in various complex configurations in preparation for the arrival of the biological animal. Second, there are the finishing processes in which the newly formed individual is perfected by various changes and additions which take place in *it*. During the preparatory processes the individual does not yet exist, and during the finishing processes the individual already fully exists.

The antigradualist, in other words, seems to be committed to the totally instantaneous and catastrophic (in the mathematical sense) introduction into the world of the new individual. Let's call this sudden existential leap the 'pop.' The gradualist finds the idea that artifacts and human beings pop into existence extremely artificial and implausible. On his view, gradual and continuous phenomena have been radically misrepresented in the interest of logical neatness and simplicity. Of course, the antigradualist has a reply. The pop, he will insist, while indeed implausible, is not implied by his theory. For the *vagueness* of the substance sortal under which the new individual is individuated (for example, 'house' or 'human being') makes it impossible to identify any precise temporal point as the first moment of its existence. The beginning of all individuals, biological or artificial, is shrouded in vagueness, and that, according to the antigradualist, is why we are intuitively set against the idea of the pop.

The letter of the objection has been attended to, the gradualist will respond, but not its spirit. The pop is implausible not because of vagueness but because of our clear intuition that the coming to be of a new individual is the passive equivalent of the making process. If a builder's making a house or mother nature's making a human being are genuine processes taking time then so too are the coming to be of a house or human being. The vagueness that protects the antigradualist's account has nothing whatever to do with the fact that a thing is coming to be. Vagueness surrounds our concepts in all directions. It arises from a natural desire that our standard vocabulary be learnable and applicable in ordinary epistemic contexts and not from an attempt to accommodate our metaphysical intuitions. To see this, consider the sometimes heard logicist proposal to reconstruct a version of our language more free from ambiguity and vagueness than what we now have, so as to be able to think about the world with greater precision. Suppose we were to succeed in doing so for at least that range of discourse describing fetal development and the beginnings of human existence. Our revised language might then have the resources to represent the pop that was formerly hidden by the vagueness of our unrevised language.[14] But would having the existential pop really be one of the gains in this reconstruction of our ordinary notions? The gradualist finds it implausible to think so. He will say that the 'improved' concepts are in this respect really no improvement, not because they give definite answers where our old, familiar concepts could give none at all, but because they give the wrong answer where the old ones gave the right answer. Where the status of a shack or a hut is concerned our concept of 'house' may simply fail to provide for a definite decision. But where a house under construction is concerned our concept provides us with a definite characterization. The thing in question is very definitely a *house under construction*, and is definitely neither a completed house nor a mere assemblage of materials for the building of a house. And as the construction progresses the object's right to be called a house increases accordingly. The gradualist supposes that our ordinary concepts recognize and make room for processes in which things come into existence and that the motivation behind this is to be

[14] Perhaps our concept of 'human being' would have been lost in the process of reducing vagueness. But this would only mean that our old concepts had been doing us the disservice of misrepresenting the true character of the newly emerging individual. When put into sharp focus the situation presents us with the instantaneous coming to be of an individual K where 'K' replaces our previous vague concept of a human being.

distinguished from the very general linguistic considerations that produce vagueness.[15]

The thought that the process theory is *logically* incoherent comes from two sources. First, it is undeniable that its adoption will involve nontrivial logical complications of various sorts. We will need a predicate admitting of degrees for existence or reality; we may, depending on how the logic is worked out, also need a graduated notion of identity; and, as I shall suggest below, our conception of the extension of a predicate will certainly have to be revised. One may well complain of such complications, but from a certain philosophical perspective such complaints do not themselves constitute objections. Logic may well have to be complicated to accommodate the unruly character of our actual thought rather than our thought rendered simpler to fit an elegant logic.

The second source of worry seems even less creditable. The process theory posits a special kind of noninstantaneous change. Ordinary change over time is nothing more than the gradual acquisition by an already fully existing individual of new attributes. If this were the only variety, it would of course follow that any individual undergoing noninstantaneous change would have to be as fully real at the beginning as at the end of it. But the process theory explicitly denies that all noninstantaneous change is like this, insisting that there is a fundamentally different kind of constitutive change in which an individual gains or loses attributes as part of the process of gradually coming to be. And given that this is its distinctive claim, its defenders should not be daunted by objections that arise from attempts to model coming to be on some other kind of change. For example, if one tries to picture something coming into being as like someone coming into a room, the former idea will immediately lose its distinctive character and collapse into a species of mere change of attributes.[16] But it is all too evident that such picturing begs the question against the claim that coming to be is a unique kind of change.

Although it is no part of the present project to devise a complete conceptual scheme for the gradualist ontology of becoming, a few remarks in that direction may make clear what is at issue. A more or less Aristotelian version of the process theory would assume that any individual object or

---

[15] Vagueness will, of course, confront the gradualist if he should try to pinpoint precise moments when the process of coming into existence begins and ends. But it will also face the antigradualist with respect to the precise beginnings and endings of what he regards as the preparatory and finishing processes.

[16] The example is borrowed from Roderick M. Chisholm whose objections to the idea of gradual coming to be seem to me to involve this kind of modeling. See 'Coming into Being and Passing Away,' in Stuart Spicker and H. Tristram Engelhardt (eds.), *Philosophical Medical Ethics: Its Nature and Significance* (Dordrecht: Reidel, 1977), 169–82.

being is basically individuated as the individual thing it is by one of the sortal predicates that hold of it. For Smith, this individuating *substance sortal* is (*pace* the first theory) 'human being' while for his house it is the sortal 'house.' The idea that some human beings or houses are incompletely real at a given time is tantamount to the idea that individuals of these kinds may fall under their substance sortals in two different ways. This means that the extensions of these substance sortals must divide into two distinct classes—one containing the fully realized individuals and the other containing the only partly realized individuals of the kind in question. We may call sortals with this kind of two-part extensional structure *complex* to mark the contrast with *simple* sortals having a one-part extension.

Several other kinds of related sortals should be mentioned. First there are those complex sortals each of whose extension classes includes the corresponding extension class of the substance sortal. These are the *generic sortals* of the substantial kind in question. 'Mammal' and 'animal' are, in this sense, generic sortals of human beings, while 'building' and 'dwelling' seem to be generic sortals for houses. Generic sortals preserve the distinction between partial and full reality found within the substance sortal. Thus a partly actual house is only a partly actual building while a fully actual house must be a fully actual building.

True generic sortals, which are complex, must be distinguished from those simple sortals which apply to all the individuals, whether fully or partially real, falling under the substance sortal. Let's call such simple sortals *mock-generic*. 'Construction,' in one recognizable sense, is a mock-generic sortal for houses. Every house *and* every house under construction is equally, in this sense, a construction. 'Construction' thus clearly differs from the true generic 'building.' For while every partly actual house is no more than a partly actual building, every such house is already a full-fledged construction.[17] Another type of important simple sortal comprises the stage sortals that apply exclusively to *partly* real individuals of a given kind. We may call these *proto-stage sortals*. 'House under construction' is clearly a proto-stage sortal of houses, for an incipient house can be a full-fledged house under construction without being a fully real individual house. Unlike substance sortals and true generics, both mock-generic and proto-stage sortals fail to provide within their own extensions for the distinction between full and partial reality. Partly real individuals can fully and unambiguously satisfy the criteria associated with such sortals. The simplicity of these sortals can therefore be misleading. We must be on guard not to infer from the fact that

---

[17] When 'S' is a simple sortal, the claim that 'x is a full-fledged S' means that S clearly and unambiguously includes x in its extension.

we have found a full-fledged S that we have found a fully real individual. For 'S' may turn out to be a mock-generic or a proto-stage sortal for a substantial kind that admits of gradual coming and ceasing to be.

We must now consider how all of this is to be applied to the fetus. There seem to be three choices. The fetus could be identified with the collection of biological materials in the process of being transformed into a human being; it could be identified with the human being that is coming into existence; or it could be seen as yet some third kind of object that either gradually ceases to exist as the human being becomes increasingly realized or that continues to exist throughout the human being's life as a constituent entity. Both versions of the third possibility seem implausible for reasons that have been discussed in connection with the stage theory. The developmental succession of fetal stages does not strike us, as the transformation of the caterpillar into the butterfly strikes some, as involving the gradual ceasing to be of an independent biological organism. Nor, if we reject the view of body as component subentity, are we left with any constituent part of the later human being with which the fetus could plausibly be identified. The first possibility seems even less plausible. A fetus does not seem to *be* a collection of anything, even biological materials, although it is of course in some sense composed of such a collection.

But it may also seem unacceptable to identify the fetus with the human being who is coming into existence. The fetus is perfectly definite—it can be seen, touched, probed, and measured. It has a fully determinate, although constantly changing, morphology and histology. All this makes it seem fully and not just partially realized. Nevertheless, there is something wrong with this objection. There is nothing in the way I have defined gradualism that commits it to the absurd view that objects in the process of coming into being should be empirically indeterminate. A house under construction can, at a given moment, be characterized with every bit as much precision as a fully built house. Its incompleteness lies only in its relation to the special sortal that best indicates the kind of thing it is, namely, 'house.' Thus there is no reason in the kind of full empirical reality that the fetus possesses to reject the claim that it is the human being in the making. And this is indeed the position that the gradualist who applies his process theory to human becoming ought, I think, to take.

The resulting picture is this: The fetus is a human being in the making, a partly but not fully real individual human being. However, the fetus is also a full-fledged fetus, fully satisfying the appropriate criteria. There is no contradiction in this because 'human being' is the substance sortal for the individual in question while 'fetus' is what I have called a protostage sortal. As the stage theory insisted, the fetus changes and acquires new attributes. But the process theory has the resources to enable it to deny the stage theory's claim that such change is merely a change of attributes. According to it, the fetus is most tellingly described as a partly existent individual human being, and its acquisition of new forms is best seen as part of the process of coming to be. A similar reinterpretation of the status of the human organism is also possible. While it is correct to see a full-fledged biological organism from conception on, it is wrong to interpret 'biological organism,' in this sense, as a substance sortal. It is more naturally seen, the process theory will insist, as a mock-generic sortal that stands to 'human being' in the way that 'construction' stands to 'house.' A fetus is indeed a full-fledged organism, but this is quite consistent with the claim that such a full-fledged organism is not a fully real individual. One must not be misled by the fact that the incipient human being gets a secure status as a coherent continuing object of biological interest before it is a fully real individual.

Of course, this identification of the fetus as a partly real human being will help sustain my initial moral intuitions only if it can be made immediately or very soon after conception. But conception seems an eminently plausible candidate for the role of starting point of the becoming process. Given that human beings are biological beings and given that the first theory was correct in rejecting the conception of the body as brutish subentity, the beginning of the formation of our bodies would seem to be the beginning of our own formation. And the embryological evidence is clear that the processes of cell differentiation and migration in which the various parts of the body come to be differentiated begin almost immediately after conception.[18] As to the question when the becoming process is over and the human being fully realized, the tentative remarks made earlier about the counterpart question of the first theory seem equally appropriate. It is natural to think that the becoming process is over when the higher nervous system is developed enough for the organism to start learning, in the fashion of the normal neonate, the ways of the world.

III

We can now see that both the stage theory and the process theory secure the existential ambiguity we were seeking and that they do so in quite different ways. On the stage theory, the normal fetus will some day be a human being even though it cannot now be correctly described as one. On the process theory, the normal fetus is already to some extent but not fully a human

---

[18] The earlier qualifications about twinning will have to be made here as well.

being. Either of these theories does better justice, I would argue, to our biologically informed, extramoral intuitions than either the extreme anti-abortionist's view that a fetus is, even in its earliest stages, a fully existent human being or the extreme proabortionist's view that in early pregnancy the human being is in no way already in the picture. But I would like now to consider what the positive aspects of these theories, the way that each sees the human being as already present, imply about the fetus's capacities to be touched by good and evil. Both theories regard the fetus as something that will, under favorable circumstances, come or continue to exist as a human being. Whether we see it as a human organism or as an incipient human being, the normal fetus that is not going to be aborted may have great *human* goods and evils, indeed a whole human life, in *its* future. And a fetus that is going to be aborted might well have had that life were it not for the abortion. So to the extent that having a human life is a good, abortion can be, it would seem, a bad thing or *loss* for the fetus.[19] It should not, however, be seen as an intrinsically bad thing. If it is bad, it must be so extrinsically, bad in the difference it makes to the being's future. Events are extrinsically bad, in this sense, when they affect one's prospects for the worse. Some extrinsic evils make things worse by causing the future to contain positive intrinsic evils, for example, pain and suffering. But this is by no means necessary. Losing one's inheritance, for example, may not cause impoverishment; indeed it may leave one with a perfectly agreeable life. But it may still be seen as a very bad thing when one reflects on the really splendid life one might have had.

What we thus need to know when we assess an event as extrinsically good or bad is the way the future *would have been* but for the event. The metaphysical status of such conditional states of affairs is, of course, philosophically problematic, and to the extent that my conditional future really is indeterminate at a given time, events that occur then lack this kind of positive or negative extrinsic value for me. But we ordinarily assume that the future is not, relative to different things that might occur, completely indeterminate. Winning the lottery, getting married, being cured of cancer, are thus seen as good things, while failing the bar exam, being jilted, and losing one's wallet are seen as evils. Of course we may be wrong. Value

[19] In 'The Evil of Death,' *Journal of Philosophy*, 77 (1980), 401–24, Harry Silverstein argues that 'loss' in the literal sense implies subsequent existence in a deprived condition. It is clear, on the other hand, that those who with me speak of 'loss' of life through, for example, accident or illness mean to call attention to the difference for the worse from the point of view of the subject that the accident or illness makes by causing it to be true that he will not have the life he would otherwise have had, and do not mean to imply that the subject will subsist in some existentially deprived state. Since it seems perfectly intelligible, it is perhaps not important to establish whether this usage constitutes a metaphor or an ordinary sense.

judgments of the type in question, because they presuppose some knowledge of the counterfactual future, may go wildly astray. The apparent misfortune may turn out to be a blessing in disguise and the seeming stroke of luck the very stuff of tragedy. This risk of error, however, does not and should not stop us from making judgments of extrinsic value as best we can and from shaping our prudential and moral choices in light of them.

Abortion is an event in the history of a human organism (on the first theory) or incipient human being (on the second theory) that has tremendous impact. In most cases the creature thereby loses the whole human life it would otherwise have come to have. For this reason abortion can be, from the point of view of the fetus, a far from inconsiderable extrinsic evil.[20] Or can it? At this point a number of objections will come to mind.[21] And the best way to proceed is to consider them one by one. Perhaps it will seem to some that a loss cannot constitute a real evil unless what is lost is already wanted—or, if this is too strong, something the creature would have wanted were it to have considered the matter. Whichever condition of actual or potential desire is selected, it is clear that a totally unconscious fetus cannot qualify. It neither wants nor envisions a future; nor, in any relevant sense, is it able to. But one must say in response to this objection that it is extremely implausible to insist on desire or foreknowledge as a requirement for the

[20] My defense of this proposition against certain objections will recall points made by Thomas Nagel in 'Death,' *Nous*, 4 (1970), 73–80.

[21] Silverstein, in 'The Evil of Death,' discusses the Epicurean objection to the idea of death as an evil, namely that as long as we exist death is not with us and when it comes we no longer exist. He thinks the root of the objection is the idea that one's future death does not now timelessly exist and is therefore not now available as an object of those negative attitudes that would constitute it as an evil. My guess, however, is that Epicurus could admit the timeless presence of one's future death, but would still hold that it is irrational to think that it could be evaluated from the point of view of one's welfare. Nagel's discussion in 'Death' (pp. 76–8) suggests to me a relevant distinction between temporally indexed and temporally vague conceptions of human good. Some datable conditions (for example, pain) affect one's welfare at a precise time (often at the very time they occur) while other perhaps equally datable conditions (for example, being unable to live up to one's early promise) seem to affect one's good in a much less datable and more general way. Epicurus's assumption, I suspect, is that future nonexistence, if it were to be an evil at all, would have to be an evil of the first sort, affecting our welfare at the very time it occurs. But since all such evils presuppose the subject's existence, the idea that nonexistence is such an evil is absurd. If this is the Epicurean assumption, it is by no means easily discredited. The basic difference between such a skeptic about death and his critics is that he is unimpressed by the fact that most of us seem to find it quite possible to consider the alternatives of staying alive and being dead and to form a decided preference for the former. He finds this preference irrational, not because nonexistence isn't available as an object to consider, but because it cannot be assigned any value that could make sense of the preference. His critics, however (and I am clearly among them), find the apparent fact of the preference sufficient reason to believe that death can be assigned a value (presumably a nonpositive value) that makes sense of the strong preference for life. And, it must be added, when we reflect on whether death is preferable to life, we cannot be supposing that our preference itself will constitute the evaluative difference. Otherwise we would have nothing to reflect on. That attitudes, and even the possibility of attitudes, are not the whole story about the evil of death is something I shall be arguing for in what follows.

possibility of extrinsic evil. Suppose some fiendish experimenter surgically deprives a fetus of the possibility of future sexual activity.[22] Should the fetus survive to maturity as a fully existent human being, he can rightly regard that long past experimental surgery as having been a very bad thing for him indeed. And in so doing he need not suppose that, as a fetus, he had any conception or attitude toward his future. Of course, in this case, the evil event would bring suffering. And this may lead someone to suggest that, where fetuses are concerned, an event can be extrinsically evil only by bringing *positive* future evils, for example pain and suffering. But this is equally implausible. For suppose the researcher had deprived the fetus not only of its sexual potential but also of the emotional and intellectual potential it would need to understand and regret its condition. Far from having set things right, this would only have made the harm done by the experimentation greater.

Of course, the case of abortion is quite different, for what is lost there is not some particular kind of future good but future life itself. So perhaps what failed to be true in general will be true here, and death will be a loss only when it frustrates future directed desires and plans. On this view, it is an adult's interest in his future that gives him something to lose in death.[23] And a child or infant, having little perspective on its future, will have correspondingly little to lose. One is bound to admit that there is an important element of truth in this modification of the first objection; what we have planned and hoped for may constitute an especially important kind of loss. But it must also be said that this is certainly not the whole story even for adults. The future that one now dead had planned and hoped for might, after all, have turned out to be very unsatisfying to him, and good might have come to him from changes in his life that he never imagined. And even if the hoped for future would have proved to be as good as expected, it seems odd to explain the badness of its loss by reference to the hope rather than to the good things the future would have contained. Consider a person who finds himself with all his ambitions fulfilled and interests secured. Or, even better, someone who, *much* more than most of us, lives for the present, taking little interest either in what his future will be like or whether it will exist at all. Do we regard death as less of a loss for him than for the rest of us? In some ways, perhaps, yes. But in some important ways, no. And I would not find it absurd for someone to suggest that in dying such a one loses more than we do. In any case, if the good lost in death may bear little relation to what the

---

[22] This is like an example of Michael Tooley's in 'A Defense of Abortion and Infanticide,' in Joel Feinberg (ed.), *The Problem of Abortion* (Belmont, Calif.: Wadsworth, 1973), 64.

[23] See John Perry's 'The Importance of Being Identical,' in Amélie Rorty (ed.), *The Identities of Persons* (Berkeley: University of California Press, 1976), 67–90.

deceased envisioned and desired for his future, the fetus's present incapacity to envision a future at all is no objection to its possible vulnerability to that same kind of loss.

It should be noted here that it is possible to speak of a human being as having come into possession of a new life. This may be, as when a student graduates, no more than a pleasant metaphor. But it is possible to take the idea with a certain philosophical seriousness, not unlike the seriousness some philosophers have attached to the idea that a prisoner may emerge from prison as a new person.[24] The common philosophical idea is to split the concept of a person or, in this case, of a person's life into two subconcepts. In one broad sense we each have one and only one life. In the other narrow sense we may have many. And this idea of lives within a life might be thought to have relevance to the present issue. For someone might suggest that death can deprive us only of the life (in the narrow sense) that we now have. One might think of life in this sense as a kind of artifact, something we, in part, make for ourselves out of the circumstances luck has thrown our way. This 'artifact' consists partly in a network of ongoing associations and activities and partly in the current personality, character, interests, and abilities that shape our experience of them. It consists in what we do and can do, what we know and love, where we go and why. And it is this and only this present network of possibilities that we stand to lose in death.

This objection is relevantly different from the last one. It is not our anticipations and projects that make us vulnerable. Rather it is our current possession of the as yet unexhausted good of our present life, a good that the fetus cannot possess and therefore cannot lose. But despite its attractiveness, this idea seems to me to express at best an incomplete picture of what one loses in death. It likens loss of life to the loss involved in extreme dislocation or exile, as when a child, having lost its parents, suddenly finds itself in an orphanage with no one and nothing the same. In such cases one loses almost all of the life one has had, and this indeed can be tragic. But surely part of the special evil of death lies in its final foreclosure of all possibilities of change and growth—not the least important of which is the possibility of coming into possession of new lives. It is, of course, true that the only life we now know that we can lose in death is the life we already have. But in the

[24] In 'Later Selves and Moral Principles,' in Alan Montefiore (ed.), *Philosophy and Personal Relations* (Montreal: McGill-Queen's University Press, 1973), 137–69, Derek Parfit describes *alternative* 'Simple' and 'Complex' views of personal identity with different moral implications attaching to each. It seems to me possible, however, to regard the two views not as competing explications of the same concept but as marking off two different relations each of which may have its own moral relevance.

death of anyone, and particularly of an infant, one central mystery lies in our sense that we mourn a loss of which we can know very little.[25]

Still, the child and even the infant loses at most *part* of its life, while the fetus is alleged to lose *all* of it. For although the fetus is alive it has not yet come into possession of the human life we are here speaking of, nor can it until it is already a full human being. And this fact may itself be thought to show that any talk of the fetus losing its human life is incoherent. For it may be said that when a person's life is cut short the evil is done in the first instance *to his life* and only derivatively to him. To die in childhood or infancy is to be deprived of a natural life span; such a death makes one's life a stunted and unshapely affair. And even death in middle age denies one the chance to find the right finish, the right way of tying things up and rounding things off for the best. But the fetus, as we have seen, has no human life already under way that can be spoiled or even made slightly worse by death. So on this view, abortion cannot be regarded as an evil for it.

In reply it must be said that the generalized version of this claim, the idea that a lost future good must be one that would have added to the intrinsic value of a person's life as already in progress, seems false. At times, life offers us a prospect that is in some clear sense intrinsically good (like the prospect of an extramarital affair with someone deeply loved) but that cannot, because of what it is in itself, add to the intrinsic value of our life as already established.[26] Consider, for example, the case of an old man about to die. He has had a normal life, has no outstanding plans and projects, and is not terrified or troubled by the thoughts of death. Suppose a doctor can give this man an additional six months of life by administering some new drug still in the experimental stage. And suppose further that although the old man is now understandably indifferent to the prospect of the reprieve, he would in the end be glad of it if it arrived despite the fact (let us also suppose) that it would not contain any achievements, personal discoveries, reconciliations, or insights and would unfortunately contain more discomfort and less

---

[25] Consider the death of Mozart and the musical mystery it poses. Supposing that he would have lived as long as Michelangelo but for the attack of rheumatic fever that claimed him at thirty-five, he would have worked into the period of Schumann and Chopin. What the masterpieces we would now have would be like is something we can know almost nothing about, save that they would have been incalculably great and that the whole course of nineteenth-century music would have been very different.

[26] The problem in the case of the affair may well be more than just a matter of consequences. Certain intrinsically good states of affairs may fail to fit the value system of a given life and may tend therefore, simply by their occurrence, to spoil or make nonsense of it. The determinate character of our actual history may make it impossible to intrinsically enhance our lives by the addition of certain indisputable intrinsic goods. G. E. Moore provides for this point in his notion of 'organic wholes.' See *Principia Ethica* (Cambridge: Cambridge University Press, 1903), esp. 27–31.

pleasure than he is used to. Far from having the character of final *coda*, the added six months would, if he got them, be anticlimactic, detracting a bit from the beauty of his life as a whole. And for these reasons, it may well be that the extension cannot be seen as one which would add to his life's overall intrinsic goodness. But even so, since the man would be glad to have had the additional six months, there seems to be a very good reason to give him the drug. For in so doing, the doctor would be doing the *man* a real service, although not the special service of enhancing the long-term project we call his *life*. The moral of this for the case of abortion seems clear. If the old man can sustain a real loss (should the doctor decide not to give the drug) that is not to be explained as a blow to his life, then the fetus may be able to lose its whole future in just this way.

The objector may reply that I have underestimated the significance of the fact that the human life of the fetus has not yet begun, for it consists not in the fact that all injuries are injuries to lives but in the bedrock fact that the limits of a life (in what I before called the broad sense) are the limits of a creature's capacity to lose its future. To convince us, he may ask us to imagine a possible world in which the biological facts of human life are quite different. Instead of dying in old age, the human being lapses into a coma and gradually shrinks to the size and condition of a fetus. At this point some womb, artificial or natural, must be provided until it is born again. In its second life it remembers nothing of its first and may even have, within the limits of its continuing genetic makeup, a somewhat different appearance and personality. Lives are repeated several times until the organism finally wears out and really dies. Now let us suppose that Jones is a being in such a world currently in his first life. Let us further suppose that Jones cares only for his present life and is unwilling to take the necessary steps to ensure his survival to the next. He holds in effect that, whatever the underlying metaphysics, the boundaries of the life he is now living in some sense individuate a unique subject of goods and evils with which he psychologically identifies and in which he takes an exclusive prudential interest. That he is a human organism or human being that will be able to lead other lives seems to him to have no relevance to his present interests. And, the objector will conclude, Jones's attitude is intuitively correct, for it is just the attitude we should have were we suddenly to find ourselves in such a world.

But surely extreme caution is required in thinking about such bizarre possibilities. For our immediate intuitive reactions, having been formed in a world in which the real possibilities are very different, may prove inadequate. We must try to imagine what such a creature's intuitions would be, all other intuitions being suspect as parochially irrelevant. Of course, we must first be sure that the imaginary biological facts really do the intended job, that is, that we really have before us a case in which one and the same individual survives through various human lives. Let us suppose therefore that something like a genetic blueprint for the entire series is present in the original fetus and that the tendency to develop through the entire series is part of its nature. But whatever fact it is about these creatures that inclines us to think them capable of multiple lives, their own recognition of this fact and their own thought of themselves as having this capacity would surely have a special evaluative significance for them. Since it would be natural for them to see each of their successive lives as something like a reincarnation, they would be bound to feel, and would be encouraged to take, an interest in their past and future lives that would be, even more than our interest in the lives of our parents and siblings, quasi-prudential in character. They would be consoled by learning that their past lives had been happy, and they would be disturbed by the thought that their future lives might be unhappy. In short, in at least one strand of their evaluative thinking, they would surely be inclined to think in terms of a common subject of all their lives, a subject to which all the various goods and evils in them could be attributed. The Jones the objector has pictured in such a world would thus be something of a skeptic, and it is doubtful that his skepticism would have more power to threaten the natural intuitions of his own kind than the analogous skepticisms of our world have to threaten ours.[27]

It is now possible to see that the objections we have been canvassing make a common charge. They claim and argue that it is only when the fetus's present and the future it would have had but for our choice to destroy it are connected by relations stronger (more specific) than that of being different parts of a possible history of one being that its death can be seen as an extrinsically regrettable loss. In each case, I have in effect accepted the idea that the stronger connection proposed is relevant—that it does create the possibility of a special kind of loss. But I have tried to show that there is a type of loss that remains even when all of these special connections are absent. This is the loss whose possibility is provided by the fact of individual continuity itself, by the fact that the very same human organism or incipient human being here present would later have enjoyed a human life but for the abortive procedure that destroys it. It is nothing other than the fact of this loss, I think, that makes abortion a moral problem.

---

[27] Which is not to say that it would have none.

84   WARREN QUINN

IV

In this final section I want to try to sort out some of the moral implications of the kind of metaphysical status the two theories have assigned to the fetus with particular attention to the kind of moral constraints that arise from the fact that the fetus has something important to lose in being aborted. Specifically, I will try to state how it is that the second negative intuition, the idea that early abortion cannot be regarded either as a violation of a mature right to life like our own or even as comparable in moral gravity to infanticide, is satisfied. And I will also, of course, try to sustain the first intuition by motivating the idea that the fetus's susceptibility to loss brings it under some important moral protections.

To do this, I will need to invoke some version of the common division of morality into what are often called the spheres of 'justice' and 'benevolence' (although, as will become apparent, I think these particular headings can be misleading). I follow a Kantian tradition here in thinking that one important part of morality is made up of constraints on our behavior toward others that spring from our recognition of others as mature agents on an equal moral footing with ourselves.[28] The fundamental attitude underlying virtuous action of this type seems to be respect for what can be thought of as the moral authority of others. Defining the scope of this authority amounts to specifying the rights that mature moral agents have over each other. But what is characteristic, interesting, and important about these rights for our purposes is that they exert their force on others only in virtue of actual (or in some situations, counterfactual) exercises of will. Take, for example, the well-known rights of life, liberty, and the pursuit of happiness. Among the several moral reasons you may have not to kill me, take me captive, or subject me to your idea of the good life, perhaps the most important lies in the simple fact that I *choose*, or would choose were I to consider the matter, that you do not. Viewed in this way these rights are nothing other than equally distributed moral powers to forbid and require behavior of others, and violations of them are nothing other than refusals to respect the exercise of these powers.

The picture of morality as a nexus of independent spheres of authority to permit, forbid, and require is, in one special use of the term, a picture of

---

[28] I am also clearly drawing here on H. L. A. Hart's conception of natural rights. See 'Are there any Natural Rights?', *Philosophical Review*, 64 (1955), 175–91. In some respects Hart's 'Bentham on Legal Rights,' in A. W. B. Simpson (ed.), *Oxford Essays in Jurisprudence*, 2nd ser. (Oxford: Clarendon Press, 1973), repr. in David Byons (ed.), *Rights* (Belmont, Calif.: Wadsworth, 1979), gives a clearer picture of the type of right in question, although here in a legal rather than a moral setting.

'justice.' But while justice in the more ordinary and contemporary sense enters into the definition of these spheres, especially with regard to property, most violations of these rights are not altogether naturally described as injustices. I propose therefore to call this first part of morality the *morality of respect* and the rights that it includes *rights of respect*. These rights are marked by an often mentioned common grammatical feature whose presence is easily explained. Since what is constrained by someone's choice is in a perfectly obvious sense constrained by *him*, the constraints generated by rights of respect are obligations owed *to* individuals and not merely obligations to act in various ways with respect to individuals.

The other relevant area of morality is quite different and, in one way, much easier to understand. The constraints that arise in it are not grounded in the will of others but in consideration of the good and evil that our actions may do to them. Since the basic motivation of virtuous action here is concern for the well-being of others, I shall call this the *morality of humanity*. This part of morality, unlike the morality of respect, extends its protections to immature human beings and other creatures presently or permanently incapable of joining the community of moral agents. In fact, it seems tempting to think that it especially serves to protect them and not us. As a young person becomes an adult and more responsible for his own successes and misfortunes he tends, I suspect, to exchange some protection under the morality of humanity for protection of his developing authority under the morality of respect. This may be why our humane obligation to look after the abandoned child seems so much more obvious and pressing than any similar obligation to look after the derelict even though each be in equal danger without our aid. However, the name 'humanity,' like 'benevolence,' must not be allowed to obscure the fact that the obligations of humanity are sensitive to special natural and institutional relations that exist between moral agents and those toward whom they act. For example, parents have a much weightier obligation under what I am calling humanity to avoid harming the interests of their own infants than they have to avoid harming the interests of those of their neighbor.

It is interesting to ask whether there are rights in this part of morality and if so what the propriety of speaking in this way can consist in. People are sometimes tempted to think that the obligations that remain once we have subtracted those of respect are in some unique way grounded in the purely self-referential necessity of promoting virtue and avoiding vice. This conception is fundamentally unsound, I think, and speaking of rights here is one way of expressing one's objection to the error. Any part of morality can be practiced with an eye to one's own virtue, justice as well as benevolence. The humane part of morality, no less than the other parts, gives rise to obligations and prohibitions in large part grounded in relevant facts about others. And it is for this reason that the discharge of one's obligations under humanity is a matter in which the community or even the law may take an interest.

The rights of animals provide a good illustration of this. When animal lovers speak of animal rights (say, a right against wanton abuse or torture) they mean to be reminding us of three things: (a) that prima facie we *must not* subject animals to certain forms of suffering and pain, (b) that the law ought to take an interest in enforcing these prohibitions, and (c) most important, that the ground of the moral constraint that is here active is the welfare of the animal itself (and not the moral virtue of the human agent). In these ways the morality of respect and humanity are alike. In both we look to something about the creatures our action affects and to our connections with them to find the ground of the requirement or prohibition. The difference, as we have seen, is that in the one the obligation, grounded in the will of the other creature, is therefore owed to it whereas in the other the obligation is not grounded in the other creature itself, that is, in its will, but in its well-being.[29] For this reason an obligation under benevolence may sometimes require us to do what is neither willed nor wanted by the affected party, as parents educating their children well know.[30]

But what are the implications of all this for the abortion issue? One thing is evident. Neither fetuses nor infants are yet in posession of rights of respect. And this explains my original intuition that abortion cannot be seen as a violation of the kind of full-fledged right to life that we possess. Fetuses, like animals, do not *require* us to do anything; nor do they have any wills to contravene. They are incapable of the authority that is the ground of the respect owed to others. Here it must be stressed that one does not constrain others in the relevant way simply by disliking or reacting negatively to what they do. Such a reaction may well create strong reasons of humanity to desist. But one is not showing respect for a creature in expressing humane concern over its discomfort. (This distinction can also be seen when one reflects that a person may explicitly refuse to activate rights at his disposal

[29] With rights of respect, x's obligation *to* y matches y's right *against* x. But while rights under humanity do not give rise to obligations *to* the right-holder, I am inclined to think that such rights can properly be said to be *against* those specific individuals whom morality requires to take a special interest in the right-holder's welfare. Thus a child may have special rights under humanity against its parents.

[30] In this kind of case it would not be natural to speak of the child's right to the unwanted benefit as what constrains the parent. Still the child does have a right to the benefit and there would be no impropriety in speaking of that right constraining the parent in cases where the benefit is not unwanted. The constraints of humanity are brought under the idea of 'rights' only insofar as the benefits are not unwanted or disliked. Here we perhaps hear an echo of the connection between rights and will found in the morality of respect.

while continuing to show extreme displeasure at the very action he has the authority to prevent, as when a lender makes it clear both that he is very distressed by the nonpayment of a debt and that he nevertheless does not yet demand payment.)

Nor should we let the absurdity of crediting the fetus or infant with rights of respect be obscured by the fact that the prohibitions created by these rights are typically in force unless the right-holder has explicitly indicated otherwise. It is true that one cannot defend removing life-sustaining equipment from an unconscious adult on the ground that he never explicitly said (supposing him never to have considered the matter) that one must not. But this is because one must presume that the injured man's will is in a general way set against actions that would lead to his death and that he would not make an exception in this case. But we cannot make sense of the idea, and therefore cannot be obliged to presume, that the fetus's will is set in a general way against anything; and we cannot therefore respect any such will in refusing to abort it.[31]

If this is right and fetuses do not fall under the morality of respect, they must therefore lack an important right to life which we possess. And, although I will argue shortly that they do fall under the morality of humanity, it is possible to see why even their protectedness there should seem to fall short of the infant's. The obligations of humanity are, as noted above, sensitive to various natural and institutional relations that exist between the agent and the being toward which he acts. It is one thing to foreclose on the mortgage of a brother or a friend, another to foreclose on a colleague or a neighbor, and yet another to foreclose on a stranger (supposing, of course, that none of them had any right of respect against the action). That we think such relations make a difference is one of the more important ways in which most of us are not utilitarians. Of course, relations of friendship and kinship matter very little where, for example, the killing of infants is concerned; we are simply not to kill any infant whether our own or a stranger's. But while it is true that these kinds of particular relationships seem irrelevant to the inhumanity of killing fully actual human beings it does not follow that the very special relationship of acting toward such a fellow human being is

[31] Here someone might suggest that we are able to respect the future retrospective will the fetal being would come to have were the abortion not to occur. Although I am doubtful that such a strategy could plausibly bring abortion under the morality of respect, a similar strategy does have some attractiveness in the case of the fetus who is not killed but who is deprived, for example, by an experiment, of normal future human intelligence and volition. That the future will of the creature would have been retrospectively set against such interference can seem not irrelevant to the character of the offense. For a discussion of these kinds of moral situations see Joel Feinberg's 'Is there a Right to be Born?', in his *Rights, Justice, and the Bounds of Liberty: Essays in Social Philosophy* (Princeton: Princeton University Press, 1980), 183–216, esp. 214.

irrelevant to the inhumanity of killing. Most people would think it matters very much whether we kill a retarded member of our own species or an equally intelligent chimpanzee. And so it is not surprising that it should also seem to matter whether a fetus is unequivocally a human being, as the extreme antiabortionist insists or something less, as on our two theories. For if our most psychologically salient conception of the human community is as a community of fully actual human beings, it will naturally make a difference whether the fetus is one of us in this full sense.

But if the fetus has no rights of respect and it is not yet a full-fledged member of the human community, why should we have to take it into account at all, morally speaking? Here I would answer that the question of whether a creature's good or ill needs to be taken seriously cannot be wholly separated from the question of what that good or ill consists in. This, I think, is one of the most important truths in classical utilitarianism. According to both our theories, the fetus is a being to some extent capable of losing a fully human future life, the very kind of life we now enjoy. And it is hard for me to see how the loss of an object of this significance, the loss of the very thing that for ourselves we hold most important in the world, could have no moral weight. In any case, there is surely no precedent for thinking that it could be ignored, for there are simply no other situations in which such losses are at issue where a morally sensitive agent ignores them. The fetus, I feel, must have a right that its future welfare count for something and thus that there be a sufficiently strong moral case for sacrificing its good. And to the extent that the ties of biological kinship themselves add special weight, it will have an especially strong version of this right against its parents.

In this regard, the process theory gives a somewhat different result from the stage theory. To the extent that the human being already exists it is susceptible to the loss of future life and its rights under humanity come into play. But to the extent that it does not yet fully exist it cannot, it would seem, suffer this or any other loss and is to that extent removed from moral consideration. But what in this regard the process theory loses in moral impact, it seems to gain back in its implication that abortion directly concerns a creature with some claim already to *be* a human being. Abortion on this view therefore falls under the part of humane morality that looks after the welfare of human beings, or at least that special part of it that treats of the transitions in the course of which human beings move into and out of existence. For if, as I have already indicated, the morally binding force of humane considerations varies according to various dimensions in which the object affected is nearer to or further from us, the fact that the fetus is to some extent already a human being, already to some extent one of us, can only make its loss, however qualified, count for more. And as the fetus becomes more fully human the seriousness of aborting it will approach that of infanticide. In this way the process theory, unlike the stage theory, validates the third moral intuition that later abortions are more objectionable than earlier ones.

It is clear then that the two ontologies point to a limited, if important, moral consequence. Even the early fetus is a creature whose status arguably brings it at least within the fringes of the morality of humanity. How powerful its rights are against other competing moral forces is the very important problem of casuistry that I have gladly left aside. Women have rights of respect over their own bodies and rights of humanity concerning their own happiness, rights which cannot be ignored. How the complex web of moral forces vectors out in particular situations is, as Aristotle would say, what the wise man knows.

PART II

END OF LIFE

4

TERMINATING LIFE-SUSTAINING TREATMENT OF THE DEMENTED

DANIEL CALLAHAN

Some subjects in ethics elicit a far greater degree of emotional discomfort than others. It is not the delicacy or complexity of the subject as such that seems to be the problem. It is, instead, a tacit recognition that, try as we might, it is especially hard to disentangle our personal response from the issues themselves. And this makes it especially hard to avoid self-deception and self-interest in our analysis.

Terminating life-sustaining treatment for demented patients is such an issue. Dementia is universally feared, more so than almost any other disease. Few of us can tolerate the thought that we might become its victim. Even if we can bring love and devotion to the care of those with dementia, they can in turn elicit in us the fear that we might someday be ourselves so afflicted, and they can incite a sense of loathing and horror, usually despite ourselves. We cannot easily distinguish our own feelings about the condition from what is the actual good of the patient. The harder it is for us to imagine life as tolerable in such circumstances, the harder it will be to determine what is beneficial for the patient.

This same troubling dimension will, analogously, almost surely begin playing itself out in the years to come on the social and economic level, as a combination of increased numbers and likely higher costs for the care of those afflicted with dementia becomes a more explicit agenda item for resource allocation. Will society show the same kind of ambivalence, self-questioning, and anguish felt by many individuals as it further develops policies and spending patterns? If so, how will it incline in its values and predilections, with increased generosity or discreet withdrawal?

The general question I want to pursue is this: under what circumstances should life-sustaining treatment for dementia patients be ended and the

From Daniel Callahan, 'Terminating Life-Sustaining Treatment of the Demented,' *Hastings Center Report*, 25/6 (Nov.–Dec. 1995), 25–31. This article is derived from a chapter written by the author for Leslie S. Libow, Ellen M. Olson, and Eileen R. Chichui (eds.), *Controversies in Ethics in Long Term Care* (New York: Springer, 1994).

I want to thank The Greenwall Foundation for support of a project on Alzheimer's disease at The Hastings Center.

patients allowed to die? The more specific, troubling, question is: ought the fact of dementia make a difference in our decision, distinguishing it from other termination situations? These questions would have been much easier to deal with ten or fifteen years ago. They are harder now for three reasons—reasons which, vexingly enough, move in different, conflicting directions. The first reason is that recent research on Alzheimer disease is beginning to show that much more can be done for its sufferers than was previously possible and that a viable, even if crippled, self may endure far later into the disease process than was earlier believed. The second reason is that new sensibilities about disabled populations have emerged over the past few decades that have alerted us to the possibility of stigmatizing and demeaning the demented, thus worsening their situation. The third reason is that, one way or another, health care resources will become more limited in the future, and the explicit, open rationing of health care more certain; dementia is not likely, nor should it be spared from scrutiny in that process. It would be ideal to develop a way of thinking about Alzheimer that managed to take on all three of these problems simultaneously despite their potential conflict, seeing if they can be dealt with in a way that is integrated and coherent.

I will initially sketch a context to help situate the care of dementia patients and the termination of their treatment. Then I will move on to develop some criteria to make termination decisions.

A CONTEXT FOR ANALYSIS

The pertinent context here is threefold: (1) our knowledge of the inner life, and selfhood, of those suffering from dementia (by which I will primarily mean Alzheimer disease); (2) the messages, symbolic and literal, about dementia that could be conveyed to society by alternative kinds of policies and practices; and (3) the economic considerations involved in making decisions about the good of individual patients.

Dementia and the Self

Two major problems need to be noted. One of them, to which I will not devote much attention, bears on the place and force of advance directives in the care of the demented. Ideally, people should draw up advance directives, either a living will or the appointment of a surrogate to act in their behalf should they become incompetent. Those advance directives should stipulate what one wants done in the case of dementia (and I will take it for granted that most, but not all, people are not likely to want aggressive life-saving or life-extending treatment with advanced dementia).

Yet there is a potential puzzle here, nicely brought out in the writings of Ronald Dworkin and Sanford H. Kadish, both distinguished legal scholars. At issue is whether the patient's earlier advance directive or the patient's presently expressed or implied desires (assuming the latter differ from the former) should be the determining consideration in decisions to terminate treatment. This situation presents no dilemma if the patient cannot express desires at all, but does if the patient states a desire to continue living, or if behavioral evidence suggests that the patient is satisfied enough with his present condition and seems to have no urge to be dead.

Dworkin distinguishes between a patient's 'experiential' interests—the patient's present state of experienced pleasure, pain, or satisfaction—and the patient's 'critical' interests—those interests expressive of a patient's long-standing, settled convictions about what he values in life.[1] An advance directive signed while a patient was in good health and that reflects some carefully thought out personal values could come into conflict with the actual condition and inclinations of a patient at a critical moment. If I have stated while in good health, and after careful reflection, that I would not care to have my life extended if I become demented, should that declaration be respected even if, when the time comes, I seem to be happy enough in my demented state? Dworkin takes the position that the critical interests should be determinative, representing the settled convictions of a patient, and thus that the advance directive should be respected.

Kadish takes the other side, and I believe has the better argument.[2] His reasons bear on the selfhood of the demented person—a self he presumes continues to exist, even if incompetent. It is perfectly possible that we may now find acceptable a life we had earlier judged to be unacceptable, and that we could not have known in advance that such a change in our judgment was possible. As such, it would seem unduly rigid, even doctrinaire, to deny evidence of a dementia patient doing better than he could have anticipated. But what if a patient had foreseen exactly this kind of a possibility and still wanted termination? Doesn't the 'critical interest' position encompass just this possibility? Even so, we are still left with a problem: how can someone in any rational way irrevocably determine well in advance what they will want in a situation they have never experienced before? We would do well to be suspicious of such earlier declarations when the evidence before our eyes is

[1] Ronald Dworkin, *Life's Dominion: An Argument about Abortion, Euthanasia, and Individual Freedom* (New York: Alfred A. Knopf, 1993), 195.
[2] Sanford H. Kadish, 'Letting Patients Die: Legal and Moral Reflections,' *California Law Review*, 80 (1992); 857–88.

that of a patient doing reasonably well and not obviously seeking death. A second reason for resisting Dworkin's position is that a key feature in the development of advance directives has been to stress the possibility of changing or revoking those directives at any time while capacitated, not to assume that they are to function in a fixed, unchangeable way. That same reasoning could be extended to include behavior of the incapacitated that would imply either a change of mind or an implicit unwillingness to see the original criteria of the advance directives invoked in actuality. But I will not explore the problem of advance directives any further here other than to note that how we analyze the problem will, in great part, turn on our interpretation of the selfhood of demented patients, and what various states of that selfhood might morally entail.

I will instead focus my analysis on what should be done when we have no prior knowledge of a person's wishes about termination or even about the person's values. I am thus taking on a hard but not uncommon kind of case, where it is left entirely to us to decide what to do based on our own values or, more precisely, on those values we conscientiously believe should apply in these cases. This focus also helps to bring in sharp relief how we might best think about dementia and termination of treatment. The tendency in much of the discussion of termination is to focus on patient wishes, known or inferred. Obviously that is important but, in the long run, what patients and would-be patients decide is in their best interests, or their ideas of the kind of life best worth living, will be a function of how we come to think of a life weighted down with dementia. What *ought* I to want when I am dying of dementia? That question will also hover just below the surface. We cannot achieve a perfect dissociation of our judgment about ourselves and our judgment about other people; and it would be insensitive to accept a perfect bifurcation.

I begin with my first background question: How are we best to understand the selfhood of the demented person and understand it at different stages in the development of dementia? In what sense can it be said that the demented person has a self? I will here define full selfhood as the capacity to have feelings and to be aware of them, to reason and be able to make decisions, and to enter into relationships with other persons. A person who has even one of those capacities can be said to have a self, even if limited and impaired.

The moral corollary of this definition of selfhood is that, unlike the person in a persistent vegetative state (PVS), a person with even a minimal self should be assumed to have the same desire to live as those of us more fortunate to have a full self. We have no reason to think otherwise. There should be, that is, the same presumption in favor of treatment as would be the case with anyone else. I stress 'presumption' here to indicate that there can be reasons to overturn that presumption, including inferred evidence from the emotional or other expressions of the patient himself, a point to which I will return later.

What can be said of the selfhood of those suffering dementia? Recent scientific evidence and more careful patient analysis is beginning to show that the reality may be more complex, less wholly destructive, and more open to intervention than was previously believed, especially if strong efforts are made to work therapeutically with the patient. Joseph Foley strikes a note of caution about the conventional pessimism in this respect. 'We too often assume,' he writes, 'that the absence of emotional display means that no emotion is being experienced. We too often assume that because communication is absent, internal mental process has stopped.'[3] Foley does not claim that we know what is going on inside the mind of the demented person. He stresses instead two important points. The first is the lack of good research on the insight of the demented person into his own condition. This deficit in our knowledge is striking when compared with the emphasis on self-understanding found, for example, in psychiatry or psychology more generally. The second is the importance of recognizing the variability, from patient to patient and time to time, in the dementia of the individual patient. No less significant, 'it is important to identify functions that are lost, but even more so to identify functions that are preserved.' Rebecca Dresser, in her masterful explanation of the possibility of insight into the mind of demented persons, concludes that 'we can achieve adequate evidentiary ground for judgments on the nature of life from the patient's point of view.'[4]

Tom Kitwood and Kathleen Bredin, of the Bradford Dementia Group at Bradford University in England, strike an even more optimistic note. They emphasize a number of points: that there can be a considerable reversal of even severely deteriorated patients when their social relationships and conditions of life are changed; that the condition can be stabilized in those given an intensive program of activities; and that some animal studies show the significant positive effect of companionship and activity and an improved environment.[5] They conclude that 'Evidence from the care context, then, is

[3] Joseph M. Foley, 'The Experience of being Demented,' in Robert Binstock, Stephen Post, and Peter Whitehouse (eds.), *Dementia and Ageing; Ethics, Values, and Policy Choices* (Baltimore: Johns Hopkins University Press, 1992), 30–43.

[4] Rebecca Dresser, 'Missing Persons: Legal Perceptions of Incompetent Patients,' *Rutgers Law Review*, 46/2 (1994), 690.

[5] Tom Kitwood and Katheleen Bredin, 'Toward a Theory of Dementia Care: Personhood and Well-Being.' *Ageing and Society*, 12 (1992), 269–87.

beginning to suggest that a dementing illness is not necessarily a process of inevitable and global deterioration.'

In still another study, Steven R. Sabat and Rom Harré provide evidence to show that the self of personal identity 'persists far into the end stage of the disease.' The self, they contend, can be lost, 'but only indirectly as a result of the disease. The primary cause of the loss of self is the ways in which others view and treat the Alzheimer sufferer.'[6] Victoria Cotrell and Richard Schulz add still another dimension, focusing on the active role of patients in shaping a response to their condition. 'The inherent message,' they write, 'is that individuals with dementia are important actors responding and adapting to the disease, rather than passive individuals who are succumbing to deficits.'[7] Taken together, these two perspectives have the potential to transform common attitudes toward those with dementia. How we as family and friends and caretakers think about and respond to the demented patient will make a difference in the self-perception of the patient, and that self-perception is itself potentially amenable to alteration by the patient herself.

The evidence cited in these articles is not definitive, and the authors do not make such a claim. But it is surely sufficient to suggest that, for ethical purposes, the sufferer of dementia cannot decisively be declared either out of touch with himself or definitively out of the human community (especially since communication, however rudimentary, with dementia patients remains possible almost to the very end). As outside observers, we may be appalled by the kind of self we observe, even fearful; but this is *our* reaction, not necessarily that of the demented person to herself. A distinction must of course be made between the earlier and later stages of the condition, and it is surely possible that by the last stages the deterioration is so far advanced that the familiar stereotype is realized; that of a person whose deterioration has destroyed both her body and her self. Even then we may not know exactly when the self was irretrievably lost, when some significant borderline was crossed.

I draw from this analysis one simple conclusion. There is no self-evident reason why, based on the selfhood of the dementia victim, he or she should be treated in any significantly different way from any other incapacitated patient. In early stages of the disease, there is less and less reason now to write off the patient as beyond useful therapy or to excuse caretakers from making vigorous efforts to promote the most supportive environment for the patient. Even as the disease progresses, the possibility of useful intervention

[6] Steven R. Sabat and Rom Harré. 'The Construction and Deconstruction of Self in Alzheimer's Disease,' *Ageing and Society*, 12 (1992); 443–61.
[7] Victoria Cotrell and Richard Schulz, 'The Perspective of the Patient with Alzheimer's Disease: A Neglected Dimension of Dementia Research,' *The Gerontologist*, 33/2 (1993), 206.

remains. Only when the patient is in the late stages of the disease, wholly out of contact with those around him, is it legitimate to change course; and then comfort care only is appropriate. Even at the latest stage, however, the demented patient should clearly be distinguished from the (carefully diagnosed) PVS patient, when all possibility of selfhood has almost certainly been lost. It is doubtful there could ever be a comparable level of certainty with dementia patients.

This conclusion presupposes a partial answer to a question posed at the outset, whether the fact of dementia, as distinguished from other medical conditions, should make a difference in our decisions to terminate treatment. If the most important issue is the selfhood of a patient, then dementia poses problems no different in kind from those posed by other medical conditions or situations where the disease is degenerative, the future bleak, and the patient increasingly incompetent. We can well understand the special fear that we all have about becoming demented and the profound assault of dementia upon the integrity of the self. Yet I find it hard to identify a feature of dementia that makes it singularly different from other diseases that can bring about a destruction of the mind and then the body such that some special standards are needed.

At the same time, however, something about the constellation of symptoms and losses seems to make the whole of the illness greater than the sum of the parts; therein may lie its special horror. That horror, nonetheless, is not sufficient to justify some idiosyncratic dementia standards for termination of treatment. On the contrary, because of the fear and dread the disease inspires, every effort should be made to work against these fears and to treat the dementia patient similarly to other patients.

Public Meaning and Public Symbols

In the case of dementia, we face an old public dilemma. There is an ancient theological saying that we should love the sinner but not the sin. Paraphrased for my purposes, our public dilemma is this; how are we to work against dementia as a disease while not at the same time coming to slight or demean those who suffer from it or to create excessive anxiety on the part of those who might one day come down with it? A fear of dementia already seems to be a potent force behind the desire of many to legalize euthanasia and physician-assisted suicide. A death in the throes of Alzheimer disease is seen as the mark of a 'death without dignity,' with first the self destroyed and then the body, leaving only a wreck of a person to go to his death.

The policies we come to adopt about the termination of treatment of the demented will come to play both a literal role in the way we care for them and a symbolic role in indicating how we have come to situate and value them. The symbolism could develop in three possible directions.

First, if we make it much easier to terminate treatment of the demented than other classes of incompetent patients, we will be underscoring our social loathing of the condition and our consequent devaluing of a life burdened with that condition. We will also, on the other side of the ledger, be signaling our desire to reduce the anxiety of those in the earlier stages of the condition, as well as that of family members, about their last days (or months). We will be saying that *this* condition deserves special relief. The dilemma is that the price of reducing the anxiety about having dementia is paid by stigmatizing the condition all the more—and thus possibly, very possibly, making it more difficult to engender the attitudes of social acceptance necessary to make the life of the demented (and their families, who will share in the stigmatization) more tolerable and to attract adequate social resources.

Second, if we treat dementia just like other conditions, giving the benefit of any doubt to the continuation of standard medical treatment, then we will inevitably provoke a continuing (and possibly escalating) terror as the number of demented patients increases with the rise in the proportion of the elderly. More and more of us will see ourselves at risk, particularly if we have been healthy enough to stay alive into our eighties. The source of the terror will be obvious enough: there will be no ready or quick release from the dementia, and the body will be treated as if the self of which it is a part is to be preserved at all costs.

To follow the latter course would be to accept the notion that a self remains almost to the end. And how could we not treat that self, even though diminished, much like other selves? The dilemma here is clear enough: the price of recognizing an ongoing self may be to (a) undergird the usual forces of technological medicine, which work with the simple rule 'when in doubt, treat,' while (b) at the same time enhancing the fear of the condition by seeming to close off a fast release from it.

Third, we could develop some kind of compromise position, aiming to minimize further stigmatization of dementia while simultaneously reducing the widespread fear that the life of the demented will be unconscionably prolonged. That will not be easy to do, but I will propose an approach below that may strengthen the possibilities in that direction.

Economics: Priorities and Standards

There can be little doubt that the United States, like all other developed countries, faces increasingly heavy economic pressures on its health care system. The growing number of elderly, particularly those over age eighty, and the growing number of demented patients as a direct result of that demographic change, must force some unpleasant choices about the future care of this population. Increasingly, it is possible to hear people say that, given a shortage of resources, it makes no sense to invest in extended care for demented patients, who are a burden upon themselves, their families, and society. Alternatively, some would say that demented patients should be treated like all other patients and that, in any case, no price can be put on a human life, damaged or not. If the former view is too crude and insensitive, the latter is increasingly unrealistic and potentially unjust to other sick people who may be deprived of needed resources due to an imbalance of care given to the demented.[8] How can we try to think about this problem?

We can begin by not looking at dementia independently of other grave medical conditions. It is no longer reasonable to consider the economic dimensions of medical conditions and diseases one at a time, in isolation from each other. That is, to ask how much money we should spend on dementia apart from all other medical conditions will get us nowhere (any more than we can say how much should be spent on cancer apart from any other disease). A health care system must respond to the aggregate ensemble of conditions, and it must do so by putting them next to each other so that their claims can be seen in a comparative way. The economists are right with their concept of an opportunity cost, which reflects an evaluation of how any amount of money spent on one medical condition might more usefully or fairly (or both) be spent on some other medical condition.

The hard problem is to find a way to implement that insight, in this case to decide what counts as a reasonable expenditure on the demented population in comparison with spending comparable funds on other patient populations. Here again we encounter another problem about assigning a unique status to dementia. Is it so uniquely oppressive and fearful that we should *therefore* spend more money on those in its last stages than on other fatal conditions, perhaps simply to avoid the appearance of an invidious comparison between the worth of this life and some other life? Or is its downward course so inevitable and destructive that we should *therefore* spend less life-prolonging money on it, spending our money where it could do more

---

[8] Richard C. Adelman. 'The Alzheimerization of Aging,' *The Geronotologist*, 35/4 (1995), 526–32.

good? Given the impact on families, I would be inclined toward the latter course, but I cannot find anything specific to dementia that would support this bias, though the burden on the family, an extrinsic but hardly irrelevant consideration, provides a nudge in that direction,

A priority-setting approach, of the kind used in the state of Oregon with its Medicaid program, appears as the most feasible way of managing this problem. How can we rank the different medical conditions, physical and psychological, that afflict people? Which are comparatively more or less important? Such a ranking would encompass public opinion, some form of cost-benefit analysis, the likelihood of efficacious treatment, the degree of pain and suffering a condition brings about, and the like. This is not the place to develop a full theory of priority-setting. My own guess is that public opinion would give a high priority to providing decent nursing and palliative care for demented patients but a much lower priority to the use of expensive medicine to prolong life.

I would argue, in any case, that the expenditure of large amounts of money deliberately to prolong the life of the late-stage demented person would not pass an opportunity cost test or qualify as a high priority matter. The inevitable downhill course of the disease would be one reason: death could not be averted, only delayed; and neither cure of the dementia nor amelioration of its effect could be achieved by deliberate efforts to prolong life. The increasingly diminished selfhood of the patient would be another reason: the more diminished the self, as part of a trajectory of gradual diminishment, the less likely that prolongation would be able even significantly to maintain, much less restore, the selfhood that had been lost. On the contrary, it would seem a perfect example of prolonging an irreversible death. I conclude that society would, under any comparative analysis, most likely conclude that expensive life-extending care for the severely demented—as for any late-stage terminally ill patient—could not compete well in the face of other medical needs. Nor should it. I add here one caveat: to the extent that further research can find ways to improve the life of those with early-stage dementia the claim to resources to do just that would be strong.

DEVISING CRITERIA FOR TREATMENT TERMINATION

In proposing three contextual and background considerations, I have tried to elaborate on those aspects of dementia that should most concern us in thinking about termination of life-sustaining treatment. The welfare of the demented person must, however, take precedence over other considerations (though not wholly to override them), and thus the question of selfhood is central. But since economic forces will impinge on treatment decisions, and since any policy affecting the demented will telegraph social meaning and symbols, they cannot go unconsidered.

I want now to focus on individual treatment decisions, indicating along the way where the economic and social dimensions might make a difference in the analysis. I will assume that individuals differ in their response to dementia, and that any criteria must have sufficient flexibility to take that into account. I will also assume that the degree to which the disease has advanced will be an important variable; late-stage dementia is not the same as early-stage dementia and that difference counts. I will assume, finally, that whoever is making the termination decision will have done everything possible to take into account the bias of his or her own emotional responses to the patient's condition, recognizing that it is the good of the patient, not that of the decisionmaker, that matters.

Just because of the problem of bias, it would be unwise to use the notion of 'quality of life,' commonly used in this kind of a context. Since we do not have good insight into the mind of the demented person, we cannot assume *a priori* that dementia is inevitably and necessarily *experienced* by the person himself as a poor quality of life. That may be the case early on with the condition but, ironically, perhaps not so much when the disease is far advanced and the patient is perhaps less aware of his own deterioration. As mentioned above, our lack of insight into the consciousness of the demented person should make us hesitate about quality-of-life judgments. Here in particular lies the temptation to mistake our own distress for and recoil from the patient's condition for that of the patient; the patient may or may not feel the same, and we will have no definitive way of knowing. To the extent that we learn better how to gain such insight, the possibility for a firmer judgment will increase.

Three standards can be proposed for making decisions to terminate treatment: (1) No one should, in the modern world, have to live longer in the advanced stages of dementia than he would have in a pre-technological era; (2) the more advanced the damage of the dementia, the more legitimate it is to overturn the usual bias in favor of treatment; (3) whoever is making the decision has as strong an obligation to prevent a painful and degrading death as to promote health and life. I will discuss each standard in turn.

No one should now have to live longer in the advanced stages of dementia than he would have in a pre-technological era. Every person suffering from dementia should be given adequate care, comfort, and palliation. That standard should never be changed and always be honored. It has been an enduring goal of medical practice for 2,500 years in the Western world and is particularly pertinent here given the chronic, degenerative nature of the condition. But what about the use of those medical skills and technologies that are the mark of modern medicine and that are ordinarily used to cure disease and to extend life? Are they equally required? They range from the inexpensive, painless use of antibiotics to the more elaborate and expensive techniques of open-heart surgery, dialysis, and organ transplantation.

There can be no obligation, in the later stages of dementia, to prolong with technology—even simple, nonburdensome technologies—the life of someone whose course is most likely going to be steadily downhill, steadily worse. If at all possible, a patient should be spared that likelihood, and thus opportunistic infections, organ failures, and other life-threatening conditions should not be opposed with technology (whose use should be restricted to palliation). It is hard to imagine how the use of modern technologies that extend life could be more beneficial for the advanced-stage patient, since such use actually enhances the likelihood of an even worse outcome than its omission. Modern medicine should be an option for severely deteriorated patients only if it promises clear benefit; it should not be an imposed burden. Moreover, the costs of high-technology terminal care are not a trivial consideration. Such costs can be justified only if some clear benefit is to result; and there seems to be none here.

The likely deterioration in a late-stage demented patient should lead to a shift in the usual standard of treatment, that of stopping rather than containing treatment. The ordinary standard of treatment with an incompetent patient is, lacking specific instructions otherwise, to treat rather than not to treat, with the burden of proof on those who would want to stop the treatment. With advanced dementia—as with any irreversible terminal illness in its later stages—that burden should be reversed; that is, the presumption should be against aggressive treatment unless there are some compelling reasons to continue the treatment. The traditional reasoning behind the older and ordinary rule is that most people prefer to go on living rather than dying; thus, it is a not-surprising standard. In this case, where the effect of continuing treatment would be simultaneously to prolong the life and the deterioration of the patient, there can be no obvious benefits. The treatment paves the way for further deterioration, not improvement or even stability. That would seem to be a strange way of honoring the remaining selfhood of the patient, if selfhood there is.

Should, however, there be some degree of reasonable uncertainty about the prognosis of the patient, then there is a middle-way option between aggressive treatment and none at all. In her illuminating and enormously sensible recent book, *Choosing Medical Care in Old Age*, Dr. Muriel Gillick develops the option of 'intermediate-level care,' by which she means conservative, low-technology treatment, and often at home rather than in a hospital. This gives the patient a chance for improvement if the basic biological resiliency is there, but at the same time does not invasively and artificially try to increase the low odds. 'We need,' she writes, 'to accept that a *chance* of recovery is not a sufficient reason to embark on a treatment course if the chance is small, the hazards great, and the patient irreversibly demented.'[9] Intermediate-level care provides a prudent way of dealing with those ambiguous situations in which the chance may not be too low. The value of this approach has been partially confirmed in a study comparing outcomes in Dementia Special Care Units, which concentrate on patient comfort, with those in traditional long-term care facilities, which are more open to interventions. The former units, the study found, resulted in both a lower level of patient discomfort and lower costs as well (though there was a higher mortality rate, as might be expected).[10]

There is as great an obligation to prevent a lingering, painful, or degrading death as there is to promote health and life. Among the important goals of medicine are those of preserving life, sustaining health, and relieving pain and suffering. I propose one other goal: the duty to seek, within moral means, a decent, peaceful death, which is an aspect of the duty to try to relieve suffering. A death that is lingering, painful, or psychologically degrading is not a good death. If medicine fails to do what it can within moral limits to avoid such a death, it has failed in an important part of its mission. This means avoiding a technological obsessiveness that would seek to maintain the body and its organs well past the point of any benefit. It also means encouraging efforts to understand how the continuation of treatment may affect the quality of the death it might make possible or likely.

In thinking about the likely downhill course of the disease, ought the diminished self of the patient make a difference? I am ambivalent on this point. I argued above that, since the demented person has a residual, though severely impaired self, he should be treated like any other impaired person, and treatment continued. But there is a side of me, and of most others I would surmise, that wants to say that the degree of impairment of the self should somehow make a difference in our reckoning. This impulse no doubt

[9] Muriel R. Gillick, *Choosing Medical Care in Old Age: What Kind, How Much, Where to Stop* (Cambridge, Mass.: Harvard University Press, 1994), 41.

[10] Ladislav Volicer, Ann Collard, Ann Hurley *et al.*, 'Impact of Special Care Unit for Patients with Advanced Alzheimer's Disease on Patients' Discomfort and Costs,' *Journal of the American Geriatric Society*, 42/6 (1994), 597–603. See also Jill A. Rhymes and Laurence B. McCullough, 'Nonaggressive Management of the Illnesses of Severely Demented Patients: An Ethical Justification,' *Journal of the American Geriatric Society*, 42/6 (1994); 686–87.

springs from a common reaction to the deteriorated self of the demented person: I do not want to end *my* life like that. Though understandable as an impulse, I can find no good reason to allow it to overcome the previously stated principle that, if there is any self at all, the demented person should not be singled out on the basis of special criteria related to her dementia.

No physician can guarantee a peaceful death, but many things can be done to increase its possibility. The most important is simply to promote a responsibility to balance the possible benefits of continued treatment with the possible harms of worsening the process of dying. Those two possibilities should be set in fruitful tension with each other. This will require asking not simply about the immediate benefit that treatment will bring (for it might reduce a fever or thwart a spreading infection), but also about the long-term consequences of the intervention. A treatment that provides an immediate benefit only to set the patient up for a worse death in the future should not be considered a value for the patient. Nor, economically, can it be considered a desirable social value.

APPLICATION OF THE CRITERIA

What I am looking for with these criteria is to address three major problems of decisions to terminate treatment: how and when to use available technologies that could sustain the life of the patient; how and when to turn upside down the traditional standard that when in doubt treatment should be provided; and how to determine when to invoke the duty of the physician to help the patient avoid a poor death. At present, treatment is often initiated or sustained because of a pervasive belief that potentially effective treatment should be used, that doubt should be resolved in favor of treatment, and that the physician's primary duty lies in improving or maintaining a decent quality of life rather than in promoting a peaceful death. I do not claim that this belief exists everywhere, or that the principles I am suggesting are not already at least tacitly used. The existence of a hospice movement shows that there are other extant standards (even though hospice care is too infrequently available or used by the dying demented). I only want to note what appear to be the prevailing standards and why they need to be significantly modified in the case of those patients dying with dementia (though not uniquely with them).

There still remain some problems with the proposed criteria. The most obvious is in trying to determine when the time has come to invoke them: when is the deterioration sufficient to invoke the criteria? No precise moment can be specified; like much else in medicine it will be a matter of judgment. But some indicators can be suggested. One of them would be the emotional state of the patient. If there is evidence that the patient is suffering, whether evinced by the ordinary sounds of suffering (moaning, for instance) or by the body language of discomfort and agitated restlessness, then that apparent, suffering should be taken seriously. If demented patients continue to have some kind of a self, they should be accorded all the usual deference given to someone who, apparently suffering, cannot verbally express himself. Thus evidence of suffering, verbal or nonverbal, should be a significant signal to terminate (or not to initiate) life-sustaining treatment.

Another indicator would be the degree of probability, based on clinical experience, that further treatment will enhance the likelihood of a poor death rather than an improved quality of life. Since this is a matter of probabilities, it will often not be easy to calculate. But, since the general course of dementia is downhill, there should be as much care to avoid increasing the odds of a poor death as care not to terminate treatment too quickly. Thus the standard for when the time has come to terminate treatment should not be set so high that the risk of a poor death is increased.[11]

STIGMATIZATION AND ECONOMICS

I have sought here to find a middle way between the hazard of treating the demented too aggressively, as if their dementia counted for nothing in our judgment, and failing to give them sufficient treatment, on the grounds that their dementia removes them from the human community. The suggested standards for terminating treatment are meant to reassure those suffering from dementia in its early stages that we will not medically sustain their lives only to allow them a worse death; nor will we allow our horror of dementia to lead us to ignore or deny the self that may remain, even if damaged and all but hidden from our sight. I have looked for a stance that signals to demented patients and their families that we can and will terminate treatment if at all possible before total deterioration has taken place. But we will not do so in a way that suggests we have a special horror of the condition, creating criteria that allow us to stop treatment well before what would he acceptable with other patients. An approach of this kind could help to neutralize or at least reduce the hazard of stigmatization, which is likely to draw its force from a general dread of the disease exacerbated by policies

[11] See Daniel Callaban, *The Troubled Dream of Life: In Search of a Peaceful Death* (New York: Simon & Schuster, 1993), 187–219.

suggesting the need to rush the demented out of their life and our midst. It may be hard to do much about the former, but we can at least ameliorate the potential hazards of the latter.

If for economic reasons it becomes necessary and desirable to give a low priority to the use of expensive life-extending technologies for late-stage terminal illness, including dementia, there is one place where a stronger stand should be taken. What does set dementia apart from other chronic and terminal illnesses is the impact upon families. Their lives can be crippled and harmed, even ruined, by the demands made upon them, at times cruel and inhuman. They need support of all kinds, economic and social and personal, and that costs money. If it is useless and wasteful and socially imprudent to extend marginally the life of the late-stage dementia patient, the same cannot be said of their families. Their lives will go on, and it is important that we help them to go on as well as possible.

5

WHICH WAY DOWN THE SLIPPERY SLOPE? NAZI MEDICAL KILLING AND EUTHANASIA TODAY

RUTH MACKLIN

A TROUBLING CASE

A case that came before a recent meeting of a hospital ethics committee was troubling, but not uncommon. The patient, about 70 years old, had been brought to the emergency room with a fever of 107°. Following her admission to the hospital seven months earlier, she was given a diagnosis of 'status epilepticus.' Now she is in the Intensive Care Unit, on a respirator from which she cannot be weaned. Brain damage is far-reaching. The doctors are having difficulty gaining access for the insertion of intravenous lines. The patient does not respond to stimuli, has already developed large decubitus ulcers, and requires regular suctioning and turning. A private duty nurse carries out these tasks of daily maintenance.

The patient's family—her husband and two daughters—were told of the bleak prognosis from the beginning. Yet they insist that this level of care be continued. The husband refuses to consider the physician's suggestion to write a 'Do Not Resuscitate Order' for the patient. Contrary to expert medical evaluations, the family believes the patient is communicating with them. They refuse to believe the prognosis and hold out hope that the patient will recover.

I said this case is not uncommon. The relatives of patients often demand treatment beyond the point where physicians are able to prevent death or restore functioning.

Families sometimes maintain false hope—in their grief or denial—that a miracle will occur. Doctors are reluctant to ignore or override the wishes of a patient's family in such cases, not only out of fear of being sued but also out of respect for the next of kin as surrogate decision-makers for patients who lack decisional capacity. One good reason for deferring to family members is that they are the ones most likely to know what the patient would

From Ruth Macklin, 'Which Way Down the Slippery Slope? Nazi Medical Killing and Euthanasia Today,' in Arthur L. Caplan (ed.), *When Medicine Went Mad* (Totowa, NJ: Humana Press, 1992).

have wanted regarding continuation or cessation of life supports. A less compelling reason, ethically speaking, is that doctors are unwilling to offend family members. When the patient can no longer participate in decisions, it is the family the physician must deal with.

Yet there was a troubling aspect to this case, which was the reason the physician sought the help of the ethics committee. The doctor has been pressured by the hospital administration to discontinue this level of therapy because of financial costs. The hospital is paying for the private duty nurse, and a bed in the ICU costs considerably more than one on a regular hospital floor. The patient is being given antibiotics, as well as artificial food and fluids to maintain her life. The physician believes he should be an advocate for the family of his patient, and that the right course of action is to honor their wishes about the level of care being provided. Yet he is being criticized, even threatened by his superiors for refusing to make financial considerations the overriding factor. The message is clear that this patient is absorbing a disproportionate share of the hospital's resources.

The physician told the ethics committee that the patient and her husband are Holocaust survivors, having spent years in a concentration camp. The family's experience under the Nazis underscores their unwillingness to forgo life-prolonging treatments. Some members of the ethics committee wonder whether it is ethically relevant that these people are Holocaust survivors. No one makes the explicit suggestion that lowering the level of care would constitute euthanasia. Everyone agrees that continued biological life could not benefit the patient herself. Yet some committee members are deeply worried about the justification for withdrawing treatment. The patient is costing the hospital too much money. She has become a 'useless eater.'

Would it be an act of euthanasia to deny this patient her private duty nurse and to reduce the level of care by removing her from the ICU? The answer depends on the definition of 'euthanasia.' Physicians at the ethics committee meeting were in unanimous agreement that the patient's death would be hastened if she received anything less than her current level of care. Yet the intention of lowering the level of care is to save money, not to cause the death of the patient. But her imminent death could be foreseen, even if not directly intended. Nonetheless, death would not relieve the suffering of this patient, since she is unresponsive and the extent of brain damage precludes the possibility of any awareness. However, according to one viewpoint, people who are comatose 'are benefited by euthanasia, even though they are not relieved of suffering.'[1]

---

[1] T. L. Beauchamp and A. I. Davidson, 'The Definition of Euthanasia,' in S. Gorovitz *et al.* (eds.), *Moral Problems in Medicine*, 2nd edn. (Englewood Cliffs, NJ: Prentice-Hall, 1983), 453.

One member of the ethics committee suggested that the family be told that the hospital simply does not have the resources to continue to provide this level of care for this patient. Is the patient's family mistaken in thinking that withdrawal of care bears any resemblance to what happened in Nazi Germany?

EUTHANASIA UNDER THE NAZIS AND TODAY: THREE APPROACHES

No ethical indictment is more devastating than the charge of 'Nazi practices.' Yet the temptation to issue that indictment often surfaces when euthanasia is mentioned. Although it is hard to remain dispassionate in any discussion relating to the Holocaust, several questions deserve sober reflection: Were there any aspects of the euthanasia program under the Nazis that could legitimately be described as 'euthanasia' in our sense of the term? Is there a clear and unequivocal meaning of the concept of euthanasia today? Are there any relevant similarities between 'medical killing' during the Holocaust and recent biomedical practices involving termination of treatment? If there are such similarities, does ethical consistency require that we accept or condemn both?

Three general approaches to this set of questions can be discerned. To be sure, there are differences in style and method among adherents of any one approach. But to understand and analyze the overall debate, it is useful to draw the boundary lines with broad brushstrokes. The first approach finds all too many similarities between the Nazi 'euthanasia program' and what goes on in hospitals today. The second approach argues against the meaningfulness and accuracy of alleged similarities. The third approach is not an intermediate position between the first two, but rather, one that sounds a cautionary alarm about the dangers of the slippery slope.

In the first group are those who find current practices involving termination of life-sustaining treatment unacceptable. Some in this group hold that euthanasia, *by definition*, is morally wrong, and that today's practices are all examples of euthanasia. A more nuanced view claims that a great many contemporary biomedical practices have ideological roots similar to those of the Nazis. Proponents of both viewpoints use Nazi allusions and comparisons to buttress their account.

An example of the definitional indictment is an inflammatory article entitled 'Hitler's Euthanasia Program—More Like Today's than you might Imagine.' It begins by asserting: 'Today we are faced with the prospect that our society will accept and legalize, the crime of euthanasia, for which Nazi doctors hanged at Nuremberg.'[2]

The article uses the phrase 'today's Death Lobby' to refer to advocates of patients' right to refuse life-prolonging treatment, and identifies a 'whole breed of "medical ethicists" in the service of death . . . whose vocation is to tell doctors, hospitals, families and clergymen that it is highly moral to kill helpless patients in American hospitals.'[3]

Less inflammatory but nonetheless issuing a similar indictment is an article by Nat Hentoff, who argues that even with the very best of intentions, it is possible 'to think and plan in a way that would bring about results that were also the goals of the Nazis—from different motivations.'[4] Hentoff picks out several targets. One is Daniel Callahan, for implying in his book, *Setting Limits*, that 'the lives of the elderly are worth less—in terms of prolonging them—than other lives,' a view Hentoff assimilates to the Nazis' *'lebensunwertes Leben,* "life unworthy of life." '[5] Another target is Ronald Crawford, along with others who argue that when individuals are in a persistent vegetative state, 'personhood' has vanished, and 'without personhood, there could be no act of murder,' that is, wrongful killing.

A lengthy, more nuanced article by Richard John Neuhaus serves as an example of the view that active euthanasia is morally prohibited, and moreover, it is always wrong to withhold or withdraw certain medical treatments. Entitled 'The Return of Eugenics,' this article argues that Nazi Germany's doctrines and practices 'effected but a momentary pause in the theory and practice of eugenics . . . [T]oday, . . . eugenics is back . . . '[6] Neuhaus asserts that 'the question of euthanasia is . . . an integral part of the progress of the eugenics project.'[7] The meaning of 'eugenics' is broadened here to include new ways of using and terminating 'undesired human life,'[8] as well as other biomedical practices the author deplores. One such practice, abortion, is likened by Neuhaus to the killing of Jews, gypsies, homosexuals, and Slavs by the Nazis.[9] Here, Neuhaus claims that the justifications offered for

[2] M. H. Kronberg, in N. B. Spannaus, M. H. Kronberg and L. Everett (eds.) *How to Stop the Resurgence of Nazi Euthanasia Today*, EIR Special Report (1988), 129.

[3] Ibid. 130, 131.

[4] N. Hentoff, 'Contested Terrain: The Nazi Analogy in Bioethics,' *Hastings Center Report*, 18 (1988), 29.

[5] Ibid.

[6] R. J. Neuhaus, 'The Return of Eugenics,' *Commentary* (July 1988), 15.

[7] Ibid. 20.

[8] Ibid. 15.

[9] Richard John Neuhaus, 'The Way they Were, the Way we Are,' in Caplan (ed.), *When Medicine Went Mad.*

abortion and research with human embryos in our society 'are very much like the arguments employed in the Holocaust . . .'[10]

The second approach is at the opposite end of the spectrum. Writers in this group seek to deny either definitional equivalence or factual similarities between the Nazis' euthanasia program and today's examples of forgoing life-sustaining treatment.

First is the attempt to sever the very meaning of the concept of euthanasia from the Nazi program that went by that name. In an article whose purpose is simply to define the term 'euthanasia,' Beauchamp and Davidson dismiss an entire range of examples, claiming that 'some actions which have commonly been denominated euthanasia—such as the overused Nazi examples—would not be euthanasia on our definition.'[11] Seeking to provide a 'definition . . . which dictates no moral conclusions', these authors argue that the concept of euthanasia 'includes no inherently evaluative component. "Murder" entails wrongful killing, and therefore possesses both prescriptive and descriptive force; but "euthanasia" is not analogous.'[12]

Not only is the concept of euthanasia devoid of a negative evaluative component according to this account; it also lacks a positive evaluative component, despite its derivation from the Greek word for 'good death.' Thus, Beauchamp and Davidson argue, it is not a contradiction to say 'an act of euthanasia is immoral.'[13] Correctly describing an act as an instance of euthanasia is one thing; evaluating a particular act described as euthanasia is quite another.

Beauchamp and Davidson are correct in observing that the term 'euthanasia' need not entail either a positive or a negative evaluation of the act. The concept can be defined and used in a purely descriptive way, denoting a means of bringing about death but neither praising nor condemning it. However, most people who talk or write about euthanasia do not use the term in that purely descriptive way. Beauchamp and Davidson are telling us how people ought to use the concept, what the term euthanasia 'really' means. Most people haven't read their scholarly article, though, and will continue to use the term with its built-in value connotations.

A variant of this second approach to the question of comparisons between the Nazi euthanasia program and today's medical practices takes the position that not only do certain concepts used by the Nazis differ in meaning from their current usage; but also, there are great factual dissimilarities between what the Nazis were about and what goes on today. This denial

---

[10] Ibid., MS, fo. 26.
[11] Beauchamp and Davidson, 'The Definition of Euthanasia,' 448.
[12] Ibid. 456.
[13] Ibid. 457.

takes several forms. One focuses not directly on euthanasia, but on other concepts, most notably, 'quality of life.' In an article entitled ' "Quality of Life" and the Analogy with the Nazis,' Cynthia Cohen provides a detailed explication of how the Nazis used that phrase, arguing that their use was radically different from our own. The Nazis viewed the quality of life of individuals only in terms of their social worth, how they were of service to the *Volk*. In contrast, Cohen maintains, 'a coherent "quality of life" position is grounded in a theory of the value of humans as beings with a capacity for self-reflective deliberation and action. It explicates the meaning of "quality of life" of human beings in terms of standards of individual well-being, rather than in terms of social worth.'[14]

Yet even when its meaning is confined to standards of individual well-being, the phrase 'quality of life' poses the problem of determining how high or low a standard of individual well-being is acceptable. In a long-standing debate surrounding the ethics of allowing handicapped newborns to die, standards have been proposed that many people consider unacceptably high. An example is the criterion used by John Lorber, a British pediatrician: 'The ability to work or marry.'[15]

A more direct form of this approach focuses on the term 'euthanasia' itself. Such terms, when applied to the Nazi experience 'do not have our meaning. These terms and the programs they stood for were integral aspects of Nazi racism. Nazi racism derived from a theory about the ultimate value of the purity of the *Volk* . . . '[16] This observation, by Lucy Dawidowicz, makes only half of the comparison, however. It fails to specify *our* meaning—assuming that there is a single meaning, which there is not—of the term 'euthanasia.'

THE CONCEPT OF EUTHANASIA

Before proceeding to the third approach—one that finds both similarities and differences between the Nazi program and today's practices—this is a suitable place to pause for the obligatory conceptual inquiry. Although there is not a single definition of euthanasia, there is a core meaning common to a number of leading candidates. To cite only a few of the definitions that have been offered:

[14] C. B. Cohen, ' "Quality of Life" and the Analogy with the Nazis,' *Journal of Medical Philosophy*, 8 (1983), 114. See also Cohen's commentary in 'Contested Terrain: The Nazi Analogy in Bioethics,' *Hastings Center Report*, 18 (1988), 32, 33.

[15] J. Lorber, 'Ethical Problems in the Management of Myelomeningocele and Hydrocephalus,' *Journal of the Royal College of Physicians*, 10/1 (1975), 47–60.

[16] L. Dawidowicz, in H. Kuhse and P. Singer (eds.), *Should the Baby Live?* (New York: Oxford University Press, 1985), 94.

1. 'The painless inducement of a quick death;'
2. 'An act or practice of painlessly putting to death persons suffering from incurable conditions or diseases;'
3. 'The intentional putting to death by artificial means of persons with incurable or painful disease;'
4. 'An act . . . in which one . . . kills another person . . . for the benefit of the second person, who actually does benefit from being killed.'[17]

Not only do these definitions differ substantially from one another; they also are open to 'fatal counterexamples.'[18] Definition 1. could be applied to a simple case of murder, such as injecting a quick-acting poison into a sleeping person whom one hates. This definition also permits accidental death to be an instance of euthanasia.[19] Definition 2. could also be a simple case of murder, such as injecting a quick-acting poison into a rich relative who has a mild case of multiple sclerosis (an incurable disease) without the relative's consent and for the purpose of inheriting his wealth. Definition 3. includes the vague and problematic term 'artificial,' and like 1. and 2., also omits mention of the central intention, namely to end suffering or to benefit the person whose death is intended. Definition 4. comes closer to our intuitive understanding of the concept of euthanasia. But cast in terms of one person *killing* a second person, it rules out, by definition, situations in which suffering patients are passively 'let die,' rather than actively killed.

One attempt to summarize the relevant differences between the Nazis' use of the term 'euthanasia' and what is assumed to be our current meaning appears in a historical study of Nazism.[20] It is worth quoting the long opening paragraph of the chapter entitled 'The "Euthanasia" Programme 1939–1945'.

In current parlance the term *euthanasia* refers to the practice of so-called 'mercy killing,' that is of painlessly ending the life of a person who is terminally ill at his or her request or, if they are no longer capable of making such a request, then with the consent of their relatives. It is a highly controversial issue, but it should not be confused with the Nazi 'euthanasia' policy. For, although the Nazis used the term to describe their own programme of killing over one hundred thousand mentally sick and handicapped persons from 1939 to 1945, their practice had little in common with the term as it is normally understood. In the first place, the decision to terminate the life of a patient under the Nazi programme was taken not by the individual concerned or by his or her relatives but by an official body. Secondly, the criterion for the 'mercy killing' was not the welfare of the individual patient but whether or not the patient's life was judged to be of 'value' or 'worth,' and of value not to the individual

[17] Beauchamp and Davidson, 'The Definition of Euthanasia,' 446, 447, 457.
[18] Ibid. 446.
[19] Ibid. 449.
[20] J. Noakes and G. Pridham (eds.) *Nazism 1919–1945*, iii: *Foreign Policy, War and Racial Extermination*, Exeter Studies in History, no. 13 (Exeter: Exeter University Publications, 1988).

concerned (although the Nazis sometimes used this as an additional justification) but to the community.[21]

The first condition—that the decision to terminate the life of a patient be made either by the individual concerned or by his or her relatives—is not part of the *meaning* of the term 'euthanasia;' nor does it fully and accurately describe current or proposed practices. The second condition—that the criterion for mercy killing be the welfare of the individual patient—does capture the central feature of the concept of euthanasia, but whether or not the sufferer must be terminally ill remains a matter of conceptual and ethical dispute. There is great uncertainty and consequently, much ethical controversy about how to determine the welfare or 'best interest' of individuals who are incapable of speaking for themselves.

A classification scheme often used to elucidate the concept of euthanasia distinguishes four categories: Active, passive, voluntary, and involuntary. Each category can be marked by a paradigm case, yet conceptually and practically, these distinctions are easily blurred. In the following examples, assume that the intention in causing the death of the individual is to end suffering or to benefit the patient.

A clear case of active euthanasia is the injection of a lethal substance into a patient with advanced, metastatic cancer, who is suffering extreme pain and discomfort. The act would count as *voluntary*, active euthanasia if the patient knew she was in the advanced stage of incurable cancer, requested the injection, and believed the injection would cause her death. It would be *involuntary*, active euthanasia if the patient were not consulted and her wishes were not known.

Paradigm cases of *passive* euthanasia are ones in which a life-sustaining treatment is withheld. These are cases of 'letting die,' rather than 'killing.' A patient who requests to be allowed to die rather than being intubated and placed on a ventilator might be said to seek voluntary, passive euthanasia. The case becomes more convincing as relief of suffering if the patient had already been on a ventilator, found that mode of existence intolerable, and after being weaned requests that she not be reintubated even if necessary to prolong her life. To ensure that death by this means would be painless as well as quick, the patient requests that she be adequately sedated.

An example of involuntary, passive euthanasia would be withholding renal dialysis from an irreversibly comatose patient whose kidneys have failed. The act is involuntary because the patient has not requested that dialysis be withheld. Since on virtually all accounts continued life would not be a benefit to an irreversibly comatose individual, this case could qualify conceptually as euthanasia.

But here is where definitional uncertainty begins, leading to the conceptual debate. Does a 'good death' require that the patient be relieved of suffering? Can death itself count as a benefit to a person who is comatose or in a persistent vegetative state? Reasonable people disagree on the answers to these concepual questions, yet without agreement on that point, the boundaries of euthanasia remain fuzzy.

According to one view, patients in a coma or persistent vegetative state (PVS) 'are benefited by euthanasia, even though they are not relieved of suffering.'[22] An opposing view holds that 'no definition [of euthanasia] is acceptable which includes under its instances persons who are comatose . . .'[23] This is because the concept of euthanasia should apply only in cases where the intent is to benefit a person by relieving that person's suffering. It is important to see this as a conceptual dispute, not an ethical disagreement. There is virtually no controversy over whether individuals who are in a coma or in the unresponsive condition known as PVS are experiencing suffering. Opponents in the conceptual dispute might disagree about whether withholding life supports from comatose individuals counts as euthanasia; yet they may still agree on whether it is morally permissible to forgo the respirator.

Conceptual debate is even more intense when it comes to drawing a line between 'active' and 'passive' means. Is the removal of life supports already in place active or passive? Many physicians insist that withdrawing treatment counts as 'active' euthanasia. They argue that if they fail to institute life-prolonging treatment, it is the disease that kills the patient; but if life supports already in place are withdrawn, it is the doctor who kills the patient. This conceptual maneuver rests on an underlying ethical stance: Allowing to die is morally permissible, but killing is not.

Yet that proposition is problematic. It brings to mind the rationalization used by Nazi doctors involved in the Child Euthanasia Program. Some left their institutions without heat, allowing the children to die of exposure. This enabled the doctors to offer the rationale that they were not engaged in murder, since 'withholding care' was simply 'letting nature take its course.'[24] This shows that ethical permissibility cannot rest simply on whether the means leading to death are 'active' or 'passive.'

Indeed, it is suggested by proponents of active euthanasia that active

---

[22] Beauchamp and Davidson. 'The Definition of Euthanasia,' 453.

[23] Ibid.

[24] R. N. Proctor, *Racial Hygiene: Medicine under the Nazis* (Cambridge, Mass.: Harvard University Press, 1988). 187.

killing is sometimes more humane, and therefore, more ethically acceptable than allowing to die. When performed under limited, specified circumstances and with adequate safeguards, a painless lethal injection is more humane, they argue, than letting the cancer patient die a slow, agonizing death. Among those who believe that active killing, under certain circumstances, can be ethically permissible are physicians who practice active euthanasia in the Netherlands, along with their supporters; and members of the Hemlock Society in the United States, along with those who signed a petition seeking to place a referendum legalizing active euthanasia on the California ballot in 1988. Both the existing practice in Holland and the proposed plan in California permit only *voluntary* euthanasia, and both require that the patient who requests euthanasia be terminally ill at the time the request is made. Additional safeguards, designed to prevent abuses, are also built into the practice.

At the other extreme are those who oppose any and all withholding of life-sustaining treatment, whether active or passive, voluntary or involuntary; and a more moderate group who draw the moral line at withholding food and fluids, or more generally, at the boundary between 'ordinary' and 'extraordinary' treatments or 'routine' and 'heroic' measures. Withholding food and fluids amounts to 'starving people to death,' it is argued. What could be more like the Nazi euthanasia program?

THE NAZI EUTHANASIA PROGRAM

The case that is said to have precipitated the first phase of the Nazi euthanasia program, known as the 'children's "euthanasia" program,' occurred in late 1938 or early 1939 and involved a handicapped child. As recalled by Hitler's personal physician, Karl Brandt, in his testimony at the Nuremberg Medical Trial, the child was born blind, with one leg and part of one arm missing, and in Brandt's words 'appeared to be an idiot.'[25] In that case, the father had written to Hitler 'and asked for this child, or this creature, to be put down.'[26] From that 'small beginning,' Hitler launched the 'children's euthanasia program,' authorizing Brandt and another official, Philipp Bouhler, to deal with similar cases in the same way.[27]

Could it plausibly be argued that this was not a 'life worth living,' as judged from the infant's point of view? Using Lorber's criterion of an

---

[25] Noakes and Pridham (eds.), *Nazism*, 1005; see also R. J. Lifton, *The Nazi Doctors* (New York: Basic Books, 1986), 50, 51.
[26] Noakes and Pridham (eds.), *Nazism*, 1005 (statement of Karl Brandt from Nuremberg Trial).
[27] Ibid. 1005.

acceptable quality of life, 'the ability to work or marry,' this child would fall below the line. Is it even possible to make an assessment of the value that child's life could have for him?

Jumping to a recent case, that of Baby Doe born in April 1982 in Bloomington, Indiana, we find that the infant's father did seek to make that assessment for him. Baby Doe was born with a correctable intestinal defect—an improperly formed esophagus. But he was also born with Down's syndrome, the chromosomal anomaly formerly known as mongolism. In the court proceeding that later ensued, the baby's father told the Circuit Court that 'he was a schoolteacher and had sometimes worked closely with Down's syndrome children. He said that he and his wife were of the opinion that such children never had a minimally acceptable quality of life.'[28] The parents decided that 'it was in the best interests of Baby Doe, and also of their family as a whole' to forgo the life-preserving surgery. They understood that although efforts would be made in the hospital to keep the infant comfortable and free of pain, he would die within a short time, either from starvation and dehydration—since he could not be fed by mouth—or from complications leading to pneumonia.[29]

In August 1939, a circular issued by the Reich Interior Ministry mandated a 'duty to report deformed births.' All newborn infants 'suspected of suffering from the following congenital defects' were to be registered: (1) Idiocy and Mongolism (particularly cases that involved blindness and deafness); (2) Microcephalie; (3) Hydrocephalus of a serious or progressive nature; (4) Deformities of every kind, in particular, the absence of limbs, spina bifida, and so on; (5) Paralysis, including Little's disease.[30] Some of these infants were identified by 'assessors' (who did not actually examine them) and marked for death. This group was transferred to special 'pediatric clinics,' where they were either starved to death, given lethal injections, or died of diseases caused by malnutrition.[31]

Thus, some of these children marked for death were actively killed, whereas others were simply allowed to die. Their parents were pressured to allow the infants to be transferred to these special clinics on the grounds that they would be given 'optimum treatment.' The stated reason was an obvious falsehood, clearly intended to deceive the parents about the purpose of the transfer.[32] Although it was possible for parents to refuse, they had to sign a declaration committing themselves to remove the children from the hospital,

[28] Kuhse and Singer (eds.), *Should the Baby Live?*, 12.
[29] Ibid.
[30] Noakes and Pridham (eds.), *Nazism*, 1006.
[31] Ibid. 1007.
[32] Lifton, *The Nazi Doctors*, 54.

and provide supervision and care.[33] Again in order to deceive, the cause of death was listed as 'a more or less ordinary disease such as pneumonia, which could even have [a] kernel of truth . . . '[34]

THE SLIPPERY SLOPE

This account of the 'Children's Euthanasia Program' brings us to the third, and ultimately the most interesting approach to comparisons between the Nazi euthanasia program and current practices of withholding or withdrawing life supports: commentators on the slippery slope. Adherents of this approach cite the description by Leo Alexander, who worked with the United States Counsel for War Crimes in Nuremberg. Alexander wrote that the Nazi euthanasia program

started from small beginnings. The beginnings at first were merely a subtle shift in emphasis in the basic attitude of the physicians . . . that there is such a thing as a life not worthy to be lived. This attitude in its early stages concerned itself merely with the severely and chronically sick. Gradually the sphere of those to be included in this category was enlarged to encompass the socially unproductive, the ideologically unwanted and finally all non-Germans. But it is important to realize that the infinitely small wedged-in lever from which this entire trend of mind received its impetus was the attitude towards the nonrehabilitable sick.[35]

Assessing the slipperiness of the slope are three camps. One group contends that there are simply not enough similarities between the Nazis' euthanasia program and today's practices to cause concern that we have begun the dangerous slide down that slope. An example appears in a book by Helga Kuhse and Peter Singer, who write:

When the Nazis talked of 'a life not worthy to be lived' they meant that the life was unworthy because it did not contribute to the health of that mysterious racial entity, the *Volk*. Since our society does not believe in any such entity, there is no real prospect that allowing active euthanasia of severely handicapped newborn infants would lead to Nazi-style atrocities.[36]

A member of the opposite camp contests that assessment of the likelihood of sliding down the infamous slope. David Lamb writes:

An immediate reaction to Kuhse and Singer here is that racism in our culture is very much alive and that the homogeneity presupposed by the expression 'our society' simply does not exist. However, it may be the case that despite the existence of racism in Western society, contemporary medicine does not have notions of the 'Volk' at its

[33] Noakes and Pridham (eds.), *Nazism*, 1007.
[34] Lifton, *The Nazi Doctors*, 55.
[35] Kuhse and Singer (eds.), *Should the Baby Live?*, 93.
[36] Ibid. 95.

core. But there is an increasing concern with social utility which may turn out to be not that far removed from the Nazi standpoint.[37]

How far removed a current concern might be from the Nazi standpoint is difficult to determine. Consider a statement made in 1984 by a physician, following the passage of amendments to the Child Abuse and Neglect Prevention and Treatment Act and ensuing federal regulations: 'The law now states that in obstetric units, babies must be fed and given full support regardless of how extensive and hopeless their congenital malformations . . . These [issues] must be viewed not only in the light of the individual's right to life, but in that of society's right for its members to have pleasant and productive lives, not to be lived mainly to support the growing numbers of hopelessly disabled, often unconscious people whose costly existence is consuming so much of the gross national product . . . '[38]

The author of this article is careful to point out that he is not referring to defects that can be treated (harelips, spina bifidas, or deformities of the extremities). He does include, however, 'totally incurable and accurately diagnosable brain defects' such as Down's syndrome: 'No child with Down's syndrome ever grew up to be self-sustaining.'

The author is surely not endorsing active euthanasia of Down's syndrome infants or other groups for whom 'there should be no reason to support life artificially,' such as 'oldsters with mental deterioration from stroke or Alzheimer's disease [who have] become totally incompetent to care for themselves . . . ' However, he does assert that 'there should be no support from the community or the state' to keep such people alive. It is worth recalling that in 1939, under the children's euthanasia program fashioned by the Nazis, it was possible for parents to refuse to have their children transferred to special 'pediatric clinics' if they signed a declaration committing themselves to remove the children from the hospital, and provide supervision and care.

Those who are quick to dismiss all attempts to compare the Nazi euthanasia program with current attitudes and practices should reflect soberly on whether society has a 'right' for its members to have pleasant and productive lives. The driving force behind the Nazi program was the perception of 'growing numbers of hopelessly disabled people who consume so much of the gross national product.'

Hitler's adult euthanasia program had a separate organization and history from the children's program. It began with a statement in August, 1939 by Philipp Bouhler, then head of the Party Chancellery, that the purpose of

---

[37] D. Lamb, *Down the Slippery Slope: Arguing in Applied Ethics* (New York: Croom Helm, 1988), 28, 29.
[38] G. Crile, Jr., 'The Right to Life,' *Medical Tribune* (19 Dec. 1984), 27.

eliminating persons having a 'life unworthy of life' was not only to continue the 'struggle against genetic disease' but also to free up hospital beds and personnel for the coming war.[39] At a meeting of the 'steering group' in October, 1939, this statement of purpose was translated into a cost-benefit assessment of how many would be killed:

The number is arrived at through a calculation on the basis of a ratio of 1000:10:5:1. That means out of 1,000 people 10 require psychiatric treatment; of these 5 in residential form. And, of these, one patient will come under the programme. If one applies this to the population of the greater German Reich, then one must reckon with 65–75,000 cases.[40]

The program proceeded according to schedule, and by the end of August, 1941, when the gassing phase was ended, 70,273 people had been killed.[41]

The focus of the adult euthanasia program was on adult chronic patients, especially mental patients. Implementation of the program involved virtually the entire psychiatric community, as well as physicians from the general medical community.[42] In a later phase of the program—referred to in Nazi documents as 'wild euthanasia'—physicians were empowered to act on their own initiative regrarding who would live or die.[43]

When the question was posed of how the killings would be done, the initial answer was again arrived at by a cost-benefit analysis.

The number referred to by Party Comrade Brack also tallies with [Heyde's] own estimation. It makes the proposed method of injections put forward by Professor Nitsche unviable. For the same reason, the use of doses of medicine is also impossible . . . The question has been discussed with the director of the Reich Criminal Police Department . . . We are in agreement with him that CO (Carbon Monoxide) is the best method.[44]

As for just which inmates of psychiatric asylums were to be selected for the euthanasia program, 'the criteria for assessment were . . . periodically adjusted.'[45] Initially, patients who could perform useful work were to be excluded from this action, as well as people who had had a stroke and had become 'mentally defective,' and 'war disabled who had suffered some kind of mental damage.'[46] By 1941, the exclusion criterion of war service was eliminated.

The final set of criteria for assessment of candidates for the adult

[39] Proctor, *Racial Hygiene*, 182.
[40] Noakes and Pridham (eds.), *Nazism*, 1010.
[41] Proctor, *Racial Hygiene*, 191.
[42] Lifton, *The Nazi Doctors*, 65.
[43] Ibid. 96.
[44] Noakes and Pridham (eds.), *Nazism*, 1010, 1011.
[45] Ibid. 1017.
[46] Ibid. 1013.

euthanasia program was issued in March, 1941, before the official ending of the program. The document explicitly excluded senility as a criterion: 'Extreme caution in cases of senility. Only urgent cases, e.g., criminals or asocials are to be included ... This reference to senile patients does not apply to aged patients with psychoses, such as schizophrenia, epilepsy, etc. who are basically included in the programme.'[47] The exclusion of senility as a criterion is interesting in light of the Nazi analogy often invoked when it is suggested today that life prolonging resources be withheld from the elderly based on their chronological age. Not only did the Nazis reject advanced age as a criterion for euthanasia, but they also urged extreme caution in cases of 'ordinary' senility.

Hitler issued a 'halt' order in August of 1941, but in practice, it applied only to the large-scale gassing of mental patients. After Hitler's order, the focus shifted to the concentration camps and began to include Jewish prisoners who were neither mentally nor physically sick and thus unable to work. They were selected simply on the basis of race.[48]

A different approach to slippery slope arguments contends that even avowed opponents of that form of argument may have unwittingly begun the slide themselves. Thus, Neuhaus, citing Daniel Callahan's rejection of the Nazi analogy in his discussion of quality of life, observes that Callahan himself has already said:

Daniel Callahan is a spirited opponent of the slippery-slope metaphor ... but his own emotional preparedness with respect to the treatment of the dependent and incapable has undergone a remarkable development ... In ... 1983 ... he wrote forcefully against withdrawing food and water ... Four years later, Callahan invites us ... to discard that moral emotion.[49]

According to Neuhaus, Callahan has slid because to hold that nutrition and hydration may ethically be withheld 'requires the erasure of two distinctions of long standing in medical ethics and practice. The first distinction is between "ordinary" and "extraordinary" means ... and the second distinction is between medical treatment and providing food and water.'[50]

Vast literature on the vagueness and ambiguity of the ordinary/ extraordinary distinction, and recent work by the President's Commission,[51] seem finally to have laid to rest its utility for the purpose of making ethical judgments. Moreover, one feature of the oft-quoted statement of Pope Pius

[47] Ibid. 1018.
[48] Ibid. 1043.
[49] Neuhaus, 'The Return of Eugenics,' 24.
[50] Ibid. 22.
[51] President's Commission for the Study of Ethical Problems in Medicine and Biomedical and Behavioral Research, *Deciding to Forgo Life-Sustaining Treatment* (Washington, DC: US Government Printing Office, 1983), 82–90.

XII has the potential for being morally pernicious. The 1957 statement holds that 'normally one is held to use only ordinary means—means that do not involve any grave burden for oneself or another.'[52]

Now what might constitute a grave burden for *another?* A great expenditure of money required to sustain hospitalization and life supports? The agony of a family watching a loved relative linger for months in an intensive care unit? The provision of frequent and unpleasant nursing chores to an incontinent, bedridden, elderly parent with Alzheimer's disease? This feature of the ordinary/extraordinary distinction makes it a criterion for forgoing treatment that is not exclusively patient centered. This opens the door to far wider abuses than abandonment of a distinction found to be unhelpful in medical practice today. To erase the distinction appears to have been a moral gain, rather than a slide down the slope.

Still, it is easy to see how withholding food and water can be assimilated to Nazi practices. The Nazi doctor, Hermann Pfannmuller, was credited with the policy of starving to death those selected for the children's euthanasia program, rather than wasting medication on them.[53] According to the account of a visitor to the institution Pfannmuller directed, he said:

We do not kill . . . with poison, injections, etc. . . . No, our method is much simpler and more natural, as you see. . . . The murderer explained further then, that sudden withdrawal of food was not employed, rather gradual decrease of the rations. A lady who was also part of the tour asked—her outrage suppressed with difficulty—whether a quicker death with injections, etc., would not at least be more merciful.[54]

The irony of the visitor's question is a reminder of a core ingredient in the meaning of euthanasia. A lethal injection might very well bring about a more 'merciful' death than starvation for these children. But unlike patients in the last throes of terminal illness, the children in the Nazi euthanasia program were deliberately selected to die. It is a cruel irony to voice an ethical indictment of the *mode* of death, when it is the very fact of death that constitutes the moral outrage. The same moral judgment applies to the cases of Baby Doe in Bloomington, Indiana, and the Johns Hopkins baby more than 15 years ago. The fact that they were not fed, and hence starved to death, addresses the lesser of the moral evils. Both infants would have lived if their parents had not refused to consent to surgery to correct their intestinal malformation. And both would have lived had a court order been granted to override parental refusal. There is every reason to believe that these infants suffered.

But there is no reason to believe that irreversibly comatose patients or those in PVS suffer when artificial nutrition and hydration are withheld.

[52] Cited in President's Commission, 85 n. 122 (italics added).
[53] Lifton, *The Nazi Doctors*, 62.   [54] Ibid.

These patients have no awareness of their surroundings, nor do they experience sensations. They do not respond to any stimuli, even deep pain. The part of their brain that enables them to have experiences has ceased to function. Therefore, they cannot suffer, either from starvation, dehydration, or continued medical treatment. Whether withdrawal of life supports from such patients should be termed euthanasia is a conceptual question. Whether withdrawal of medical treatment, including artificially administered nutrition and hydration, is ethically acceptable is a separate and distinct question.

There is a third group that remains camped at the base of the slippery slope, watching and waiting. Gregory Pence is prepared to wait and see whether what is for many people the most worrisome practice—active euthanasia, as currently practiced by a few Dutch physicians—will precipitate the slide:

What will happen in the future is difficult to predict. A statute won't solve all problems because it can't be drafted broadly enough to cover all patients and precisely enough to close loopholes ('terminal condition,' 'unbearable suffering'). In any case, the Dutch experience may show whether mercy killing leads to Auschwitz, civilized death, or somewhere in between.[55]

Another writer in this camp observes that there's more than one slope to slide down. Laurence McCullogh argues that the accuracy of the comparison between the Nazi euthanasia program and our own biomedical practices depends on which features are taken to be relevantly similar or different:

We see that what got German society on the slippery slope, indeed what characterized the slope, was the racist attitudes already in place. It is a reasonable defence and distinguishes our case from theirs, for us to say that we don't have those attitudes . . . *Our* slippery slope might yet be analogous to Germany's in a more abstract way. If we consider the rationale which gives social utility or economic returns precedence over individual freedom, then we might see how our society could approach the kind of thinking that underlay the Nazi experience. There, racism overrode personal autonomy; here, it might be an economic rationale—the attitude that we won't spend so much per year to keep somebody alive on the slim chance of recovery.[56]

This view is echoed and reinforced by Alan Weisbard and Mark Siegler, who observe that one slide has already begun, and now is the time to be vigilant. Their concern is the acceptance of withholding of food and fluids from dying patients, conjoined with recent furious efforts to control the costs of medical care:

---

[55] G. E. Pence, 'Do not Go Slowly into that Dark Night: Mercy Killing in Holland,' *American Journal of Medicine*, 84 (1988), 141.
[56] L. McCullogh, cited in Lamb, *Down the Slippery Slope*, 29.

We have witnessed too much history to disregard how easily society disvalues the lives of the 'unproductive'—the retarded, the disabled, the senile, the institutionalized, the elderly—of those who in another time and place were referred to as 'useless eaters.' The confluence of the emerging stream of medical and ethical opinion favoring legitimation of withholding fluids and nutrition with the torrent of public and governmental concern over the costs of medical care ... powerfully reinforces our discomfort.[57]

These different worries about the prospect of sliding down a slippery slope are instructive. Each reveals a somewhat different value bias about euthanasia—what practices are unacceptable, what we have most to fear, or which of several slopes are most dangerous.

For Neuhaus, it matters not whether euthanasia is 'passive' or 'active,' 'voluntary' or 'involuntary.' All are morally wrong. Using the technique known as 'persuasive definition,' Neuhaus subsumes all forms of euthanasia under his broader heading, the 'eugenics project.'

For Pence, it appears to be both the continued voluntariness of the Dutch practice of euthanasia, and its success in maintaining the limited conditions under which active, voluntary euthanasia may be performed that would permit the practice to be ethically acceptable.

For McCullogh, the slide down the slope can be halted so long as personal autonomy remains paramount, and is not overridden by economic considerations.

For Callahan, the key lies in paying strict adherence to an acceptable standard for assessing quality of life. So long as 'borderline cases' are not excluded from the human community, and denied life-preserving therapies on the grounds that they are lives 'not worth living' according to some comparative social standard, we can avoid the murderous tendencies of the Nazi regime.[58]

For Lamb, it is only the ability of our pluralistic society to resist the growing tendencies to violence and increased tolerance of aggression that can successfully halt a precipitous slide.[59]

For Weisbard and Siegler, the danger lies in two trends that are reinforcing one another: Monomaniacal concern over the costs of medical care, and acceptance by physicians and society of the ethical acceptability of withholding food and fluids from patients. Weisbard and Siegler state their worries about the slippery slope partly in response to their expressed concern about methods of cost control:

[57] A. J. Weisbard and M. Siegler, 'On Killing Patients with Kindness: An Appeal for Caution,' in J. D. Arras and N. K. Rhoden (eds.), *Ethical Issues in Modern Medicine*, 3rd edn. (Mountain View, Calif.: Mayfield Publishing, 1989), 218.

[58] D. Callahan, *Setting Limits* (New York: Simon & Schuster, 1987), 179.

[59] Lamb, *Down the Slippery Slope*, 37–40.

It may well prove convenient—and all too easy—to move from recognition of an individual's 'right to die' . . . to a climate enforcing a socially obligatory 'duty to die,' preferably quickly and cheaply.[60]

Concern about still another slippery slope is sometimes voiced about the role physicians are asked to play in voluntary, active euthanasia. If doctors begin to perceive an obligation to kill patients who request it, in addition to their long-standing obligation to heal their patients, they could readily develop an indifference to human beings. Robert Jay Lifton identifies a psychological process he calls 'doubling,' whereby Nazi doctors could function in their evil role. Lifton describes the process as follows:

the division of the self into two functioning wholes, so that a part-self acts as an entire self. An Auschwitz doctor could, through doubling, not only kill and contribute to killing but organize silently, on behalf of that evil project, an entire self-structure (or self-process) encompassing virtually all aspects of his behavior.[61]

Whether 'doubling,' or becoming indifferent to the value of human life, is an inevitable consequence of physicians performing active euthanasia in response to patients' requests is an empirical question, one that can only be answered by observation and experience.

Similarly, a parallel slope envisaging a slide from physicians performing voluntary euthanasia to engaging in involuntary euthanasia requires empirical support. Indeed, some critics of the practice in the Netherlands claim that already there are numerous instances of involuntary euthanasia, and more will no doubt follow, despite the strict safeguards designed to permit only voluntary euthanasia with terminally ill patients.

Anyone who tentatively accepts the ethical permissibility of voluntary, active euthanasia would almost certainly reject its incorporation into social policy if it became evident that any of these predictions about the slippery slope were beginning to be realized. Some actions might be morally right in an ideal world, but should be ruled out in the real world, given human fallibility and other practical deterrents to attaining the ideal.

THE MOST DANGEROUS SLOPE

Critics of today's practices contend that what is afoot is at least the inception of a programmatic effort to terminate the lives of some patients. Kronberg refers to the 'modern Euthanasia Movement,' claiming that it 'is scarcely

---

[60] Weisbard and Siegler, *On Killing Patients*, 218, 219.
[61] Lifton, *The Nazi Doctors*, 418.

different from its Nazi predecessor.'[62] Neuhaus refers to 'the eugenics project,'[63] which he takes to include cessation of life-sustaining treatment. More
circumspect and less polemical critics, such as Weisbard and Siegler, assert
that the '"death with dignity" movement has now advanced to a new
frontier: the termination or withdrawal of fluids and nutritional support.'[64]

Whether today's medical practices regarding termination of treatment are
referred to as a 'project' or 'movement,' or described in morally neutral
terms, numerous writers remind us that the Holocaust did not begin with a
'euthanasia program.' Not only did it start from 'small beginnings;' it was
preceded by a period in which resources were scarce, when 'there was a
temptation to adopt a narrowly materialistic perspective for the establishment of priorities and to seek savings through shortcuts at the expense of
those who were weak and less able to defend themselves.'[65] It is just such
considerations that lead to worries about where we are headed today.

Without specific reference to Nazi practices, that worry is voiced by Leslie
Steven Rothenberg, one of the contributors to the Hastings Center's Project
on Termination of Treatment Guidelines. Rothenberg writes:

> The ethical distinction between 'terminating treatment' and 'terminating life'
> (whether called active euthanasia, mercy killing, assisted suicide, or 'medical killing')
> may be more important to me than to others, particularly because the health care
> system is preoccupied with cost containment and because society undervalues persons
> with disabilities (including those that accompany advanced age).[66]

For these reasons, Rothenberg dissents from several sections of the *Guidelines*. He expresses the fear that the *Guidelines* 'may be used to give a moral
"imprimatur" to undertreating or failing to treat persons with disabilities,
unconscious persons for whom accurate prognoses are not yet obtainable,
elderly patients with severe dementia, and others whose treatment is not
believed . . . "costworthy." '[67]

Withholding or withdrawing life-sustaining therapy from patients whose
continued treatment is not 'costworthy' bears a much greater similarity to
the Nazi euthanasia program than does the current practice of active euthanasia in the Netherlands. The 'costworthy' rationale also bears a greater
similarity to the Nazis' purpose than does the current practice of complying
with patients' requests to forgo life supports or following their advance directives regarding medical treatment once they have lost decisional capacity.

---

[62] Kronberg, in Spannaus (ed.), *How to Stop the Resurgence of Nazi Euthanasia Today*, 129.
[63] Neuhaus, 'The Return of Eugenics', 20 and passim.
[64] Weisbard and Siegler, *On Killing Patients*, 215.
[65] Noakes and Pridham (eds.), *Nazism*, 1001.
[66] L. S. Rothenberg, *Guidelines on the Termination of Life-Sustaining Treatment and Care of the Dying* (Briarcliff Manor, NY: The Hastings Center, 1987) App. 158.
[67] Ibid.

A careful reading of the Hastings Center's *Guidelines on the Termination of Life-Sustaining Treatment* reveals a good deal of caution. There is an admonition 'to avoid discriminating against the critically ill and dying, to shun invidious comparisons of the economic value of various individuals to society, and to refuse to abandon patients and hasten death to save money.'[68] There is a concerted effort in the section entitled 'The Use of Economic Considerations in Decisions concerning Life-Sustaining Treatments' to retain a patient-centered ethic in medicine.[69]

Yet despite these cautions and concerns, the *Guidelines* acknowledge the relevance and importance of considerations of costworthiness. One statement begins with the prohibition: 'The health care professional caring for an individual patient should *not* be involved in cutting costs or rationing scarce resources at the bedside for the benefit of society,' yet ends with the proviso: 'unless it is in accordance with institutional or governmental policy.'[70]

This brings us back to the case with which we began—the family of Holocaust survivors who were unwilling to reduce the level of care being provided. The patient's physician did not want to be the one to ration resources at the bedside. There was no institutional policy in place. One ethics committee member questioned whether the hospital ought to have such a policy, making it easier for physicians to tell patients or families that an official policy required care to be withdrawn. The Hastings Center's *Guidelines* state that 'when such policies have been developed according to procedures and standards that are reasonable and just by government or by institutions, it is ethically justifiable for health care professionals to follow such policies and to refuse to provide this treatment.'[71]

In this case, the physician did continue to provide treatment and the patient lived for another seven months, though she never awakened to recognize her family or interact with her environment. Despite the pressure exercised by hospital administration, it is the physicians, not the administration, who retain final authority in patient management decisions in that hospital.

Whether it is accurate to call reducing the level of care for this patient 'euthanasia' is not the moral issue. Terminating treatment would not count as 'euthanasia' according to several of the definitions discussed earlier, but might fit other definitions. It is ironic to note that on one account, it would not count as euthanasia but would fit the description of the Nazi program: '[T]he decision to terminate the life of a patient under the Nazi programme was taken not by the individual concerned or by his or her relatives but by an official body . . . [T]he criterion . . . was not the welfare of the individual

---

[68] Ibid. 120.   [69] Ibid. 118–126.   [70] Ibid. 120.   [71] Ibid. 126.

patient but whether or not the patient's life was judged to be of 'value' or 'worth' . . . to the community.'[72]

Some find the possibility of allowing active euthanasia—even the voluntary kind—to be the most worrisome prospect. Others fear that from an ethical standpoint, the most dangerous practice is withdrawing or withholding treatment involuntarily, that is, from patients who lack decisional capacity. I maintain that a far greater danger lies in the use of an economic rationale.

When the justification offered for terminating treatment is that it is not 'costworthy,' or that it is consuming a disproportionate amount of society's or an institution's resources, the slide down one of the slopes to the Nazi program has already started. As one scholar has observed, 'the argument for the destruction of life not worth living was at root an economic one.'[73]

This is not to overlook the salient fact that racial ideology was a driving force behind Nazi policies. Is our society so free of racism that we are in no danger of sliding down that slope, as well? I think that danger may lurk in the background, but it is likely to arise in an indirect fashion, rather than directly. Although racial prejudice in our society undeniably exists, it does not assume the proportions of an ideology except in the case of fringe sects and fanatic groups. However, since disproportionate numbers of the poor are members of racial or ethnic minorities, a *de facto* pattern of discrimination can be detected.

The pressure to ration health care or to deny access to the health care system to certain members of society is greatest when tax dollars are used to fund services for the poor or indigent. A case in point is refusal by the federal government and a number of states to allow the use of public funds to finance abortions. To the extent that this pattern of health care spending continues, the poor, largely a minority population, are likely to be more negatively affected by schemes to limit the use of life-prolonging measures. Even when government-supported programs pay for all who are in need of a medical treatment, as in the case of end-stage renal disease, it is striking that many more whites receive these life-preserving therapies than do blacks and other minorities.

I do not suggest that efforts cannot be made to halt a slide that has begun. But when a society regularly and systematically confuses economics with ethics, and uses cost-benefit analysis as its only tool in forging health policy, it will fail to recognize the most dangerous slope of all.

---

[72] Noakes and Pridham (eds.), *Nazism*, 997.
[73] Proctor, *Racial Hygiene*, 183.

6

ADVANCE DIRECTIVES AND THE PERSONAL IDENTITY PROBLEM

ALLEN BUCHANAN

THE VALUE OF ADVANCE DIRECTIVES

Recent years have seen a marked increase in the use of and enthusiasm for advance directives for medical care. Perhaps the most familiar type of advance directive is the living will, a document whereby a person when competent issues more or less specific instructions as to which forms of care or treatment she wishes to have or not to have under certain circumstances, when she is no longer competent to decide. The other main type of advance directive, usually called a durable power of attorney, is the designation of a proxy, a trusted individual or committee of individuals who are to make decisions for a person after she becomes incompetent. It is possible to combine the two: a person may designate a proxy but also lay down instructions that place limits on the proxy's discretion to decide.

What is the value of advance directives—or, more precisely, what values are they supposed to serve? Either of two answers is usually given. First, advance directives are said to protect us from unwanted, virtually futile medical interventions that at best may prolong a miserable or meaningless existence. Second, some contend that advance directives are valuable because they allow self-determination, which is said to be valuable for its own sake. These answers, though correct as far as they go, are seriously incomplete. Indeed, they give a foreshortened picture not only of the value of advance directives, but also of the moral life.

In addition to protecting its author from unproductive bodily invasions and allowing her to exercise self-determination, an advance directive can allow her to relieve emotional and financial burdens that would otherwise fall on others. By issuing an appropriate advance directive one can *do good to*

From Allen Buchanan, 'Advance Directives and the Personal Identity Problem,' *Philosophy & Public Affairs*, 17/4 (1988), 277–302.

I am grateful to Dan W. Brock, Joel Feinberg, Deborah Mathiu, and Daniel I. Wikler for helpful comments on an earlier version of this article.

others.[1] Viewing advance directives in this broader way can be liberating. Instead of being seen simply as devices for protecting the patient or for exercising autonomy for its own sake, they might in addition become, vehicles for *new forms of altruism*, new ways of exercising the virtue of charity. For example, instead of specifying that if one comes to be in a persistent vegetative state all means of life support are to be withdrawn, a person with a strong sense of social obligation might instead request to be sustained in such a condition until his organs and other transplantable tissues are needed to save or enhance the lives of others. For several reasons, then, advance directives are of great potential value. Nevertheless, serious objections can be raised against their use, as we shall see.

THE MORAL AUTHORITY OF ADVANCE DIRECTIVES

Those who have shown unreserved enthusiasm for the use of advance directives have perhaps made the following assumption: if, as the courts and most bioethicists now agree, the competent individual has a virtually unlimited right to refuse treatment, even life-sustaining treatment, then the same choice ought to be respected when a competent individual makes it concerning a future decision situation through the use of an advance directive.

I have argued elsewhere that this assumption is dubious because it overlooks several morally significant asymmetries between the contemporaneous choice of a competent individual and the issuance of an advance directive to cover future decisions.[2] For example, even if at the time an advance directive was issued an individual was well informed about the options available should she develop a particular disease or be in a certain condition,

---

[1] For a person who takes a direct interest in the well-being of others who will be affected by what is done to her after she becomes incompetent, an advance directive can make a significant contribution to its author's own good in two ways. First, the issuance of an advance directive can contribute to its author's well-being *while she remains competent* by reducing her anxiety about the distress her loved ones would experience in making difficult decisions without her guidance, and by assuring her that they will not be subject to crushing and wasted financial costs. Second, there is a sense in which our interest can survive us. I have an interest in how my family will fare after my death, and that interest survives me in the sense that whether or not it is satisfied will depend upon events that occur after I am gone. An advance directive can help me ensure that my 'surviving interests' are satisfied. To the extent that one's well-being, or at least the goodness or success of one's life, depends on how one's interests in general fare—including one's surviving interests—an advance directive can make an important contribution to it.

[2] Allen Buchanan, with Dan W. Brock and Michael G. Gilfix. *Surrogate Decision-Making for Elderly Individuals who are Incompetent or of Questionable Competence*, report prepared for the Office of Technology Assessment, U.S. Congress (1986), ch. 3. See also Allen Buchanan and Dan W. Brock. 'Deciding for Others.' *Milbank Quarterly*, 64, suppl. 2 (1986), 17–94.

therapeutic options and hence prognosis may change between the time the directive was issued and the time at which it is to be implemented. A second morally relevant difference is that the assumption that a competent person is the best judge of her own interests is weakened in the case of a choice about future contingencies under conditions in which those interests have changed in radical and unforeseen ways.

A third and equally significant asymmetry is that important informal safeguards that tend to restrain imprudent or unreasonable contemporaneous choices are not likely to be present, or if present, to be as effective, in the case of an advance directive. If a competent patient refuses life-sustaining treatment, those responsible for her care can and often do urge the patient to reconsider her choice, and in some cases this can prevent a precipitous and disastrous decision. This safeguard, if it occurs at all, is unlikely to come into play as forcefully during the process of drawing up an advance directive. For when the decision to forgo life-sustaining treatment is a remote and abstract possibility it is less likely to elicit the same protective responses that are provoked in family members and health care professionals when they are actually confronted with a human being who they believe can lead a meaningful life but who chooses to die.

Once these three asymmetries are appreciated, it should be clear that even if the competent patient has a virtually unlimited right to refuse life-sustaining treatment, it does not immediately follow that a refusal of life-support ought always to be respected if it is expressed in an advance directive. After more complex argumentation, however, we might well conclude that in spite of these asymmetries the law ought to regard valid advance directives as having the same force as a competent patient's contemporaneous choice. For we might be persuaded that attempts to limit the authority of advance directives would in practice lead to their being ignored by paternalistic physicians or families, thus robbing them of their value. The well-documented persistence of unjustified paternalistic behavior by physicians indicates that this is a significant danger.[3]

LOSS OF PERSONAL IDENTITY

There is, however, a much more profound and potentially grave threat to the moral authority of advance directives which remains even if we conclude

---

[3] Allen Buchanam, 'Medical Paternalism,' in Rolf E. Sartorious (ed.) *Paternalism* (Minneapolis: University of Minnesota Press, 1983), 61–81; Buchanan, Brock, and Gilfix, *Surrogate Decision-Making for Elderly individuals*, ch. 3; Charles W. Lidz *et al.*, *Informed Consent* (London: Guilford Press, 1984), esp. 8–9.

that, all things considered, the asymmetries cited above do not provide sufficient grounds for limiting that authority. This is the objection that the very process that renders the individual incompetent and brings the advance directive into play can—and indeed often does—destroy the conditions necessary for her personal identity and thereby undercut entirely the moral authority of the directive.

This challenge rests upon the assumption that whatever the correct theory of personal identity turns out to be, it will include the claim that psychological continuity is (at least) a *necessary condition* for personal identity. In what follows I will accept this assumption for the sake of argument. Though I believe it can be adequately defended, I shall not attempt to do so here. I think it is also fair to say that this view about personal identity is already so widely held and well supported in the philosophical literature that the threat it appears to pose to advance directives ought to be taken seriously.[4]

The notion of psychological continuity, of course, is inherently vague, since the continuity between mental states (including memories, affective states, and dispositions) admits of degrees. Thus the question arises: just how 'close' must various types of interconnections among such states and dispositions be to support an ascription of psychological continuity?

Nevertheless, the fact that there is a twilight does not show that we can not distinguish between noon and midnight. There are some cases in which human beings suffer permanent neurological damage so severe that psychological continuity is utterly destroyed—cases in which there is no psychological continuity regardless of how low we set the standard of continuity necessary for the preservation of personal identity. This is so because some neurological damage causes the permanent extinction of all psychological properties and states, while stopping just short of the point at which (according to the whole-brain or brain death criterion) the individual ceases to live.[5] An individual who is in a 'persistent vegetative state,' an irreversible deep coma, fits this description, as do infants born with no cerebral cortex (anencephalics). In such cases the being has no psychological states or properties, only 'vegetative,' that is, autonomic, ones. For present purposes, such cases are wholly unproblematic, because on the conception of personal identity

---

[4] For an influential recent discussion of the psychological continuity view see Derek Parfit, *Reasons and Persons* (New York: Oxford University Press, 1986), 204–9. See also H. P. Grice, 'Personal Identity,' in John Perry (ed.), *Personal Identity* (Los Angeles and Berkeley: University of California Press, 1975), 73–95.

[5] For a detailed explanation of the whole-brain death criterion, according to which death occurs when there is a permanent cessation of all functioning throughout the brain (including lower and higher brain centers), see *Defining Death*, Report of the President's Commission for the Study of Ethical Problems in Medicine and Biomedical and Behavioral Research (Washington, DC: US Government Printing Office, 1981).

we are investigating, which I shall call the psychological continuity view, such patients have without question suffered a loss of personal identity. Difficulties arise, however, when irreversible neurological damage falls short of permanent unconsciousness but is nonetheless so severe as to call into question the persistence of enough psychological continuity to preserve personal identity.

The most troubling sort of case might seem to be the following: advanced Alzheimer's dementia has resulted in such extensive, permanent neurological damage that the patient's memory has been destroyed, his cognitive processes have been virtually obliterated, and all that remains is basic perceptual awareness. Unlike the persistently vegetative patient, the profoundly demented Alzheimer's patient can see and hear or at least has visual and auditory sensations (though this is not to say that he can distinguish conceptually and label appropriately what he sees and hears). In addition, the patient in question (again, unlike the permanently unconscious patient) is capable of pain and even of physical pleasure, though of fleeting and rudimentary sorts.[6]

Such cases have seemed to some to rob advance directives of their moral authority.[7] Their argument may be reconstructed as follows:

(i) One person's advance directive has no moral authority to determine what is to happen to *another person*.

(ii) In some cases of severe and permanent neurological damage, for example, that due to advanced Alzheimer's dementia, psychological continuity is so disrupted that the person who issued the advance directive no longer exists.[8]

Therefore

(iii) In such cases the advance directive has no moral authority to determine what is to happen to the individual who remains after neurological damage has destroyed the person who issued the advance directive.

Let us call this the slavery argument, since it portrays advance directives, not

[6] Office of Technology Assessment, US Congress, *Losing a Million Minds: Confronting the Tragedy of Alzheimer's Disease and Other Dementias* (Washington, DC: US Government Printing Office, 1987), 68–83. This chapter also contains a bibliography on Alzheimer's disease.

[7] Rebecca Dresser, 'Life, Death, and Incompetent Patients: Conceptual Infirmities and Hidden Values in the Law,' *Arizona Law Review*, 28/3 (1986), 379–81.

[8] Premise (ii) in the slavery argument is *not* offered as a claim about which individuals *the law* presently considers to be persons. Instead, the argument is intended to express a severe limitation on the *moral* authority of advance directives, a limitation which the law, if it is to be morally sensitive, *ought* to recognize.

as vehicles for self-determination, but as sinister devices to subjugate other persons.

The slavery argument, however, is invalid—conclusion (iii) does not follow from the conjunction of premises (i) and (ii). To make it valid, another premise must be added:

(ii′) The individual who remains after neurological damage has destroyed the person who issued the advance directive is a (different) *person*.

Although the addition of premise (ii′) renders the argument valid, it also makes it vulnerable to the charge that it is unsound, because the truth of premise (ii′) can be challenged.

The key to appreciating the force of this challenge is to understand what sort of judgment we are making when we judge that the psychological continuity necessary for personal identity no longer exists. Psychological continuity, as we have already noted, admits of degrees, just as the decision-making capacities that constitute competence are a matter of degree.[9] Further, just as *where* we set the threshold for competence is a matter of choice, not a decision uniquely determined by the facts of the case, so also a choice must be made as to what degree of psychological continuity we will regard as necessary for personal identity and how much diminution of psychological continuity we will regard as the destruction of the person. As with the threshold of decision-making capacity for competence, however, our choice of a degree of psychological continuity necessary for preservation of the person (or a degree of psychological discontinuity sufficient for the loss of personal identity) need not be *arbitrary*. There may be sufficient reasons for setting the threshold at one level rather than another, just as there are sufficient reasons for setting the threshold of decision-making capacities required for competence at one level rather than another.[10]

[9] *Making Health Care Decisions*, Report of the President's Commission for the Study of Ethical Problems in Medicine and Biomedical and Behavioral Research (Washington, DC: US Government Printing Office, 1982), 55–62. For a more detailed analysis of competence, see Buchanan, Brock, and Gilfix, *Surrogate Decision-Making for Elderly Individuals*, ch. 2.

[10] In particular, it can be argued that, other things being equal, the greater the risk and the more complex the information that a reasonable person would want to take into account in making a given decision, the higher the level of decision-making capacities the individual should have in order to be considered competent to make the decision. See Buchanan, Brock, and Gilfix, *Surrogate Decision-Making for Elderly Individuals*, ch. 2.

HOW MUCH PSYCHOLOGICAL CONTINUITY IS ENOUGH?

It must be emphasized that the psychological continuity view does not itself answer the question 'Just how much psychological continuity is necessary for the preservation of personal identity?' If the degree of psychological continuity necessary for preservation of personal identity is set rather *low* or, conversely, if the degree of diminution of psychological continuity compatible with the preservation of personal identity is set rather *high*, then *there will be very few if any real-world cases in which we would be justified in concluding that neurological damage has destroyed one person but left a living, different person.* For reasons that will soon become clear, a conception which sets the level of psychological continuity necessary for personal identity rather low may be called a *conservative* criterion of personal identity.

The crucial point is this: if we adopt a conservative (low threshold) criterion of psychological continuity, then those cases in which we can confidently conclude that the person, Jones, has ceased to exist (because neurological damage has so severely diminished psychological continuity) will be cases in which neurological damage is so catastrophic that we would be equally confident in concluding that the living being who remains is *not a person at all* and hence, *a fortiori*, not a *different* person, Jones II.

Although there is dispute about precisely which properties are jointly necessary and sufficient for personhood, there is considerable consensus in the philosophical literature as to what at least some of the necessary conditions are.[11] The following cognitive capacities are among the strongest candidates for necessary conditions:

(*a*) The ability to be conscious of oneself as existing over time—as having a past and a future, as well as a present;

(*b*) the ability to appreciate reasons for or against acting; being (sometimes) able to inhibit impulses or inclinations when one judges that it would be better not to act on them;

(*c*) the ability to engage in purposive sequences of actions.

If any of these three, or anything even roughly similar to any of them, is at least a necessary condition of being a person, then it appears that the profoundly demented patient described above is not a person. It must be emphasized, however, that lack of personhood does not imply lack of moral

[11] Joel Feinberg, 'The Problem of Personhood,' in Tom L. Beauchamp and LeRoy Walters, (eds.), *Contemporary Issues in Bioethics*, 2nd edn. (Belmont, Calif.: Wadsworth, 1982), 108–16, and Mary Ann Warren, 'On the Moral and Legal Status of Abortion,' in ibid. 25–60.

status altogether. The very fact that a being can experience pleasure and pain may itself impose significant limitations on how we may act toward it.

It might be objected that this reasoning is flawed by an equivocation on 'person', because that term, as it occurs in debates about personal identity, embodies a *metaphysical* concept of persons, while the term 'person' is used in a *moral* sense when it is said that features (a)–(c) are necessary conditions for being a person. Thus even though the living being that remains after neurological damage produces a drastic diminution of psychological continuity may not be a person in the moral sense, it does not follow that that being is not a person in the metaphysical sense, and hence that he is not a different person who issued the advance directive. And if he is a different person, then the advance directive of another person has no moral authority concerning how he is to be treated.

There are two difficulties with this objection. The first is that it rests on the very dubious assumption that a metaphysical and a moral sense of 'person', or a metaphysical and a moral concept of person, can be neatly distinguished. The fact that philosophers typically appeal to our intuitions about responsibilities and commitments—that is, to basic *moral* concepts—in order to support their metaphysical theses about the criterion of identity for persons casts serious doubt on this assumption. Second, and more important, unless the concept of a person implicated in the psychological continuity view is in some sense the concept of *moral* personality, it is difficult to see why showing that psychological continuity has not been so severely diminished as to result in a loss of personal identity would establish that an advance directive still has moral authority. In other words, if the concept of a person implicated in the psychological continuity view is a purely metaphysical, nonmoral concept, then it is hard to understand why certain marks on paper made by a person in *this* (metaphysical) sense should *ever* be thought to create obligations or confer authority, since obligations can be created and authority conferred only by persons in the moral sense.

Indeed, it is not surprising that it is difficult, if not impossible, to distinguish a purely metaphysical, nonmoral sense of 'person', at least if we are looking for a criterion of personal identity that articulates or builds upon our ordinary, pretheoretical concept of personal identity. For surely our ordinary judgments typically, if not exclusively, are motivated by moral concerns—in particular, the ascription of responsibility, the recognition of rights and obligations, and the acknowledgment of commitments.

I suggested earlier that if the degree of psychological continuity necessary for the preservation of personal identity is set rather low, the cases in which we should be most confident in declaring that neurological damage has destroyed personal identity (without causing death) will *not* be cases in which we would judge that one person (Jones) is replaced by another person (Jones II). Instead, they will be cases like that of the profoundly and permanently demented individual with Alzheimer's dementia, where neurological damage has destroyed a person, and all that survives is a terminally ill nonperson with what we may call radically truncated interests. If this is so, then we will not be faced with a choice between implementing a formerly existing person's advance directive and protecting the rights and interests of another person who will be harmed, indeed destroyed, if the first person's advance directive is implemented. Instead, our task will be that of deciding whether following a formerly existing person's instructions is compatible with discharging whatever obligations we may have toward a living being whose existence will probably be brief no matter what we do and whose mental capacities are much less sophisticated than those of a small child or of a nonhuman animal such as a dog, and who virtually always suffers debilitating and painful physical ailments as well.[12] Should we follow the advance directive and terminate support for the surviving individual, or should we ignore the advance directive (now that its author has ceased to exist) and attend only to the interests of the surviving individual?

The nature of the surviving being's interests provides an answer to this question. These consist solely in the interest in avoiding pain and the interest in having whatever fleeting, fragmentary, and unanticipated experiences of simple physical pleasure his or her damaged nervous system still allows. The crucial point is that our obligations to such a being are at best quite limited because of the radically truncated character of its interests. In the case of those 'primitive' species of nonhuman animals who have such radically truncated interests, it is hardly controversial to conclude that our obligation is simply the negative one of not inflicting suffering (or that at most we are obligated to give them pleasure if we can do so at little cost to ourselves and without compromising the interests of other beings with more robust interests).[13]

It is tempting to believe that in such a case there is no moral conflict at all—no question of weighing the authority of the advance directive against the interests of the surviving being. For if the person who issued the advance directive no longer exists, then it would appear that her advance directive would be wholly irrelevant to the question of how we may treat this other

[12] Office of Technology Assessment, *Losing a Million Minds*, 77–8.
[13] The fact that a profoundly and permanently demented Alzheimer's patient is a *human being* with radically truncated interests certainly makes a difference to most of us, psychologically speaking. Our greater sense of identification with members of our own species, unbolstered by any arguments of principle, may even be sufficient to justify behaving differently toward human beings with truncated interests simply because they are human beings, if we *choose* to do so. But none of this shows that we have robust, positive *obligations* toward them.

individual. According to this line of thought, there is no conflict because the advance directive becomes *inapplicable*—null and void—with the extinction of its author. The advance directive exerts no moral pull whatsoever; all that is morally relevant is whatever moral status accrues to the (radically truncated) interests of the surviving individual.

This conclusion, however, will not stand scrutiny. A person who issues an advance directive may do so not only to exercise control over what happens to her*self* after she becomes incompetent, but also to protect certain interests she has in what happens to her body after she, the particular person who she is, no longer exists.

Persons often have interests that survive them. Most persons, for example, have an interest in the well-being, both financial and personal, of their loved ones, and many have an interest in how their mortal remains are treated. These are 'surviving interests' in the sense that whether they are satisfied or thwarted depends upon events that occur or do not occur after the person no longer exists.

Suppose that you have issued an advance directive including the instruction that if you become permanently and profoundly demented—that is, if you are 'succeeded' by a terminally ill nonperson with truncated interests—all life-support efforts are to be withdrawn. Presumably you have a legitimate interest in what happens to your living remains under these circumstances, just as you have a legitimate interest in what happens to your body after you are pronounced dead. Your advance directive is a tool for protecting that interest.

Your interest in not having your remains sustained by life-support systems may be based on your notion of personal dignity or fittingness, or it may be based on your commitment to avoiding what you believe to be unjustifiable burdens on your family or on society. Part of what makes advance directives so attractive to many people is that they can serve as a device for securing such surviving interests.

Just as the interest in the treatment of one's corpse is a legitimate interest of persons, so is one's interest in what happens to one's living remains. We would be justified in thwarting the latter interest only if satisfying it required the thwarting of other, morally weightier interests. In the type of case under discussion, however, following an advance directive will not thwart morally weighty interests. Instead, it will only result in the earlier death of a severely physically debilitated, suffering, terminally ill being who possesses only radically truncated interests.

So the advance directive is applicable and does override whatever extremely limited obligations we may have to sustain the life of the surviving individual in such cases. The legitimate interest one has in determining what happens to one's living remains makes the advance directive applicable, even though the person who authored it no longer exists. And in the absence of countervailing weighty moral interests that would speak in favor of sustaining those living remains, we should acknowledge the legitimacy of the person's interest by following the advance directive.

The preceding argument establishes that *if* the degree of psychological continuity necessary for the preservation of personal identity is set very low, then three conclusions follow. First, adoption of the psychological continuity view of personal identity does *not* undercut the moral authority of advance directives because the slavery argument is invalid or, if modified to achieve validity, unsound. Even if the person who issued the advance directive no longer exists, it does not follow that following the advance directive is inflicting one person's will upon *another person*. Second, if the being that remains after neurological damage undercuts personal identity is not a person but a being with radically truncated interests, our obligations toward that being are quite limited. Following an advance directive to achieve a painless termination of life support for a being with such radically truncated interests need not involve the violation of any obligations toward that being. Third, whether neurological damage that results in the diminution of psychological continuity presents us with a choice between following one person's advance directive and preserving another person's life will depend upon the degree of psychological continuity required for the preservation of personal identity. If it is set quite low, such choices will only rarely, if ever, be necessary.

This is an important result. For if faced with such a choice we would have to disregard the advance directive. To do otherwise would be to give one person a wholly illegitimate, nonconsensual power of life and death over another person. So if the threshold for psychological continuity were set so high that loss of personal identity was a frequent occurrence, then the authority of advance directives would be frequently undercut. If the threshold is set low, however, the mere possibility of loss of personal identity will not threaten the legitimacy of advance directives. However, nothing said so far supports the further claim that the degree of psychological continuity *ought* to be set so low.

ATTEMPTS TO RAISE THE THRESHOLD

Indeed, some proponents of the psychological continuity view have adduced hypothetical examples calculated to convince us that we do or should set the threshold rather high—or, conversely, that we do or should regard some disruptions of psychological continuity far less drastic than those wrought by advanced Alzheimer's dementia as constituting a loss of personal identity.[14] The two examples that follow have been used to support the high threshold (that is, radical as opposed to conservative) view in the following fashion. First, those who offer them surmise that most thoughtful and morally discerning people would respond to the cases in a certain way. Then they suggest that the explanation, or at least the best explanation, of these moral responses, or at least the best way to render them principled and consistent, is to acknowledge a concept of personal identity that sets the threshold of psychological continuity necessary for persistence of personal identity quite high.

The first case is that of a young nineteenth-century Russian nobleman who is, he sincerely professes, committed to socialist ideals. Since he knows that later in life he will inherit vast wealth and may be tempted to abandon his socialist ideals, he extracts a promise from his young wife. If, after he inherits the fortune, he attempts to renege on his commitments to redistributing it to the poor (freeing his serfs, and so on), she is to prevent him from doing so. Those who employ this example first conclude that we think it proper for the woman to resist her middle-aged husband's attempts to keep the wealth for himself or that at the very least we recognize that she faces a serious conflict of moral obligations.[15] This first conclusion seems unexceptionable. However, those who employ the example go on to contend that this moral assessment presupposes or at least is best explained by the judgment that we regard the young nobleman and the middle-aged husband as *different persons*.

This latter conclusion, however, is as unconvincing as it is gratuitous. To understand the wife's predicament we need only recognize that the obligations a person acquires through a promise made to another can sometimes conflict with other obligations she has toward *him*, and that a person may find it advisable to use a promise extracted from another to prevent *himself* in the future from abandoning his current commitments.

This is not to say that the wife would or should choose to honor the promissory obligation at the price of other values or obligations. She might, for example, conclude that her youthful husband had been deluded, brainwashed by leftist friends, and that his commitment had been formed under duress or at a time when he lacked competence to make it. (Similarly, we might conclude that a particular advance directive for medical treatment was

[14] Donald Regan, 'Paternalism, Freedom, Identity, and Commitment,' in Sartorious (ed.), *Paternalism*, 113–38.
[15] Derek Parfit, 'Later Selves and Moral Principles,' in A. Montefiore (ed.), *Philosophy and Personal Relations* (London: Routledge & Kegan Paul, 1973).

invalid because issued under duress and hence fails to confer authority or create obligations.) If, on the other hand, the wife believed that her youthful husband's commitment to socialist ideals and his decision to ask her to make the promise were ones he was competent to make and were substantially voluntary, then she might conclude, with justification, that she should resist his current pleas. Clearly, one obvious condition for being released from a promise does not apply here; the wife cannot justify not acting on the promise on the grounds that the promisee failed to foresee the current situation and would not have wished the promise to be carried out in it. His whole point in asking her to make the promise, rather, is that he did foresee that he would be tempted to abandon his ideals.

Moreover, if we were to take literally the proposal that the man who extracted the promise no longer exists, we would get a dissolution, not an explanation, of the wife's serious *moral* conflict. For now her current husband is simply making the outrageous and immoral claim that he is entitled to her former husband's property. Though the 'widow' may, for prudential reasons or out of love for her second husband, *prefer* to misuse the money her first husband entrusted to her, she can view this a conflict of *moral obligations* only if she is either confused or self-deceiving. In sum, the first example does nothing to support the claim that the threshold of psychological continuity either is or should be set so high as to wreak havoc with the moral authority of advance directives.

The second example is no more persuasive. It concerns an elderly saintly man who is for good reason awarded the Nobel Peace Prize. After the prize is awarded it comes to light that some sixty years earlier a very young man— who not only bore the same name as the Nobel laureate, but also had a body and brain identical with those of the laureate—ferociously attacked and injured a policeman in a brawl.[16] Purveyors of this example contend that it supports their claim that we do or at least should conclude that the young rowdy and the saintly laureate are different persons, that the links of psychological continuity stretching from the former to the latter are sufficiently tenuous as to fall short of the appropriate degree of continuity necessary for the persistence of a single person.

This conclusion, as in the Russian nobleman case, is supposed to provide an explanation, or the best explanation, of our moral responses to the case. Presumably the relevant moral response would be an unwillingness to punish the saintly elderly laureate for the crime of the rowdy youth. But it should be obvious that there is another way of explaining this response that is at least equally plausible as an explanation and that does not require us to

---

[16] Parfit, *Reasons and Persons*, 326.

embrace the radical conclusion that the young man and the laureate are different persons.

We may, instead, conclude that *mercy*—which presupposes guilt and hence the preservation of identity—is appropriate in this case, for several reasons. First, in this case punishment would not serve at least two of the goals that are usually thought to justify it: it could neither *reform* the person on whom it would be inflicted (since he has already not only reformed himself, but become saintly), nor *deter* or *prevent* him from committing further crimes (since he is not now the sort of person who will ever commit any crime). Second, to the extent that we think of the criminal as having incurred through his crime a 'debt to society,' we may decide not to punish him because we believe that through the extraordinary efforts that earned him the Nobel Peace Prize the laureate has more than discharged that debt.

It might be objected that even if his debt to *society* has been discharged, the crime the young man committed wronged a *particular person*, the policeman, and that *this* debt has neither been paid to nor forgiven by that individual. To show mercy would be to fail to appreciate the nature of the criminal act—the fact that it was the wronging of a particular person. Consequently, the objection goes, we cannot explain the judgment that the laureate should not be punished by saying that it is an appropriate exercise of mercy. Instead, we can explain our judgment that he should not be punished—or at least justify it—only on the assumption that the laureate and the youth are different persons.

This objection contains a grain of truth, but it is nonetheless spurious. All it establishes is that showing mercy by not punishing the laureate is one thing, while deciding not to require him to render compensation for his wrong to the policeman is another. If, as seems appropriate, we view the offense as both a public and a private wrong, *we* may show mercy for the former, while acknowledging that it is up to the *victim* whether to forgive the latter.

Suppose the policeman has remained seriously incapacitated and wracked with pain since the injury. To the extent that we feel that the laureate owes him compensation, this belief *supports* the conclusion that the youth and the laureate are the same person. And, as we have seen, our feeling that the laureate should not be punished does *not* presuppose that he and the youth are not one and the same person. So it seems that the second example, like the first, fails to provide solid support for the conclusion that we do or should set the threshold of psychological continuity necessary for the preservation of personal identity quite high. Therefore, neither of these examples supports the claim that there will be a significant number of cases in which neurological damage is severe enough to undercut the moral authority of an advance directive by destroying its author while leaving in his place another *person*.

It might also be argued that a healthy and reasonable conservatism weighs heavily in favor of setting the threshold of psychological continuity required for the persistence of personal identity rather low. Some of our most important social practices and institutions—those dealing with contracts, promises, civil and criminal liability, and the assignment of moral praise and blame—apparently presuppose a view of personal identity according to which a person can survive quite radical psychological changes and hence a high degree of psychological *discontinuity*. If this is so, then given the value of these practices and institutions, we would have to have extraordinarily weighty reasons for giving up the view of personal identity upon which they are founded. But as we have seen, examples like those of the Nobel laureate and the Russian nobleman do not supply such reasons, since our responses to them can be explained quite well without assuming loss of personal identity. Nor, it should be recalled, does adoption of the psychological continuity view itself commit us to setting the threshold lower (or higher) than our social practices and institutions presuppose. That view is simply neutral as to what degree of psychological continuity is required for the persistence of the person. It appears, then, that since the value of preserving some of our most basic institutions and practices speaks in favor of setting the threshold of psychological continuity necessary for personal identity low, and there is nothing of comparable weight on the other side of the balance, we clearly ought to set (or rather leave) the threshold low.

The issue may not be quite so clear-cut as this, however. Consider what would occur if a much higher threshold of psychological continuity were *consistently* employed so that our expectations would adapt to it. Ponder, in particular, how such a change would affect the practice of issuing advance directives and more generally our practices of caring for incompetents.

If people knew that the degree of psychological continuity considered necessary for the preservation of personal identity was rather high and if they were confident that there were reliable methods for ascertaining when such a degree of continuity had been lost, they would take this into account. I would know, for example, that after I became incompetent I might suffer sufficient neurological damage so that others would judge that *I* no longer existed, but without the damage (at least for a time) being so catastrophic that what remained was not a person at all. I would know that if this occurred, I would be declared dead and my will would be read. The declaration of my death would have definite and predictable social, moral, and legal implications: my family would no longer be responsible (morally or legally) for the care of the different person who remained after I ceased to exist. Nor, presumably, would they have any special standing in decisions concerning the treatment or nontreatment of that person.

What I am suggesting is that it is a mistake simply to assume that a significant raising of the threshold of psychological continuity necessary for the preservation of personal identity would be incompatible with some of our most valuable social practices and institutions. It is also a mistake to assume that such a shift would undermine the practice of issuing advance directives. Instead, what might occur would be a revision of those institutions and practices and a narrowing of the scope of the authority of advance directives. There would be no conflict between honoring one person's advance directive and preserving the life of the different person who succeeded him because the authority of the advance directive would be understood by all concerned to begin with the onset of incompetence and to terminate with the loss of personal identity.

Nevertheless, it is worth contemplating what the cost—both moral and financial—of such a shift would be. There would, of course, be *transition costs*. Greater or lesser degrees of confusion, lack of coordination, and anxiety might result, depending upon how the new conception of personal identity—along with the new legal definition of the death of a person it requires—is implemented. But even after the transition had been achieved there would be major social, legal, and moral problems to deal with. The new system would result in the 'births' of large numbers of 'new persons' who would as it were spring full-blown into the world and who would not, strictly speaking, be the sons, daughters, husbands, wives, or friends of anyone. Such 'new persons' would have no financial assets (or debts), nor would any individual or family be legally responsible for them. Of course, it might be possible to restructure our practices concerning family responsibility to include 'quasi obligations' of family members to the 'successor persons' of their deceased loved ones. Indeed we might fashion legal obligations of a limited sort and impute them to the 'predecessor person' himself. The price of setting the threshold for psychological continuity high is that doing so enormously complicates and magnifies the problem of intergenerational justice.

The strangeness and complexities of the arrangements needed to cope with the new problem of intergenerational justice—and the potential for conflicts of obligations they generate—numb the mind. I sketch them here only to emphasize that those who have advocated adopting a view of personal identity that significantly raises the threshold of psychological continuity necessary for the preservation of the person simply have not thought through the disturbing implications of their proposal. Even worse, as I have already argued, they have given us no good reasons for undertaking the

radical revision of our practices, institutions, and ways of thinking of ourselves and our relationships with one another that taking their proposal
seriously would require.

A COMPROMISE POSITION

I have argued that even if the psychological continuity view is accepted, it
does not follow that we should recognize a high threshold of psychological
continuity as necessary for personal identity. And from this it follows that we
have no reason to fear that the moral authority of advance directives will
dissolve with or soon after the onset of incompetence, thus rendering them
useless.

Even if I am correct in this, however, there is another thesis, held by Derek
Parfit, the most prominent proponent of the psychological continuity view,
which remains unscathed by my criticisms thus far. This is the claim that
since psychological continuity is a matter of degree, we should acknowledge
in our morality and social practices and institutions the implications of the
fact that personal identity is not an all-or-nothing affair, but rather a matter
of degree. In other words, the moral and social significance we attach to
personal identity should reflect the fact that being the same person is not an
either/or proposition, but a matter of more or less.

According to Parfit, not only philosophers but also ordinary people have
tended to assume that personal identity is or depends upon some deeper,
metaphysical fact. This, he believes, is a mistake. Psychological continuity is
all there is to personal identity. There is no deeper (or other) fact of the
matter. And the importance we attach to personal identity should reflect the
fact that there is no deeper fact.

I propose to understand this latter thesis as follows. In real-life situations,
the judgment that A is the same person as B typically has moral implications. Once we see that personal identity depends on psychological continuity (and not on any further or deeper fact) we should acknowledge that the
character and force of the judgment that A is the same person as B *vary* with
the degree of psychological continuity between the psychological states (or
psychological properties) of A and those of B. For example, we ordinarily
think that if A, the man we now see before us, is the same person as B, the
cold-blooded killer who assassinated the president a year ago, then A is
culpable for that killing. But, Parfit suggests, if personal identity depends
upon psychological continuity, then the lesser the degree of psychological
continuity, the lesser the culpability.

The application of this general thesis to the case of advance directives is straightforward. The greater the degree of psychological continuity between A, the competent person who issued the advance directive, and B, the (incompetent) individual whose body (and brain) are spatiotemporally continuous with A's, the greater the moral authority of the advance directive, that is, the more *weight* A's wishes, as expressed in the advance directive, should be accorded in determining what is to be done to or for B.

If taken at face value, this proposal does not represent a mere revision, even a radical revision, of our conception of personal identity. Rather, it is a proposal to do away with personal identity judgments as we ordinarily understand them and to replace them with judgments about differing degrees of psychological continuity and the differing moral weights that correspond to them. Once we accept the psychological continuity view, the thesis that psychological continuity is necessary for personal identity, along with the seemingly unexceptionable claim that psychological continuity is a matter of degree, the replacement of 'all-or-nothing' moral judgments (A is responsible or he is not, A's wishes should be dispositive or they should not count at all) with varying moral weight judgments may seem inescapable.

But this is not so. There are powerful pragmatic reasons for maintaining a social consensus according to which degrees of psychological continuity which meet or exceed a particular threshold are sufficient for an *unqualified* judgment of personal identity, a judgment which carries with it *maximal moral force*. And this is so even if the moral weights corresponding to degrees of psychological continuity below the threshold may vary, diminishing as the degree of psychological continuity decreases. Similarly, being a competent adult depends on a complex of skills and capacities, and the possession of these skills and capacities is always a matter of degree. Nevertheless, there may be decisive pragmatic reasons for recognizing a certain threshold of the relevant skills and capacities as necessary for maturity and for ascribing, in an *all-or-nothing* fashion, a distinctive social and legal status to persons whose skills and capacities fail to meet that threshold. So from the claim that the psychological continuity upon which personal identity depends is a matter of degree, it does *not* follow that personal identity judgments should be replaced by judgments about varying degrees of psychological continuity and corresponding moral judgments concerning the varying weights of rights and obligations.

What sorts of pragmatic considerations might count in favor of the social recognitions of a threshold of psychological continuity that might be used to make 'all-or-nothing' personal identity judgments? First of all, any other approach faces daunting epistemic obstacles. Attempts to make numerous fine-grained judgments about degrees of psychological continuity would require far richer data than we ordinarily have or could acquire, even with great cost and effort. The various moral weights to be assigned to interests, rights, or obligations on the basis of these judgments of psychological continuity would be correspondingly ill founded and unreliable. Second, even if these epistemic difficulties could be surmounted, tailoring the ascriptions of rights and responsibilities to reflect such fine-grained distinctions would require institutions whose constituent rules would be so complex as to preclude most if not all people from mastering them well enough to achieve a stable framework for legitimate expectations and the efficient social coordination that depends upon such a framework.

Again, an analogy may help. Being designated a mature person (or competent adult), as opposed to a minor, carries with it a fairly clear-cut bundle of legal rights and social privileges and responsibilities. Of course, it is theoretically possible to fragment this bundle, by distinguishing different rights and obligations (or giving the same rights and obligations different weights) and mapping them onto varying degrees of the several skills and capacities which together constitute maturity. But here, as in the case of attaching different moral weights to rights, obligations, or interests in such a way that the weights correspond to different degrees of psychological continuity, greater sensitivity may come at a prohibitive price—costly information gathering that results nonetheless in inaccurate judgments and inefficiently complex institutions.

One of the attractions of a system that designates thresholds as markers for ascriptions of status (such as that of competent adult) and assigns bundles of rights (and obligations) indiscriminately to all who enjoy the status in question is that it facilitates coordination by sharply limiting the number and sensitivity of judgments upon which people must agree if their expectations are to be sufficiently congruent. It has long been noted that the social recognition of rights minimizes the need for complex consequentialist reasoning (and the potential for disagreement, error, and lack of coordination which such reasoning carries with it). Indeed, the appeal to rights typically avoids consequentialist reasoning by declaring consequences to be irrelevant. Similarly the use of a threshold of psychological continuity in the making of personal identity judgments not only reduces the number of estimates of degrees of psychological continuity, it also simplifies the ascription of rights and obligations by bundling them together and avoids the problem of recognizing different weights for rights and obligations corresponding to different degrees of psychological continuity.

If, as I am suggesting, a strong pragmatic case can be made for singling out a threshold of psychological continuity for personal identity judgments, there is nevertheless a way in which the (alleged) fact that personal identity is *really* a matter of degree could still be accommodated. We might attach full moral force to the rights and obligations that we ascribe to those who clearly meet or exceed the socially recognized threshold, while attaching diminishing moral significance to those obligations and rights (or to the interests that the rights serve) as we move 'downward' from the threshold.

In the case of advance directives, this would amount to the following procedure. So long as the degree of psychological continuity which we take to be necessary for the preservation of personal identity is present, the advance directive has full moral authority. (Recall, however, my earlier argument that this 'full authority' may *not* be as robust as the authority of the competent patient's contemporaneous decision.) As we move 'downword' from this threshold, through lessening degrees of psychological continuity, the moral authority or force of the advance directive diminishes correspondingly. In other words, for cases that fall *below* the threshold—and only for those—the weaker the degree of psychological continuity, the more readily the advance directive may be overridden by competing moral considerations, including our concern for the well-being of the incompetent individual. Presumably a point is eventually reached at which the degree of psychological continuity between the author of the advance directive and the incompetent individual is so small that the advance directive of the former has no authority at all over the latter, at least if the incompetent individual can be said to have interests of any morally significant sort.

Thus even where diminution of psychological continuity is great enough to lead us to conclude that the incompetent individual is not the person who issued the advance directive, we might nevertheless conclude that there is enough psychological continuity to give the wishes expressed in the advance directive *some weight* in our decison concerning the treatment of the incompetent individual. This would amount to recognizing as morally significant the especially intimate relationship between these individuals while at the same time acknowledging that they are distinct individuals.

The virtue of the compromise view is that it acknowledges both the value of our current institutions and practices, which to a large extent do treat personal identity as an all-or-nothing affair, *and* the implications of the view that personal identity depends upon something, namely, psychological continuity, which admits of degrees.

That such a strategy is coherent is again made clear by the analogy used earlier. We can (1) admit that maturity (being a competent adult) depends upon skills and capacities that admit of degrees (and that there is no 'deeper fact' about maturity), (2) single out a threshold level of these skills and capacities as necessary for maturity, (3) ascribe a bundle of moral rights and obligations only to those who meet or exceed the threshold level, and (4) ascribe successively more restricted (less weighty, more easily overridden) rights and obligations to those who fall further and further below the threshold. Thus nascent obligations and rights (or morally considerable interests) would ripen as the individual moves toward the threshold of maturity.

CONCLUSIONS

The results of our investigation of the claim that a proper understanding of personal identity poses a serious challenge to the authority of advance directives can now be summarized. The thesis that psychological continuity is at least a necessary condition for personal identity is plausible and widely held. Yet on any reasonable interpretation of this thesis it is undeniable that there can be and indeed are some cases in which neurological damage results in loss of personal identity without being so complete as to result in death, as defined by the widely accepted whole-brain death criterion. Since those who are permanently unconscious have no *psychological* states or properties, there has been loss of personal identity in these cases, no matter how high or low we set the degree of psychological continuity necessary for the preservation of personal identity. Such cases pose no radical challenge to the moral authority of advance directives, however, because they are not cases in which following one (formerly existing) person's advance directive will end another, different person's life, since the permanently unconscious are not persons at all.

Nor do cases of profound and permanent dementia pose such a challenge, for in these cases neurological damage, though it falls short of permanent unconsciousness, destroys at least some of the necessary conditions for personhood. Here, too, as in the case of the permanently unconscious being, we are not faced with a choice between respecting the wishes of one (formerly existing) person and protecting the interests or rights of another person. There is this important difference, however: the profoundly demented individual, though not a person, is by virtue of her capacity for pleasure and pain a being with morally considerable interests. For this reason a genuine conflict may arise—between implementing the advance directive and acting in morally appropriate ways toward the profoundly demented individual. Such a conflict, however, is neither so fundamental nor so intractable as a conflict between the rights of two persons. One reason for this is that the profoundly and permanently demented Alzheimer's patient is not like a happy and otherwise normal individual who has simply lost some of his cognitive functions. On the contrary, the advanced Alzheimer's patient not only has radically truncated interests, but also has a very limited life expectancy and typically suffers a number of serious and often painful physical ailments as well. Our obligations toward such beings are to minimize their pain and to provide comfort, not to prolong their lives by costly medical interventions.

The psychological continuity view of personal identity does not itself provide an answer to the question: Where should we set the threshold for psychological continuity—what degree of psychological continuity is necessary for the preservation of personal identity? If the threshold is set high, then we will be forced to conclude that there will be many cases in which neurological damage destroys that person who issued an advance directive but leaves in his place a different person, over whose fate the advance directive can have no authority. If it is set low, the cases in which we are confident that loss of personal identity has occurred will be those in which what remains is not a person and, *a fortiori*, not a different person.

Some philosophers have adduced hypothetical examples to support the conclusion that we ought to set the threshold very high. These examples do not succeed, however, because our moral responses to them can be explained just as well (or better) by alternative hypotheses that do not presuppose loss of personal identity.

Setting the threshold high might not be incompatible with the existence of some of our most valued social practices and institutions—those involving commitment and responsibility—nor even with a coherent practice of implementing advance directives. For such institutions, as well as the practice of advance directives, may be flexible enough to adapt to a new conception of personal identity. However, the moral and social costs of the restructuring of our practices and institutions which such a shift in the threshold would mandate would be very high, and as yet we have no good reasons to incur them. Thus the fact that neurological damage can destroy the psychological continuity necessary for personal identity does not, as some have argued, undermine the moral authority or value of advance directives as a basic tool for dealing with problems of decision making for those who are incompetent.

A quite different implication of the psychological continuity view is that the very attempt to locate a threshold of psychological continuity (whether high or low) reveals a failure to understand that personal identity judgments, understood as all-or-nothing claims, ought to be replaced with judgments concerning degrees of psychological continuity, along with corresponding judgments concerning the moral weight of rights, obligations, or interests— including the moral weight to be accorded to interests expressed in advance directives. We have seen, however, that the thesis that the psychological continuity upon which personal identity depends admits of degrees does *not* entail that we should abandon the use of all-or-nothing personal identity judgments, any more than the fact that maturity depends upon skills and capacities that are a matter of degree entails that it is a mistake to designate as mature only those who possess the skills and capacities in question to a certain degree. There is nothing incoherent about designating a certain degree of psychological continuity as necessary for the persistence of personal identity *and* recognizing that psychological continuity is a matter of degree *and* admitting that psychological continuity is all there is to personal identity.

Nor is there any inconsistency in combining the threshold approach with social practices and institutions that recognize the diminishing moral authority of an advance directive as the degree of psychological continuity decreases below the threshold. Moreover, I have indicated why such a way of thinking about personal identity—which I have labeled the compromise position—may be advisable. It allows us to preserve the core of some of our most valuable practices and institutions, those which presuppose the use of all-or-nothing personal identity judgments, while acknowledging that personal identity is simply a matter of psychological continuity and does not depend on some deeper, metaphysical fact. This compromise approach allows us to make a significant place for advance directives among our social institutions and practices without presupposing a dubious metaphysical theory of personal identity. For cases in which justified all-or-nothing personal identity judgments can be made, valid advance directives have their full moral force. For cases in which psychological continuity has diminished to points below the threshold that grounds all-or-nothing personal identity judgments, the moral force of advance directives is correspondingly weakened and may disappear altogether.

This is not to say, however, that advance directives are never morally problematic. Perhaps the most troubling case for according an advance directive absolute authority would *not* be one in which we think that there has been a loss of personal identity. Instead, it might be of the following sort. An apparently valid advance directive specifies that no life-sustaining treatments, including antibiotics, are to be used on the individual if she suffers loss of cognitive function. The patient does suffer a serious loss of cognitive function due to a discrete neurological injury, such as a stroke. She is now a mentally handicapped person, but clearly a person—and indeed the same person—nonetheless. Moreover, the patient is otherwise healthy, is apparently quite happy, and wants to live. Then she develops a life-threatening pneumonia. Following the advance directive will result in the easily avoidable death of a happy and reasonably healthy, though mentally handicapped, person. Suppose also that she is judged not to be competent to rescind the advance directive. There is clearly a sense in which a decision to ignore her advance directive would interfere with her earlier autonomous choice.

Cases like this challenge the depth of our commitment to individual autonomy and with it the assumption that the moral authority of advance directives may never be limited on paternalistic grounds. I am not convinced that it is possible to provide a conclusive argument to show that paternalism is never in principle justified in any such case. My aim here, however, is not to evaluate paternalistic challenges to advance directives but rather to evaluate a more fundamental objection rooted in the problem of personal identity.

It is important to emphasize, however, that the combination of factors that makes cases such as this so disturbing will probably be quite rare. And it is worth repeating that the challenge such cases pose to the authority of advance directives does not rest on the assumption that there has been a loss of personal identity.[17] The fact that neurological damage can result in loss of personal identity without death is not, I have argued, a serious challenge to the moral authority of advance directives.

[17] For a more comprehensive treatment of advance directives, see Allen Buchanan and Dan W. Brock, *Deciding for Others: The Ethics of Surrogate Decision-Making* (Cambridge: Cambridge University Press, 1990).

PART III

THE VALUE OF LIFE

7

WHAT IS SACRED?

RONALD DWORKIN

PART 1: WHAT IS SACRED?

Scientists sometimes cannot explain their observations about the known universe except by assuming the existence of something not yet discovered—another planet or star or force. So they assume that something else does exist, and they look for it. Astronomers discovered the planet Neptune, for example, only after they realized that the movements of the planet Uranus could be explained only by the gravitational force of another celestial body, yet unknown, orbiting the sun still farther out.

I have been arguing that most of us—liberals as well as conservatives—cannot explain our convictions in the way that many politicians, self-appointed spokesmen, moralists, and philosophers think we can. They say that the different opinions we have about when and why abortion is morally wrong, and about how the law should regulate abortion, all follow from some foundational conviction each of us has about whether a fetus is a person with rights or interests of its own, and, if so, how far these trump the rights and interests of a pregnant woman. But when we look closely at the kinds of convictions most people have, we find that we cannot explain these simply by discovering people's views about whether a human fetus is a person. Our convictions reflect another idea we also hold, whose gravitational force better explains the shape of our beliefs and our disagreements.

I have already said what that different idea is. We believe that it is *intrinsically* regrettable when human life, once begun, ends prematurely. We believe, in other words, that a premature death is bad in itself, even when it is not bad for any particular person. Many people believe this about suicide and euthanasia—that a terrible thing has happened when someone takes his own life or when his doctor kills him at his own request even when death may be in that person's own best interests. We believe the same about abortion: that

From Ronald Dworkin, 'What is Sacred?' and 'Dying and Living,' in his *Life's Dominion* (London: HarperCollins, 1993).

it is sometimes wrong not because it violates a fetus's rights or harms its interests, but in spite of a fetus's having no rights or interests to violate. The great majority of people who have strong views about abortion—liberal as well as conservative—believe, at least intuitively, that the life of a human organism has intrinsic value in any form it takes, even in the extremely undeveloped form of a very early, just-implanted embryo. I say 'at least intuitively' because many people have not related their views about abortion or euthanasia to the idea that human life has intrinsic value. For them, that idea is the undiscovered planet that explains otherwise inexplicable convictions.

The idea of life's intrinsic value may seem mysterious, and I must try to make it seem less so. I shall have to overcome, first, an objection that philosophers have raised, which denies the very possibility that *anything* has intrinsic value. David Hume and many other philosophers insisted that objects or events can be valuable only when and because they serve someone's or something's interests. On this view, nothing is valuable unless someone wants it or unless it helps someone to get what he does want. How can it be important that a life continue unless that life is important for or to someone? How can a life's continuing be, as I am suggesting, simply important in and of itself?

That may seem a powerful objection. But much of our life is based on the idea that objects or events can be valuable in themselves. It is true that in ordinary, day-to-day life people do spend most of their time trying to get or make things they value because they or someone else enjoys or needs them. They try to make money and buy clothes or food or medicine for that reason. But the idea that some events or objects are valuable in and of themselves—that we honor them not because they serve our desires or interests but for their own sakes—is also a familiar part of our experience. Much of what we think about knowledge, experience, art, and nature, for example, presupposes that in different ways these are valuable in themselves and not just for their utility or for the pleasure or satisfaction they bring us. The idea of intrinsic value is commonplace, and it has a central place in our shared scheme of values and opinions.

It is not enough, however, simply to say that the idea of intrinsic value is familiar. For we are concerned with a special application of that idea—the claim that human life even in its most undeveloped form has intrinsic value—and that application raises unique puzzles. Why does it not follow, for example, that there should be as much human life as possible? Most of us certainly do not believe that. On the contrary, it would be better, at least in many parts of the world, if there were less human life rather than more. Then how can it be intrinsically important that human life, once begun, continue? Those are important questions, and in answering them we will discover a crucial distinction between two categories of intrinsically valuable things: those that are *incrementally* valuable—the more of them we have the better—and those that are not but are valuable in a very different way. I shall call the latter *sacred* or *inviolable* values.

There is another, quite independent puzzle. I claim not only that most of us believe that human life has intrinsic value, but also that this explains why we disagree so profoundly about abortion. How can that be? How can a shared assumption explain the terrible divisions about abortion that are tearing us apart? The answer, I believe, is that we interpret the idea that human life is intrinsically valuable in different ways, and that the different impulses and convictions expressed in these competing interpretations are very powerful and passionate.

It is obvious enough that the abstract idea of life's intrinsic value is open to different interpretations. Suppose we accept this abstract idea, and also accept that in at least some circumstances a deliberate abortion would show a wrongful contempt for the intrinsic value of life. Which circumstances are these? The list of questions we must pose in deciding this is very long. Is an abortion at a late stage of pregnancy a worse insult to the intrinsic value of life than one at an early stage? If so, why? What standard of measurement or comparison do and should we use in making that kind of judgment?

What else, besides abortion, fails to show the required respect for human life? Does a doctor show respect for life when he allows a mother to die in order to save a fetus? Which decision that a doctor might make in such circumstances would show more and which less respect for the intrinsic value of human life? Why? Suppose a pregnancy is the result of rape: which decision then shows greater respect for the intrinsic value of human life—a decision for or against abortion? Suppose a fetus is horribly deformed: does it show respect or contempt for life to allow it to be born? What standard of measuring respect or contempt for human life should we use in making these judgments?

Different people with sharply different convictions about a range of religious and philosophical matters answer these various questions differently, and the different answers they give in fact match the main divisions of opinion about abortion. If we can understand the abortion controversy as related to other differences of religious and philosophical opinion in that way, then we shall understand much better how and why we disagree. We shall also be in a better position to emphasize how we agree, to see how our divisions, deep and painful though they are, are nevertheless rooted in a fundamental unity of humane conviction. What we share is more fundamental than our quarrels over its best interpretation.

RONALD DWORKIN

THE IDEA OF THE SACRED

What does it mean to say that human life is intrinsically important? Something is *instrumentally* important if its value depends on its usefulness, its capacity to help people get something else they want. Money and medicine, for example, are only instrumentally valuable: no one thinks that money has value beyond its power to purchase things that people want or need, or that medicine has value beyond its ability to cure. Something is *subjectively* valuable only to people who happen to desire it. Scotch whiskey, watching football games, and lying in the sun are valuable only for people, like me, who happen to enjoy them. I do not think that others who detest them are making any kind of a mistake or failing to show proper respect for what is truly valuable. They just happen not to like or want what I do.

Something is intrinsically valuable, on the contrary, if its value is *independent* of what people happen to enjoy or want or need or what is good for them. Most of us treat at least some objects or events as intrinsically valuable in that way: we think we should admire and protect them because they are important in themselves, and not just if or because we or others want or enjoy them. Many people think that great paintings, for example, are intrinsically valuable. They are valuable, and must be respected and protected, because of their inherent quality as art, and not because people happen to enjoy looking at them or find instruction or some pleasurable aesthetic experience standing before them. We say that we want to look at one of Rembrandt's self-portraits because it is wonderful, not that it is wonderful because we want to look at it. The thought of its being destroyed horrifies us—seems to us a terrible desecration—but this is not just because or even if that would cheat us of experiences we desire to have. We are horrified even if we have only a very small chance of ever seeing the painting anyway—perhaps it is privately owned and never shown to the public, or in a museum far away—and even if there are plenty of excellent reproductions available.[1]

We treat not just particular paintings or other works of art that way, but, more generally, human cultures. We think it a shame when any distinctive form of human culture, especially a complex and interesting one, dies or languishes. Once again, this cannot be fully explained merely in terms of the

---

[1] I do not mean to take any position on a further, very abstract philosophical issue not pertinent to this discussion: whether great paintings would still be valuable if intelligent life were altogether destroyed forever so that no one could ever have the experience of regarding paintings again. There is no inconsistency in denying that they would have value then, because the value of a painting lies in the kind of experience it makes available, while still insisting that this value is intrinsic because it does not depend on any creatures' actually wanting that kind of experience.

contribution that cultural variety makes to the excitement of our lives. We create museums to protect and sustain interest in some form of primitive art, for example, not just because or if we think its objects splendid or beautiful, but because we think it a terrible waste if any artistic form that human beings have developed should perish as if it had never existed. We take much the same attitude toward parts of popular or industrial culture: we are troubled by the disappearance of traditional crafts, for example, not just if we need what it produced—perhaps we do not—but because it seems a great waste that an entire form of craft imagination should disappear.

Is human life subjectively or instrumentally or intrinsically valuable? Most of us think it is all three. We treat the value of someone's life as instrumental when we measure it in terms of how much his being alive serves the interests of others: of how much what he produces makes other people's lives better, for example. When we say that Mozart's or Pasteur's life had great value because the music and medicine they created served the interests of others, we are treating their lives as instrumentally valuable. We treat a person's life as subjectively valuable when we measure its value to him, that is, in terms of how much *he* wants to be alive or how much being alive is good for him. So if we say that life has lost its value to someone who is miserable or in great pain, we are treating that life in a subjective way.

Let us call the subjective value a life has for the person whose life it is its *personal* value. It is personal value we have in mind when we say that normally a person's life is the most important thing he or she has. It is personal value that a government aims to protect, as fundamentally important, when it recognizes and enforces people's right to life. So it is understandable that the debate about abortion should include the question of whether a fetus has rights and interests of its own. If it does, then it has a personal interest in continuing to live, an interest that should be protected by recognizing and enforcing a right to life. I have argued that an early fetus has no interests and rights, and that almost no one thinks it does; if personal value were the only pertinent kind of value at stake in abortion, then abortion would be morally unproblematic.

If we think, however, that the life of any human organism, including a fetus, has intrinsic value whether or not it also has instrumental or personal value—if we treat any form of human life as something we should respect and honor and protect as marvelous in itself—then abortion remains morally problematical. If it is a horrible desecration to destroy a painting, for example, even though a painting is not a person, why should it not be a much greater desecration to destroy something whose intrinsic value may be vastly greater?

We must notice a further and crucial distinction: between what we value incrementally—what we want more of, no matter how much we already have—and what we value only once it already exists. Some things are not only intrinsically but incrementally valuable. We tend to treat knowledge that way, for example. Our culture wants to know about archaeology and cosmology and galaxies many millions of light-years away—even though little of that knowledge is likely to be of any practical benefit—and we want to know as much of all that as we can.[2] But we do not value human life that way. Instead, we treat human life as sacred or inviolable. (As I said in chapter 1, I use those terms—and also the terms 'sanctity' and 'inviolability'—interchangeably.) The hallmark of the sacred as distinct from the incrementally valuable is that the sacred is intrinsically valuable because—and therefore only once—it exists. It is inviolable because of what it represents or embodies. It is not important that there be more people. But once a human life has begun, it is very important that it flourish and not be wasted.

Is that a peculiar distinction? No: we make the same distinction about other objects or events that we think are intrinsically valuable. We treat much of the art we value as sacredly rather than incrementally valuable. We attach great value to works of art once they exist, even though we care less about whether more of them are produced. Of course we may believe that the continued production of *great* art is tremendously important—that the more truly wonderful objects a culture produces the better—and we believe the same about great lives: even those who are most in favor of controlling population growth would not want fewer Leonardo da Vincis or Martin Luther Kings. But even if we do not regret that there are not more works by a given painter, or more examples of a particular artistic genre, we insist on respecting the examples we do in fact have. I do not myself wish that there were more paintings by Tintoretto than there are. But I would nevertheless be appalled by the deliberate destruction of even one of those he did paint.

Something is sacred or inviolable when its deliberate destruction would dishonor what ought to be honored. What makes something sacred in that way? We can distinguish between two processes through which something becomes sacred for a given culture or person. The first is by association or designation. In ancient Egypt, for example, certain animals were held sacred to certain gods; because cats were associated with a certain goddess, and for no other reason, it was sacrilegious to injure them. In many cultures, people take that attitude toward national symbols, including flags. Many Americans consider the flag sacred because of its conventional association with the life

---

[2] Of course, we may have competing reasons for wanting something *not* to be known: how to blow up the universe, for example. But even in this sort of case, we believe that deliberately avoiding knowledge sacrifices something of intrinsic importance.

of the nation; the respect they believe they owe their country is transferred to the flag. Of course, the flag's value to them is not subjective or instrumental. Nor is the flag incrementally valuable; even the most flag-reverent patriot does not believe that there must be as many flags as possible. He values the flag as sacred rather than incrementally valuable, and its sacred character is a matter of association.

The second way something may become sacred is through its history, how it came to be. In the case of art, for example, inviolability is not associational but genetic: it is not what a painting symbolizes or is associated with but how it came to be that makes it valuable. We protect even a painting we do not much like, just as we try to preserve cultures we do not especially admire, because they embody processes of human creation we consider important and admirable.

We take a parallel attitude, we must now notice, toward aspects of the natural world: in our culture, we tend to treat distinct animal species (though not individual animals) as sacred. We think it very important, and worth considerable economic expense, to protect endangered species from destruction at human hands or by a human enterprise—a market in rhinoceros tusks, valued for their supposed aphrodisiac power; dams that threaten the only habitat of a certain species of fish; or timbering practices that will destroy the last horned owls. We are upset—it would be terrible if the rhinoceros ceased to exist—and we are indignant: surely it is wrong to allow such a catastrophe just so that human beings can make more money or increase their power.

Why are individual species so valuable that it would be dreadful if some useful enterprise destroyed one or a few of the many thousands of species in the world? Someone might say: we protect endangered species because we want the pleasure of continuing to see animals of each species, or because we want the useful information we might gain by studying them, or because it is more interesting for us that there be more rather than fewer species. But none of these arguments rings true. Many—perhaps most—of the people who consider endangered species important are very unlikely ever to encounter any of the animals they want to protect. I doubt that many who have labored to protect the horned owl have any plans to visit the habitat of those birds or to look them up in zoos, nor do I think they believe that in keeping horned owls alive we will learn enough useful information to justify the expense. These people struggle to protect the species simply because they think it would be a shame if human acts and decisions caused it to disappear.

So this is another important example of something many of us take to be of intrinsic rather than instrumental value. It is also an example of sacred rather than incremental value: few people believe the world would be worse if there had always been fewer species of birds, and few would think it important to engineer new bird species if that were possible. What we believe important is not that there be any particular number of species but that a species that now exists not be extinguished by us. We consider it a kind of cosmic shame when a species that nature has developed ceases, through human actions, to exist.

I put the point that way—about not destroying what nature has created—to emphasize the similarity I claim between our reverence for art and our concern for the survival of species. Both art and species are examples of things inviolable to us not by association but in virtue of their history, of how they came to exist. We see the evolutionary process through which species were developed as itself contributing, in some way, to the shame of what we do when we cause their extinction now. Indeed, people who are concerned to protect threatened species often stress the connection between art and nature themselves by describing the evolution of species as a process of creation.

For most Americans, and for many people in other countries, the evolutionary process is quite literally creative, for they believe that God is the author of nature. On that assumption, causing a species to disappear, wholly to be lost, is destroying a creative design of the most exalted artist of all. But even people who do not take that view, but who instead accept the Darwinian thesis that the evolution of species is a matter of accidental mutation rather than divine design, nevertheless often use artistic metaphors of creation. They describe discrete animal species as not just accidents but as achievements of adaptation, as something that nature has not just produced but wrought. The literature of conservation is studded with such personifications of nature as creative artist. They are part of the fertile ground of ideas and associations in which the roots of conservationist concern are buried. Indeed, so thoroughly have the metaphors of artistic and cultural creation come to dominate pleas for the preservation of species that the analogy is now used in reverse. An anthropologist recently pleaded that we should treat the threatened death of a primitive language with as much concern and sympathy as we show snail darters and horned owls and other near-extinct species of animal life.[3]

Our concern for the preservation of animal species reaches its most dramatic and intense form, of course, in the case of one particular species: our own. It is an inarticulate, unchallenged, almost unnoticed, but nevertheless

---

[3] See John N. Wilford, 'In a Publishing Coup, Books in "Unwritten" Languages,' *New York Times*, 31 Dec. 1991.

absolute premise of our political and economic planning that the human race must survive and prosper. This unspoken assumption unites the two different examples of sanctity we have so far identified. Our special concern for art and culture reflects the respect in which we hold artistic creation, and our special concern for the survival of animal species reflects a parallel respect for what nature, understood either as divine or as secular, has produced. These twin bases of the sacred come together in the case of the survival of our own species, because we treat it as crucially important that we survive not only biologically but culturally, that our species not only lives but thrives. That is the premise of a good part of our concern about conservation and about the survival and health of cultural and artistic traditions. We are concerned not only about ourselves and others now alive, but about untold generations of people in centuries to come.

We cannot explain our concern about future humanity, of course, as concern for the rights and interests of particular people. Suppose that through great stupidity we were to unleash radioactivity whose consequence was that human beings were extinct by the twenty-second century. It is absurd to argue that we would then have done terrible injury or injustice to people who would otherwise have lived, unless we think that in some very crowded mystical space people are waiting to be conceived and born. We sometimes talk that way, and may even fall into ways of thinking that would make sense only if there were such mystical worlds of possible people with a right to exist. But in fact our worries about humanity in centuries to come make sense only if we suppose that it is intrinsically important that the human race continue even though it is not important to the interests of particular people.

We also consider it important that people live well, and we therefore think we have a responsibility not only not to destroy the possibility of future generations but also to leave them a fair share of natural and cultural resources. That is the presupposition of what philosophers call the problem of justice between generations: the idea that each generation of people must in fairness leave the world fit for habitation not only by their children and grandchildren, whom they already know and love, but for generations of descendants whose identity is in no way yet fixed, at least in ways we can understand, but depends on what we must consider billions of independent accidents of genetic coupling. Philosophers speak of this as a matter of justice, and so do politicians and columnists: they argue, for example, that the huge national debt that the government has allowed the United States to develop in recent decades is unfair to generations yet unborn. But that way of putting it is misleading, because our concern for the future is not concern for the rights or interests of specific people. The decisions we now make about conservation and the economy will affect, in ways we cannot understand, let alone anticipate, not only what resources our descendants will have but which people they will be. It hardly makes sense to say that we owe it to some particular individual not selfishly to squander the earth's resources if that individual will exist only if we do squander them. Or, for that matter, only if we don't. Our concern for future generations is not a matter of justice at all but of our instinctive sense that human flourishing as well as human survival is of sacred importance.

Through this canvass of things, events, and processes that many people take to be inviolable, I have tried to show how general the idea of the sacred really is, and therefore to forestall the objection that the principle that I believe is at the root of most people's convictions about abortion—the principle that human life, even the life of a very early embryo, is inviolable—is bizarre or odd. But the examples have the further value of suggesting that at least in many of the most familiar cases, the nerve of the sacred lies in the value we attach to a process or enterprise or project rather than to its results considered independently from how they were produced. We are horrified at the idea of the deliberate destruction of a work of art not just because we lose the art but because destroying it seems to demean a creative process we consider very important. Similarly, we honor and protect cultures, which are also, more abstractly, forms of art, because they are communal products of the kinds of enterprise we treat as important. Our attitudes toward individual works of art and discrete cultures, then, display a deep respect for the enterprises that give rise to them; we respect these enterprises independently of their particular results.

Our concern for the preservation of animal species is also based on respect for the way they came into being rather than for the animals considered independently of that history. The natural processes of evolution and development themselves have a normative significance for us, and this is not because the species they generated—the rhinoceros or the horned owl, for example—are superior on some independent test of animal worth to others that might have evolved if they had not, but because we consider it wrong, a desecration of the inviolable, that a species that evolution did produce should perish through our acts. Geneticists have created plants that we find instrumentally valuable: they produce food and may save lives. But we do not think that these artificially produced species are intrinsically valuable in the way that naturally produced species are.

For many people, as I said, the respect we owe nature is respect for God conceived as the divine creator. We respect all God's creatures, on this view, not one by one, not each robin or horse or horned owl or snail darter, but as imaginative designs produced by God's inspired genius, to be honored as such, as God commanded Noah to honor his designs by keeping species, not individual animals, alive in the ark. Some conservationists who do not think of themselves as religious may nevertheless hold a powerful, intuitive conviction that nature is *itself* alive, a mysterious, inexorable force unifying all life in Life itself. Walt Whitman was the poet of that conviction—in *Leaves of Grass* and *Song of Myself* he celebrated the 'procreant urge of the world'[4]— and another poet, David Plante, speaks of an elemental 'pulse in the mud' as the mysterious source of all life. People with either of these views—the conventionally religious one or some version of the idea that nature itself is purposive—believe that destroying a species is wrong because it wastes an important and creative achievement of God or the procreant world. They mean that we should regret the loss of a species just as—though to a much greater degree than—we would regret the foundering of some project on which we or others had long labored. We regret the waste of a creative investment not just for what we do not have, but because of the special badness of great effort frustrated.

But many people who wish to protect endangered animal species or other important or beautiful natural products do not believe in a creative God or in a mysterious intelligence guiding nature. For them, the analogy between nature and art is only an analogy: they speak of nature as creative only as a metaphorical way of reporting their primitive but strong conviction that nature and art are both processes whose products are, in principle, inviolable. They believe that it is a shame for human beings to destroy what was created over aeons of natural selective evolution, not because some divine or cosmic artist created it but just because, in some primal way, it *is* a shame, an intrinsically bad thing to do. When they say that the extinction of a species is a waste of nature's investment, they mean not that nature is a conscious investor but that even unconscious natural processes of creation should be treated as investments worthy of respect.[5] Perhaps future generations will mock the idea as ridiculously sentimental. But it is nevertheless very wide-spread now, and there is nothing irrational or disreputable about it. It is no more sentimental to treat what nature has created as an investment we should not waste than it is to take the same view of an ancient work of art,

---

[4] 'Song of Myself,' in Oscar Williams (ed.), *A Little Treasury of American Poetry* (New York: Scribners, 1948), 108.

[5] The idea of respect for natural processes has other dramatic consequences. When a London fertility clinic announced in 1993 that it would allow certain parents to choose the sex of their test-tube baby, for example, many British politicians quickly declared their outrage: several of them said that their objection was based not on 'rational' grounds but on an instinctive distaste for interfering with the 'mysteries of nature.' Even if we think that their reaction was premature, or insufficiently sympathetic toward some parents, most of us understand and share the impulse behind it.

whose unknown author perished many centuries ago, or of some ancient language or craft created by people who never thought they were investing in anything.

I must emphasize, finally, two further features of our convictions about the sacred and inviolable. First, for most of us, there are degrees of the sacred just as there are degrees of the wonderful. It would be sacrilegious for someone to destroy a work by a minor Renaissance artist but not as bad as destroying a Bellini. It is regrettable when a distinctive and beautiful species of exotic bird is destroyed, but it would be even worse if we stamped out the Siberian tiger. And though we would no doubt regret the entire extinction of pit vipers or sharks, our regret might be mixed; we might think it not as bad when a species is destroyed that is dangerous to us. Second, our convictions about inviolability are selective. We do not treat everything that human beings create as sacred. We treat art as inviolable, but not wealth or auto-mobiles or commercial advertising, even though people also create these. We do not treat everything produced by a long natural process—coal or petrol-eum deposits, for example—as inviolable either, and many of us have no compunction about cutting down trees to clear space for a house or slaughter-ing complex mammals like cows for food. And we consider only some species of animals as sacred: few people care when even a benign species of insect comes to an end, and even for those who believe that viruses are animals, the eradication of the AIDS virus would be an occasion for celebration untinged by even a trace of regret.

So in different ways we are selective about which products of which kinds of creative or natural processes we treat as inviolable. As we would expect, our selections are shaped by and reflect our needs and, in a reciprocal way, shape and are shaped by other opinions we have. We honor human artistic effort, for example, because it can produce marvelous things, like great paint-ings of beauty and insight and wonder, and then, because we honor that form of human creative enterprise, we respect everything it produces, includ-ing paintings we do not find marvelous. We honor nature because it has produced striking geological formations and majestic plants and living crea-tures we find extraordinary, including us, and we protect examples of that production—mountains or rivers or forests or animals—in a special and more intense way because they are natural. The reciprocity between our admiration for processes and our admiration for product is complex, and its result, for most people, is not a single overarching principle from which all their convictions about the inviolable flow, but a complex network of feelings and intuitions.

It is not my present purpose to recommend or defend any of these wide-spread convictions about art and nature, in either their religious or secular form. Perhaps they are all, as some skeptics insist, inconsistent superstitions. I want only to call attention to their complexity and characteristic structure, because I hope to show that most people's convictions about abortion and euthanasia can be understood as resting on very similar, though in some important ways different, beliefs about how and why *individual* human life, in any form, is also inviolable.

THE SANCTITY OF EACH HUMAN LIFE

An obscure nineteenth-century Austrian philosopher, Joseph Popper-Lynkeus, said that the death of any human being, except of a murderer or a suicide, was 'a far more important happening than any political or religious or national occurrence, or the sum total of the scientific and artistic and technological advances made throughout the ages by all the peoples of the world.'[6] He added that anyone tempted to regard this extraordinary claim as an exaggeration should 'imagine the individual concerned to be himself or his best beloved.' His addition confuses the intrinsic value of human life with what I called its personal value. My life may be personally more important to me than anything else, but it does not follow that it is intrinsically more important, and once that distinction is made, it is ludicrous to suppose that even a premature and tragic death, let alone a natural death after a long life, is intrinsically a worse event than the destruction of all human art and knowledge would be. But Popper-Lynkeus's claim does capture, in hyperbolic form, a conviction that must now be our main concern: that in some circumstances the deliberate ending of a single human life is intrinsically bad—objectively a shame—in the same way as the destruction of great art or the loss of important knowledge would be.

We are now in a better position to appreciate that conviction. I said that we treat the preservation and prosperity of our own species as of capital importance because we believe that we are the highest achievements of God's creation, if we are conventionally religious, or of evolution, if we are not, and also because we know that all knowledge and art and culture would disappear if humanity did. That combination of nature and art—two traditions of the sacred—supports the further and more dramatic claim that each individual human life, on its own, is also inviolable, because each individual life, on its own, can be understood as the product of both creative traditions. The first of these traditions—the idea that nature is creative—has had a

---

[6] See Paul Edwards (ed), *The Encyclopedia of Philosophy*, vi (New York: Macmillan, 1967; New York: Free Press, 1972), 403.

prominent role as a basis for that claim. The dominant Western religious traditions insist that God made humankind 'in His own image,' that each individual human being is a representation and not merely a product of a divine creator, and people who accept that article of faith will understandably think that each human being, not just the species as a whole, is a creative masterpiece. A secular form of the same idea, which assigns the masterpiece to nature rather than God, is also a staple of our culture—the image of a human being as the highest product of natural creation is one of Shakespeare's most powerful, for example. 'What a piece of work is a man!' says Hamlet, and James Tyrrel, who arranges the murder of the princes in the Tower for Richard III, quotes a killer as being appalled at realizing that he has 'smothered the most replenished sweet work of Nature that from the prime creation e'er she framed.' In these and other ways, the idea that human beings are special among natural creations is offered to explain why it is horrible that even a single human individual life should be extinguished.

The role of the other tradition of the sacred in supporting the sanctity of life is less evident but equally crucial: each developed human being is the product not just of natural creation, but also of the kind of deliberative human creative force that we honor in honoring art. A mature woman, for example, is in her personality, training, capacity, interests, ambitions, and emotions, something like a work of art because in those respects she is the product of human creative intelligence, partly that of her parents and other people, partly that of her culture, and also, through the choices she has made, her *own* creation. The Greeks used two words for life that bring out the distinction: *zoe*, by which they meant physical or biological life, and *bios*, by which they meant a life as *lived*, as made up of the actions, decisions, motives, and events that compose what we now call a biography.[7]

The idea that each individual human life is inviolable is therefore rooted, like our concern for the survival of our species as a whole, in two combined and intersecting bases of the sacred: natural *and* human creation. Any human creature, including the most immature embryo, is a triumph of divine or evolutionary creation, which produces a complex, reasoning being from, as it were, nothing, and also of what we often call the 'miracle' of human reproduction, which makes each new human being both different from and yet a continuation of the human beings who created it. Levin—Tolstoy's fictional self-projection in *Anna Karenina*—is struck by wonder, in spite of himself, at the birth of his son:

---

[7] This distinction is emphasized in James Rachels and William Ruddick, 'Lives and Liberty,' in John Christman (ed.), *The Inner Citadel: Essays on Individual Autonomy* (New York: Oxford University Press, 1989), and explored in James Rachels, *The End of Life* (Oxford: Oxford University Press, 1986), 24–7.

Meanwhile, at the foot of the bed, in Lizaveta Petrovna's skillful hands flickered the life of a human being, like the small uncertain flame of a night-light—a human being who had not existed a moment ago but who, with the same rights and importance to itself as the rest of humanity, would live and create others in its own image ... Whence, wherefore had it come, and who was it? He could not understand at all, nor accustom himself to the idea. It seemed to him too much, a superabundance, to which he was unable to get used for a long time.[8]

The natural miracle that so moved Levin begins much earlier than birth: it begins in the genetic identity of an embryo. The second form of sacred creation, the human as distinct from the natural investment, is also immediate when pregnancy is planned, because a deliberate decision of parents to have and bear a child is of course a creative one. Any surviving child is shaped in character and capacity by the decisions of parents and by the cultural background of community. As that child matures, in all but pathological cases, his own creative choices progressively determine his thoughts, personality, ambitions, emotions, connections, and achievements. He creates his life just as much as an artist creates a painting or a poem. I am not suggesting, as some nineteenth-century Romantic writers did, that a human life is literally a work of art. That is a dangerous idea, because it suggests that we should value a person in the same way that we value a painting or a poem, valuing him for beauty or style or originality rather than personal or moral or intellectual qualities. But we can—and do—treat leading a life as itself a kind of creative activity, which we have at least as much reason to honor as artistic creation.

The life of a single human organism commands respect and protection, then, no matter in what form or shape, because of the complex creative investment it represents and because of our wonder at the divine or evolutionary processes that produce new lives from old ones, at the processes of nation and community and language through which a human being will come to absorb and continue hundreds of generations of cultures and forms of life and value, and, finally, when mental life has begun and flourishes, at the process of internal personal creation and judgment by which a person will make and remake himself, a mysterious, inescapable process in which we each participate, and which is therefore the most powerful and inevitable source of empathy and communion we have with every other creature who faces the same frightening challenge. The horror we feel in the willful destruction of a human life reflects our shared inarticulate sense of the intrinsic importance of each of these dimensions of investment.

[8] See Leo Tolstoy, *Anna Karenina*, trans. Rosemary Edmonds (New York: Penguin, 1978), 749.

THE METRIC OF DISRESPECT

I must now try to show how this understanding of the sacredness of human life allows us better to explain the two opposing attitudes toward abortion than does the traditional account, which supposes that these attitudes are based on different views about whether and when a fetus is a person with a right to life. I shall assume that conservatives and liberals all accept that in principle human life is inviolable in the sense I have defined, that any abortion involves a waste of human life and is therefore, in itself, a bad thing to happen, a shame. And I shall try to show how that assumption explains why the two sides both agree and disagree in the ways that they do.

I begin with their agreement. Conservatives and liberals both suppose, as I said, that though abortion is always morally problematic and often morally wrong, it is worse on some occasions than on others. They suppose, in other words, that there are degrees of badness in the waste of human life. What measure are they assuming in those judgments? Let us put that question in a more general form. We all assume that some cases of premature death are greater tragedies than others, not only when we are puzzling about abortion, but in the context of many other events as well. Most of us would think it worse when a young woman dies in a plane crash than when an elderly man does, for example, or a boy than a middle-aged man. What measure of tragedy are we assuming when we think this? What measure should we assume?

This is not the question moral philosophers and medical ethicists often write about—the question of what *rights* different sorts of people have to live, or of how relatively wicked it is to deny them lifesaving resources or to kill them. We might believe that it is worse—that there has been a greater waste of life—when a young person dies than when an old one does, or when an emotionally healthy person dies than a suicidal one, or when a man with young children dies than a bachelor, without suggesting that it would be any less wicked to kill an old than a young person, or a depressive than a happy one, or a bachelor than a father. Nor even—though this is obviously a different and harder question—that it would be any fairer to deny an old man scarce lifesaving resources, like kidney machines, when there is not enough for everyone who needs them, or to deny those resources to depressives and bachelors so that they could be used for spirited fathers of six. \

These judgments about murder and fairness belong to the system of rights and interests, the system of ideas I said could not explain our most common convictions about abortion. Most people think (and our laws certainly insist) that people have an equal right to life, and that the murder of a depressive handicapped octogenarian misanthrope is as heinous, and must be punished as seriously, as the murder of anyone younger or healthier or more valuable to others. Any other view would strike us as monstrous. It is more complicated, as I just conceded, how these differences between people should affect the distribution of scarce medical resources. Doctors in most countries assume that such resources should be devoted to younger rather than older people, and for many doctors, quality of life and value to others come into the equation as well. But even these questions of fairness are different from the question of the intrinsic goodness or badness of events that we are considering. We might insist, for example, that the interests of a seriously depressed and gravely handicapped person should be respected just as much as those of an emotionally healthy person in allocating scarce medical resources, and yet think (as some people might, though many do not) that it is a greater tragedy when the latter dies young than the former. I am now asking, then, not about justice or rights or fairness, but about tragedy and the waste of life. How should we measure and compare the waste of life, and therefore the insult to the sanctity of life, on different occasions?

We should consider, first, a simple and perhaps natural answer to that question. Life is wasted, on this simple view, when life is lost, so that the question of how much has been wasted by a premature death is answered by estimating how long the life cut short would probably otherwise have lasted. This simple answer seems to fit many of our intuitive convictions. It seems to explain the opinion I just mentioned, for example: that the death of a young woman in an airplane crash is worse than the death of an old man would be. The young woman would probably otherwise have had many more years left to live.

The simple answer is incomplete, because we can measure life—and therefore loss of life—in different ways. Should we take into account only the duration of life lost with no regard to its quality? Or should we take quality into account as well? Should we say that the loss of the young woman who died in the crash would be greater if she had been looking forward to a life full of promise and pleasure than if she was physically or psychologically handicapped in some permanent and grave way? Should we also take into account the loss her death would cause to the lives of others? Is the death of a parent of young children, or of a brilliant employer of large numbers of people, or of a musical genius, a worse waste of life than the death at the same age of someone whose life was equally satisfying to himself but less valuable to others?

We should not puzzle over these alternatives, however, because this simple answer, which measures waste of life only in terms of life lost, is unacceptable whether we define that loss only as duration of life or include quality of life or benefit to others. It is unacceptable, in any of these forms, for two compelling reasons.

First, though the simple answer seems to fit some of our convictions, it contradicts other important and deeply held ones. If the waste of life were to be measured only in chronological terms, for example, then an early-stage abortion would be a worse insult to the sanctity of life, a worse instance of life being wasted, than a late-stage abortion. But almost everyone holds the contrary assumption: that the later the abortion—the more like a child the aborted fetus has already become—the worse it is. We take a similar view about the death of young children. It is terrible when an infant dies but worse, most people think, when a three-year-old child dies and worse still when an adolescent does. Almost no one thinks that the tragedy of premature death decreases in a linear way as age increases. Most people's sense of that tragedy, if it were rendered as a graph relating the degree of tragedy to the age at which death occurs, would slope upward from birth to some point in late childhood or early adolescence, then follow a flat line until at least very early middle age, and then slope down again toward extreme old age. Richard's murder of the princes in the Tower could have no parallel, for horror, in any act of infanticide.

Nor does the simple interpretation of how death wastes life fit our feelings better in the more elaborate forms I mentioned. Our common view that it is worse when a late-stage fetus is aborted or miscarries than an early-stage one, and worse when a ten-year-old child dies than an infant, makes no assumptions about the quality of the lives lost or their value for others.

The simple view of wasted life fails for a second, equally important reason. It wholly fails to explain the important truth I have several times emphasized: that though we treat human life as sacred, we do not treat it as incrementally good; we do not believe abstractly that the more human lives that are lived the better. The simple claim that a premature death is tragic only because life is lost—only because some period of life that might have been lived by someone will not be—gives us no more reason to grieve over an abortion or any premature death than we have to grieve over contraception or any other form of birth control. In both cases, less human life is lived than might otherwise be.

The 'simple loss' view we have been considering is inadequate because it focuses only on future possibilities, on what will or will not happen in the future. It ignores the crucial truth that waste of life is often greater and more tragic because of what has already happened in the past. The death of an adolescent girl is worse than the death of an infant girl because the adolescent's death frustrates the investments she and others have already made in her life—the ambitions and expectations she constructed, the plans and projects she made, the love and interest and emotional involvement she formed for and with others, and they for and with her.

I shall use 'frustration' (though the word has other associations) to describe this more complex measure of the waste of life because I can think of no better word to suggest the combination of past and future considerations that figure in our assessment of a tragic death. Most of us hold to something like the following set of instinctive assumptions about death and tragedy. We believe, as I said, that a successful human life has a certain natural course. It starts in mere biological development—conception, fetal development, and infancy—but it then extends into childhood, adolescence, and adult life in ways that are determined not just by biological formation but by social and individual training and choice, and that culminate in satisfying relationships and achievements of different kinds. It ends, after a normal life span, in a natural death. It is a waste of the natural and human creative investments that make up the story of a normal life when this normal progression is frustrated by premature death or in other ways. But how bad this is—how great the frustration—depends on the stage of life in which it occurs, because the frustration is greater if it takes places after rather than before the person has made a significant personal investment in his own life, and less if it occurs after any investment has been substantially fulfilled, or as substantially fulfilled as is anyway likely.

This more complex structure fits our convictions about tragedy better than the simple loss-of-life measure does. It explains why the death of an adolescent seems to us worse in most circumstances than the death of an infant. It also explains how we can consistently maintain that it is sometimes undesirable to create new human lives while still insisting that it is bad when any human life, once begun, ends prematurely. No frustration of life is involved when fewer rather than more human beings are born, because there is no creative investment in lives that never exist. But once a human life starts, a process has begun, and interrupting that process frustrates an adventure already under way.

So the idea that we deplore the frustration of life, not its mere absence, seems adequately to fit our general convictions about life, death, and tragedy. It also explains much of what we think about the particular tragedy of abortion. Both conservatives and liberals assume that in some circumstances abortion is more serious and more likely to be unjustifiable than in others. Notably, both agree that a late-term abortion is graver than an early-term one. We cannot explain this shared conviction simply on the ground that fetuses more closely resemble infants as pregnancy continues. People believe that abortion is not just emotionally more difficult but morally worse the later in pregnancy it occurs, and increasing resemblance alone has no moral significance. Nor can we explain the shared conviction by noticing that at some point in pregnancy a fetus becomes sentient. Most people think that abortion is morally worse early in the second trimester—well before sentience is possible—than early in the first one (several European nations, which permit abortion in the first but not the second trimester, have made that distinction part of their criminal law). And though that widely shared belief cannot be explained by the simple lost-life theory, the frustration thesis gives us a natural and compelling justification of it. Fetal development is a continuing creative process, a process that has barely begun at the instant of conception. Indeed, since genetic individuation is not yet complete at that point, we might say that the development of a unique human being has not started until approximately fourteen days later, at implantation. But after implantation, as fetal growth continues, the natural investment that would be wasted in an abortion grows steadily larger and more significant.

HUMAN AND DIVINE

So our sense that frustration rather than just loss compromises the inviolability of human life does seem helpful in explaining what unites most people about abortion. The more difficult question is whether it also helps in explaining what divides them. Let us begin our answer by posing another question. I just described a natural course of human life—beginning in conception, extending through birth and childhood, culminating in successful and engaged adulthood in which the natural biological investment and the personal human investment in that life are realized, and finally ending in natural death after a normal span of years. Life so understood can be frustrated in two main ways. It can be frustrated by premature death, which leaves any previous natural and personal investment unrealized. Or it can be frustrated by other forms of failure: by handicaps or poverty or misconceived projects or irredeemable mistakes or lack of training or even brute bad luck; any one of these may in different ways frustrate a person's opportunity to redeem his ambitions or otherwise to lead a full and flourishing life. Is premature death always, inevitably, a more serious frustration of life than any of these other forms of failure?

Decisions about abortion often raise this question. Suppose parents discover, early in the mother's pregnancy, that the fetus is genetically so deformed that the life it would lead after birth will inevitably be both short and sharply limited. They must decide whether it is a worse frustration of life if the gravely deformed fetus were to die at once—wasting the miracle of its creation and its development so far—or if it were to continue to grow in utero, to be born, and to live only a short and crippled life. We know that people divide about that question, and we now have a way to describe the division. On one view, immediate death of the fetus, even in a case like this one, is a more terrible frustration of the miracle of life than even a sharply diminished and brief infant life would be, for the latter would at least redeem some small part, however limited, of the natural investment. On the rival view, it would be a worse frustration of life to allow this fetal life to continue because that would add, to the sad waste of a deformed human's biological creation, the further, heartbreaking waste of personal emotional investments made in that life by others but principally by the child himself before his inevitable early death.

We should therefore consider this hypothesis: though almost everyone accepts the abstract principle that it is intrinsically bad when human life, once begun, is frustrated, people disagree about the best answer to the question of whether avoidable premature death is always or invariably the most serious possible frustration of life. Very conservative opinion, on this hypothesis, is grounded in the conviction that immediate death is inevitably a more serious frustration than any option that postpones death, even at the cost of greater frustration in other respects. Liberal opinion, on the same hypothesis, is grounded in the opposite conviction: that in some cases, at least, a choice for premature death minimizes the frustration of life and is therefore not a compromise of the principle that human life is sacred but, on the contrary, best respects that principle.

What reasons do people have for embracing one rather than the other of these positions? It seems plain that whatever they are, they are deep reasons, drawn consciously or unconsciously from a great network of other convictions about the point of life and the moral significance of death. If the hypothesis I just described holds—if conservatives and liberals disagree on whether premature death is always the worst frustration of life—then the disagreement must be in virtue of a more general contrast between religious and philosophical orientations.

So I offer another hypothesis. Almost everyone recognizes, as I have suggested, that a normal, successful human life is the product of two morally significant modes of creative investment in that life, the natural and the human. But people disagree about the relative importance of these modes, not just when abortion is in question but on many other mortal occasions as well. If you believe that the natural investment in a human life is transcendently important, that the gift of life itself is infinitely more significant than anything the person whose life it is may do for himself, important though that may be, you will also believe that a deliberate, premature death is the greatest frustration of life possible, no matter how limited or cramped or unsuccessful the continued life would be.[9] On the other hand, if you assign much greater relative importance to the human contribution to life's creative value, then you will consider the frustration of that contribution to be a more serious evil, and will accordingly see more point in deciding that life should end before further significant human investment is doomed to frustration.

We can best understand some of our serious disagreements about abortion, in other words, as reflecting deep differences about the relative moral importance of the natural and human contributions to the inviolability of individual human lives. In fact, we can make a bolder version of that claim: we can best understand the full range of opinion about abortion, from the most conservative to the most liberal, by ranking each opinion about the relative gravity of the two forms of frustration along a range extending from one extreme position to the other—from treating any frustration of the biological investment as worse than any possible frustration of human investment, through more moderate and complex balances, to the opinion that frustrating mere biological investment in human life barely matters and that frustrating a human investment is always worse.

If we look at the controversy this way, it is hardly surprising that many people who hold views on the natural or biological end of that spectrum are fundamentalist or Roman Catholic or strongly religious in some other orthodox religious faith—people who believe that God is the author of everything natural and that each human fetus is a distinct instance of his most sublime achievement. Our hypothesis explains how orthodox religion can play a crucial role in forming people's opinions about abortion even if they do not believe that a fetus is a person with its own right to life.

That is a significant point. It is widely thought that religious opposition to abortion is premised on the conviction that every human fetus is a person with rights and interests of its own. It is therefore important to see that religious opposition to abortion need not be based on that assumption. I said that many religious traditions, including Roman Catholicism for most of its history, based their opposition to abortion on the different assumption that human life has intrinsic value. The present hypothesis shows how that assumption can ground very fierce, even absolute, opposition to abortion. A strongly orthodox or fundamentalist person can insist that abortion is

---

[9] Many people who hold that view will make exceptions: for capital punishment, for example, and for killing the enemy in war. I cannot consider, in this book, the large and important question of how far these exceptions contradict the principle. But people who believe that the natural contribution to life is paramount for a particular reason—that God has created all life—will obviously not count these as contradictions if they also believe that executing murderers or killing enemy soldiers in a just war is also God's will.

always morally wrong because the deliberate destruction of something created as sacred by God can never be redeemed by any human benefit.

This is not to suggest, however, that only conventionally religious people who believe in a creator God are conservatives about abortion. Many other people stand in awe of human reproduction as a natural miracle. Some of them, as I said, embrace the mysterious but apparently powerful idea that the natural order is in itself purposive and commands respect as sacred. Some prominent conservationists, for example, though hardly religious in the conventional sense, seem to be deeply religious in that one and may be drawn a considerable distance toward the conservative end of the spectrum of opinion I described. They may well think that any frustration of the natural investment in human life is so grave a matter that it is rarely if ever justified—that the pulse in the mud is more profound than any other source of life's value. They might therefore be just as firmly opposed to aborting a seriously deformed fetus as any religiously orthodox conservative would be.

Nor does it follow, on the other hand, that everyone who is religious in an orthodox way or everyone who reveres nature is therefore conservative about abortion. As we have seen, many such people, who agree that unnecessary death is a great evil, are also sensitive to and emphatic about the intrinsic badness of the waste of human investment in life. They believe that the frustration of that contribution—for example, in the birth of a grievously deformed fetus whose investment in its own life is doomed to be frustrated—may in some circumstances be the worse of two evils, and they believe that their religious conviction or reverence for nature is not only consistent with but actually requires that position. Some of them take the same view about what many believe to be an even more problematic case: they say that their religious convictions entail that a woman should choose abortion rather than bear a child when that would jeopardize her investment in her *own* life.

I described extreme positions at two ends of the spectrum: that only natural investment counts in deciding whether abortion wastes human life, and that only human investment counts. In fact, very few people take either of these extreme positions. For most people, the balance is more complex and involves compromise and accommodation rather than giving absolute priority to avoiding frustration of either the natural or the human investment. People's opinions become progressively less conservative and more liberal as the balance they strike gives more weight to the importance of not frustrating the human investment in life; more liberal views emphasize, in various degrees, that a human life is created not just by divine or natural forces but also, in a different but still central way, by personal choice, training, commitment, and decision. The shift in emphasis leads liberals to see the crucial creative investment in life, the investment that must not be frustrated if at all possible, as extending far beyond conception and biological growth and well into a human being's adult life. On that liberal opinion, as I have already suggested, it may be more frustrating of life's miracle when an adult's ambitions, talents, training, and expectations are wasted because of an unforeseen and unwanted pregnancy than when a fetus dies before any significant investment of that kind has been made.

That is an exceptionally abstract description of my understanding of the controversy between conservative and liberal opinion. But it will become less abstract, for I shall try to show how the familiar differences between conservative and liberal views on abortion can be explained by the hypothesis that conservatives and liberals rank the two forms of frustration differently. We must not exaggerate that difference, however. It is a difference in emphasis, though an important one. Most people who take what I call a liberal view of abortion do not deny that the conception of a human life and its steady fetal development toward recognizable human form are matters of great moral importance that count as creative investments. That is why they agree with conservatives that as this natural investment continues, and the fetus develops toward the shape and capacity of an infant, abortion, which wastes that investment, is progressively an event more to be avoided or regretted. Many people who hold conservative opinions about abortion, for their part, recognize the importance of personal creative contributions to a human life; they, too, recognize that a premature death is worse when it occurs not in early infancy but after distinctly human investments of ambition and expectation and love have been made. Conservatives and liberals disagree not because one side wholly rejects a value the other thinks cardinal, but because they take different—sometimes dramatically different—positions about the relative importance of these values, which both recognize as fundamental and profound.

CONSERVATIVE EXCEPTIONS: RECONSIDERING THE NATURAL

I am defending the view that the debate over abortion should be understood as essentially about the following philosophical issue: is the frustration of a biological life, which wastes human life, nevertheless sometimes justified in order to avoid frustrating a human contribution to that life or to other people's lives, which would be a different kind of waste? If so, when and why? People who are very conservative about abortion answer the first of these questions No.

There is an even more extreme position, which holds that abortion is never justified, even when necessary to save the life of the mother. Though that is the official view of the Catholic church and of some other religious groups, only a small minority even of devout Catholics accept it, and even Justice Rehnquist, who dissented in *Roe* v. *Wade*, said that he had little doubt that it would be unconstitutional for states to prohibit abortion when a mother's life was at stake. So I have defined 'very conservative' opinion to permit abortion in this circumstance. This exceedingly popular exception would be unacceptable to all conservatives, as I have said, if they really thought that a fetus is a person with protected rights and interests. It is morally and legally impermissible for any third party, such as a doctor, to murder one innocent person even to save the life of another one. But the exception is easily explicable if we understand conservative opinion as based on a view of the sanctity of life that gives strict priority to the divine or natural investment in life. If either the mother or the fetus must die, then the tragedy of avoidable death and the loss of nature's investment in life is inevitable. But a choice in favor of the mother may well seem justified to very conservative people on the ground that a choice against her would in addition frustrate the personal and social investments in her life; even they want only to minimize the overall frustration of human life, and that requires saving the mother's life in this terrible situation.

The important debate is therefore between people who believe that abortion is permissible *only* when it is necessary to save the mother's life and people who believe that abortion may be morally permissible in other circumstances as well. I shall consider the further exceptions the latter group of people claim, beginning with those that are accepted even by people who regard themselves as moderately conservative about abortion and continuing to those associated with a distinctly liberal position.

Moderate conservatives believe that abortion is morally permissible to end a pregnancy that began in rape. Governor Buddy Roemer of Louisiana, for example, who has declared himself in favor of a ban on abortion, nevertheless vetoed an anti-abortion statute in 1991 because it excepted rape victims only in a manner that he said 'dishonors women . . . and unduly traumatizes victims of rape.'[10] On the a-fetus-is-a-person view, an exception for rape is even harder to justify than an exception to protect the life of the mother. Why should a fetus be made to forfeit its right to live, and pay with its life,

---

[10] See 'Nation's Strictest Abortion Law Enacted in Louisiana over Veto,' *New York Times*, 19 June 1991. The Louisiana legislature overrode Governor Roemer's veto, and the strict anti-abortion law it enacted has been held unconstitutional by two federal courts. See 'Court Backs Overturning of Strict Abortion Law,' *New York Times*, 23 Sept. 1992. In 1992, the Supreme Court refused to review a lower-court decision striking down a similar Guam statute. See Linda Greenhouse, 'Guam Abortion Law; High Court Reaffirms Right to Regulate, but not to Ban,' *New York Times*, 6 Dec. 1992, D2.

for the wrongdoing of someone else? But once again, the exception is much easier to understand when we shift from the claim of fetal personhood to a concern for protecting the divine or natural investment in human life. Very conservative people, who believe that the divine contribution to a human life is everything and the human contribution almost nothing beside it, believe that abortion is automatically and in every case the worst possible compromise of life's inviolability, and they do not recognize an exception for rape. But moderately conservative people, who believe that the natural contribution normally *outweighs* the human contribution, will find two features of rape that argue for an exception.

First, according to every prominent religion, rape is itself a brutal violation of God's law and will, and abortion may well seem less insulting to God's creative power when the life it ends itself began in such an insult. Though rape would not justify violating the rights of an innocent person, it could well diminish the horror conservatives feel at an abortion's deliberate frustration of God's investment in life. In his opinion in *McRae* v. *Califano*, the Hyde amendment case I described in chapter 2, Judge John Dooling summarized testimony by Rabbi David Feldman: 'In the stricter Jewish view abortion is a very serious matter permitted only where there is a threat to life, or to sanity, or a grave threat to mental health and physical well-being. Abortion for rape victims would be allowed, using a field and seed analogy: involuntary implantation of the seed imposes no duty to nourish the alien seed.'[11]

Second, rape is a terrible desecration of its victim's investment in her own life, and even those who count a human investment in life as less important than God's or nature's may nevertheless recoil from so violent a frustration of that human investment. Rape is sickeningly, comprehensively contemptuous because it reduces a woman to a physical convenience, a creature whose importance is exhausted by her genital use, someone whose love and sense of self—aspects of personality particularly at stake in sex—have no significance whatsoever except as vehicles for sadistic degradation.

Requiring a woman to bear a child conceived in such an assault is especially destructive to her self-realization because it frustrates her creative choice not only in sex but in reproduction as well. In the ideal case, reproduction is a joint decision rooted in love and in a desire to continue one's life mixed with the life of another person. In Catholic tradition, and in the imagination of many people who are not Catholics, it is itself an offense against the sanctity of life to make love without that desire: that is the basis of many people's moral opposition to contraception. But we can dispute

[11] 491 F. Supp. 630 (1980), 696.

that sex is valuable only for reproduction, or creative only in that way—as most people do—while yet believing that sex is maximally creative when reproduction is contemplated and desired, and that reproduction frustrates creative power when it is neither. Of course, people in love often conceive by accident, and people not in love sometimes conceive deliberately, perhaps out of a misguided hope of finding love through children. Rape is not just the absence of contemplation and desire, however. For the victim, rape is the direct opposite of these, and if a child is conceived, it will be not only without the victim's desire to reproduce but in circumstances made especially horrible because of that possibility.

Moderate conservatives therefore find it difficult to insist that abortion is impermissible in case of rape. It is sometimes said that conservatives who allow the rape exception but not, for example, an exception for unmarried teenagers whose lives would be ruined by childbirth must be motivated by a desire to punish unmarried women who have sex voluntarily. Though some conservatives may indeed believe that pregnancy is a fit punishment for sexual immorality, our hypothesis shows why conservatives who make only the rape exception do not necessarily hold that appalling view. The grounds on which I said conservatives might make an exception for rape do not extend so forcefully to pregnancies that follow voluntary intercourse. Though many religious people do think that unmarried sex also violates God's will, few consider it as grave as rape, and the argument that an unwanted pregnancy grotesquely frustrates a woman's creative role in framing her own life is weaker when the pregnancy follows voluntary sex. Of course, the difference would not be pertinent at all, as I said, if a fetus were a person with rights and interests of its own, because that person would be completely innocent whatever the nature of level of its mother's guilt.

LIBERAL EXCEPTIONS: PROTECTING LIFE IN EARNEST

Other, more permissive exceptions to the principle that abortion is wrong are associated with a generally liberal attitude toward abortion, and we should therefore expect, on the basis of the hypothesis we are testing, that they will reflect a greater respect for the human contribution to life and a correspondingly diminished concern with the natural. But we must not forget that people's attitudes about abortion range over a gradually changing spectrum from one extreme to the other, and that any sharp distinction between conservative and liberal camps is just an expository convenience.

Liberals think that abortion is permissible when the birth of a fetus would

184 RONALD DWORKIN

have a very bad effect on the quality of lives. The exceptions liberals recognize on that ground fall into two main groups: those that seek to avoid frustration of the life of the child, and those that seek to prevent frustration of the life of the mother and other family members.

Liberals believe that abortion is justified when it seems inevitable that the fetus, if born, will have a seriously frustrated life. That kind of justification is strongest, according to most liberals, when the frustration is caused by a very grave physical deformity that would make any life deprived, painful, frustrating for both child and parent, and, in any case, short. But many liberals also believe that abortion is justified when the family circumstances are so economically barren, or otherwise so unpromising, that any new life would be seriously stunted for that reason. It is important to understand that these exceptions are not based, as they might seem to be, on concern for the rights or interests of the fetus. It is a mistake to suppose that an early fetus has interests of its own; it especially makes no sense to argue that it might have an interest in being aborted. Perhaps we could understand that latter argument to mean that if the fetus does develop into a child, that child would be better off dead. But many liberals find abortion justified even when this is not so. I do not mean to deny that sometimes people would be better off dead—when they are in great and terminal pain, for example, or because their lives are otherwise irremediably frustrated. (We shall be considering the problems posed in such cases later in this book.) But this is rarely true of children born into even very great poverty. Nor is it necessarily true even of children born with terrible, crippling handicaps who are doomed shortly to die; sometimes such children establish relationships and manage achievements that give content and meaning to their lives, and it becomes plain that it is in their interests, and in the interests of those who love and care for them, that they continue living as long as possible. The liberal judgment that abortion is justified when the prospects for life are especially bleak is based on a more impersonal judgment: that the child's existence would be intrinsically a bad thing, that it is regrettable that such a deprived and difficult life must be lived.

Sometimes this liberal judgment is wrongly taken to imply contempt for the lives of handicapped children or adults, or even as a suggestion, associated with loathsome Nazi eugenics, that society would be improved by the death of such people. That is a mistake twice over. First, as I insisted earlier in this chapter, the general question of the relative intrinsic tragedy of different events is very different from any question about the *rights* of people now living or about how they should be treated. The former is a question about the intrinsic goodness or evil of events, the latter about rights and fairness. Second, in any case, the liberal opinion about abortion of deformed fetuses in no way implies that it would be better if even grievously handicapped people were now to die. On the contrary, the very concern the liberal judgment embodies—respect for the human contribution to life and anxiety that it not be frustrated—normally sponsors exactly the opposite conclusion. The investment a seriously handicapped person makes in his own life, in his struggle to overcome his handicap as best he can, is intense, and the investment his family and others make is likely to be intense as well. The liberal position insists that these investments in life should be realized as fully as possible, for as long and as successfully as the handicapped person and his community together can manage; and liberals are even more likely than conservatives to support social legislation that promotes that end. One may think that in the worst of such cases it would have been better had the life in question never begun, that the investment we are so eager to redeem should never have been necessary. But that judgment does not detract from concern for handicapped people; on the contrary, it is rooted in the same fundamental respect for human investment in human life, the same horror at the investment being wasted.

The second distinctly liberal group of exceptions, which take into account the effects of pregnancy and childbirth on the lives of mothers and other family members, are even harder to justify on any presumption that includes the idea that a fetus is a person with rights and interests. But the popularity of these exceptions is immediately explicable once we recognize that they are based on respect for the intrinsic value of human life. Liberals are especially concerned about the waste of the human contribution to that value, and they believe that the waste of life, measured in frustration rather than mere loss, is very much greater when a teenage single mother's life is wrecked than when an early-stage fetus, in whose life human investment has thus far been negligible, ceases to live. That judgment does not, of course, depend on comparing the quality of the mother's life, if her fetus is aborted, with that of the child, had it been allowed to live. Recognizing the sanctity of life does not mean attempting to engineer fate so that the best possible lives are lived overall; it means, rather, not frustrating investments in life that have already been made. For that reason, liberal opinion cares more about the lives that people are now leading, lives in earnest, than about the possibility of other lives to come.

The prospects of a child and of its mother for a fulfilling life obviously each depend very much on the prospects of the other. A child whose birth frustrates the chances of its mother to redeem her own life or jeopardizes her ability to care for the rest of her family is likely, just for that reason, to have a more frustrating life itself. And though many people have become superb parents to disabled or disadvantaged children, and some extraordinary ones have found a special vocation in that responsibility, it will sometimes be a devastating blow to a parent's prospects to have a crippled child rather than a normal one, or a child whose bearing and care will seriously strain family resources.

This is only another instance of the difficulty any theoretical analysis of an intricate personal and social problem, like abortion, must face. Analysis can proceed only by abstraction, but abstraction, which ignores the complexity and interdependencies of real life, obscures much of the content on which each actual, concrete decision is made. So we have no formulas for actual decision but only, at best, a schema for understanding the arguments and decisions that we and other people make in real life. I have argued that we do badly, in understanding and evaluating these decisions and arguments, if we try to match them to procrustean assumptions about fetal personhood or rights. We do better to see them as reflecting more nuanced and individual judgments about how and why human life is sacred, and about which decision of life and death, in all the concrete circumstances, most respects what is really important about life.

There will be disagreement in these judgments, not only between large parties of opinion, like those I have been calling conservative and liberal, but within these parties as well. Indeed, very few people, even those who share the same religion and social and intellectual background, will agree in every case. Nor is it possible for anyone to compose a general theory of abortion, some careful weighing of different kinds or modes of life's frustration from which particular decisions could be generated to fit every concrete case. On the contrary, we discover what we think about these grave matters not in advance of having to decide on particular occasions, but in the course of and by making them.

Where do we stand? I began by suggesting that we must redesign our explanation of the great abortion controversy, our sense of what the argument is an argument about. I have now completed my proposal for that redesign. I said that our new explanation would have important implications for political morality and for constitutional law. I said that it would allow us to see the legal argument about the role of the United States Constitution in a new light, and even cautiously to raise our hopes that Americans and people in other countries where liberty is prized might find a collective solution to the political controversy that all sides could accept with dignity. I shall try to redeem those high promises in the next three chapters. But I shall anticipate my most important conclusion. Seeing the abortion controversy in the fresh light I described will not, of course, end our disagreements about the morality of abortion, because these disagreements are deep and may be perpetual.

But if that fresh light helps us to identify those disagreements as at bottom *spiritual*, that should help bring us together, because we have grown used to the idea, as I said, that real community is possible across deep religious divisions. We might hope for even more—not just for greater tolerance but for a more positive and healing realization: that what we share—our common commitment to the sanctity of life—is itself precious, a unifying ideal we can rescue from the decades of hate.

PART 2: DYING AND LIVING

DEATH AND LIFE

It is a platitude that we live our whole lives in the shadow of death; it is also true that we die in the shadow of our whole lives. Death's central horror is oblivion—the terrifying, absolute dying of the light. But oblivion is not all there is to death; if it were, people would not worry so much about whether their technical, biological lives continue after they have become unconscious and the void has begun, after the light is already dead forever. Death has dominion because it is not only the start of nothing but the end of everything, and how we think and talk about dying—the emphasis we put on dying with 'dignity'—shows how important it is that life ends *appropriately*, that death keeps faith with the way we want to have lived.

We cannot understand what death means to people—why some would rather be dead than existing permanently sedated or incompetent, why others would want to 'fight on' even in terrible pain or even when they are unconscious and cannot savor the fight; why so few people think that whether they live or die once they fall permanently unconscious does not matter to them at all—we cannot understand any of this, or much else that people feel about death, unless we turn away from death for a while and back to life.

In almost every case, someone who is permanently unconscious or incompetent was not born into that condition: the tragedy lies at the end of a life that someone has led in earnest. When we ask what would be best for him, we are not judging only his future and ignoring his past. We worry about the effect of his life's last stage on the character of his life as a whole, as we might worry about the effect of a play's last scene or a poem's last stanza on the entire creative work. That is the familiar but mysterious worry we must now try to analyze.

So far as we know, Socrates was the first philosopher to make prominent the question of how to live well. But both before and after him, philosophers, moralists, priests, prophets, novelists, psychiatrists, poets, and busybodies have also speculated about the circumstances and signs of a good life: about what makes one life successful or meaningful or enviable and another impoverished or wasted or pointless. Those wise and foolish people have given very different answers. Socrates said that a good life consists in self-knowledge, Aristotle that it consists in the perfection of skill and talent, the Catholic philosophers that it consists in devotion and the love of God, Hume in the satisfaction of what one genuinely and naturally wants, Bentham in as much pleasure as possible. Others have taken a more negative view of the idea of a good life. Skeptics say that the very idea that one life could really be any better than another is sanctimonious nonsense.

Few of us are skeptical in that way, but most of us have only ramshackle ideas, not philosophical theories, about what kinds of lives are good ones. We almost all think material comfort well worth having. Dedicated ascetics aside, and all else equal, we consider a life of pain or poverty much worse than a comfortable one, and many people's picture of the most satisfactory life for them includes very great wealth. But even for them, material comfort is only part of the story. For many people, for example, achievement also plays an important part. We want (as people often say) to *do* something with our lives, to leave the world a better place for our having been in it. There are grand forms of that ambition: people aim to invent or discover something marvelous, write great music or poetry or philosophy, liberate a nation or make one just. There are less grand forms: many people want nothing more than to play their part well in a cooperative enterprise like a family or a farm or a team, to have contributed to something important rather than to have done it all themselves. Some people think 'experience' an important component in a good life: they want to have traveled, perhaps to exotic places, to have lived in different ways, to have tried everything. Others take pride in almost the opposite: in rootedness, in belonging to a place, and to national or ethnic or religious traditions into which they believe they have been born, traditions of faith or humor or food or culture. Almost everyone thinks family and friends are an important part of a good life: that a life without special and intense concerns for particular people would lack something crucial.

Most of these different ideas about a good life we hold intuitively and in the background; we do not reexamine them except in moments of special crisis or drama. But these background ideas are always there, guiding decisions and choices that may seem to us automatic, and accounting for at least some part of the exhilaration or boredom or shame or sadness we find ourselves feeling, from time to time, about the way our lives are going. It is absolutely crucial to notice, however, that these various opinions and convictions, however inarticulate or submerged, are *critical* in the sense that they concern what makes a life successful rather than unsuccessful—when someone has made something of his life, not just wasted it. They are not, that is, opinions only about how to make life pleasant or enjoyable minute by minute, day by day.

I want to capture that difference by pointing out a distinction between two kinds of reasons people have for wanting their lives to go one way rather than another. First, everyone has what I shall call *experiential* interests. We all do things because we like the experience of doing them: playing softball, perhaps, or cooking or eating well, or watching football, or seeing *Casablanca* for the twelfth time, or walking in the woods in October, or listening to *The Marriage of Figaro*, or sailing fast just off the wind, or just working hard at something. Pleasures like these are essential to a good life—a life with nothing that is marvelous only because of how it feels would be not pure but preposterous. But the value of these experiences, judged one by one, depends precisely on the fact that we do find them pleasurable or exciting *as experiences*. People who do not enjoy an activity I do—who are bored by my enthusiasm for televised football, for example—are not making a *mistake*; their lives are not worse for not sharing my tastes. My own life would not be worse, or defective in some way, if I found watching football as unpleasant as my wife does. Football—and working hard and eating well—seem good to me, add something to my life, because and when they feel good.

Of course, a great many things are bad as experiences, too: pain, nausea, and listening to most politicians. We take pains to avoid these experiences, and sometimes we dread them. But we do not disapprove of people, if there are any, who don't much mind dental pain or listening to politicians. Nor are these the kinds of experiences, at least within limits, that make a life as a whole worse. My life is not a worse life to have lived—I have nothing to regret, still less to take shame in—because I have suffered in the dentist's chair. That is shown, among other ways, by the fact that our attitude toward these forms of suffering is dramatically time sensitive: we are indifferent about pain we suffer in the dentist's chair once the pain is past.

But most people think that they also have what I shall call *critical* interests: interests that it does make their life genuinely better to satisfy, interests they would be mistaken, and genuinely worse off, if they did not recognize. Convictions about what helps to make a life good on the whole are convictions about those more important interests. They represent critical judgments rather than just experiential preferences. Most people enjoy and want close friendships because they believe that such friendships are good, that people *should* want them. I have many opinions about what is good for me in that critical sense. I feel that it is important that I have a close relationship with my children, for example, that I manage some success in my work, and—what I despair of achieving—that I secure some grasp, even if only desperately minimal, of the state of advanced science of my era. I do think my life would have been worse had I never understood the importance of being close to my children, for example, if I had not suffered pain at estrangements from them. Having a close relationship with my children is not important just because I happen to want the experience; on the contrary, I believe a life without wanting it would be a much worse one.[12]

I do not mean that experiential interests are characteristically frivolous or critical interests inevitably profound. There is nothing frivolous about Mozart or particularly profound about my laughable attempts to understand cosmology. Nor am I trying to contrast supposedly elite, reflective, philosophical lives with more ordinary or mundane ones. I mean to identify what is elite, in the sense of aspirational, within most lives. Nor am I saying that people who do not consciously reflect on how their lives are going as a whole, who just get on with living, taking things as they come, are defective or not living well. Lives like that can be extremely attractive, even enviable, and they are plainly preferable to lives ruined by detailed planning and constant trial-balance-sheet assessments of progress. I do believe, however, that even people whose lives feel unplanned are nevertheless often guided by a sense of the general style of life they think appropriate, of what choices strike them as not only good at the moment but in character for them.

We need the distinction between experiential and critical interests to understand many of our convictions about how people should be treated. We need it, for example, to explain why we think that mind-changing drugs or other forms of brainwashing that produce long-lasting pleasure and contentment are not in their victims' interests: we mean they are not in their *critical* interests. Understanding the difference between experiential and critical interests is also essential to understanding a certain kind of tragedy, in life as well as in fiction. It is tragic when someone looks back on his life, near the end, and finds it wasted, empty of any real significance, with nothing in which he can take any pride at all. The classic literary exposition of that sense of waste is Tolstoy's account of the death of Ivan Ilyich.

Worse than his physical sufferings were his mental sufferings, which were his chief torture . . . 'What if in reality my whole life has been wrong?' It occurred to him that

---

[12] The distinction between critical and experiential interests raises a number of interesting philosophical questions, and though we do not need to consider them in this discussion I shall mention two. First, do rational people always have either a critical or an experiential reason for wanting something for themselves? Is it rational for someone to want to do something—collect stamps, succeed in business, or travel, for example—even though he does not expect to enjoy doing it, and does not think his life will be a better one for having done it, but only because it is a goal he has set himself, for instance, or for no reason at all? Second, if someone's experiential interests— what he enjoys doing—conflict with what he takes to be his critical interests, does it make sense for him to ask what he should do *all things considered*, what would be in his best interests *overall*? I have discussed these and other similar issues in my 'Foundations of Liberal Equality.'

what had appeared utterly impossible the night before—that he had not lived his life as he should have done—might after all be true. It struck him that those scarcely detected inclinations of his to fight against what the most highly placed people regarded as good, those scarcely noticeable impulses which he had immediately suppressed, might have been the real thing and all the rest false. And his professional duties, and his ordering of his life, and his family, and all his social and official interests might all have been false. He tried to defend it all to himself. And suddenly he realized the weakness of what he was defending. There was nothing to defend. 'But if that is so,' he said to himself, 'and I am leaving this life with the consciousness that I have lost all that was given me and there's no putting it right—what then?'[13]

We cannot explain that terrible kind of regret if we think, as some philosophers have, that the only interests people have are experiential ones. The converted hedonist, or man of property and power, who enjoyed his life fully day by day may now regret the enjoyment, too. He may say that his pleasure was superficial or thin or incomplete. But that is a critical judgment made now, in retrospect, from the perspective of his new convictions, not a new discovery about the actual felt quality of the experiences he had then.

It is not at all puzzling why we all care about our experiential interests. Nothing is more natural than any animal's desire to put itself in the way of pleasure and out of the way of pain. If lying in the sun or listening to music gives us great pleasure, and dental drills and electrical shocks and nausea are very disagreeable, then it is hardly surprising that we seek out the former and try to avoid the latter. But it might seem puzzling why people should also care about their critical interests or even have the concept of such interests. Why should Ivan Ilyich, who in the past had exactly what gave him pleasure, despair at the end of his life that he has made a mistake, that he should have chosen a radically different kind of life? Why should some people—saints and some artists—deliberately choose lives of discomfort, even poverty, in order to do something they regard as more valuable than simple enjoyment? Why should people care about not 'wasting' their lives? Why should they care about anything except having as good a time as possible?

Jeremy Bentham and other utilitarian philosophers denied that people ever do care about anything else. Bentham might have said that Ivan Ilyich was really worried that he might have had even more pleasure than he did if he had devoted himself less to profit and status. But that is a very poor account of the regret people feel when they think they have led the wrong kind of life. They feel not that they could have had a more enjoyable time leading a different life but that having a good time is not, after all, as important as they thought. They want, suddenly, to have made something,

---

[13] Leo Tolstoy, *The Death of Ivan Ilyich and Other Stories*, trans. Rosemary Edmonds (New York: Penguin, 1960), 157.

or contributed to something, or helped someone, or been closer to more people, not just because these were missed opportunities for more pleasure but because they are important in themselves. And even people who do regret missed opportunities for pleasure do so as *critical* hedonists: they believe that the experience of pleasure is a kind of achievement.

Can we explain critical interests? I do not mean a Darwinian theory that explains, if any evolutionary account can explain, why the species developed the beliefs that some lives are more worth living than others and that it is a matter for regret when the wrong life has been lived, even if it was a pleasant one. Nor do I mean a biological account that explains how people are genetically disposed to these ideas, or a social-scientific one that shows how these ideas are carried in or restricted by culture. We need an *intellectual* explanation of critical interests, so that we may better understand these ideas from the inside, understand introspectively how they connect with other large beliefs we have about life and death and why human life has intrinsic value.

Is it merely a brute fact that some of us happen to want friendship or achievement for its own sake, not just as a pleasurable experience? That we sometimes change our minds about what we want for its own sake, and then regret our previous choices? That flat account greatly understates the psychological complexity of the matter, viewed from the inside, because it leaves mysterious why we should be *puzzled* about what kind of life is best for us. And puzzled we often are.

Think of someone—yourself, if you can—facing an important self-defining decision. If you are a woman with a chance to begin a demanding career that intrigues you, but only by sacrificing time with your young children, which choice do you make? Or, if you are a law-school graduate with an offer from an established firm, do you reject it for a less challenging offer that is more likely—but by no means certain—to lead to a political career later? Or, if you are a Jew, should you abandon your comfortable life in Los Angeles and emigrate to Israel to identify yourself firmly with that nation's fate?

People do not make momentous decisions like these by trying to predict how much pleasure each choice might bring them. We sometimes say that we discover our own identities through such decisions. But we do not mean that we discover how we have already been wired, as, we might say, a computer 'discovers' its own programming. We can search our past for clues about what satisfies us or makes us happy, but life-shaping decisions are also occasions for imaginative fantasy and, above all, for commitment. People are often deeply uncertain about which decision is right: we shift and change before we settle, if we ever do, into the comfort of firm conviction. Some of us believe that each person's nature is fixed by biology or society, that whatever ambitions we have are built into us by genetics or culture. But even so, our built-in ambitions are more complex and abstract than merely to lead one particular kind of life or another. We have the abstract ambition to lead a *good* life, and we worry, some of us all our lives, about what that is.

People think it important not just that their life contain a variety of the right experiences, achievements, and connections, but that it have a structure that expresses a coherent choice among these—for some, that it display a steady, self-defining commitment to a vision of character or achievement that the life as a whole, seen as an integral creative narrative, illustrates and expresses. Of course, this ideal of integrity does not itself define a way to live: it presupposes substantive convictions. No one who thinks his life has been based on mistake will take comfort from seeing that it was based on only one mistake. But integrity nevertheless has great independent importance in life as it does in art and science. We admire the person who does it his way, even if that is very much not our way. Integrity is closely connected to dignity, moreover: we think that someone who acts out of character, for gain or to avoid trouble, has insufficient respect for himself.[14]

Recognizing the independent importance of integrity helps us to understand much that would otherwise be puzzling in the idea of critical interests. When we reflect about what makes a person's life good, we are torn between what seem to be antagonistic beliefs. On the one hand, a person's critical interests seem very much to depend on his personality. The commitment someone makes to a given conception of virtue or achievement—to his Jewish roots, for example—is part of what makes a life organized around that commitment right for him. But that appealing idea is hard to reconcile with an even more fundamental conviction we also have—that a person's thinking a given choice right for him does not make it so, that the sometimes agonized process of decision is a process of judgment, not just choice, that it may go wrong, that one may be *mistaken* about what is really important in life. That belief is indispensable to the basic distinction between critical and experiential interests, and to the challenge and tragedy most people feel. It is at the very foundation of our ethical lives.

The first of these two ideas—that our critical interests are personal— seems to pull us toward the annihilating idea that critical interests are only subjective, only matters of how we feel. The second seems to pull us toward the equally unacceptable idea that everyone's critical interests are the same, over all history, that there is only one truly best way for anyone to live. The remedy is to embrace neither of these extreme positions but instead to

---

[14] See Bernard Williams, 'A Critique of Utilitarianism,' in J. J. C. Smart and Bernard Williams, *Utilitarianism: For and Against* (Cambridge: Cambridge University Press, 1973).

194   RONALD DWORKIN

remind ourselves of how it feels to believe that a given life is the right one. We feel this not as a discovery of a timeless formula, good for all times and places, but as a direct response to our own specific circumstances of place, culture, and capacity. The response, however, includes conviction: it is important both that we find a life *good* and that we *find* it good. Integrity plays two parts in this story: it is the mark of conviction, of commitment, not just past choice; it also reflects investment, the idea that the value of a life lies in part *in* its integrity, so that its having already been established as one kind of life argues, though of course far from conclusively, that it should go on being that kind of life.

As I said, some philosophers are deeply skeptical about the whole idea that people have critical interests, that there is any inherent difference between a 'good' or a 'bad' life beyond how pleasant or enjoyable it is. They say that there is nothing for people to be agonized about, that Ivan Ilyich was silly or demented, that the illusion of critical interests is just what the Oxford biologist Richard Dawkins has called religion—a computer virus passed from one human brain to another down many centuries[15]—that from the point of view of the universe, it makes no difference whatsoever how people live. My purpose, here as throughout this book, is not to defend the various ethical or religious convictions I am describing from skeptical attacks of this sort but to observe how widespread and powerful these convictions are, and how pervasive an influence they have over our various moral and political beliefs, including those about abortion and euthanasia.

But it might be helpful to distinguish two forms the skeptical attack takes, because the difference is important. The first we might call an external form. It purports to criticize the way people think about their lives on the basis of some general philosophical position about metaphysics or the ultimate nature of reality. The British philosopher John Mackie, for example, said that there could not be objective values in the universe, because they would be such 'queer' kinds of entities.[16] That form of skepticism is disengaged from the human enterprise it criticizes: it bases its criticism on an a priori and wholly general assumption about the kinds of entity or truth or knowledge that are metaphysically possible. It aims to change not how we lead our lives but the philosophical claims we make. External skepticism always fails, in my view, because it cannot characterize the external claims it criticizes, except in uncashable metaphors about 'queer' entities and the like.[17] But in

[15] *The Independent*, 16 Apr. 1992.
[16] J. L. Mackie, *Ethics: Inventing Right and Wrong* (New York: Penguin, 1977).
[17] See R. Dworkin, 'Pragmatism, Right Answers, and True Banality,' in Michael Brint and William Weaver (eds.), *Pragmatism in Law and Society* (Boulder, Colo.: Westview Press, 1991).

any case, external skepticism is unthreatening, because we can embrace it, if we wish, and continue to live and feel as we have before.

The second kind of skepticism—internal skepticism—is a very different matter. It is the disabling substantive skepticism of the person who is suddenly gripped by the implications, as he thinks, of discovering that there is no God; or of someone like Goncharov's gray hero, Oblomov, who suddenly sees no point in anything, no reason to leave his bed; or of most of us, sometime, in the black hours, when the idea that it is important how we live—when anyway we will soon be dead—suddenly seems irretrievably preposterous. This skepticism is dangerous exactly because it plays the same structuring role for people in its grip, except in a draining, negative way, that positive convictions play for those who embrace them.

The philosophical standing of internal skepticism is no different from that of the positive convictions it challenges; it, too, claims authority only on the basis of what we cannot but think when we ask the questions it answers. If it is true, it is true in exactly the same way, and with no more independent foundation in an objective world, than the positive opinions it mocks. That is why it is so dangerous. There is no answer to internal skepticism once it has taken hold except to test it again by measuring the conviction it finally brings. Most people then find that it has loosened its grip.[18]

DEATH'S MEANING

We have explored the complex idea of critical interests because we cannot think about whether death is in someone's best interests unless we understand this dimension of the interests people have. It would be easy to decide whether it was in the best interests of Lillian Boyes or Nancy Cruzan or Janet Adkins to live or die if we had only their experiential interests in mind. Lillian Boyes had only pain to look forward to, and no pleasurable experiences that could possibly compensate for its experiential horror, so it was plainly in her interests, measured that way, to die as soon as possible. Nancy Cruzan would never have any experience, good or bad, again, so her experiential interests would not be affected by a decision either way. Janet Adkins probably had more to gain in pleasant experience by living on until a natural death—she would have remained capable of simple pleasures for

---

[18] I do not mean that while internal skepticism is true, we should try to shake it off and live in delusion. We have no more reason for thinking that it does not matter how we live, if we feel that it does, than the other way around. If we believe that it does matter, then that is what we think is true, even though others disagree, and it would be silly, and contradictory, to say that it isn't really true, or that we are just pretending it is.

several years, and many demented people do not suffer at all—so she was wrong to kill herself when she did if her experiential life was all that mattered.

Several opinions in the House of Lords decision in the *Bland* case I mentioned simply assumed that only experiential interests can matter, at least legally, and therefore had no difficulty in deciding that it could be neither in *nor* against Anthony Bland's interests that his life support be discontinued. Lord Mustill, for example, considered and rejected the argument that it was against Bland's interests that his body was full of tubes to no point or that his family's happy recollections of him were being replaced by horrific ones or that his situation was causing them great misery; that cannot be so, Mustill said, because 'he does not know what is happening to his body and cannot be affronted by it; he does not know of his family's continuing sorrow. . . . The distressing truth which must not be shirked is that [discontinuing life support] is not in the best interests of Anthony Bland, for he has no best interests of any kind.'[19]

If we accept this view that only experiential interests count, we can make no sense of the widespread, near, universal, view I described: that decisions like those we have been reviewing are often personally problematic and racking. We agonize about these decisions, for ourselves when we are contemplating living wills, or for relatives and friends, only or mainly because we take our and their critical interests into account. We must therefore begin by asking: how does it matter to the critical success of our whole life how we die? We should distinguish between two different ways that it might matter: because death is the far boundary of life, and every part of our life, including the very last, is important; and because death is special, a peculiarly significant event in the narrative of our lives, like the final scene of a play, with everything about it intensified, under a special spotlight. In the first sense, when we die is important because of what will happen to us if we die later; in the second, how we die matters because it is how we *die*.

Let us begin with the first, less theatrical, of these ideas. Sometimes people want to live on, even though in pain or dreadfully crippled, in order to do something they believe important to have done. They want to finish a job, for example, or to learn something they have always wanted to know. Gareth Evans, a brilliant philosopher who died of cancer at the age of thirty-four, struggled to work on his unfinished manuscript as long as medicine could keep him in a condition in which he could work at all.[20] Many people want to

---

[19] *Airedale Trust (Respondents)* v. *Bland*, 45–6.

[20] *The Varieties of Reference* (Oxford: Oxford University Press, 1982) was finished and revised by his colleague John McDowell, now a professor of philosophy at the University of Pittsburgh, and it has become a classic in the philosophy of language.

live on, as long as they can, for a more general reason: so long as they have any sense at all, they think, just being alive is *something*. Though Philip Roth had persuaded his eighty-six-year-old father to sign a living will, he hesitated when his father was dying and the doctors asked whether Roth wanted him put on a respirator. Roth thought, 'How could I take it on myself to decide that my father should be finished with life, life which is ours to know just once?'[21]

On the other hand, people often think they have strong reasons of a comparable kind for *not* staying alive. The badness of the experiences that lie ahead is one: terrible pain or constant nausea or the horror of intubation or the confusions of sedation. When Roth thought about the misery to come, he whispered, 'Dad, I'm going to have to let you go.' But people's reasons for wanting to die include critical reasons as well; many people, as I said, think it undignified or bad in some other way to live under certain conditions, however they might feel if they feel at all. Many people do not want to be remembered living in those circumstances; others think it degrading to be wholly dependent, or to be the object of continuing anguish. These feelings are often expressed as a distaste for causing trouble, pain, or expense to others, but the aversion is not fully captured in that other-regarding preference. It may be just as strong when the burden of physical care is imposed on professionals whose career is precisely in providing such care, and when the financial burden falls on a public eager to bear it. At least part of what people fear about dependence is its impact not on those responsible for their care, but on their own dignity.

I must emphasize that this is *not* a belief that every kind of dependent life under severe handicaps is not worth living. That belief is disproved not only by dramatic examples, like the brilliant life of Stephen Hawking, the almost wholly paralyzed cosmologist, but by the millions of ordinary people throughout the world who lead engaged, valuable lives in spite of appalling handicaps and dependencies. It is, however, plausible, and to many people compelling, that total dependence is in itself a very bad thing, quite apart from the pain or discomfort it often but not invariably entails. Total or near-total dependence with nothing positive to redeem it may seem not only to add nothing to the overall quality of a life but to take something important from it. That seems especially true when there is no possibility even of understanding that care has been given, or of being grateful for it. Sunny von Bulow still lies wholly unconscious in a hospital room in Manhattan; every day she is turned and groomed by people willing and paid to do it. She will never respond in any way to that care. It would not have been odd for her

---

[21] Philip Roth, *Patrimony* (New York: Simon & Schuster, 1991), 232–3.

to think, before she fell into her coma, that this kind of pointless solicitude was insulting, itself an affront to her dignity.

When patients remain conscious, their sense of integrity and of the coherence of their lives crucially affects their judgment about whether it is in their best interests to continue to live. Athletes, or others whose physical activity was at the center of their self-conception, are more likely to find a paraplegic's life intolerable. When Nancy B., the Canadian woman who won the right to have her respirator turned off, said that all she had in her life was television, she was saying not that watching television was painful, but that a wholly passive life, which watching television had come to symbolize, was worse than none. For such people, a life without the power of motion is unacceptable, not for reasons explicable in experiential terms, but because it is stunningly inadequate to the conception of self around which their own lives have so far been constructed. Adding decades of immobility to a life formerly organized around action will for them leave a narrative wreck, with no structure or sense, a life worse than one that ends when its activity ends.

Others will have radically different senses of self, of what has been critically important to their own lives. Many people, for example, would want to live on, almost no matter how horrible their circumstances, so long as they were able to read, or understand if read to them, the next day's newspaper. They would want to hear as many chapters as possible of the many thousands of stories about science and culture and politics and society that they had been following all their lives. People who embrace that newspaper test have assumed, and cannot easily disown, that part of the point of living is to know and care how things are turning out.

So people's views about how to live color their convictions about when to die, and the impact is intensified when it engages the second way in which people think death is important. There is no doubt that most people treat the manner of their deaths as of special, symbolic importance: they want their deaths, if possible, to express and in that way vividly to confirm the values they believe most important to their lives. That ancient hope is a recurrent theme of Shakespearean drama. (Siward, for example, learning that Macbeth has killed Young Siward at Dunsinane in that poor boy's first battle, says: 'Had I as many sons as I have hairs, I would not wish them to a fairer death.') When the great British political columnist Peter Jenkins realized on his deathbed that any conversation might be his last, he insisted on talking, though his nurses warned him not to, and on talking about political philosophy and the latest threats to free speech.

The idea of a good (or less bad) death is not exhausted by how one dies—whether in battle or in bed—but includes timing as well. It explains the premium people often put on living to 'see' some particular event, after which the idea of their own death seems less tragic to them. A woman dying of cancer, whose life can be prolonged though only in great pain, might think she had good reason to live until the birth of an expected grandchild, or a long-awaited graduation, or some other family milestone. The aim of living not just until, but actually for, an event has very great expressive power. It confirms, in a fashion much exploited by novelists and dramatists, the critical importance of the values it identifies to the patient's sense of his own integrity, to the special character of his life. If his has been a life rooted in family, if he has counted, as among the high peaks of his life, family holidays and congresses and celebrations, then stretching his life to include one more such event does not merely add to a long list of occasions and successes. Treating the next one as salient for death confirms the importance of them all.

Many people have a parallel reason for wanting to die if an unconscious, vegetable life were all that remained. For some, this is an understandable worry about how they will be remembered. But for most, it is a more abstract and self-directed concern that their death, whatever else it is like, express their conviction that life has had value because of what life made it possible for them to do and feel. They are horrified that their death might express, instead, the opposite idea, which they detest as a perversion: that mere biological life—just hanging on—has independent value. Nietzsche said, 'In a certain state it is indecent to live longer. To go on vegetating in cowardly dependence on physicians and machinations, after the meaning of life, the right to life, has been lost, that ought to prompt a profound contempt in society.' He said he wanted 'to die proudly when it is no longer possible to live proudly.'[22] That concern might make no sense for unconscious patients in a world where everyone treated the onset of permanent unconsciousness as itself the event of death, the final curtain after which nothing else is part of the story. But in such a world, no one would be kept alive in permanent unconsciousness anyway. No one would need worry, as many people in our world do, that others will feed or care for his vegetating body with what he believes the ultimate insult: the conviction that they do it for *him*.

The relatives I mentioned, who visit permanently unconscious patients regularly, and feel uncomfortable or anxious when they cannot, do not necessarily have that conviction. They come because they cannot bear not to see and touch someone they love so long as that is possible and not bad for him, and because they think that closing the final door before he is biologically

---

[22] Friedrich Nietzsche, 'The Twilight of the Idols,' in *The Complete Works of Friedrich Nietzsche*, ed. Oscar Levy and trans. Anthony M. Ludovici (Russell & Russell, 1909–11; repr. 1964), xvi. 88.

dead and buried or cremated—before they can *mourn* him—would be a terrible betrayal, a declaration of indifference rather than the intense concern they still feel. There is no contradiction, but great force and sense, in the views of parents who fight, in court if necessary, to have life support terminated but who will not leave their child's side until it is. But some people do believe—as Mr. Wanglie believed about his wife—that it *is* in a patient's best interests to be kept alive as long as possible, even in an unconscious state. For such people, contemplating themselves in that position, integrity delivers a very different command. The struggle to stay alive, no matter how hopeless or how thin the life, expresses a virtue central to *their* lives, the virtue of defiance in the face of inevitable death. It is not just a matter of taste on which people happen to divide, as they divide about surfing or soccer. None of us wants to end our lives out of character.

Now we can better answer the question of why people think what they do about death, and why they differ so dramatically. Whether it is in someone's best interests that his life end in one way rather than another depends on so much else that is special about him—about the shape and character of his life and his own sense of his integrity and critical interests—that no uniform collective decision can possibly hope to serve everyone even decently. So we have that reason of beneficence, as well as reasons of autonomy, why the state should not impose some uniform, general view by way of sovereign law but should encourage people to make provision for their future care themselves, as best they can, and why if they have made no provision the law should so far as possible leave decisions in the hands of their relatives or other people close to them whose sense of their best interests—shaped by intimate knowledge of everything that makes up where their best interests lie—is likely to be much sounder than some universal, theoretical, abstract judgment born in the stony halls where interest groups maneuver and political deals are done.

SANCTITY AND SELF-INTEREST

Let us turn now to what I said was a separate issue: how far euthanasia in its various forms—suicide, assisting suicide, or withholding medical treatment or life support—may be wrong even if it *is* in a patient's best interests. In discussing abortion, I defended a particular understanding of the sanctity of life: that once a human life has begun, it is a waste—an inherently bad event—when the investment in that life is wasted. I distinguished between two different dimensions of the investment in a human life that a decision for death might be thought to waste—what I called the natural and the human dimensions—and I used that distinction to construct a distinctly conservative view about abortion: that the natural investment in a human life is dominantly more important than the human investment, and that choosing premature death is therefore the greatest possible insult to life's sacred value. We can use the same distinction to construct a distinctly conservative view about euthanasia. If we adopt the view congenial to many religious traditions, that nature's investment in a human life has been frustrated whenever someone dies who could be kept technically alive longer, then any human intervention—injecting a lethal drug into someone dying of a painful cancer or withdrawing life support from a person in a persistent vegetative state—cheats nature, and if the natural investment, understood in that way, dominates the sanctity of life, then euthanasia always insults that value. That argument, I believe, forms the most powerful basis for the strong conservative opposition to all forms of euthanasia throughout the world. It is not, of course, the only argument: people worry about practical and administrative issues, and they are terrified lest they license the death of someone who might have been restored to a genuine life. But the instinct that deliberate death is a savage insult to the instrinsic value of life, even when it is in the patient's interest, is the deepest, most important part of the conservative revulsion against euthanasia. Justices Rehnquist and Scalia, as we saw, both relied on that instinct in their decisions in the *Cruzan* case.

The instinct is central to many religious traditions. In its most straightforward formulation, as we saw, the appeal to the sanctity of life uses the image of property: a person's life belongs not to him but to God. But some religious leaders and scholars have put the point more formally: by distinguishing, as I have, between the question of when keeping someone alive is good for him and when it is good because it respects a value he embodies. Richard Neuhaus, for example, in an influential article in *Commentary*, aligned himself with critics of 'rational quality-of-life measurement' who contend 'that the question whether life is good for the person gets things backwards.' 'The argument of the critics,' he said, 'is that life is a good *of* the person.'[23] An article on Jewish views of euthanasia said, 'According to Jewish law, life is to be preserved, even at great cost. Each moment of human life is considered to be intrinsically sacred. Preserving life supersedes living the "good life." '[24]

We know, however, that the idea that human life is sacred or inviolable is both more complex, and more open to different and competing

[23] Richard John Neuhaus, 'The Return of Eugenics,' *Commentary* (Apr. 1988), 22.
[24] Byron L. Sherwin, 'Jewish Views of Euthanasia,' in M. Kohl (ed.), *Beneficent Euthanasia* (Buffalo, NY: Prometheus Books, 1975), 1, 7.

interpretations, than its religious use sometimes acknowledges, and we can construct other interpretations of that idea that ground more liberal attitudes toward euthanasia. Even people who accept the dominance of the natural investment in life (and who hold very conservative views about abortion for that reason) may nevertheless disagree that euthanasia inevitably frustrates nature. They may plausibly believe that prolonging the life of a patient who is riddled with disease or no longer conscious does nothing to help realize the natural wonder of a human life, that nature's purposes are not served when plastic, suction, and chemistry keep a heart beating in a lifeless, mindless body, a heart that nature, on its own, would have stilled.

That is a less conservative view because it denies that biological death always cheats nature. But suppose we also deny that the natural contribution to life is dominant, and insist that the human contribution is important as well, and that it, too, should not be frustrated or wasted. Then we will have a much stronger reason for denying that euthanasia always insults the sanctity of life: we will then insist that sometimes euthanasia *supports* that value. In order to see this, we must now elaborate—and qualify—a distinction that I have emphasized throughout this book: the distinction between the question of what acts or events are in some creature's interests and the question of what acts or events respect the sanctity of that creature's life. The idea I introduced in this chapter—that people have critical as well as experiential interests—complicates that distinction.

Anyone who believes in the sanctity of human life believes that once a human life has begun it matters, intrinsically, that that life go well, that the investment it represents be realized rather than frustrated. Someone's convictions about his own critical interests are opinions about what it means for his *own* human life to go well, and these convictions can therefore best be understood as a special application of his general commitment to the sanctity of life. He is eager to make something of his own life, not simply to enjoy it; he treats his own life as something sacred for which *he* is responsible, something *he* must not waste. He thinks it intrinsically important that he live well, and with integrity. That objective, intrinsic importance is just what the internal form of skepticism threatens; that is why it sometimes seems so irresistible.

Someone who thinks his own life would go worse if he lingered near death on a dozen machines for weeks or stayed biologically alive for years as a vegetable believes that he is showing more respect for the human contribution to the sanctity of his life if he makes arrangements in advance to avoid that, and that others show more respect for his life if they avoid it for him. We cannot sensibly argue that he must sacrifice his own interests out of respect for the inviolability of human life. That begs the question, because he thinks dying is the best way to respect that value. So the appeal to the sanctity of life raises here the same crucial political and constitutional issue that it raises about abortion. Once again the critical question is whether a decent society will choose coercion or responsibility, whether it will seek to impose a collective judgment on matters of the most profound spiritual character on everyone, or whether it will allow and ask its citizens to make the most central, personality-defining judgments about their own lives for themselves.

I have not defended any detailed legal scheme for deciding when doctors may hasten the death of patients who understandably want to die or of unconscious patients who cannot make that choice. My main concern has been to understand why people hold the apparently mysterious opinions they do about their own deaths, and to show what is really at stake in the heated public discussion of euthanasia. Part of the public discussion, as I have emphasized, centers on difficult and important administrative questions I have not considered. But much of it concerns moral and ethical issues, and that part of the debate has been seriously compromised by two misunderstandings that we have noticed but which it would be wise to mention again by way of summary.

The first is a confusion about the character of the interests people have in when and how they die. Many arguments against euthanasia presuppose that patients who are not suffering great pain, including patients who are permanently unconscious, cannot be significantly harmed by being kept alive. That assumption underlies, as we saw, the procedural claim that relatives urging that an unconscious patient would have wanted to die must meet an especially severe standard of proof, the 'slippery slope' argument that the law should license no euthanasia because it may end by licensing too much, and the claim that doctors will be corrupted and their sense of humanity dulled if they are asked and allowed to kill. When we understand how and why people care about their deaths, we see that the assumption on which each of these arguments depends is fallacious and dangerous.

The second misunderstanding arises from a misapprehension about an idea we have been studying throughout this book and which we just considered again: the sanctity of life. It is widely supposed that active euthanasia—doctors killing patients who beg to die—is always offensive to that value, and should be prohibited for that reason. But the question posed by euthanasia is not whether the sanctity of life should yield to some other value, like humanity or compassion, but how life's sanctity should be understood and respected. The great moral issues of abortion and euthanasia, which bracket life in earnest, have a similar structure. Each involves decisions not just about the rights and interests of particular people, but about the intrinsic, cosmic importance of human life itself. In each case, opinions divide not because some people have contempt for values that others cherish, but, on the contrary, because the values in question are at the center of everyone's lives, and no one can treat them as trivial enough to accept other people's orders about what they mean. Making someone die in a way that others approve, but he believes a horrifying contradiction of his life, is a devastating, odious form of tyranny.

8

TAKING AND SAVING LIVES

ERIC RAKOWSKI

INTRODUCTION

Sometimes it is morally imperative, or at any rate morally permissible, to keep alive as many people as possible. If rescue workers must choose between groups of thirty and five equally blameless people trapped in mine shafts, or caught in a burning apartment building, or floundering in the sea, most people think they ought to save the larger group straightaway. Or at least most think that the rescuers earn no censure if they aid the larger group simply because that will save more lives. The same is generally true if a runaway trolley will kill five workers unless a bystander shunts it onto a side track, where it will kill but one: the right course—certainly in most cases an irreproachable course—is to divert the train. But the number of lives saved is not always all that matters. Suppose that a surgeon can anesthetize a healthy visitor to her office and remove his vital organs to save five dying patients. Nobody, to my knowledge, would condone trading one life for five.[1]

From Eric Rakowski, 'Taking and Saving Lives,' *Columbia Law Review*, 93/5 (June 1993), 1063–1156.

For helpful written comments. I would like to thank Roger Crisp. Meir Dan-Cohen, Kent Greenawalt, Sanford Kadish. Robert Post, Judith Thomson, and Jeremy Waldron. I am also grateful to participants in Columbia Law School's Legal. Theory Workshop for criticisms and suggestions.

[1] The so-called 'trolley problem'—the problem of explaining why it is morally permissible to turn the trolley toward the single worker even though it is ordinarily impermissible to kill one person to save five others, as in the organ transplant case—has generated a voluminous literature. See generally Judith Jarvis Thomson, 'The Trolley Problem,' *Yale Law Journal*, 94 (1985), 1395, 1409 (advocating saving the greater number when the means do not violate the victim's right not to be killed); Judith Jarvis Thomson, *The Realm of Rights* (1990), 177–202 (appealing to the parties' antecedent advantage in deciding how to act); Philippa Foot, 'The Problem of Abortion and the Doctrine of the Double Effect,' in *Virtues and Vices and Other Essays in Moral Philosophy* (Oxford: Blackwell, 1978) (emphasizing the moral difference between positive and negative duties); Michael J. Costa, 'The Trolley Problem Revisited,' *S. J. Phil.*, 24 (1986), 437 (defending the Principle of Double Effect); 'Another Trip on the Trolley,' *Journal of Philosophy*, 25 (1987), 461 (modified defense of the Principle of Double Effect); F. M. Kamm, 'Harming Some to Save Others,' *Philosophical Studies*, 57 (1989), 227 (claiming that the causal proximity of acts to harms and benefits is morally crucial); James A. Montmarquet, 'On Doing Good: The Right and the Wrong Way,' *Journal of Philosophy*, 79 (1982), 446–9 (stressing the moral difference between

Why may, or must, the number of survivors be maximized in some instances but not others? The answer, I suggest, is fundamentally the same for cases in which one or more people must be killed so that others may live and cases in which only some of those imperiled can be saved but none must be slain to preserve the rest, as when a rescue ship can save the passengers of only one of two capsized boats. The killing of an innocent human being ordinarily cannot be justified, in my view, by reference to some greater good that his death might accomplish.[2] However, if somebody would reasonably have favored killing under certain circumstances—because, for example, that course would tend to maximize the number of lives saved and thus antecedently reduce her own risk of dying—then killing that person to save others is morally permissible, or even commendable.

In addition, people may, I argue, be killed to save a larger number of others if several conditions are met: (1) a majority of those affected by a life-saving decision either endorsed a policy maximizing the number of lives saved or would have welcomed that policy in the circumstances in which they found themselves were they aware of their moral and religious beliefs, their desires and aversion to risk, and their personal abilities and history, but ignorant of whether they would be killed or saved under the policy; (2) those who dissent or who would have dissented for either moral or religious

originating and redirecting threats); Warren S. Quinn, 'Actions, Intentions, and Consequences: The Doctrine of Doing and Allowing,' *Philosophical Review*, 98 (1989), 287 (stressing the moral distinction between initiating and permitting harm); Warren S. Quinn, 'Actions, Intentions, and Consequences: The Doctrine of Double Effect,' *Philosophy & Public Affairs*, 18 (1989), 334 (analyzing the moral appeal of the Doctrine of Double Effect); Don Locke, 'The Choice among Lives,' *Philosophy*, 57 (1982), 453 (defending a version of the Doctrine of Double Effect); Michael Gorr, 'Thomson and the Trolley Problem,' *Philosophical Studies*, 59 (1990), 91 (criticizing Thomson and Montmarquet's distinction between redirecting and creating harmful forces); B. C. Postow, 'Thomson and the Trolley Problem,' *S. J. Phil.*, 27 (1989), 529 (criticizing Thomson's account of the right not to be killed); John M. Fischer, 'The Trolley and the Sorites,' *Yale Journal of Law and Humanities*, 4 (1992), 105 (attempting to 'dissolve' the trolley problem by denying the moral difference between switching the trolley and compelling lethal organ transplants).

John Harris dissents from this philosophical enterprise. He argues that mandatory organ transplant schemes that effect a net saving of lives can be justified in certain circumstances if donors are selected randomly. See John Harris, *Violence and Responsibility* (London: Routledge & Kegan Paul, 1980), 82; 'The Survival Lottery,' repr. in Bonnie Steinbock (ed.) *Killing and Letting Die* (Englewood Cliffs, NJ: Prentice Hall, 1980). A doctor's haphazard choice of a donor from among the people in her waiting room, however, would probably not be random enough to win Harris's approval.

[2] Nevertheless, the defense of oneself or of those for whom one has special concern, even were it not to secure an objectively greater good, would often justify or excuse killing. The line between justification and excuse is frequently hazy and not one I wish to explore here. For helpful discussion, see Kent Greenawalt, 'The Perplexing Borders of Justification and Excuse,' *Columbia Law Review*, 84 (1984), 1897, 1898 (arguing that 'Anglo-American criminal law should not attempt to distinguish between justification and excuse in a fully systematic way'); George P. Fletcher, 'The Right and the Reasonable,' *Harvard Law Review*, (1985), 949, 954–7 (comparing the concepts of justification and excuse in the civil law and common law traditions).

reasons (and not so that they could ride free) under the counterfactual condition just described, and who would be killed if the greater number were saved, could not fairly have been excluded from the benefits of a maximizing scheme; and (3) the dissenters' chances of staying alive would have been boosted by the prior adoption of a maximizing policy.[3]

This view evinces a deep respect, Kantian in inspiration,[4] for people's freely formed preferences consistent with the demands of fairness to all whose lives are threatened. Acting towards those in danger as they would have wanted one to act—not as imaginary rational people with programmed wishes would have chosen, but as these actual persons would have preferred—is, I maintain, the appropriate way to recognize their individuality and autonomy as responsible agents. The principles and reasoning that underlie mainstream accounts of the acceptable limits to paternalistic intervention may be extended to justify acting towards a person in the manner he would have chosen had he been free from the pressures of his life-threatening predicament. Individual autonomy is not, however, the sole value at stake in deciding whether to kill some to save others. Allowing a majority's reasonable preference for a policy that would maximize the number of lives saved to subordinate the contrary preferences of others, if those others cannot be exempted without abandoning the policy, seems to me a disquieting but unavoidable implication of people's moral equality.

Similar considerations should guide decisions to save one of two or more groups of people when no one need be killed but some must be left to die. If a majority of the smaller groups' members would for good reason have supported a policy of saving the most lives before they recognized their plight, and if moral or religious dissenters could not fairly be exempted from a maximizing scheme, rescuers ought to save the greater number.[5] Respect for the threatened people's uncoerced wills, together with the constraints fairness imposes in recognition of people's equality as moral subjects, compels this result. What distinguishes this case from situations in which killing is necessary to save lives is the correct default rule. If some of those facing death would reasonably have opposed a maximizing rule because its

---

[3] See below, Sects. 5.3–4. In the far rarer case in which all members of a group will be killed unless an agent kills some smaller subset, I argue that killing people chosen randomly from among the entire group's membership is justified so long as at least one member of the group favors that course.

[4] See Immanuel Kant, *Groundwork of the Metaphysics of Morals* (1785), trans. H. J. Paton (1964), 95–6.

[5] Qualifications are needed if rescuers are subject to special obligations or duties, such as those imposed on health care providers by medical insurance contracts. The same is true if special moral permissions exist—for example, where somebody the rescuer loves dearly would die if he saved the biggest group.

application would not have improved their prospect of survival or the expected quality of their lives, rescuers should choose randomly among the imperiled groups, regardless of differences in the groups' sizes. Only by giving each person the same prospect of survival are all treated as equally deserving. Because most life-saving decisions that do not involve killing arise in situations in which those whose lives are at stake would have wanted a maximizing convention to be applied to persons in their predicament, reasonable opposition to saving the greater number in life-saving cases will rarely occur.

What are the legal implications of these moral conclusions? The law, I contend, should remain roughly as it is in most American jurisdictions. Failing to kill some people to save additional others in circumstances in which those one might have killed would have approved of a rule maximizing the number of survivors ought not to make somebody eligible for criminal punishment. Judgments about when those conditions are met are frequently too difficult, the inconsistency with the law's refusal to criminalize failing to *save* people too striking, and the imposition on people who are conscientiously opposed to killing too considerable to warrant criminal sanctions for not taking human life.

Killing in these circumstances should, however, be exempt from criminal liability. Whether this recommendation conflicts with the choice-of-evils or necessity defense most states provide is uncertain, given the vagueness of statutes setting forth the defense and the paucity of cases construing them. An explicit statutory statement making the choice-of-evils or necessity defense available to defendants who kill when the preceding conditions are met would therefore be desirable, although the nature of the permission and the rareness of justified kill might lead lawmakers to shun codification. Whether or not the general defense is amended or judicially interpreted to apply specifically to life-saving situations, the killer should, if prosecuted, bear the burden of producing evidence supporting his claim to have acted in the reasonable belief that the circumstances necessary to license killing obtained. This preliminary burden would be equivalent to the threshold requirements most states prescribe for invoking the necessity defense. If a defendant discharges this burden, the prosecution would then have to prove beyond a reasonable doubt that it was unreasonable for him to believe that killing was warranted and that the other elements of a crime were all present. Although the risk of prosecution and the defendant's threshold evidentiary requirement supply some disincentive to do what morality, apart from the law, requires, relieving the agent of an initial showing of the reasonable likelihood that his action would save more lives than it cost would predictably have worse consequences.

The route to these conclusions is relatively direct. After setting out various simplifying assumptions in Section 1, I consider in Section 2 several attempts to justify and circumscribe killing some people to save a greater number of others by reference to Kant's imperative that people are to be treated as ends in themselves, never merely as means to another person's goals. All these arguments fail, because their implications in life-saving cases are counterintuitive and the principles they invoke are ultimately at odds with the notions of equality and individual worth that infuse Kant's imperative. In Section 3, I contend that Frances Kamm's Principle of (Im)Permissible Harm cannot solve the trolley problem either, because it fails the test of intuition and lends a false prominence to the directness of the causal relations between an action and its beneficial and harmful effects. Section 4 is devoted to Judith Thomson's evolving approach to the trolley problem. It completes the critical section of this Article by exposing the inadequacies of Thomson's initial attempt to justify turning the trolley toward the lone worker by reference to what she alleged was a fundamental moral difference between creating and redirecting an injurious force. Section 4 also points to ambiguities and flaws in her most recent appeal to what people would, if acting rationally, antecedently have preferred be done to them in situations in which some can be slain to spare others.

In Section 5, I attempt to build, on a foundation similar to that supporting Thomson's new reliance on antecedent rational advantage, a more solid, comprehensive account of the moral propriety of taking and saving lives. This account, grounded in notions of hypothetical consent and fairness, will, I hope, also prove useful in formulating theories of political obligation and secession, and in defining individual moral duties.

1. PRELIMINARIES

Several assumptions will help channel discussion of the relative merits of the appeal to hypothetical consent and fairness that I endorse and of rival approaches to judging the morality of taking lives to help others and choosing among persons in distress.

First, all of the people considered—victims and beneficiaries alike—are the same age, are in identical health, enjoy equal rights as members of the rescuer's community, and are equally blameless or blameworthy, except when deviations are noted. Relaxing this assumption would complicate the argument considerably, particularly with respect to choices between persons who will all die without help. How these differences should affect conclusions formed independently of varying personal attributes and political allegiance will for many people turn on the correctness of broad theories of distributive justice and political obligation that resist brief examination.[6]

Second, none of the cases reviewed presents the question of whether somebody should disregard an agreement to govern the disposition of aid that was entered into voluntarily, with full information, by those in danger or those whose lives might be sacrificed. Apart from constraints imposed by paternalistic concerns and by considerations of fairness in reaching agreement, there seems no persuasive reason for rescuers to ignore an express arrangement for selecting survivors formed freely by persons in need, either before or after they discovered their plight.[7] My focus is instead on situations in which the person choosing survivors is unaware of any explicit agreement intended to guide her decision by those she might save or kill and situations in which no agreement exists.

Third, I assume that, with the exception of certain lifeboat scenarios discussed in Section 5.5 the person forced to choose whom to save or compelled to decide whether to kill some to save others is not herself in danger. I further suppose that none of those she might harm or benefit is a friend or a relative or somebody towards whom she has special obligations (because, for instance, she is responsible for the plight of someone she might rescue). I share the common belief that morality does not require people to act with strict impartiality when their most salient interests are in peril.[8] But because people might dispute this claim, I sidestep cases in which this issue might arise, to better spotlight the moral problems posed by saving and killing when different numbers of people stand to gain or lose.

Fourth, I shall assume in Section 5 that, in the absence of an explicit compact among those in danger or their fair hypothetical consent, there is no moral reason to prefer or to act to secure the deaths of one group of

---

[6] My views on the relevance of various characteristics to choices between lives are set forth in Eric Rakowski, *Equal Justice* (Oxford: Clarendon, Press, 1991), 310–32.

[7] I abstract from the question of whether potential rescuers not bound by contract may or should auction their services to people in need, allowing them to bid for help. The question is familiar to many health care providers. For example, dialysis machines that can keep alive many more acute patients than chronic patients are sometimes in short supply. Should the machines go to the chronic patients if they can and will pay more to use them than the eligible acute patients collectively offer? For some thoughts on this question, see ibid. 88–92, 313–24, 331–32.

[8] What Samuel Scheffler calls 'agent-centered prerogatives' are part of any acceptable moral theory, in my view, and they undeniably come into play when life-saving or life-taking choices must be made. See, e.g., Samuel Scheffler, *The Rejection of Consequentialism* (Oxford: Clarendon Press, 1982), 5, 17–21 (agent-centered prerogatives deny 'that one is always required to produce the best overall states of affairs,' although they permit one to do so); see also Samuel Scheffler, 'Prerogatives without Restrictions' *Philosophical Perspectives*, 6 (1992), 377 (same); Thomas Nagel, *The View from Nowhere* (Oxford: Oxford University Press, 1986), 166–75 (offering a similar account of agent-relative reasons). For a sustained attack on Scheffler's claim that morality incorporates agent-centered restrictions, see Shelly Kagan, *The Limits of Morality* (Oxford: Clarendon, Press, 1989), 204–16, 381–85.

persons rather than the deaths of another, smaller group of relevantly similar persons so long as the second group is not a subset of the first. I have defended this view elsewhere, borrowing in some measure from John Taurek's spirited arguments on its behalf.[9] I shall not repeat that defense here. Because this view is unpopular, my criticisms of competing approaches in Sections 2 through 4 do *not* deny that numbers are morally significant. Rather than take issue with that prevalent assumption, I concentrate in those Parts on exhibiting the intuitive shortcomings of opposing views in a range of cases and the unattractiveness of several principles they invoke. Those who, like Taurek, believe that numbers have no moral significance over and above any role they might play in motivating actual or hypothetical consent to a rule endorsing their relevance will have an additional ground for rejecting most of the alternative views I examine.[10]

Finally, I should underscore a significant limitation of my inquiry. As the preceding remarks suggest, my approach to moral choices is not consequentialist. I regard people as endowed with rights against one another and encumbered by duties towards one another by virtue of their independence and equality as moral subjects, rather than by virtue of a careful calculation of how best to achieve impersonally valuable ends, such as the maximum satisfaction of people's preferences. In determining what rights people have, we must, of course, pay attention to the consequences that might flow from alternative assignments of rights. But consequences enter as considerations that autonomous, morally equal persons would credit in adopting reciprocal restrictions on the means they might use to advance their interests, not as independently valuable moral counters.[11] It may be that a sophisticated consequentialist approach to life-saving decisions, one that derived rights and duties directly from consequences characterized in some non-moral manner,

[9] See Rakowski, *Equal Justice*, 277–309; John Taurek, 'Should the Numbers Count?', *Philosophy & Public Affairs*, 6 (1977), 293.

[10] Appeals to people's hypothetical preferences and fundamental moral convictions of the sort I favor will often, though not always, render numbers decisive in life-saving situations. Those appeals do not, assume, however, that the value of lives can be summed for the purpose of moral decisionmaking. I describe instances in which my view offers prescriptions that diverge from the thesis that numbers have direct moral relevance below, Sect. 5.10.

[11] Many consequentialist theories can be described in ideal contractarian terms. Utilitarian views, for example, can be derived from some notion of an original congress as easily as can John Rawls's theory of distributive justice. See, e.g., John C. Harsanyi, 'Morality and the Theory of Rational Behaviour,' in Amartya Sen and Bernard Williams (eds.) *Utilitarianism and Beyond* (Cambridge: Cambridge University Press, 1982), 39 R. M. Hare, 'Rawls' Theory of Justice', in Norman Daniels (ed.) *Reading Rawls* (Oxford: Blackwell, 1974), 81. Insofar as these views regard moral prescriptions as issuing from the hypothetical choices of people whose knowledge, desires, and reasoning are constrained to ensure that their choices fairly reflect their moral equality, I discuss them below in arguing for a rival conception of hypothetical consent. See below, Sects. 5.2–3. Here, I merely signal my intention to ignore consequentialist theories that have other grounds, as hedonistic utilitarianism is generally thought to do.

could justify many of the prescriptions I advance in Section 5. There are, for example, strong consequentialist arguments against compelling organ donation.[12] Whether a consequentialist theory could account satisfactorily for every instance in which it seems appropriate to depart from choice according to numbers seems to me doubtful, although much would depend upon the moral importance attached to various consequences described in non-normative ways. Standard accounts of hedonistic or preference-satisfaction utilitarianism would almost surely fail. Make the numbers sufficiently lopsided and the trade-off rare enough and utilitarians of these stripes will, for instance, urge us to push innocents in front of trains to save others farther down the track, even if the victims had been promised safety by the multitude they might save.[13] But I shall not attempt, in any systematic fashion, to refute possible consequentialist theories that would justify substantially the same verdicts as my approach. There is no point in arguing abstractly against theories whose prescriptions converge in the relevant situations. I therefore leave their construction and defense to those who find consequentialist moral reasoning attractive and who desire to show its intuitive appeal in the range of cases I discuss.

2. TREATING PEOPLE AS ENDS AND NOT MERELY AS MEANS

That people should be treated as ends in themselves, not merely as means to an agent's objectives, is a commonplace of much contemporary moral reasoning. As an abstract principle, Kant's injunction seems unexceptionable. Not only does it appeal to deontologists, who place respect for people's rights above the achievement of worthy goals defined without regard to people's moral claims. Kant's maxim could likewise be endorsed (although in fact it is rarely invoked explicitly) by consequentialist thinkers who see the principle of maximizing the world's good as that which equally deserving individuals would fairly choose if asked to agree on moral standards. Like

[12] Philosophers who are strongly drawn to consequentialist reasoning commonly acknowledge the importance of an individual's responsibility for his medical condition, for example. See, e.g., Kagan, *The Limits of Morality*, 26; Harris, 'The Survival Lottery,' 152.
[13] I offer a series of objections to utilitarianism as an account of distributive justice in Rakowski, *Equal Justice*, 23–39. In the case of utilitarian and related consequentialist approaches to life-saving, it seems to me likely that they will run aground of adamantine intuitions about how much sacrifice people are morally obligated to make for the sake of others, and of popular conceptions of rights to be free from harm even when invading those rights would benefit others. Alternatively, they assume so protean a form that they can almost invariably be made to match resilient intuitions, in which case the theories have little independent justificatory force. I shall not, however, sketch these objections more fully.

the vague though suggestive imperative to treat people as equals entitled to the same concern and respect from a moral point of view, the force and attraction of Kant's principle depend upon how it is glossed.

Several proposed answers to the question of when one may kill to save lives rely crucially upon the notion that a person is used impermissibly as a means to enhance the welfare of others when he is intentionally made a causal antecedent of their salvation. Sometimes this notion stands on its own as a justificatory principle.[14] More frequently, it is portrayed as partly or wholly coincident with, or as flowing from, some superficially different moral idea, such as the Principle of Double Effect,[15] or a distinction between doing and allowing,[16] or the division between positive and negative duties.[17] The common conclusion of views showing this family resemblance is that killing somebody in a way that makes him *direct* instrument for saving one or more other persons is impermissible, except perhaps if the number of lives saved or the good achieved is very much greater than the evil of using somebody as a means by killing him. Killing somebody *incidentally* or *indirectly* in the course of saving others is allowable, however, provided that the aggregate gains exceed the total losses by the proper amount. The background thought is that turning someone to purposes he will not consent to serve is evil, but achieving some worthy goal in a way that will inevitably, regrettably, but inessentially harm somebody is less bad. An action earns no reproach, according to this view, if the net gains are large enough and if an injury to one person is not a necessary condition of the benefit to others. It is not a necessary condition if the good action would have been performed anyway, with greater satisfaction, had the person not been harmed.

Approaches that share these features I refer to as endorsing the 'ends not means' principle. They comprise a subset of the many views that occasionally invoke Kant's maxim against treating people as means only, not also as ends in themselves. Section 3 considers a different, more intricate conception of the causal connections that define the impermissible 'means' relation; Section 4 examines the claim that a person is wrongly used as a means not in all cases in which she is killed in a way that makes her death a cause of others' survival, but only when her death becomes such a cause because the person saving the others created rather than diverted the dangerous force that killed her. Thus, writers who rely upon what I call the 'ends not means'

[14] See, e.g., Postow, 'Thomson and the Trolley Problem,' 530, 534 (arguing that the thesis that '[u]sing a person merely as a means is impermissible' best solves the trolley problem).
[15] See, e.g., Costa, 'Another Trip on the Trolley,' 465 (the Principle of Double Effect requires 'that the act by means of which the good is produced not itself be an evil').
[16] See generally Quinn, 'Actions, Intentions, and Consequences: The Doctrine of Doing and Allowing.'
[17] See, e.g., Foot, 'The Problem of Abortion and the Doctrine of the Double Effect.'

principle are not the only philosophers who draw inspiration from Kant or who believe that the causal role that victims play in preventing the deaths of others determines whether their killing is permissible. They are those who defend a relatively expansive definition of the 'means' relation, tying it to a minimally qualified conception of necessary cause.

This entire class of views presupposes that the value of lives can be summed for purposes of moral appraisal;[18] insofar as that premise is rejected, they can be dismissed as unsatisfactory. My criticisms in this Section, however, originate in a different quarter. When their implications are fully sketched, these constructions of the 'ends not means' principle cannot match resilient intuitions about how we should act in crucial test cases. And the attraction of the abstract notions supporting these views is not strong enough to lead us to modify or abandon the intuitions against which they are measured. What the shortcomings of these approaches reveal, I argue, is that the fundamental conceptions of equality and individual worth that animate the 'ends not means' principle, as well as nurture the closely related views discussed in Sections 3 and 4, demand one of two quite different interpretations. Either those conceptions should be read as favoring a strict prohibition on killing, except perhaps to save a vastly greater number of lives.[19] Or they should be seen as supporting an unadulterated consequentialist position that bids people maximize the number of lives or life-years saved subject to other constraints justified on consequentialist grounds—a position that appears too tolerant of homicide. The 'ends not means' principle represents an unstable equilibrium that can be maintained, if at all, only if our intuitive judgments in certain paradigm cases can resist the centrifugal forces shoving the principle's interpretation toward these two extremes. But that, I argue, our intuitions lack strength to do.

Michael Costa's views exemplify many theories that regard the 'ends not means' principle, interpreted as a deontological constraint that ignores hypothetical consent, as the key to the trolley problem's solution. Costa argues that the morally relevant difference between switching the trolley headed for five workers so that it kills one instead and using one patient's organs against his will to keep five other patients alive is that the surgeon kills the one *in order* to save the others, whereas the person who turns the

---

[18] This assumption yields an easy prescription in cases in which an agent must decide whether to save a larger or a smaller group and killing *cannot* boost the number of lives saved: rescue the greater number. Whether an agent's personal projects, affections, affiliations, or special duties or obligations may or should take precedence in certain cases, and whether the guilt or innocence of the endangered persons matters, are separate questions.

[19] I later argue that this prohibition may be modified by appeals to hypothetical consent and fairness; in the absence of these modifications, it appears too frequently to condemn killing some people to save others.

trolley does not.[20] Why does this difference matter morally, given that the results are the same and equally foreseeable in both cases and that the agents' motives are identical? Killing somebody as a means to save more lives is significantly worse than killing somebody incidentally but foreseeably in pursuit of the same end—enough worse to make killing wrong even though four additional people are kept alive—because, Costa says, 'treating a person as an *instrument* [is] intrinsically evil.'[21] Making his death 'actually a link in the causal chain that results in the continued life of the others'[22] is inherently wrong. This principle condemns the doctor's action, because she intentionally harms one person to save others, but it permits someone to turn the trolley because switching it does not *use* the one to save the five.[23]

Many philosophers echo Costa's analysis.[24] Typically, they offer no explanation of the moral significance of using someone as an instrument. As Don Locke says: 'Phrases such as "respect for persons", "individual

[20] See Costa, 'The Trolley Problem Revisited,' 442. Costa detects a second salient difference—the surgeon kills intentionally while the trolley-turner does not—but recognizes that this second difference is 'indirectly dependent upon the first' because the difference in intentions is best explained by 'the respective agents' perception of their actions being or not being in certain means relations.' Ibid.

[21] Ibid. 448. Costa also says that using somebody as an instrument evinces a character trait 'that is likely to produce bad consequences in other circumstances.' Ibid. This second explanation, however, fails to solve the trolley problem. One reason it falters is its implausibility. We treat one another as instruments incessantly, as they use us reciprocally. There is little reason to think that this corrupts our habits or makes us wells of evil. But perhaps all Costa is saying is that people who use others as means in the *wrong* way are, through warped characters or misbegotten convictions, likely to repeat their immoral actions and thus worsen the world. This claim is undeniable, but it is also unhelpful, for it leaves unexplained why, and in what way, it is wrong to use people as means. Even if we ignore her future ill deeds, we would shrink from allowing a doctor to kill an unwilling victim to furnish vital organs for several people. Costa's argument, like that of other partisans of the 'ends not means' principle, must ultimately rest on the intrinsic wrongness of a class of actions.

[22] Ibid. 443.

[23] I pass over the objection that, even in the transplant case, the doctor does not *intend* to kill: she would be delighted if, after removing the hapless patient's organs, the patient were to walk away from the operating table. See Jonathan Bennett, 'Morality and Consequences,' in Sterling M. McMurrin (ed.), *The Tanner Lectures on Human Values*, ii (1981), 45, 110. As Warren Quinn pointed out, the doctor does intend that her actions have *certain effects* on the donor, even though she might not intend the donor's death. In contrast, the person turning the trolley does not intend that the trolley strike the lone worker. He would attain his object if the worker were suddenly to vanish. This distinction suffices to lend substance to the distinction between killing as a means and killing incidentally, Quinn argued, once one takes account of the predictable consequences of these effects. See Quinn, 'Actions, Intentions, and Consequences: The Doctrine of Double Effect,' 337–43. This seems a promising response to Bennett's objection, although I cannot pursue the discussion further.

[24] See, e.g., Locke, 'The Choice between Lives,' 470 ('[I]t is harming one person in order to aid others which is unacceptable, where that person's death is needed as a means to saving others.'); Bruce Russell, 'On the Relative Strictness of Negative and Positive Duties,' in Steinback (ed.), *Killing and Letting Die*, 215, 228 ('To adopt a plan where someone is killed or let die for the sake of others is to treat the relevant person as a means only. To use people in that way is an affront to their worth and dignity . . . ').

autonomy and dignity", or Kant's notion of treating people as ends not means, spring readily to mind, though they seem to label the point rather than explain it.'[25] Explanations must end somewhere, of course, so these philosophers' inability to portray the ban on using people as a means to saving others as manifesting some deeper moral principle or value does not necessarily expose a deficiency in their argument. It does, however, make the defense of their view depend primarily, if not exclusively, on its capacity to yield prescriptions in particular cases that comport with our considered judgments.

Testing the 'ends not means' principle's implications against our responses to concrete cases is, unhappily, no simple feat. Its ramifications are contentious, and the principle's formulation is sufficiently elastic to accommodate a variety of constructions. Examining several ways in which the principle has been applied to difficult cases is thus unavoidable.

Two variants of the trolley case will aid in this analysis. The *Loop Variant* involves trolley tracks that diverge at the switch and then join together again in a loop. If the train proceeds straight, it will strike the five, whose bodies will prevent it from looping around and killing the one; if the trolley is switched, it will hit the one, whose body will block it from looping around and killing the five. The *Asymmetrical Variant* is the same, except in one respect: the loop is unidirectional. If the trolley is allowed to continue on its course toward the five, their bodies will stop it, but it would *not* have hit the one had they not been there because the main line continues straight. If, however, the trolley is diverted toward the one, his body *will* keep it from hitting the five, because the side track circles back into the main track, as in the Loop Variant.[26]

The Loop Variant poses a challenge to defenders of the 'ends not means' principle because it diverges from the original trolley case in precisely that respect that appears decisive for them. Turning the trolley will now save the five only if the single worker's body is used as a means to halt the train. If that worker were to step off the track just after the trolley were turned, the five would die, just as the surgeon in the transplant case could not keep the five alive if the would-be donor escaped. But, as Judith Thomson says, 'we cannot really suppose that the presence or absence of that extra bit of track

[25] Locke, 'The Choice between Lives,' 470. Warren Quinn stated that what distinguishes the agent of direct harm is that he

has something in mind for his victims—he proposes to involve them in some circumstance that will be useful to him precisely because it involves them . . . Someone who harms by direct agency must therefore take up a distinctive attitude toward his victims. He must treat them as if they were then and there *for* his purposes.

Quinn. 'Actions, Intentions, and Consequences: The Doctrine of Double Effect,' 348. This seems a fair characterization of the distinction, but it adds nothing by way of explanation.

[26] Judith Thomson first described the Loop Variant in 'The Trolley Problem,' 1402. What I call the Asymmetrical Variant originated in Costa, 'Another Trip on the Trolley,' 463.

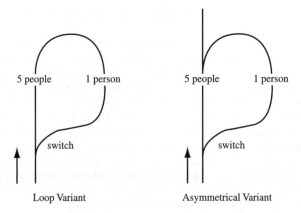

Loop Variant   Asymmetrical Variant

makes a major moral difference as to what an agent may do in these cases,'
given that both involve the foreseeable death of one person if we switch the
trolley to save five.[27]

Thomson's point exposes an important inadequacy in at least two philosophers' understanding of the 'ends not means' principle. Bruce Russell
asserts:

[O]ther things being equal, it is worse (morally) to adopt a plan where the death of
someone is needed (in a non-logical sense) to save another than it is to let that other
die regardless of whether (a) the death is brought about through an action or an
omission and whether (b) it is logically necessary or only physically inevitable, given
the successful execution of the plan.[28]

Russell construes clause (b) broadly, so that his principle appears to prohibit turning the trolley in the Loop Variant, inasmuch as saving five is not,
he thinks, an adequate justification for killing one in other contexts in
which the one is used as a means. Given this broad construction of clause
(b), Russell's argument is significantly flawed. That the one would become a
means to save five seems a poor objection to turning the trolley when the
alternative is that the five would block the train in precisely the same way to
save the one. Perhaps Russell believes that even though it is no worse deliberately to *be made* a cause of some people's salvation than accidentally to
be such a cause, and even though the beneficiaries are identical in both
cases, it is nevertheless worse *for an agent* to make somebody the cause by
which others are saved than to allow somebody to play that role without
help from the agent. But why this should be so, when an agent's motives are

[27] Thomson, 'The Trolley Problem,' 1403.
[28] Russell, 'On the Relative Strictness of Negative and Positive Duties,' 227.

above reproach and the consequences are the same in both cases, is unclear.[29]

Don Locke's qualified endorsement of the Doctrine of Double Effect— 'which forbids, not the taking of . . . innocent human life, but the *direct* killing of the innocent'[30]—seems open to the same criticism in the Loop Variant. The single worker on the side track would be killed 'directly' to save the five. Thus, Locke's understanding of the Principle of Double Effect appears to condemn turning the trolley, even though intuition approves the diversion.[31] Locke's formulation of the Principle might also be objectionable to some people because it would apparently permit blowing up the passengerless train headed for the five even if the explosion would 'indirectly' kill a couple strolling near the tracks. Identical objections could be offered to the version of the Doctrine of Double Effect that Warren Quinn has described and defended (without ultimately endorsing).[32]

The view that Quinn *does* endorse also seems to trip up on the case of the bomb that derails the train, saving the five, but killing two people nearby. Quinn's Doctrine of Doing and Allowing holds roughly that, other things being equal, greater moral opprobrium attaches to harmful 'positive' agency than to harmful 'negative' agency.[33] In a crucial passage elucidating this distinction, Quinn says that his Doctrine yields the intuitively correct result in the trolley case because allowing the trolley to barrel into five people, though passive, is actually *positive* agency:

This is because the only possibly acceptable reasons for him not to switch would be to prevent the death of the man on the side-track . . . But if the driver fails to switch for this reason, it is because he intends that the train continue in a way that will save the man. But then he intends that the train continue forward past the switch, and this leads to the death of the five. So, by my earlier definitions, his choice is really between two different positive options—one passive and one active. And that is why he may pick the alternative that does less harm.[34]

---

[29] It is also difficult to see how, in the case of a machine that in saving five people emits a lethal gas that kills someone nearby, which Russell says we may not activate, see ibid. 226–28, the death of the bystander is 'needed' any more than the death of one worker is 'needed' in the original trolley case. Both deaths are 'physically inevitable' to the same degree; in both cases one would be delighted if the lone individual somehow managed to skip out of harm's way. Russell claims that his principle prescribes different actions in the two cases, but he neglects to show how it could.

[30] Locke, 'The Choice between Lives,' 470.

[31] A defender of the Principle of Double Effect might claim that the death of the lone person was not intended: all that the bystander who switched the trolley intended was that the victim's body stop the trolley, not that he die. But if bringing the trolley to a halt by being ground under its wheels were invariably fatal, this distinction would be sophistry. That is why Bruce Russell refers to the death of the one as being 'needed (in a non-logical sense).' 'On the Relative Strictness of Negative and Positive Duties,' 227. See supra note 29 and accompanying text.

[32] See Quinn, 'Actions, Intentions, and Consequences: The Doctrine of Double Effect.'

[33] See Quinn, 'Actions, Intentions, and Consequences: The Doctrine of Doing and Allowing,' 291.

[34] Ibid. 305 (footnote omitted).

Quinn's argument is unconvincing. If the person controlling the dynamite charge refrains from blowing up the train, it is because he intends to save the couple walking near the tracks. But then he intends that the train continue on and kill five workers. So his choice is between what Quinn would call two positive actions, one passive and one active. If he may pick the less harmful alternative, he may dynamite the train, killing the pair nearby. It seems doubtful that Quinn would welcome this conclusion, for he thinks that a person who is able to stop a train that will run down somebody in its path must do so, even if halting the train to avoid hitting her will prevent the train from rescuing five people farther down the line.[35] Yet he can hardly fault the reasoning, so long as he adheres to his analysis of the standard trolley case. In trying to justify the traditional distinction between doing and allowing or acts and omissions without embracing an intuitively implausible verdict in the trolley case, Quinn swells the class of positive actions excessively.[36]

Michael Costa's approach to the Loop Variant is more inviting. He contends that turning the trolley in that case is consistent with the 'ends not means' principle, which he sees as largely if not entirely coincident with the Principle of Double Effect, because some death or deaths will *inevitably* be the means by which some other life or lives are saved. Hence, the switch operator must choose between letting one person block the train from hitting five, or letting five people prevent it from striking one. He does no wrong—indeed, he conserves the most value—if he sacrifices one for five instead of letting the trolley stay on the main rail. In contrast, the Asymmetrical Variant offers the switch operator a choice between using one person to benefit others, on one hand, and neither creating an instrumental relation nor permitting one to continue, on the other. The trolley will kill five if allowed to roll on, but the five will not be a means to saving the one, whereas turning the trolley makes the one into an instrument for saving the five. Switching the trolley is therefore impermissible.[37]

This is a superficially attractive way of handling the two cases. Declaring the decision to turn the trolley in the Loop Variant permissible, perhaps

---

[35] See ibid. 298–99.

[36] Frances Kamm offers a different criticism of Quinn's view. She claims that his account of positive agency implies that turning a trolley from one toward five is morally equivalent to refusing to turn a trolley headed for five toward one. Kamm believes, however, that these two actions are not morally on a par. The first, she says, is absolutely forbidden: the second is permissible but not obligatory. See F. M. Kamm. 'Non-Consequentialism, the Person as an End-in-Itself, and the Significance of Status,' *Philosophy & Public Affairs*, 21 (1992), 354, 369. If the position I set forth in Sect. 5 is correct, Kamm's objection is mistaken because the intuitive distinction on which she relies gives way.

[37] See Costa, 'Another Trip on the Trolley,' 462–3.

obligatory, preserves a certain consistency with Costa's verdict in the original trolley case. If the five and the one are symmetrically situated—both groups on tracks that continue straight beyond them, or both on tracks that loop back—it is permissible to choose which group will perish, and if numbers matter the one who should die. Moreover, Costa's opposite prescription in the Asymmetrical Variant appears, at least initially, to accord with a common intuitive reaction to another scenario: that in which a bystander may push somebody into the trolley's path. The apparent reason one person may not be pushed to her death to save five people farther down the line is that she would be used involuntarily as a means to keeping the five alive; refraining from pushing her will ensure that nobody is or becomes a means to saving somebody else. If that reasoning is correct, however, it seems likewise impermissible to divert the trolley in the Asymmetrical Variant because that would make the one into an instrument for saving five when the alternative is that nobody remains or becomes a means to save anybody else.

But Costa does not want to say that it is permissible to kill one person or several persons in order to save a greater number of others so long as those who will be saved would otherwise themselves have been a means to saving others. Return to the case of the woman who can be pushed onto the track to prevent the trolley from ramming the five. And suppose that the five are not positioned on a straight track, with nobody behind them. Imagine, instead, that they find themselves in the Loop Variant, along with the isolated worker stuck on the track that curves behind them. The approach one might be tempted to attribute to Costa would permit a bystander to push the woman onto the rails, because the five would have been a means to saving somebody else were the trolley allowed to hit them. It is permissible, in this view, to turn the trolley to hit one person who would otherwise not be harmed to save the five, because the five would otherwise themselves save somebody by blocking the train in the same way. It should, then, be equally permissible to put another person into harm's way—in this case, the woman beside the tracks—if by making her a means one can save more people who would otherwise save life in similar fashion. But those who would condemn pushing somebody in front of the train to save five on a straight track would not, I conjecture, change their minds if told that the deaths of the five would save another life because the track wound around behind them and a lone worker was lunching on the rails.

Costa would almost certainly share this reaction and say that shoving somebody into the trolley's path is always wrong (although the evil might sometimes be outweighed by the good it effects) because that person could not have been killed by redirecting the threat to the five, as could the lone worker.[38] This would not, for Costa, be the only limitation on killing some people to save more others. In view of his denunciation of killing in the Asymmetrical Variant, he would probably add that one person may not be made a means to saving others unless those others will be a means to saving her if the agent declines to act. But he could conjoin the two principles, which he may or may not believe to have a common root, to secure what he regards as the intuitively correct result.

This is one possible approach to explaining our steadfast intuitions in these and other cases; however, the approach seems to me seriously mistaken. I defer criticizing the distinction Costa invokes between originating and redirecting harm until I examine the views of Judith Thomson and James Montmarquet in Section 4. Here I offer further reasons to doubt Costa's understanding of the 'ends not means' principle that cannot be countered by distinguishing between originating and diverting harm.

Consider the Asymmetrical Variant again. The trolley may not be turned toward the one in this case, Costa avers, because if the trolley stays on course the five will not become a means to saving the one, while turning the trolley will make the one a means to saving the five.[39] Now alter the scene in one particular: when the bystander reaches the switch, he finds it in the *other* position, so that if he does nothing, the train will kill the single worker, whose body will stop it and thereby save the five; if the bystander switches the trolley, it will kill five, but they will not become a means to saving the one because the trolley would not have looped around had they not impeded its progress. May—or must—the bystander turn the trolley? If it would be impermissible to divert the trolley towards the one in the Asymmetrical Variant *because* that would make him a means to saving the five, and if, as Costa assumes, causing and allowing somebody physically to save others are morally on a par (which is why one can choose according to the numbers in the Loop Variant), then it seems that the bystander should equally ensure that the one not become the cause by which others are saved. Thus, he should switch the trolley, causing it to kill five when it would have killed but one. Surely this conclusion is unacceptable.

How might Costa respond? To avoid this conclusion, he must concede that *allowing* somebody to be the cause of another's survival is prima facie less iniquitous than *making* somebody into such a cause when he would

---

[38] Costa writes:

[O]ne who brings some *new* threat or source of foreseeable harm into the world is engaged in an act that is itself a *prima facie* evil and one that is more difficult to justify. This is so even if the end results are the same in terms of total harm caused versus total harm prevented. There is an important moral difference between redirecting an existing source of harm and creating a new one. ' Another Trip on the Trolley'. 464.

[39] See ibid. 463.

otherwise remain causally on the sideline. But unless Costa takes the view
that allowing somebody to become a means to saving others is not blameworthy at all, he would have to agree that there is some ratio at which it is
morally permissible or obligatory (his discussion of the trolley cases suggests
the latter) for a bystander, either in the Loop Variant or in the revised
version of the Asymmetrical Variant described in the preceding paragraph,
to divert or refrain from diverting a trolley so that more die rather than
fewer. For example, if it is twice as bad to cause somebody to die as a means
than it is to allow someone to die as a means to saving others, the person at
the switch in the Loop Variant would do no wrong—and perhaps act
commendably—if he refused to turn a trolley headed for five people down
another track where it would kill only three. This result seems a betrayal of
the imperative to extend equal regard to all, as well as a rebuke to our moral
intuitions.

If we exclude that solution, nothing remains except to claim that causing
one or more people to become a means to saving others is impermissible,
unless perhaps the number of people that can thereby be saved is much
larger, whereas allowing somebody to die so that his death saves more lives is
permissible or required. The preceding argument might tempt Costa to
accept the first half of this position. He appears to concede that if the
disparity in numbers is great enough, causing the death of one or more
persons might be justified to save others.[40] However, accepting the first part
of this view would compel Costa to abjure his verdict on the Loop Variant;
sending the trolley to kill the one would not be justified because the disparity
in numbers is slight. This result is counterintuitive. One would expect the
analysis to mirror that of the original trolley case, where the two tracks split
and do not circle back and join. Possibly, however, someone drawn to
Costa's general approach would accept that conclusion to dodge the
foregoing objections.

The second half of this position—that allowing somebody to become the
instrument by which more others are saved is morally permissible or
mandatory—should occasion more consternation. It would apparently
allow or require one to refrain from calling out to somebody about to wander onto the track if letting her be hit would save five others farther down the
track. Analogously, it would allow or require somebody to let a beggar
starve to death, or an ailing patient die, if either could provide organs for

[40] Costa says that it *might* be permissible to kill twelve to save a million lives, although he does
not say definitely that it is permissible. See id. at 466. Locke does not say when the numbers
become so lopsided as to justify killing some or letting them die to save more others, but he
suggests that in certain circumstances morality countenances this trade. See Locke, 'The Choice
between Lives,' 473.

transplantation to two or more others upon his death. One might respond, following Philippa Foot's lead, by formulating a distinction between positive and negative duties that requires intervention in these cases,[41] or drawing a distinction between doing and allowing that achieves the same end.[42] But these distinctions, if the terms in which they are cast are given their normal significations, fail to shape the inchoate notions of treating people as ends and using them merely as means in an intuitively appealing way. If, however, the distinctions are molded around specific examples to match our moral intuitions, they appear disturbingly *ad hoc*, serving no explanatory or justificatory purpose because they lack independent content against which intuitions can be measured.[43]

The claim that allowing somebody to become a means to save more others is permissible or required raises a further difficulty for Costa's approach. Suppose that a heavy weight lies atop the ceiling of a hospital room. Left alone, it will soon bring down the ceiling, killing five convalescents below. You cannot evacuate the room or move the weight onto stout floorboards. The only way to keep the ceiling from collapsing on the five is to turn on a ceiling-support machine whose poisonous exhaust fumes will inevitably dispatch the bedridden patient next door. Costa regards operating the machine as impermissible, even though the bedridden patient would not thereby be used as a means to save the five.[44] Yet if it is permissible, or even required, to allow somebody to become a means to saving others if that would maximize the number of people kept alive, even if one could easily intervene to save that person, why should it not be permissible—why should it be *worse*—to cause somebody to die in keeping the same number of people alive if that person would *not* serve as a means?

Costa cannot say that killing somebody by turning on the machine is worse than letting somebody die as a means because the first constitutes a *positive action* that takes innocent life, whereas the second is only an omission. As he recognizes, a positive action is essential in the original trolley

---

[41] See Foot, 'The Problem of Abortion and the Doctrine of the Double Effect,' 27–9.

[42] See Quinn, 'Actions, Intentions, and Consequences: The Doctrine of Doing and Allowing.'

[43] Nancy Davis notes that the distinction between positive and negative duties cannot ground claims regarding their relative stringency unless they can be identified independently of their moral force. She argues that Foot's classification of a duty to feed a starving beggar as negative if his body would be used for medical research should he be permitted to die transgresses this rule. See Nancy Davis. 'The Priority of Avoiding Harm,' in Steinbock (ed.), *Killing and Letting Die*, 172, 177–8, 190–2.

[44] See Costa, 'Another Trip on the Trolley,' 464–6. Philippa Foot introduced the gas-emitting machine case. See Foot, 'The Problem of Abortion and the Doctrine of Double Effect,' 29. Her intuitive conviction that it would be immoral to switch on the machine is widely shared. See, e.g., Costa. 'Another Trip on the Trolley,' 464; Kamm, 'Harming Some to Save Others,' 237; Jeff McMahan, 'Killing, Letting Die, and Withdrawing Aid,' *Ethics*, 103 (1993), 276; Montmarquet, 'On Doing Good: The Right and the Wrong Way,' 447; Thomson, 'The Trolley Problem,' 1407–8.

case as well. Costa's reason for distinguishing the hospital case from the original trolley case is that the former involves the *creation* of a new evil— the gas that kills the isolated patient—whereas diverting the trolley involves nothing more than the *redirection* of an existing threat.[45]

I discuss that distinction at length in Section 4. But it is worth asking here, by way of anticipation, why it should be crucially important, if people's lives have equal worth, whether one creates a new threat or rechannels an existing one, so long as the result is the same. Suppose that you can push the weight on the ceiling above an adjacent room, where it will kill only one recuperating patient when it crashes through. By analogy to the hurtling trolley, Costa's theory appears to regard shifting the weight as permissible, perhaps obligatory.[46] Yet his theory does not allow you to turn on a machine that keeps the ceiling from collapsing, even though the same five would live and the same patient would die. This result not only seems wrong intuitively. It mocks rather than exemplifies the conviction that people warrant equal regard in making decisions that profoundly affect them.

This examination of Costa's applications of the 'ends not means' principle to the trolley problem and related choices hardly exhausts the range of conceivable cases or modifications to the principle. Perhaps there is some way to revise his understanding of the principle or to marry it to some moral claim other than the distinction between originating and channeling harm so as to meet or circumvent the foregoing criticisms. There seems, however, ample reason for pessimism. The core conviction behind the 'ends not means' principle is that normal, blameless human beings are equally valuable, autonomous creatures who cannot rightly be used as the tools of other people. But this conviction points in two directions in which Costa and others who have trumpeted the principle (or some related distinction between doing and allowing or positive and negative duties) are loath to go.

On one side, it presses toward the consequentialist view that individuals' status as moral equals requires that the number of people kept alive be maximized.[47] Only in this way, the thought runs, can we give due weight to the fundamental equality of persons; to allow more deaths when we can ensure fewer is to treat some people as less valuable than others. Further, killing some to save others, or letting some die for that purpose, does not entail that those who are killed or left to their fate are being used merely as means to the well-being of others, as would be true if they were slain or left

<hr/>

[45] See Costa, 'Another Trip on the Trolley,' 464.

[46] Perhaps the hospital setting and your duties as a health worker (if you are so employed) would compel a different result, although this seems unlikely.

[47] The principle might be qualified in various ways. For example, a person's responsibility for her plight might bear on her claim to be saved before others.

to drown merely to please people who would live anyway. They do, of course, in some cases serve as means. But they do not act *merely* as means. Those who die are no less ends than those who live. It is because they are also *no more* ends than others whose lives are in the balance that an impartial decisionmaker must choose to save the more numerous group, even if she must kill to do so.

Despite the abstract appeal of this reasoning, many people, myself included, shrink from embracing it. The unqualified maximizing rule it apparently implies is intuitively unacceptable.[48] It also gives insufficient scope to people's freedom to decide which risks to run or which benefits to reap. Nonconsensual adult organ transplants, for example, are morally intolerable when people face different likelihoods of needing organs based on their voluntary behavior and no one is allowed to opt out of the transfer scheme. Those who rebel at this utilitarian recasting of the distinction between using people as means and regarding them as ends, and who accept the preceding criticisms of Costa, Locke, and others, will be pushed to its polar opposite.

This opposing view recognizes with no less force the equality of individuals as ends in themselves, by virtue of their ability to perceive, to reason, to project themselves imaginatively into the future and to steer their conduct by the light of goals and principles they choose or acknowledge freely. But it interprets more expansively the requirement that people not be used as means to promote others' objectives. This view holds that people have a right not to be killed or allowed to die simply to benefit other people, unless the victims consent to that action or omission or the costs to the agent are high.[49]

By giving backbone to the means restriction, this view risks intuitive rejection. At first blush, for example, it counsels against turning the trolley to save five at the expense of one life, because doing so would apparently violate the one's right not to be killed. But the counterintuitive implications of this approach can be reduced or eliminated in three ways: (1) by importing a principle that counts numbers and that overrides the means restriction when the disparity in lives that might be lost becomes sufficiently great; (2) by interpreting the notion of consent to include approval that somebody would reasonably have given beforehand, rather than confining consent to an individual's explicit agreement; or (3) by restricting the occasions on which

---

[48] A consequentialist could, of course, enlist a number of subsidiary principles that palliate the apparently unsavory implications of a maximizing rule. Perhaps those principles could even be shown to be entailed by whatever ends the consequentialist endorses. I shall not pursue this possibility.

[49] I leave to one side the question of how large an exception should be made for killing in self-defense and, if desirable, for killing innocent people to save or benefit oneself or somebody one loves.

rights may be exercised to thwart the contrary wishes of others. In Section 5, I fill out and fortify this reading of the 'ends not means' principle using the second and third of these modifications.

Before embarking on that project, I wish to examine two other approaches to these issues. The first is Frances Kamm's claim that what matters is not whether somebody is a direct cause of saving someone else, but whether the events that cause the loss of life bear a closer causal relation to the loss of life than to the saving of additional lives.[50] The second is the view, initially advanced by Judith Thomson and taken up by Costa and Montmarquet, that while it is permissible to divert an inevitable harm so that it kills a smaller number of people, it is impermissible to kill the smaller number by some other means because the creation of harm is especially evil.[51] The central Kantian insight about the moral importance of respecting the autonomy of rational decisionmakers, which Kamm and Thomson endorse, might well induce skepticism about the prospects for either approach. It is far from obvious what connection might obtain between the closeness of a causal relation or the distinction between creating and channeling harm, on one hand, and the moral equality of persons and the importance of not using them against their will, on the other. But part of defending any view is showing that its rivals are less comely. And in philosophy, as elsewhere, mistakes often instruct.

3. KAMM'S PRINCIPLE OF (IM)PERMISSIBLE HARM

Taking as her aim the formulation of a principle that accounts for what she regards as 'common-sense' moral intuitions better than rival moral prescriptions,[52] Frances Kamm offers a novel understanding of the impulses that inspire many familiar moral commands, such as prohibitions against using people as means, or intending injury, or putting somebody in harm's way as opposed to allowing that person to be harmed by natural forces or others' deeds. Although Kamm, like Thomson and some of the writers discussed in Section 2, believes that what is essential is that we 'not bring about a greater good *by* infringing someone's rights in a significant way,'[53] she understands the word 'by' unconventionally. For her, what matters in explicating this notion is not whether somebody intended harm or whether the violation of one person's right was a causal antecedent of a benefit to someone else.

---

[50] See Kamm, 'Harming Some to Save Others,'
[51] See Thomson, 'The Trolley Problem.'
[52] See Kamm, 'Harming Some to Save Others,' 227, 232.
[53] Ibid. 243: see ibid. 232.

What matters, she says, if our intuitions are to be vindicated, is captured by what she calls the Principle of (Im)Permissible Harm:

It is permissible to cause harm to some in the course of achieving the greater good of saving a greater number of others from comparable harm, if events which produce the greater good are not more intimately causally related to the production of harm than they are to the production of the greater good (or put another way, if events which produce the greater good are at least as intimately causally related to the production of the greater good as they are to the production of the lesser harm).[54]

A few illustrations that Kamm thinks intuition upholds will prove useful. In the original trolley case, turning the trolley causes both the five to be saved and the one to die; the act's causal relations to good and ill are equally intimate, so turning the trolley is permissible.[55] The same is true in the Loop and Asymmetrical Variants; it is irrelevant whether one or more people serve as a means to saving others. Suppose, however, that the only way to stop the trolley from hitting five workers is to push another worker in front of it. Knocking somebody onto the rails is impermissible, in Kamm's view, because harm (the death of the one) is more intimately causally related to the action being appraised (the shove) than the good that is achieved (saving the five).[56] Or suppose that the trolley can only be kept from running over the five by tossing a grenade in its path that will, regrettably, kill somebody walking nearby. We must refrain, Kamm says, from lobbing the grenade. The explosion would kill the one directly but save the five only indirectly; the explosion that killed the one would cause the trolley to stop and that in turn—another step removed—would save the five. If, by some miracle, the five could be saved by setting off the charge beneath the platform on which they are standing, so that the explosion would both lift them to safety and kill the one, then detonating the charge would be permissible.[57]

Consider also the case of the machine that spews toxic gas into the hospital ward if it is activated to keep the ceiling from collapsing.[58] As Kamm paints the scene, the toxic gas is emitted not by a ceiling-support machine but in the course of fueling a machine that is needed to perform surgery on the five. Here, the gas contributes to the survival of the five, but at some

---

[54] Ibid. 232 (footnote omitted).
[55] See ibid. 233.
[56] See ibid. 238–39.
[57] See ibid. 236. Kamm does not discuss the status of omissions within her theory. The most natural line would be to treat omissions as Kamm does actions, so that refraining from warning somebody about to stray onto the trolley track, where he will be hit by the train but save five people farther down the line, would be impermissible because the act of refraining is more closely connected causally to harm than to the eventual benefit to the five. Failure to warn would be akin to pushing the person under the trolley's wheels. The same would be true of failing to save a beggar or seriously ill patient in order to obtain multiple organs for transplant.
[58] See n. 44 above and accompanying text.

causal distance from their improved health, because it abets the surgery and it is the surgery that keeps them alive. But the causal relation between use of the gas and the death of the patient next door is snug, because the escaping fuel kills him directly. Accordingly, the surgeons must forgo use of the gas. If, however, the gas *itself* keeps the five alive but is poisonous to the one, doctors may release it, since the causal connection between that action and its good and bad consequences is equally tight and the good outweighs the bad.[59] Presumably, Kamm would say the same of shifting a weight atop the ceiling: the act of moving the weight bears an equally close causal relation to saving the five as it does to killing the one, paralleling the bystander's diversion of the trolley. Moving the weight should therefore be permissible.

Kamm's proposal is open to at least three criticisms. First, the proper description of actions and events, on which their moral evaluation depends, is underdetermined by Kamm's theory. The same events can sometimes plausibly result in inconsistent appraisals. Second, the intuitions Kamm uses to test her theory are in some cases impossible to regard sympathetically. If the Principle of (Im)Permissible Harm is lashed to them, it will founder.[60] Third, the causal relations that form the lattice of Kamm's theory are not tethered to what matters morally—what leads us to approve or condemn various actions is not the intimacy of their causal connections to harm and benefit—and Kamm produces no persuasive reason for making the Principle of (Im)Permissible Harm our benchmark.

To see the ease with which competing descriptions of an action can alter the verdicts Kamm's theory pronounces, return to the case of the noxious gas in the hospital ward. If gas is used in surgery but is not administered directly to patients on the operating table, and if that gas kills another patient next door who inhales it, then the surgery, Kamm says, is impermissible. But to defend her position, Kamm would have to show why the anchoring event from which causal chains should be measured is the release of the gas. One could as easily claim that the event that produces the greater good is the *surgery*, of which the gas leak is an unavoidable concomitant. After all, one would naturally say that the surgery, not the gas that runs some machine, is what saves the five. If one makes the surgical operation the anchoring event, however, then the benefit conferred on the five is at least as intimately related to that event as is the harm to the convalescent in the next room. So the surgery, on Kamm's theory, may go forward.

Assume, however, that Kamm's description of the events is more accur-

---

[59] See Kamm, 'Harming Some to Save Others,' 237.

[60] Of course, to the extent that the first criticism is sound, this objection may be discounted, because the more protean a theory, the more readily it can be manipulated to match whatever intuitions one has.

ate.[61] The gas that kills the one directly saves the five at one step removed, so the surgeons must lay aside their forceps. Is this result intuitively sound? Imagine that the gas is not used to run the machine, but is rather a byproduct of its operation. The benefit to the five is then at least as intimately related to the key event—presumably the operation of the machine or, more generally, the surgery—as is the harm to the one. The machine, or surgery, that gives life to the five also causes the one to die, but by an equally lengthy causal route. So by Kamm's standard, the doctors may operate. Yet this result strains credibility when juxtaposed against her conclusion regarding the gas-driven machine. Why should the moral permissibility of the surgery hinge on whether the gas is used to power the machine or is given off by the machine, when the surgeons know that in either case five will be saved and one will die?

Perhaps Kamm would agree that there should be no moral difference and respond by describing the surgery as the critical event in both cases. But if she would approve a surgical operation that killed a nearby patient because it saved five other patients, she would then need to explain why making an involuntary organ donor of somebody plucked off the street to save five terminal patients is almost universally, and rightly, condemned. Perhaps Kamm would reply that the surgical removal of the donor's organs is more intimately related to the harm he experiences than to the saving transplants the removal makes possible; so the transplants, unlike the surgical operation involving the lethal gas, may not proceed. If so, however, she would still need to say why, when five lives can be saved in both cases, it matters whether the innocent person who must die if the five are to live is killed incidentally or directly. This is the burden of explanation faced unsuccessfully by defenders of the Doctrine of Double Effect.[62] Kamm cannot, however, rely on their defense, even if it were compelling, because she endorses direct killing in a variety of instances that the Doctrine of Double Effect condemns, and therefore criticizes the Doctrine as too restrictive.[63] How she would respond to this challenge is unclear.

A second example of descriptive malleability should cement the point. For Kamm, exploding a grenade to save five from the approaching trolley is permissible even if it kills one passerby, so long as the explosion launches the five to safety; if the explosion would instead derail the trolley, the grenade should not be thrown. This distinction seems queer: why should the avenue

---

[61] How accuracy should be measured is, unfortunately, obscure. If the aim is simply to hew to intuitive judgments in particular cases, the Principle of (Im)Permissible Harm obviously does no moral work.

[62] See nn. 30–1 above and accompanying text.

[63] See Kamm, 'Harming Some to Save Others.' 244–5. Kamm also thinks the Doctrine of Double Effect too willing to permit foreseen but unintended harm in the course of doing good. See ibid. 245.

of escape make any difference, given that an innocent passerby will die from the explosion in any event? This doubt in turn makes one wonder whether Kamm's causal analysis is correct. Although Kamm does not supply a detailed description of this fantastical situation, an explosion that lifted the five off the track would presumably not operate directly on their bodies, as it would on the body of the passerby it killed. Otherwise, they too would die. One must instead imagine the blast applying considerable force to a platform or other object, which in turn boosts the five beyond harm's reach.[64] But then it seems that the benefit they derive is not as closely causally related to the explosion as is the death of the one, because the explosion must move a thick surface which, at the next stage, spirits the five to safety. So perhaps exploding the grenade would not be permissible after all.

Kamm's Principle is thus infected by indeterminacy in its description of causal chains, permitting at least some of them to be characterized in whatever way generates the intuitively proper outcome, but at the cost of depriving the theory of explanatory power. Perhaps more important, in cases in which the Principle of (Im)Permissible Harm appears to issue clear prescriptions, those prescriptions are intuitively unpalatable. Suppose, for example, that Kamm is right to say that throwing the grenade is permissible if it knocks the five to safety as it simultaneously kills the one. One could easily vary the example, so that the explosion that kills the one would have to set off a *second* explosion that rockets the five away from the juggernaut. In that case, exploding the grenade would *not* be permissible. But why should twin explosions call for a different evaluation than a single bang? Alternatively, one could drape another causal layer on the other side. Suppose that the grenade that destroys the trolley precipitates a rock slide, which kills someone strolling by. If the Principle of (Im)Permissible Harm is correct, the additional intervening event makes exploding the grenade an acceptable means to the salvation of the five.[65]

Intuition, however, tells a different story. Whether the grenade kills the oblivious walker directly or via a foreseeable rock slide is morally irrelevant. As Costa notes, 'it is hard to see how the mere number of intervening events would be *morally* relevant except insofar as it is related to epistemic issues about whether the consequence is forseen [sic] or foreseeable on the part of

---

[64] Even if there were no platform, perhaps all my argument requires is that the five wear shoes. For the force of the explosion, acting upon their shoes, drives them into the air, whereas the exploding fragments kill the one directly (or must they strike some unclothed part of her?). That one should worry about these trivial differences in sequences of causally related events (maybe one should even be counting molecular collisions) is surely absurd.

[65] See Kamm, 'Harming Some to Save Others,' 237 (confirming this conclusion in the rock slide case).

the agent.'[66] Could one seriously affirm that adding another sheet of linoleum to the platform on which the five are standing, or putting a second set of soles on their shoes, would transform a permissible explosion into an impermissible one? Or, if those changes do not count as additional causal events under Kamm's theory—though it is difficult to see why causes should be denominated in a way that precludes taking account of these changes—can putting the innocent grenade victim in a hut, where she will be killed by the collapsing walls rather than by shrapnel, render her death tolerable when otherwise it would warrant severe reproach?[67]

Multiplying examples would serve no purpose. The problem is not that the Principle of (Im)Permissible Harm wants some marginal refinement—a less arbitrary method for individuating causes, a few qualifications to align its commands and prohibitions with obdurate intuitions. The problem lies deeper. As our intuitive reactions to variations on the cases Kamm discusses reveal, the comparative lengths of the lines of causation running from some action to its good and bad consequences do not affect the action's permissibility. They are morally irrelevant, except insofar as they bear on the certainty or foreseeability of the action's consequences. We do care, at least prior to reflection, about whether an action that is likely to produce more good than bad involves using somebody against his will, how probable the good and bad consequences are, how greatly the benefit outweighs the evil, and what responsibility those affected bear for their position, perhaps among other variables. But the relevance of the fine distinctions Kamm draws by counting causal links is by no means immediately evident.

Curiously, Kamm provides only a fleeting explanation for the salience of

[66] Costa, 'The Trolley Problem Revisited,' 441. In the paragraph from which this quotation is taken, Costa questions the moral relevance of the distinction between direct and indirect killing, not Kamm's proposal. But his point applies with equal force here.

[67] The same point can be made in terms of omissions if the view attributed to Kamm, 'Harming Same to Save Others.' is correct. Suppose the trolley is headed for one worker, but you can turn it toward five. You ought not to turn the trolley because the harm from not turning the train is as intimately causally related to that omission as is the benefit to the five from keeping your hand off the switch. But now suppose the five would not be directly struck by the trolley if you turned it, but rather would die when the trolley rammed into the scaffolding on which they were standing, dropping them to their deaths. The Principle of (Im)Permissible Harm seems to tell you to *turn* the trolley, killing the five. Not doing so would save more lives, but not turning would be more intimately causally related to the harm to the one than to the benefit to the five, which is one causal link removed because of the scaffolding. If this interpretation of the Principle is right, its implications are bizarre.

Notice that it will not do to say that the mere act of *not* switching the trolley produces the benefit, and hence that it is causally equidistant from benefit and harm. For then the same should be true of not warning somebody about to wander onto the trolley tracks. Kamm could ignore the scaffolding or other intervening causes only by adopting a counterintuitive position in the failure-to-warn case and by offering an account of omissions that diverges fundamentally from her account of actions.

the causal differences she identifies. The Principle of (Im)Permissible Harm offers, she says, the best account of when we may save the greater number 'in a way that preserves morally appropriate relations between victims and beneficiaries who are moral equals.'[68] It is the most inviting expression of the idea, which also underlies the Doctrine of Double Effect, that we may not harm others as a means to some greater good.[69] Assertion cannot substitute for argument, however, and by forgoing reasoned justification at a more abstract level, Kamm rests her case on the appeal of her Principle in sorting out those acts of killing we find intuitively permissible from those we denounce. But, by that criterion, the Principle of (Im)Permissible Harm comes a cropper. It stumbles largely because, by making the permissibility of killing or letting die turn on how many intervening events separate an action from its morally significant consequences, Kamm's Principle puts an apparent irrelevancy in place of the relational factors around which our convictions are built. Any morally significant connection between the intimacy of causal relations and the duties we owe to one another as moral equals has yet to be proved.

4. THOMSON'S TWO APPROACHES TO THE TROLLEY PROBLEM

Judith Thomson's early papers on the trolley problem are responsible for much of the attention these issues have received.[70] It behooves us to consider the solution she advanced in the second of these papers, 'The Trolley Problem,' because many believe it captures a significant insight and because Thomson's proposal has been adopted, sometimes with qualifications, by other writers.[71] After describing the proposal's shortcomings, some of which Thomson has since recognized, I turn to her most recent account, in *The Realm of Rights*, of when lives may be sacrificed to save additional lives. The view I defend in Section 5 springs from the same source as Thomson's present position, but diverges from her view in several noteworthy respects.

[68] Kamm, 'Harming Some to Save Others,' 243.
[69] See ibid. 245.
[70] See Thomson, 'The Trolley Problem.' I ignore Thomson's first stab at these issues in 'Killing. Letting Die, and the Trolley Problem,' *Monist* 59 (1976), 204, because in 'The Trolley Problem' Thomson disowned her earlier suggestions and they have not been appropriated by others.
[71] See, e.g., Costa, 'Another Trip on the Trolley,' 461, 464–65; Montmarquet, 'Harming Some to Save Others,' 446–55. Kamm also believes that the 'underlying idea' of Thomson's proposal in 'The Trolley Problem' is 'sound,' and bills 'what underlies' her own Principle of (Im)permissible Harm as 'a version of Thomson's proposal.' Kamm, 231, 243.

4.1. The Significance of Redirecting Harm

In 'The Trolley Problem,' Thomson contends that two considerations explain the moral difference between turning the trolley so that one dies rather than five and cutting vital organs out of an unwilling donor to cure several other people. First, the person who shunts the trolley down the side track does not accomplish the diversion 'by means which themselves constitute an infringement of any right of the one's.'[72] Turning a trolley (viewed independently of the damage it works) does not violate a significant right of the victim; perhaps only the owner's right to control its use is violated. The surgeon's battery, in contrast, affronts the donor's physical integrity. Second, the person who turns the trolley makes something that already threatens five threaten one instead; the surgeon visits on the protesting donor a harm other than the afflictions killing the five. According to Thomson, both of these conditions—not violating a significant right and diverting an existing threat—must be met before killing one or more persons to save a larger number of other people is permissible. Thus, one may not push somebody sauntering along the tracks into the trolley's path to save five, because shoving her onto the rails would infringe one of her significant rights, even though the second requirement would be met because she would be killed by the force then threatening the five.[73] Nor can one switch on the ceiling-support machine in the hospital ward. Although doing so presumably does not infringe a significant right of the lone patient, the poisonous gas the machine emits would kill the patient by a different means than the threat—a weight atop the ceiling—already facing the five.[74]

Both of Thomson's prerequisites for killing some to save more others are flawed. Let me focus on the second, which James Montmarquet claims (and Michael Costa also appears to think) suffices by itself,[75] whatever the failings of Thomson's first requirement.[76] Anybody within what Montmarquet calls

---

[72] Thomson, 'The Trolley Problem,' 1403, 1407.
[73] See ibid. 1409.
[74] See ibid. 1407–08.
[75] See n. 38 above and accompanying text.
[76] Thomson now acknowledges the shortcomings of the first prerequisite. Turning the trolley obviously violates at least one significant right of the single worker, namely, his right not to be killed without his consent. Thomson claimed, however, that the *number* of significant rights violations matters. See Thomson, 'The Trolley Problem,' 1409–10. What distinguished the trolley case from the transplant case, in her view, was that switching the train violates one significant right of the lone worker—his right not to be killed—whereas divesting somebody of his organs involuntarily infringes two rights—his right not to be killed and his right not to have his body opened and organs taken without his consent. But making the permissibility of killing turn on the number of significant rights violations, as Thomson recently wrote, 'really will not do.' Thomson, *The Realm of Rights*, 179 n. 2. People have a claim against us that we not hit them with trolleys, whether or not the strike is fatal, as well as a right not to be killed by us. So turning the trolley and making an

the 'range' of a pre-existing threat—anybody, that is, who can be killed by pointing the threatening force wherever it is causally possible to aim it—can be killed to maximize the number of people kept alive. Contrary to Thomson's statement of her second condition, however, it does not matter, in Montmarquet's view, whether those in range are killed by the pre-existing threat or by some newly created force.[77]

Montmarquet's formulation of Thomson's second condition achieves at least one result Thomson needed her first condition to secure: it rules out pushing somebody into the trolley's path. Even though she would be killed by what threatens the five and thus would satisfy the second condition as Thomson stated it, she is out of range of the trolley inasmuch as the trolley could not have been redirected to hit her rather than the five. Montmarquet

unwilling martyr of the unlucky patient are in this respect parallel. The same is true of pushing the oblivious passerby into the path of the speeding train.

The point can be made another way. Pushing somebody onto trolley tracks ordinarily infringes a claim she has against us whether or not a train is approaching. It generally causes somebody to fall and may cause injury. But giving somebody a very slight shove, so that she catches her foot in the track for a few minutes, is not a serious violation of her rights. See Gorr, 'Thomson and the Trolley Problem,' 94. Or not calling out to somebody about to cross the tracks to remind her to check for trains typically does not infringe any important right of hers. If either the small shove or the failure to warn constitutes a serious rights violation when it causes somebody to be hit by the trolley—as it must to satisfy both of Thomson's conditions, and if those conditions are to answer to our intuitions, they must encompass these cases—it is precisely because that act or omission has the person's death as a consequence. But then the same can be said of switching the trolley in the original case. Switching a trolley ordinarily violates nobody's rights, except possibly those of its owner. But switching it when somebody is on the track infringes an important claim he has against us in just the same way as does the gentle shove or lethal silence. Thomson's first condition therefore cannot distinguish cases that are morally opposed.

[77] See Montmarquet, 'On Doing Good: The Right and the Wrong Way,' 453. Montmarquet's quibble over Thomson's formulation of the second condition—that death must come from redirecting the pre-existing threat, not one the agent brings into being—seems to me of negligible importance, and perhaps unfair. The sole example he offers to illustrate the superiority of his formulation involves a berserk gunman who can, and presumably *will*, kill each person in the crowd around him unless he is killed. In this case, Montmarquet says, one may kill the gunman with a grenade to save some of the people in danger even if one thereby kills some of the innocent people in the crowd. (I say that the gunman presumably *will* kill everybody because Montmarquet avers that a mayor would have done wrong to shoot three alleged partisans to prevent Nazis from slaying fifty children unless he 'had good reason to think that the Nazis would kill them anyway.' Ibid. 450.)

While it seems likely that Thomson would accept Montmarquet's claim that one may heave the grenade to kill the gunman, it is not clear that she would agree that his example exposes an error in her formulation of the second condition. Thomson's paper attempts to identify the circumstances in which a person may kill someone who would *not* otherwise die in order to save more lives; she does not address the question whether one may kill somebody, such as a member of Montmarquet's crowd, who would die anyway if hastening his death might save lives. She might well agree with Montmarquet's implicit assertion that one may kill somebody who will die within seconds anyway if his death would likely spare others. But she might reasonably insist that Montmarquet's formulation of the second condition should contain restrictions on the degree to which the inevitable victim's death may be accelerated or rendered more painful.

can thus regard with equanimity the shortcomings of Thomson's first condition.[78]

Nevertheless, Montmarquet's reformulated condition fails to circumvent the most critical problems that confront Thomson's original.[79] First, there is the problem of responsibility. Suppose that the larger group within range of the threat recklessly created the threat, or put themselves in range voluntarily in pursuit of thrills. In this case, it is not enough to survey the range, pick out the larger group, and ensure that the smaller group perishes instead. At the very least, maximizing the number who live must be tempered by more than the condition Thomson and Montmarquet recognize.[80]

The second problem is more serious because it cannot be met by a simple amendment: how does one explain and justify the condition's boundaries on the class of permissible victims? Why should it matter whether a person is within the small class of those inside the threat's range? Or within the narrow, but slightly wider, class of those who can be killed by whatever threatens the larger group, even if they rather than the threat must be moved? Montmarquet and Thomson (by different routes) would permit somebody to turn a trolley on an innocent person standing on a side track who would otherwise go unharmed if doing so would rescue five others. But they would not permit somebody to shove or gull an equally innocent person onto the trolley tracks to save five if she, too, would otherwise go unharmed. Nor would they allow someone to be killed by whatever destroys the threat to the five if she were not already threatened herself. The train bearing down

[78] Perhaps not with *total* equanimity: it is by no means evident how Montmarquet would handle omissions to fulfill duties when those omissions produce fewer deaths. Suppose, for example, that a deaf person is walking beside the trolley tracks. The train is chugging along and will run her down, saving five people a short distance ahead, unless you warn her of her plight. She is certainly in range, by Montmarquet's account. So it seems that you should let her be killed. Yet that seems little different from nudging her so that she gets hit by the train, if she is just inches out of range. Thomson could say that failing to warn her is morally no different from elbowing her, because both violate a significant claim that the person has against us. But there is nothing in Montmarquet's account that authorizes this reply.

[79] One minor problem might be the requirement that the pre-existing threat be able to kill the one. See Montmarquet, 'On Doing Good: The Right and the Wrong Way,' 448; Thomson, 'The Trolley Problem,' 1403, 1407. Kamm suggests that this formulation is too restrictive, because intuition draws no distinction between killing someone by diverting a threat and killing somebody by some force set in motion by diverting a threat or by the act of diverting the threat. For example, if turning the trolley will not cause it to hit the one but rather cause it to ram into a cliff where it will unleash a rock slide that will kill the one, it is no less permissible to turn it, in Kamm's view. See Kamm, 'Harming Some to Save Others.' 228–9. Likewise, if switching the trolley will render it harmless but simultaneously start up a second trolley that will kill one, it is still permissible to turn the switch. See ibid. Whether or not Montmarquet's and Thomson's use of the words 'kill' and 'make threaten' can comfortably cover these cases, their use of the words should, I think, either be understood to embrace actions such as causing the rock slide or be modified to include them explicitly.

[80] Thomson acknowledges that this modification is necessary. See Thomson, *The Realm of Rights*, 180.

on the five cannot be halted by a dynamite charge if a bystander would be killed by the explosion, unless (at least on Montmarquet's theory) the train could have been diverted to strike the one instead of the five. It is hard to see why these distinctions should make a moral difference, however, when the victims in each case are equally innocent, their losses are equally great, the gains to others are identical in all respects, and the agents' motives and intentions are exact replicas.[81]

Or consider a variation on Kamm's 'Lazy Susan' case.[82] Six people are on a giant Lazy Susan. Five are presently suspended over the trolley track, and will be killed by the train if you do nothing. You cannot stop the train, but you can spin the Lazy Susan, bringing one person over the track who is now off to the side and safe. He will be killed if you spin the Lazy Susan, but the five will live. Montmarquet and Thomson's principle enjoins you from spinning the Lazy Susan, but not from turning the train onto a side track where one person will be killed, because the trolley could not itself be redirected to kill the one on the Lazy Susan but it could be redirected to kill the lone worker. Is this distinction reasonable? If not, then what about the distinction between spinning the Lazy Susan and simply pushing somebody standing nearby onto the tracks?

Montmarquet's explanation why one cannot kill somebody outside a threat's range to save more people within it is surprisingly terse. 'The short answer is that this would be like breaking a horse's leg so to justify shooting him. If we have no right to put the unthreatened person's life into a threatened state, the fact that we could treat him differently if he were (already) threatened is of no consequence.'[83] As elucidation, this is empty. What needs explaining is *why* we have no right to move somebody within range. Why not say that the group of permissible victims is bounded by the physical limits of moving people as well as moving the threat, or that it encompasses everyone who could be killed or allowed to die to produce a net gain in lives? Bringing somebody within range is not tantamount to breaking a horse's leg gratuitously to justify shooting it without benefit to the horse or any other living

---

[81] Michael Gorr poses the same question:

[W]hy should it matter whether or not what you make threaten the one is the very same thing as what is already threatening the others? Why isn't the following set of facts all that is really morally relevant here: (i) you must choose whether or not to perform an act that will infringe the rights of innocent persons by causing their deaths in a situation in which some innocent persons will be killed somehow regardless of what you choose; (ii) neither you nor any of those persons is responsible for the existence of this choice situation; (iii) who gets killed and who does not will depend on which choice you make; (iv) fewer persons will be killed if you perform the act than if you fail to perform it; (v) the persons involved are all equally 'worthy' of living; (vi) you have no special obligations to any of these persons; and (vii) there are no other morally significant consequences of your performing (or not performing) the act in question?

Gorr, 'Thomson and the Trolley Problem,' 95. An argument similar to Gorr's is presented in Fischer, 'The Trolley and the Sorites,' 107–12.

[82] See Kamm, 'Harming Some to Save Others,' 228–9.

[83] Montmarquet, 'On Doing Good: The Right and the Wrong Way,' 449.

creature. It parallels shooting a horse to save five other horses. The question remains: why should whatever gave rise to the threat define the class of permissible victims when it is within our power to spread a wider net?

In 'The Trolley Problem,' Thomson offers no more of an answer than does Montmarquet. She admits:

I do not find it clear why there should be an exemption for, and only for, making a burden which is descending onto five descend, instead, onto one. That there is seems to me very plausible, however. On the one hand, the agent who acts under this exemption makes be a threat to one something that is *already* a threat to more, and thus something that will do harm *whatever* he does; on the other hand, the exemption seems to allow those acts which intuition tells us are clearly permissible, and to rule out those acts which intuition tells us are clearly impermissible.[84]

Thomson's first hand, however, does not give a possible justification for this exemption from the rule forbidding intentional killing. It simply restates her second condition. The other hand does offer a reason, but that reason provides no deeper insight into the exemption's foundation. It amounts to saying that we should accept the redirected threat exemption because it generates the right evaluative results, without suggesting why that coincidence exists. Perhaps Thomson would say that the coincidence cannot be explained because explanation ends here. The fact that the rule against taking life intentionally as modified by the redirected-threat exemption yields, intuitively sound prescriptions is the only justification one can give and, for that reason, a sufficient justification.

Unfortunately, this rejoinder, whether or not Thomson would have offered it, appears too easy because it seems that there ought to be some reason why pushing somebody in front of a train is worse than pushing the train into him, if indeed it is worse. Moreover, even by the test of intuition the exemption seems dubious. Recall the case of the convalescents in the hospital ward. Why may we move the weight so that it kills one rather than five, yet not switch on a machine that will keep the ceiling from crashing down if its fumes will kill the one? Our motivations, the threat, and the results would be the same in both cases, except that if we did what is forbidden—use the machine—we would not have to repair the ceiling later.

Or consider one of Montmarquet's examples. A Nazi officer tells the mayor of a Greek village that unless he kills three suspected partisans, his soldiers will execute fifty children. Montmarquet asserts, and Thomson would presumably have concurred, that the mayor may not shoot the partisans unless the Nazis would kill them anyway.[85] By shooting them himself,

---

[84] Thomson, 'The Trolley Problem,' 1408.
[85] Leave aside the possibility that the disparity in numbers is so great that the usual rule ceases to apply.

the mayor would not be diverting an existing threat, he would be creating a new one.[86] But now imagine that the Nazi officer does not offer the mayor the opportunity to shoot the alleged partisans, fearing that the mayor might turn the gun on the Germans. Instead, he gives the mayor a choice: have my soldiers shoot the three, or stand by and watch them murder fifty children. Now the three are in range, in Montmarquet's sense, and the mayor must decide whether to deflect a harmful force—the Nazis' bullets—that is headed for the children. So Montmarquet would apparently approve the mayor's choice that the three be shot. Leaving aside any considerations relating to clean hands, is there any compelling reason for the mayor to decide differently in the two cases?

To be sure, there might be a *phenomenological* difference between the two actions. It might feel more dastardly to pull a trigger while looking into a condemned man's eyes than to order someone else to shoot. Likewise, seizing somebody and shoving her to her death beneath the wheels of a train might at the time strike one as more wicked than pointing the train at a person some distance away. But our viscera are inaccurate moral barometers in these cases: only brief reflection causes these initial responses to fade, belying their moral authority. Strangling innocent enemy children with one's bare hands to induce surrender might seem more horrible than dropping bombs on babies from several miles in the air, but the evil of the two actions is, if not equivalent, then nearly so. Whatever phenomenological differences we at first experience in these situations are properly attributable to moral and emotional dispositions that appear shortsighted to the extent that they are not naturally unavoidable, rather than to any significant moral difference between the wrongness of the pairs of acts.

The distinction between redirecting an existing threat so that it kills fewer rather than more, and saving lives by killing the smaller number through some means other than the existing lethal force, is therefore bereft of a foundation in factors that seem morally pertinent. It stands detached from the moral equality of persons and their rights not to suffer harm, from intention, from motive, and from the consequential value of possible ramifications. Intuition, moreover, reveals that the redirected-threat exemption to the rule that intentional killing is forbidden is not an infallible guide, although in most cases it hugs the morally attractive course. Is it possible to explain the exception, which in a great many (if not all) cases intuition sponsors, in terms of more fundamental principles and, by reference to that explanatory ground, to hone it so that its prescriptions all pass scrutiny? In *The Realm of Rights*, Thomson claims to

---

[86] See Montmarquet, 'On Doing Good: The Right and the Wrong Way,' 446, 450.

have found a justification for the redirected-threat exception that reflection approves.

4.2. Thomson's Appeal to Rational Advantage

Thomson maintained in 'The Trolley Problem' that a bystander at the switch may turn the trolley on a single worker to save five other workers on the main track, because switching it would merely divert a pre-existing threat and lives would on balance be saved. Her current approach introduces an important distinction. The bystander, she says, should ask a question that did not occur to him before: did the six workers have an equal chance of being alone on the side track? If they did—if, for example, positions were assigned by lot each morning—then he may turn the trolley. If they did not—if the lone worker was a beam fitter and beam fitters always work alone—then apparently the bystander may not send the trolley towards the one.[87]

The reason for asking the question, according to Thomson, is that people have a claim-right not to be killed—a right people may waive and often would waive if doing so would improve their prospects for survival. Thomson's crucial contention is that if people *would* rationally have agreed to such a rule, we may act with respect to them as if they had consented, even though they never explicitly voiced their agreement. A person's claim-right not to be killed is limited by whatever rules governing killing would have been to his antecedent advantage. Thus, the bystander may turn the trolley if the workers were assigned positions randomly, for in that case they would, if rational, have agreed to a maximizing rule. If turning the trolley would kill a beam fitter who always labored alone, however, the bystander must allow the trolley to crash into the five. The beam fitters, Thomson assumes, would not have found it advantageous to waive their right not to be killed on the condition that a maximizing rule would take effect.[88]

Contrast the lone worker positioned randomly with the organ donor chosen arbitrarily by a surgeon with five dying patients in her ward. The surgeon may not proceed, Thomson says, because, in the world as we know it, many people would not have found it to their advantage to agree to this

[87] See Thomson, *The Realm of Rights*, 180–1.
[88] This is not *necessarily* true, of course. Perhaps beam fitters are paid extra to compensate them for running this additional risk, and they are happy to take the money because they are less risk-averse than other workers. Thomson presumably assumes that beam fitters receive no bonus on account of their having a greater chance than most workers of ending up in the smaller group in a world where choice trails the numbers.

life-saving procedure before they were in need. For at least some people, the scheme would be an unappealing form of insurance.[89] It would sacrifice the healthy to save the sick, thereby trading higher for lower quality life. Because health is not entirely accidental, but rather depends substantially on people's voluntary actions—their diets, their jobs, their leisure activities—insurance of this kind might have unfortunate incentive effects, removing some of the natural sanctions that attach to imprudent behavior. More important from the standpoint of someone contemplating joining the scheme, it would expose people who eat and act cautiously to the dangerous or foolish behavior of others, and could well evoke resentment when they are called to sacrifice their lives so that gluttons, chain smokers, and daredevils might live. Finally, some might hesitate to sign up because they think an involuntary donor's sudden death—the slash of the scalpel only hours after a knock at midnight—would be far worse than a slow demise from organ failure that affords time to close one's affairs. In any case, Thomson says, one can safely predict that unanimous approval would never coalesce around an organ transplant scheme in which a randomly chosen healthy person had his body plundered whenever harvesting his organs could save five sickly people. *If* people's health were independent of their voluntary actions, and *if* people were not greatly concerned about having time to bring their projects and relationships to a meaningful conclusion before dying, then we *could* imagine universal rational assent, and the transplant case would mirror the trolley case in which workers were assigned positions by lot.[90] But that fantasy world furnishes no catechism for moral appraisal here and now.

Thomson concludes that the general rule that we may not kill one to save five is therefore subject to certain exceptions.

The exceptions, I suggest, are those in which the one who will be killed, and the five who will be saved, are members of a group such that it was to the advantage of all the members that the one (whoever he or she would later turn out to be) would later be killed, and the only thing that has since changed is that it is now clear who the one was going to turn out to be. The numbers five and one have no special importance, of course; what matters, I should think, is only whether more will be saved, for that is what raises their probability of survival and (other things being equal) therefore makes proceeding later be to the advantage of all.[91]

---

[89] See Thomson, *The Realm of Rights*, 183–4.

[90] See ibid. 185–6, 195. See also Harris, *Violence and Responsibility*, 82 (describing conditions necessary for organ extraction and reconditioning lottery that does not allow for survival of the organ donor); Harris, 'The Survival Lottery,' (advocating compulsory survival lotteries under certain conditions). For a critique of Harris's view, see Rakowski, *Equal Justice*, 341–4; Peter Singer, 'Utility and the Survival Lottery,' *Philosophy*, 52 (1977), 218 (arguing that the survival lottery advocated by Harris 'removes the natural disincentive to imprudent action'): see also text accompanying nn. 160–4 below.

[91] Thomson, *The Realm of Rights*, 195.

But *ought* somebody to take another person's life in these exceptional cases if doing so would ensure that more people remain alive? Thomson thinks not. If somebody believes that chance, or fate, or some divinity should determine who lives, or if he simply feels incapable of taking a fellow human being's life, he cannot be faulted for not saving the greater number by killing fewer, even if rational persons would have favored that course beforehand. 'The view that morality requires [the bystander] to turn the trolley,' Thomson says, 'seems to me to be merely a morally insensitive descendant of the Central Utilitarian Idea.'[92]

What about flipping a coin? Thomson scoffs at the suggestion that the bystander ought to flip one. Why make that random event determine who lives when one can rely on the random sorting of people into larger and smaller groups? Indeed, flipping a coin seems an affront to the people whose lives are threatened, because it is not what they would have wanted before the situation arose. Nevertheless, Thomson declares without further argument that it is *permissible* for the bystander to flip a coin, just as it is permissible for him to stand idle as the larger group meets its end, at least if he is 'moved by the thought that he thereby gives them an equal chance at life' and is not, I suppose, acting on a whim.[93]

4.3. Doubts and Unanswered Questions

Two of Thomson's contentions seem entirely correct: first, that people, as rational, autonomous, self-conscious creatures, possess a claim against others that they not be killed, which even the lives of a great many more other people cannot ordinarily override; and second, that we may act toward others as if they had waived this claim in situations in which we can be sure that they would, with reason, have agreed to adopt a maximizing rule if asked before a choice had to be made.[94] These principles, I shall argue, offer intuitively pleasing solutions to the test cases considered above, explain the appeal of the distinction between originating and deflecting harm, and successfully challenge intuition when it dissents. Because Thomson's approach does not assume that lives have an objective value that can be

[92] Ibid. 196.

[93] See ibid. 197.

[94] It is of course unimportant (I think Thomson would agree) whether one says that a person's claim-right not to be killed is bounded by the rules licensing killing to which he would antecedently have assented, or whether one says that the right still exists in these circumstances but that there has been a constructive waiver of the right by the person whose life is in jeopardy. Some might find the first formulation more natural, because they think the notion of hypothetical waiver self-contradictory. But nothing of moral substance turns on the vocabulary.

summed for the purpose of deciding whether people's claims against us can be infringed, I find it especially congenial.[95] Before attempting to develop these points more fully than Thomson has done, however, it will be useful to probe her account for omissions, ambiguities, and doubtful claims. One may then see more clearly what expansions and corrections are needed.

One question Thomson does little more than pose is how a person should act when he is uncertain whether everybody he might kill would rationally have agreed to a maximizing rule. If, moreover, he has reason to believe that one or more people would not have assented, are there circumstances in which he may or should ignore their wishes, either because the reasons they would have given are inadequate or because the dissenters are few in number and the desires of the overwhelming majority should hold sway? Thomson says that it is hard to believe that one of the randomly positioned workers would find turning a trolley so objectionable as to outweigh his enhanced probability of survival.[96] But suppose somebody let it be known that his religious convictions barred killing in *all* circumstances and that he would rather trust God than the calculations that underpin a maximizing policy. Would morality permit our turning the trolley on him if he were in the smaller group? Certainly, some explanations for a person's refusal to go along are so irrational that they should not be credited. Is religious

---

[95] Thomson does not entirely agree with my view. Because people have, in her terms, a claim-right against us that they not be killed, numbers are, she says, irrelevant. We may not kill one to save a million. See Thomson, *The Realm of Rights*, 166–7. But when claim-rights are *not* at issue and we face 'matters of mere distribution'—when, for example, the question is whether we should rescue a larger or a smaller group of drowning sailors if we cannot save both—numbers. Thomson says, 'arguably do count.' Ibid. 167 n. 5.

It seems to me that, in themselves, and not by virtue of the role they play in determining whether people would hypothetically consent to a maximizing rule, numbers do not count in either case. We have a duty to save people in danger if we can do so at little cost to ourselves. If people matter equally from the standpoint of morality, the proper course, *in the first instance* (i.e., before consulting whatever reasoned preferences they would have expressed beforehand), is to lend each the same chance of survival, regardless of how people are spread across different sized groups. See Rakowski, *Equal Rights*, 281–91. 301–9; Sect. 5.10 below.

Why Thomson recoils from this view is unclear. She takes pains to demonstrate that people lack a claim-right to be saved. See Thomson, *The Realm of Rights*, 160–3. But her principal reason for contending that people lack this right is that recognizing it would, she thinks, entail treating a duty to save a life and a duty to refrain from killing as equally stringent, an equivalence which intuition would condemn. This conclusion does not, however, follow inexorably. One could consistently reject the premise that a right to be saved has the same force as a right not to be killed by dropping Thomson's Comparison Principle, which holds that one of two claim-rights is more stringent than another only if not honoring the first right makes things worse for the person exercising the right than does not honoring the second right. See ibid. 161. Given that Thomson also considers people who fail to save others' lives at small cost 'gravely at fault,' ibid. 163, she apparently could object to the alternative I defend only on semantic grounds. And semantic grounds offer no persuasive reason for divergent approaches to the numbers question in the context of killing some to save others and saving some rather than others.

[96] See Thomson, *The Realm of Rights*, 182.

conviction among them? Or suppose that somebody who asserted a right not to be killed would become a free rider if a maximizing rule were implemented only in situations in which he would not be made worse off. He would invariably be saved if he were in the larger group because he could not veto and might not want to veto the use of a maximizing rule in such a case. Yet he would also be protected if he were in the smaller group and the trolley would otherwise run down more people, because he has insisted on his rights. Should he be permitted this privilege?[97]

A second set of questions concerns cases Thomson discussed in her earlier article but leaves unmentioned in *The Realm of Rights*. Thomson formerly distinguished between culpably switching on the ceiling-support machine in the hospital case, which would kill the single convalescent in the next room, and permissibly re-directing toward the one a puff of lethal gas traveling up the air shaft when it would otherwise have killed five. Would she now agree that turning on the ceiling-support machine is morally allowed, assuming that the ceiling's collapse was as unexpected as the release of poisonous gas into the air shaft? What about jostling an innocent person onto the tracks to stop the train? Can we suppose that people would have consented to a maximizing rule covering these situations?

An additional problem arises when the people among whom one must choose belong to groups that might be thought to have elected to run different risks. Suppose a trolley is racing down Main Street. If a passenger does not turn it aside, it will kill five transportation workers repairing the roadway. If the passenger does swing the trolley, it will strike a smaller number of pedestrians on the sidewalk. Even if one can assume population-wide consent to a maximizing convention—and that, of course, depends on what reasons for nonparticipation one considers acceptable and on whether a sufficiently large majority can legitimately have its way—and even if one supposes that transportation workers would have agreed to such a rule too, can one simply apply a maximizing rule when one must choose between pedestrians and workers? If pedestrians would have agreed to the rule if only pedestrians' lives were at stake, how do we determine whether they would have agreed when the choice is between people who often work near trolley tracks and people who stroll by less often?

Besides not confronting what she would once have regarded as counter-

---

[97] Does it make a difference if somebody who has *not* opted out is always in the larger group? Suppose, for example, that trolley supervisors routinely accompany the larger group of workers. This case should not be troubling. Although supervisors profit from the maximizing rule relative to one that bids rescuers flip a coin or save the smaller group, the fact remains that everybody else also benefits from the maximizing rule although not as much. If everybody would favor a maximizing rule, there can be no objection to instituting it, assuming their assent is not irrational.

intuitive implications of her current view. Thomson skirts the question of
how the counterfactual situation in which rational advantage is assessed
should be imagined, and why it should be conceived of in this way.[98] With
respect to the trolley workers, she asks whether they would rationally have
agreed to a maximizing rule if questioned at the start of the day, before
positions were assigned by lot. But why should that hypothetical question be
posed daily? Why not ask whether workers would rationally have consented
at the start of each week, or each month, or each year, or at the beginning of
their careers? Thomson does not say why the hypothetical choice situation
that is morally determinative should be set at one time rather than another,
or why the information available to persons in it should be constrained in the
ways she favors.

In addition to these omissions, two features of Thomson's account seem
to me unsatisfactory. The first is Thomson's discussion of cases in which we
must choose between killing some people and watching *somebody else* kill
more people. Thomson contends, as did Foot, that we may not kill at a
villain's behest, even if we are sure that the villain will carry out his threat to
slay more people if we refuse.[99] But she does not explain why this strict
prohibition applies when we may usually divert a trolley to kill one worker
rather than five. It cannot be because another person forced us to make the
choice. If the trolley's brakes do not work because some misanthrope sabotaged them, Thomson does not suggest that our reasons for maximizing the
number of survivors evaporate. Nor is Foot persuasive when she says that if
we comply with the villain's threat, 'anyone who wants us to do something
we think wrong has only to threaten that otherwise he himself will do

---

[98] I should note that Thomson herself disdains references to 'hypothetical consent,' which she
labels an 'epiphenomenon.' Thomson, *The Realm of Rights*, 188 n. 5. She prefers to speak of what
would be to somebody's 'real advantage,' ibid., because she thinks that what we should care about
'is not that such and such people would consent if they were asked, but rather whatever it is about
them in virtue of which they would consent, if they would.' Ibid. 187. Thomson's preference for
the term 'real advantage,' however, seems not to turn on any substantive disagreement with philosophers who appeal to what people would have consented to if they were clearheaded, aware of the
risks they faced, and free from the distorting influence of strong emotion. For example, Thomson
argues that if a person's deeply held religious beliefs would impel him to refuse consent to some
action that would affect him, taking the action would be objectively bad for him. See ibid. 187–91.
If, however, a person's 'real advantage' is tethered to whatever settled preferences he has, provided
only that they are not plainly irrational, there is nothing, save a vocabulary Thomson dislikes, to
separate Thomson's approach from conventional appeals to hypothetical consent under appropriate conditions. Only if the phrase 'real advantage' denotes a person's good in a way that renders it
at least to some degree independent of what he would regard as his good in full awareness of his
situation and in calm command of his faculties would Thomson's account of a person's 'real
advantage' depart from ideal hypothetical consent accounts. But there is little evidence that she
desires this departure.
[99] See ibid. 150–3; Foot, 'The Problem of Abortion and the Doctrine of the Double Effect,' 25,
28–9.

something we think worse.'[100] Of course the creation of desirable incentives is a relevant consideration. But if we know that the villain will make good on his threat to kill five unless we kill one, then it is just as if he set a brakeless trolley in motion and left us to decide between five and one. Nor, it seems, is the relevant difference that, in the case of a villain, we would become the tool of another's malign will. That is true when we turn the sabotaged trolley, as well as when we are offered a choice between shooting Joe or watching the villain shoot Joe and Jane: if the villain has a reputation for making credible threats, it seems that we should, or at least may, shoot Joe.[101] So Thomson's assertion that we ought not to heed the villain's threat seems dubious, and in need of a justification she never supplies.

The second of Thomson's claims that I find unconvincing is her assertion that the bystander at the trolley switch may permissibly do nothing, or flip a coin, when he might turn the trolley so that one will die instead of five. Far from being 'a morally insensitive descendant of the Central Utilitarian Idea,'[102] the assertion that he *ought* to turn the trolley derives from the powerful claim of all those affected by his action to have him act as they would have wanted, when doing so does not require him to make a notable sacrifice. Unlike utilitarianism, which often dictates actions that would not have been approved by at least some of those whom the actions affect, choosing according to a maximizing policy in the situation Thomson describes would have gained the assent of everybody affected by the choice. *Not* to turn the trolley, as Thomson herself admits, would be to slight those in danger. And flipping a coin to randomize selection would be to ignore the earlier lottery that put some in the larger group and one or more in the smaller group. It would, in her words, be 'to say that [the bystander] must proceed as if the world had just been created five minutes ago, for it tells him to ignore the past history of the people now on the tracks.'[103] It therefore seems that he *should* save the greater number.

[100] Foot, 'The Problem of Abortion and the Doctrine of the Double Effect,' 25.

[101] See Davis, 'The Priority of Avoiding Harm,' 201–7, for a helpful and subtle discussion of these issues. The case of Jane and Joe is reminiscent of Bernard Williams's famous case of a South American botanist named Jim who is given the choice between shooting one blameless Indian himself and looking on as soldiers murder the Indian along with nineteen others. See J. J. C. Smart and Bernard Williams, *Utilitarianism: For and Against*, 98–9 (Cambridge: Cambridge University Press, 1973). Although Williams hesitates, it seems plain that Jim may kill an Indian who would die anyway if doing so will spare others, despite his becoming the instrument of the soldiers' evil commander. See below, text accompanying nn. 165–9. Kent Greenawalt describes a different case posing the same issue: unless a lieutenant of an invading army shoots the mayor of an embattled town, his commander will kill all the inhabitants, including the mayor. See Kent Greenawalt, 'Natural Law and Political Choice: The General Justification Defense—Criteria for Political Action and the Duty to Obey the Law.' *Catholic University Law Review*, 36 (1986), 1, 4.

[102] Thomson, *The Realm of Rights*, 196.

[103] Ibid.

Thomson seems to believe that her contrary conclusion follows at least when the bystander does *not* think the arguments from antecedent advantage that underlie the maximizing policy are correct, or when he is simply unable to do what is right.[104] But the question is not whether we should condemn somebody who acts conscientiously but wrongly or who is incapable of doing what he thinks morality requires. The question is what action is morally correct. And Thomson, so far as I can see, says nothing to cast doubt on the claim that saving the greater number is morally imperative.

5. JUSTIFICATION BY HYPOTHETICAL CONSENT AND FAIRNESS

Ordinary human beings have a powerful moral claim against their fellows not to be killed and, under certain circumstances, to be saved from death or serious harm. The scope of that right is not, of course, unrestricted. For example, it arguably does not protect, in at least some cases, innocent people who threaten others or who would be killed by the removal of what threatens others, should those in danger, or third parties who wish to assist them, use necessary lethal force to eliminate the threat.[105] That right not to be killed is also alienable. Unjustified aggression may forfeit its protection,[106] and express waivers are morally effective in some cases, even if the law does not presently recognize consent as a justification for intentional homicide. In addition, people may in certain situations be treated as though they relinquished that right—or, differently phrased, as though in those cases they did not have such a right—if they would, for good reason, have surrendered it, or if fairness to others denies them that protection. This section elucidates and defends these broad claims.

---

[104]

For mightn't [the bystander at the switch] himself think these things should be left to chance (or Fate or God)? Alternatively, mightn't [he] think these things should not be left to chance, but all the same feel incapable of killing a person, even to save five others?
Ibid.

[105] For a recent exchange on this issue, see Judith Jarvis Thomson. 'Self-Defense,' *Philosophy & Public Affairs*, 20 (1991), 283; Larry Alexander, 'Self-Defense, Justification, and Excuse,' *Philosophy & Public Affairs*, 22 (1993), 53.

[106] This is not necessarily to say (though I would) that a criminal who may lawfully be resisted or punished has no right to defend himself. Hobbes famously denied that any person may alienate the right to protect himself against invasions of his personal liberty, even if those invasions are justified. See Thomas Hobbes, *Leviathan* (1651), ed. C. B. Macpherson (1968), 199. Thomas Hobbes, *De Cive: The English Version*, ed. 'Howard Warrender' (1651; . . . 1983), 58–9. I shall avoid the question whether Hobbes was right by concentrating on situations in which it is impossible for those who might be killed to offer resistance.

5.1. Rights not to be Killed

To say that people should always be treated as ends in themselves, never just as means to enhance the welfare of others, is at a minimum to say that they may not be killed simply to satisfy another's desire. It is also to say, in my view, that they may not be killed against their will so that another person may live or so that many other people may live,[107] unless the conditions set out in Section 5.4 are satisfied or unless the victim would have been killed anyway and, to the extent possible, he was selected fairly.[108] Kant's injunction to treat people as ends and not only as means can, as I noted above, be regarded as supporting the utilitarian conclusion that people may be killed whenever more will live. But the better reading of that imperative, one more robustly supported by our intuitions in particular cases and by general moral convictions, rejects this conclusion. We know that the surgeon may not kill one of her unconsenting patients to save five others, and we know that this must be so regardless of whether a careful consequentialist calculus supports this result. Except in certain circumstances—when somebody must kill to save herself or somebody she loves, when the conditions listed above are satisfied, or perhaps in fighting a just war—killing another blameless person intentionally or foreseeably and against his will is wrong. It wrests from him everything he has for the sake of somebody who is, as his moral equal, no more worthy of continued life. People are, in a sense, treated equally if their lives are regarded as morally interchangeable, so that one can be traded for another or, if circumstances make the exchange rate favorable, for several more others. But that is not a sense that accords with the respect due them as autonomous beings not put here for the greater good of one another or some cosmic purpose outside of themselves.[109]

[107] Although this principle governs relations between normal human beings, it does not apply generally to all creatures that are wronged if killed. Any creature that possesses, or at one time possessed and might again enjoy, sufficient self-awareness for it to lose something by dying has, I think, a right not to be killed. That right, however, is not absolute. Its strength varies with a creature's ability and propensity to weave its past and future into a single life from its perspective and to distinguish itself from the world and other sentient beings by means of memory, imagination, and desire. In certain circumstances, some creatures' rights not to be killed bow before the needs or desires of people or nonhuman animals having greater self-awareness, even though the latter stand to gain something less important than life itself. See Rakowski, *Equal Rights*, 333–4, 355–63.

[108] The second qualification is one lesson of Bernard Williams's example of the botanist asked to shoot an innocent person or watch him die along with nineteen others. See above, n. 101, and below, text accompanying nn. 165–9. As noted in Section 1, I abstract from cases in which the only way somebody can protect himself or people about whom he cares is by killing someone else.

[109] Shelly Kagan argues that insupportable consequences ensue if we ascribe to people a right not to be killed for the benefit of others, and we assert that violations of this right are always wrong and cannot be rectified by paying compensation later, as one might make good an earlier violation of some property right (the starving backpacker who breaks into a cabin in the woods).

This view of a person's right not to be killed is admittedly stronger than my argument requires. A more widely accepted notion of the worth and inviolability of persons holds that individuals have a right not to be killed to save a few more others, thus precluding the surgeon from operating, but that this right gives way when the number of equally valuable lives that might be saved grows significantly larger.[110] This less stringent view is coherent, at least if the required numerical difference is a ratio of people saved to people killed rather than some fixed amount.[111] It has, however, an *ad hoc* quality,

If not killing somebody is of *incomparable* importance relative to all gains that one might thereby derive, he says, then it must also be wrong to impose even a slight risk of death on somebody for a great gain. But accepting that view would paralyze us: 'For there is absolutely *nothing* that I can do which does not carry *some* risk of harming others. Driving a car risks maiming a pedestrian, cooking supper risks harming my housemates, and turning on a light risks electrocuting my neighbors.' Kagan, *The Limits of Morality*, 89. The only acceptable alternative, Kagan says, is to make the permissible level of risk vary with the gains likely to be achieved from some activity. But that view, he thinks, would not be tolerated by at least some people who claim that individuals possess an unbending right to life. See ibid. 87–91.

This objection seems overstated. First, Kagan exaggerates the frequency with which we expose others to some risk of death. Most of what huge numbers of people do each day—sitting at a desk, strolling along a sidewalk—poses no threat to others. Moreover, those dangers we do create are ordinarily easily justified because they involve a reciprocal assumption of risk (driving on the highway, for example), see, e.g., Charles Fried, *An Anatomy of Values: Problems of Personal and Social Choice*, 189–200, 257–58; George P. Fletcher, 'Fairness and Utility in Tort Theory,' *Harvard Law Review*, 85 (1972), 537, 543–50, or are licensed by collective consent through the representative processes of government (pollution regulation; rules governing the transportation of hazardous materials; housing codes). Finally, I suppose that Kagan is right in saying that *some* people who believe that individuals have a right not to be killed, regardless of how much their death would benefit others, would balk at tying the magnitude of acceptable risks of being killed to the expected gains from which those risks are inseparable when the peril falls well short of certain death. But it seems highly unlikely that most people would take this view. The vast majority would consider risk-imposition proper to advance important ends, even if another occasionally dies as a result. Virtually everyone, for example, would deem electrical wiring in homes morally permissible, notwithstanding its potential to spark a neighborhood conflagration and even apart from the reciprocal risk homeowners typically impose on one another. Home experiments with missiles for sheer fun would not be.

[110] For example, Charles Fried, who believes that there exists a categorical moral prohibition against intentionally taking innocent life, writes: 'And even as to killing, I do not know how to answer the person who asks me whether I would be willing to kill an innocent person to save the whole of humanity from excruciating suffering and death.' Charles Fried, *Right and Wrong*, 31. This is, of course, as powerful a case for killing innocent, unwilling people as one can imagine. Perhaps Fried would kill if the balance were less uneven. Others drawn to the categorical view probably would. See above, n. 40.

[111] The non-ratio formulation of the moral importance of numbers to life-saving would be nearly impossible to sustain. According to that view, a smaller group of persons might be killed if necessary to save a group that is larger by some unvarying amount. Suppose fifty is the necessary absolute difference in the number of lives preserved. Then one person may be killed to save fifty-one (although two may not), and fifty may be killed to save one hundred. That seems to imply that the force of a person's right not to be killed, as against others' needs, varies with the number of people ranged with and against him. In some cases that right trades at fifty-one to one, in other cases at two to one, in still other cases somewhere between the two rates, or even lower than two to one. There is something unattractively odd about making the morality of killing turn on some

the result, perhaps, of trying to accommodate intuitive responses to unusual cases without recourse to a single motivating insight. Surely it is strange that one life cannot be sacrificed for five lives of equal value, yet can be taken for fifty or five hundred such lives. As with many hybrid views, the deontological and consequentialist components tend to pull apart, with each threatening to subordinate the other. I would jettison the consequentialist side of this position and affirm that nobody may *ever* be killed against his will to save another when he would not otherwise have died, unless the requirements of fairness described in Section 5.4 dictate a contrary result or the killer bears certain special relations to the person saved. This view best expresses people's independence and moral equality, in my judgment, without offending to an appreciable degree our intuitive judgments about hard cases. Nevertheless, this strict deontological thesis is not essential to my argument in this section, except for the approach to life-saving I endorse in Section 5.10. It suffices that a person's right not to be killed has *some* force against the value of however many lives killing him might save, so that it is generally impermissible to kill him against his will to save fewer than the threshold number. The question is whether that right sometimes loses the force it ordinarily has against whatever greater number of lives is otherwise insufficient to justify killing.

5.2. Conditions of Waiver: Actual and Hypothetical Consent

Volenti non fit injuria ('No wrong is done to one who consents') is an established moral principle which the law usually sanctions. Conduct that would be tortious or criminal—yanking someone's tooth, having sex with her—ceases to be so if the other party reasonably agrees. Respecting other people means allowing them to decide for themselves what harms to risk or suffer in return for what they prize. For those who share this ideal of voluntariness, rooted in both Kantian moral philosophy and the English utilitarian tradition of which Mill is representative, a person's consent to be killed for his own good or for the benefit of others will often render it morally permissible to kill him. Regard for his autonomy requires that we defer to his wishes.[112]

---

contingent fact (the happenstance that the smaller group contains one rather than fifty, whatever the size of the larger group) that is unrelated to the intrinsic wrongness of killing relative to failing to save.

[112] Laws against assisting suicide, which exist in 29 states, see David Margolick, 'Doctor who Assists in Suicides Makes the Macabre Mundane,' *New York Times*, 22 Feb. 1993, A1, and laws forbidding the taking of life even pursuant to a knowing, persistent, and rational request for voluntary euthanasia, which are even more common, might suggest that this principle is not generally accepted in the United States today. These laws do not necessarily evince popular

But consent does not always justify. A woman's consent to be killed after a villain threatens to murder her children unless she offers herself up does not absolve the villain if he kills the mother. Coerced consent cannot license wrongdoing. In addition, consent is morally effective only if it is considered rather than impulsive, the product of stable preferences and adequate reflection.[113] Consent must also satisfy certain criteria of reasonableness that are difficult to specify.[114] These requirements, intended to ensure that someone's decision faithfully reflects her values and preferences, become more stringent the larger the loss that the consent would allow.[115]

rejection of the principle, however, because their retention (whatever the reasons for their original enactment) might be motivated primarily by the fear that they will frustrate the prosecution of unjustified killings, that they will weaken the deterrent effect of laws forbidding murder, or that they will be abused by cost-conscious health care providers, misguided physicians, or self-interested family members. Narrow defeats for proposed legislation authorizing physician-assisted suicide in referenda in Washington in 1991 (Wash, Initiative 119) and California in 1992 (Cal. Proposition 161), together with widespread acceptance of discontinuing life support for apparently irreversibly comatose patients when they themselves would have favored that course, show strong public pressure for legal recognition of people's autonomy over decisions affecting the manner and timing of their deaths. See, e.g., Peter Steinfels, 'Help for the Helping Hands in Death,' *New York Times*, 14 Feb. 1993, §4, p. 1 ('In polls, large majorities of Americans express support for the proposition that doctors should help terminally ill patients commit suicide or give them lethal injections if they request them.'); cf. Marlise Simons, 'Dutch Move to Enact Law Making Euthanasia Easier,' *New York Times*, 9 Feb. 1993, A1 (78% of Dutch public support right of terminally ill to request euthanasia). To be sure, there are currents flowing the other way, visible in Michigan's enactment of a temporary law banning assisted suicide. But this law seems motivated more by the distasteful publicity that Dr. Jack Kevorkian has generated than by opposition to voluntary euthanasia, which two-thirds of Michigan voters, polls say, still support. See Isabel Wilkerson, 'Michigan Moves to Ban Doctors' Aiding in Suicides,' *New York Times*, 25 Nov. 1992, A14.

[113] The problem of defining adequate reflection is often acute in practice, especially when a person contemplates signing a living will or granting a durable power of attorney and is unable to form a vivid or accurate picture of what her life will be like if certain changes occur. For helpful discussion of the problem of adequate imagination and changes in personal identity, see Joel Feinberg, *Harm to Self* (Oxford: Oxford University Press, 1986), 354–74; Allen Buchanan, 'Advance Directives and the Personal Identity Problem,' *Philosophy & Public Affairs*, 17 (1988), 277.

[114] For example, suppose that a man's aged and domineering mother, whom he has sheepishly tended for many years, suffers kidney failure. Although she could be kept alive by dialysis for the few years remaining to her, she would probably lead a more comfortable life if she received a new kidney. Her son is the only available donor, and because he has but one functioning kidney and is himself ineligible for dialysis, donation would kill him. Even if he pleads for months with doctors to perform the transplant and says he is quite willing to die to make his mother's last years less painful, most people would doubt whether the doctors should proceed.

[115] Joel Feinberg, who skillfully defends the view that consent is the only adequate basis for interfering with adults' actions for their own good, stresses the importance of ascertaining their settled, deliberate, reasonable desires:

The more strongly we hold to the *Volenti* principle, the higher must be the standards we employ for determining the voluntariness of consent. *Volenti* is most plausible when it denies title to complain only to him whose consent was *fully voluntary*, and a person's consent is fully voluntary only when he is a competent and unimpaired adult who has not been threatened, misled, or lied to about relevant facts, nor manipulated by subtle forms of conditioning.

Joel Feinberg, *Harm to Others* (Oxford: Oxford University Press, 1984), 116.

My aim, however, is not to provide an exhaustive list of the necessary conditions for making a person's consent to be killed morally effective. Nor shall I consider how laws barring killing even when consent is given ought to affect the decision whether to kill. Instead, I wish to emphasize that a person's reasoned, informed, and uncoerced consent to an action generally suffices, as a moral if not as a legal matter, to permit one to perform the action so far as that person is concerned. When, moreover, consent is given explicitly not to die but to bear some risk of being killed that falls far short of certainty, and when the benefits seem reasonably to rival the costs, legal objections motivated by the fear that consent to suffer harm might not in some cases be completely voluntary typically fall away. We allow people to drive to work on busy highways, even though a certain number will be killed in crashes.[116] We permit people to take dangerous jobs in construction or mining. We do not ban kayaking, smoking, or stunt flying. In most if not all cases in which death might accompany some activity, we require only that participants be apprised of the risks they run and that they take minimal precautions that a large majority of persons would recognize as prudent.

Analogous considerations should apply to risks people freely assume of being killed intentionally. Situations in which killing some people might save others are rare, but in some instances one can imagine people assenting to their being killed in the unlikely event that those situations occurred. The situations most easily envisaged are those in which killing some would save many more others. In addition to runaway trolleys, examples include armed attacks on terrorists or enemy soldiers that are apt to kill innocent hostages or bystanders, or rescue efforts to save trapped miners that will inevitably collapse shafts in which fewer workers are immured.[117]

Nevertheless, explicit assent to a maximizing rule is virtually non-existent in contemporary society. Employment contracts do not include clauses specifying that as many workers as possible should be kept alive in emergencies, even if some must be killed to raise the total number of survivors.

[116] Which makes one wonder why the federal government prohibits the sale of kidneys. The increased risk of death to a healthy thirty-five-year-old from giving up a single kidney was (as of twenty-five years ago) approximately the same as the risk of fatal accident from driving sixteen miles to work each day. See Henry Hansmann, 'The Economics and Ethics of Markets for Human Organs,' *Journal of Health Politics, policy and law* 57 (1989), 72 (citing J. Hamburger and J. Crosnier, 'Moral and Ethical Problems in Transplantation,' in F. Rapaport and J. Dausset (eds.), *Human Transplantation* (1968)). I am unaware of a more recent comparative risk estimate.

[117] Jonathan Glover provides an historical example. During the Second World War, British officials were apparently able to shift German rocket attacks from London to less populous areas by sending false reports about the rockets' accuracy through a double agent. The officials did not do so, allegedly because they deemed it immoral to sacrifice one lot of citizens in place of another (larger) group. See Jonathan Glover, *Causing Death and Saving Lives* (Harmondsworth: Penguin, 1977), 102–3 (citing S. Delmer, *The Counterfeit Spy* (1971), ch. 12).

Maximizing rules find no place in regulations promulgated by labor unions, federal agencies, or state legislatures. Nor can they be said unambiguously to represent public policy as expressed in the unwritten, conventional practices of law enforcement officials, in penalties for failing to save the greater number, or in affirmative defenses to murder. In addition, informal conventions incorporating maximizing rules are difficult to locate, except perhaps among soldiers and nineteenth-century seamen.[118] Situations in which it would be possible to kill some to save more others are simply too rare, and the subject is for some people too unsettling, to make advance planning worth the trouble.

The question is therefore whether it is permissible or morally required for one to act as if people had agreed to the application of a maximizing rule when in fact they have not considered one or have not expressed their collective assent. In certain circumstances, acting as somebody would have wished if he were informed, lucid, and undistracted seems plainly appropriate if his consent to what would generally constitute an invasion of his rights cannot be obtained. Providing medical assistance to an unconscious person is the stock example. In other cases, it is appropriate even if consent could have been obtained, but for some reason was not. Borrowing a book from a friend's shelves without permission, or buying an extra bag of gravel for a neighbor that one knows he wants and requesting payment later, provide homely illustrations. Contract law supplies another example of hypothetical consent: when contracts fail to specify how some unanticipated event should be handled, arbitrators or courts typically attempt to determine what arrangements the parties would have made had they foreseen the unexpected event and accord them rights against one another on that basis.

In many other situations, however, the fact that somebody would have agreed to some proposal seems devoid of moral force if in fact he did not consent. Suppose that a colleague with an unimpeachable reputation for honesty asks me to give her $10. She had made a private bet with herself, she relates, that if a coin she flipped came up heads, she would pay me $1000, and if it came up tails, I would owe her $10. The coin, she informs me, came up tails. Even if I would have consented to bet on such favorable terms, most

---

[118] See A. W. Brian Simpson, *Cannibalism and the Common Law* (1984), 122–40 (describing an established, if sometimes dishonored, convention among starving sailors awaiting rescue at sea of drawing lots and eating the loser). Taking as an example the notorious case of *Regina* v. *Dudley & Stephens*, L.R. 14 Q.B.D. 273 (1884). Simpson describes the gulf between the moral principles espoused by the common seamen who killed and ate a weakened cabin boy to survive and the convictions of their upper-class prosecutors and judges. See ibid. 225–70; see also *United States* v. *Holmes*, 26 F. Cas. 360, 367 (E.D. Pa. 1842) (No. 15,383) (describing random choice of victims from among starving crew as rule recognized as correct by all writers).

people would say that I have no obligation to pay up because I did not actually agree to the wager.

Should the agreement somebody would have given to the imposition of a rule maximizing the number of lives saved, when assent to that rule would not have been irrational, be treated like the consent one would have manifested to medical treatment when unconscious? Or should it be treated like the wager one would gladly have made but did not?[119] Answering these questions requires that one specify the sources from which hypothetical consent draws its moral force and how far that force extends. By 'hypothetical consent' I mean the consent somebody would have given to an action that affects him and that he has a right to prevent, if he were asked under conditions in which his thinking and volition were not impaired or influenced in an untoward way, and he were aware of his beliefs, desires, and broadly

---

[119] Discussing political contractarianism, Kim Scheppele and Jeremy Waldron answer related questions concerning law's normative grounds by distinguishing consent as a basis of legitimacy from consent as a basis of obligation. See Kim L. Scheppele and Jeremy Waldron, 'Contractarian Methods in Political and Legal Evaluation,' *Yale Journal of Law and Humanities*, 3 (1991), 195. Although Scheppele and Waldron do not offer complete definitions of 'legitimacy' and 'obligation,' they describe the chief significance of distinguishing the two terms as follows:

[T]he most important difference between legitimacy and obligation is this: a person cannot be actually obligated by a *hypothetical* promise she *might have* entered into. The idea of promising requires the free assumption of an obligation that has no other basis except in the actual consent of the person assuming it. So consideration of what people would have agreed to, in circumstances where clearly they have *not* agreed to that or anything else, tells us nothing about their promissory obligations. With the consent that confers legitimacy, however, the situation is slightly different. Consent here is related rather more closely to an objective sense of *interests* than it is in the obligation case. If an unconscious person needs urgent surgical attention, the surgeon's actions may be legitimated by an affirmative answer to the question of whether the patient *would have* agreed to the operation if she had been conscious, and this hypothetical consent can be assumed more readily when something is clearly in the hypothetical consenter's *interest*. Hypothetical consent, in other words, can sometimes legitimate even though it can never actually obligate.

Ibid. 201–2.

Unfortunately, Scheppele and Waldron's distinction between legitimacy and obligation offers little guidance in the case we are considering. On one hand, being killed in accordance with a rule maximizing the number of people kept alive seems passive, like being operated upon or having taxes withheld from one's paycheck (although their article *might* be read to say that tax collection to fund welfare services is only legitimate if the taxpayer consents). See ibid. 201. On the other hand, however, the same can be said of many promissory obligations (as most people conceive of them) because many promissory obligations can easily be recast as acts of passive acquiescence when the hypothetical promisee seizes property by way of collecting on the hypothetical promise. Scheppele and Waldron's account does not indicate how the class of promissory obligations should be bounded, or why it should be limited in whatever way they favor. Referring to 'an objective sense of *interests*' is no help in tracing the divide, because everything depends on how one construes that notion, and Waldron and Scheppele do not defend one of the many contending views. They do not say, for example, whether it is in a person's objective interests to have somebody else killed so that she may live even when she believes killing morally wrong under all circumstances. In short, the distinction between obligation and legitimacy, unaccompanied by a fuller account of the bases for these two types of moral constraint, does not itself entail that killing is justified in some cases but not others, nor does it explain why and where it is permissible or morally required.

speaking, his personal situation and history.[120] This is not the consent of an imaginary rational being whose conception of his values, ambitions, and personal good is the product of some philosopher's speculation, which he might not endorse following adequate reflection free from emotional upset or duress. This is simply the consent that an actual person would give under the optimal conditions for decision.

This consent must, to be sure, be reasonable if it is to be authoritative. The consent of the insane is no warrant for harming them. But it is essential that 'reasonable' be defined elastically, so that a reasonableness requirement does not cloak the imposition upon people of values and judgments that they do not espouse and would not embrace unless they were to become people they would not recognize as themselves.[121] It is admittedly difficult to state abstractly when a person's preferences become so unreasonable that they cease to command our respect, just as it is sometimes hard to say what information we should imagine is ideally available to deliberators as they ponder. But for my purposes, precision is unnecessary. What matters is that the person whose consent is sought must be the final arbiter of his interests and values and that the recognition of putative moral or religious truths cannot be a necessary condition of the reasonableness of a choice.[122]

---

[120] A more careful, detailed account may be found in Donald VanDeVeer, *Paternalistic Intervention* (Princeton: Princeton University Press, 1986), 75–87 (discussing hypothetical individualized consent). Strikingly similar accounts of the conditions for normatively effective consent are offered by almost all the leading writers on paternalism. See, e.g., Feinberg, *Harm to Self*, 106–17; Dan Brock, 'Paternalism and Promoting the Good,' in Rolf Sartorius (ed.) *Paternalism* (Minneapolis: University of Minnesota Press, 1983), 237; Dan Brock, 'Paternalism and Autonomy,' *Ethics*, 98 (1988), 550; John Hodson, 'The Principle of Paternalism,' *American Journal of Philosophy*, 14 (1977), 61; Danny Scoccia, 'Paternalism and Respect for Autonomy,' *Ethics*, 100 (1990), 318.

This conventional formulation of ideal, hypothetical consent in terms of a person's stated preference under a number of normatively significant conditions might, of course, be challenged. One could argue, for example, that a person's overt nonverbal behavior, not his responses to set questions, is the best indication of his will. Consider philanderers who denounce fornication and adultery, or the vast number of people who say that *post mortem* organ donation is morally laudatory but who do not sign donor cards themselves.

This challenge might have merit in certain cases. But I wish here to set it to one side, along with the concomitant problem of *akrasia*. In thinking about circumstances in which people might choose to adopt a maximizing policy, it seems to me that what they would say would typically accord with what they would do, or that, if the two diverged, their considered judgment, not their ashamed inability to act on it, should prevail.

[121] See, e.g., Feinberg, *Harm to Self*, 106–13; VanDeVeer, *Paternalistic Intervention*, 81–7.

[122] As Donald VanDeVeer says: 'The guiding notion . . . is that we must respect, within limits, not only others' choices but also their prerogative to assess reasons for revising their own derivative or basic goals. Apparent or actually superior insight on the part of other competent persons does not by itself render permissible invasive intervention to promote good.' VanDeVeer, *Paternalistic Intervention*, 80. VanDeVeer offers the following helpful example:

[I]t is one thing to knock down Jones to prevent him from touching an exposed, high voltage, electric powerline and another to impose a transfusion on the Jehovah's Witness. That one ought to touch such powerlines is not likely to be a belief held by Jones. That one ought to avoid transfusions is not only a belief but an important belief in the

From what source does hypothetical consent derive its moral authority? The obvious answer is that its authority descends from its expression of an individual's autonomous will, just as express consent does when it is informed, unperturbed, and reasonable. If someone's decision to undergo surgery after being fully apprised of the risks, costs, and potential benefits deserves heeding, so too does his hypothetical consent to the operation in circumstances in which his actual consent is unobtainable. Both equally manifest his considered preferences; the advantage actual consent has as moral authorization is *evidentiary*, one of certainty not normative power, and then only insofar as the conditions for ideal choice obtain.

A deeper question is why autonomy itself has value, so that a person's status as a reasonable judge of what is right or good for him deserves respect and his choices deserve deference to the extent that they do not unjustifiably harm other people. This is a controverted question, to which there are many answers.[123] Certainly, autonomous decisionmaking has instrumental value. It contributes to our well-being, not only because of the delight we take in our own agency, but also because we are usually the best judges of what will advance our interests, if only because we tend to know ourselves better than others do.

Autonomy, however, has intrinsic value as well. We would not trade our capacity for choosing and leaving our mark in return for life on a wondrous experience-machine, even if it produced a perfect counterfeit of our *experience* of free agency.[124] More fundamentally, we not only value efficacious choice, we respect the capacity to choose in ourselves and others because ranking ends and selecting means is ultimately what defines us as persons. The construction and reworking of our higher-order desires is what

---

Witness's conception of how to live her life and is one derivable from her basic, life-defining and life-guiding, views and attitudes. To conjecture about what the Witness would choose if she believed that blood transfusions were permissible is very different from conjecturing about what Jones would choose if he believed the powerline might kill him. For Jones to come to believe that the powerline has such a potential requires no conceptual renting asunder of Jones' personality, no fundamental, imaginative, disfiguration of his outlook on life. By contrast, it is plausible to conclude that conjectures about what the Jehovah's Witness would choose if she believed transfusions were all right are close to incoherence. Rather, it is to query whether some person would choose or consent differently if she were someone else—or a radically different sort of person. But she is not, and questions about what some *particular* individual would consent to if confronted with relevant choice-affecting data are, at the very least, questions about how *that sort* of person would decide—not about what some psychologically stripped individual, similarly situated, and reclothed with quite different basic values and beliefs, would decide.

Ibid. 81.

[123] For a survey of responses, see John Christman, 'Constructing the Inner Citadel: Recent Work on the Concept of Autonomy,' *Ethics*, 99 (1988), 109, 120–1.
[124] See Jonathan Glover, *What Sort of People should there Be?* (Harmondsworth: Penguin, 1984), 95–6; Robert Nozick, *Anarchy, State, and Utopia* (Oxford: Blackwell, 1974), 42–5.

integrates us over time,[125] shaping our more immediate urges and longings and lending contour to our lives. The evident importance of autonomy to our identity and well-being is the main reason paternalism is only tolerable in exceptional situations. We resent others' choosing for us and fear tyranny that dons the mantle of benevolence. Legal and structural political limitations on paternalistic intervention into the lives of competent adults have other roots too, besides the historically justified fear of moral or religious despotism. Some see those limits as founded on skepticism about whether there is any objectively good life for people or for any particular person.[126] Others base them on the claim that even if there are objectively better or worse ways to live, one can only *lead* a good life from the inside, through conscious choice and striving; one cannot be shoved toward saintliness.[127]

For the purposes of this article, there is no reason to choose among these theories of the value of individual autonomy or the importance of safeguarding personal choice. What is crucial is the claim that competent adults' higher-order desires ought ideally to determine what may be done to them in matters that predominantly concern themselves.[128] This claim does not

---

[125] Lower-order desires are desires to do or not to do some particular thing. Higher-order desires are desires to have or not to have certain lower-order desires. They might also be thought of as those convictions and preferences about how best to live that are central to someone's conception of himself as an individual. The terminology originated over twenty years ago with Harry Frankfurt's article. See Harry G. Frankfurt, 'Freedom of the Will and the Concept of a Person,' repr. in *The Importance of what we Care About* (Cambridge: Cambridge University Press, 1988), 11. For a discussion of more recent work on this multi-tiered conception of personality and autonomy, see Christman, 'Constructing the Inner Citadel,' 112–14.

[126] See, e.g., Brock, 'Paternalism and Autonomy,' 561.

[127] This belief finds eloquent expression in John Locke's famous *Letter concerning Toleration*. A good historical account of arguments like Locke's is Preston King, *Toleration* (1976). Modern versions of this argument are common, particularly from liberals keen to deny that liberalism does not rest on agnosticism or skepticism about the existence of objectively valuable goods. See, e.g., Charles Larmore, *Patterns of Moral Complexity* (1987). The argument that attempts to coerce belief are inefficacious will find little favor among people who are more concerned with preventing bad actions (as opposed to false beliefs) or halting the spread of what they consider an ethical virus. See Brian Barry, 'How not to Defend Liberal Institutions,' in R. Bruce Douglass *et al.* (eds.), *Liberalism and the Good* (1990), 44, 47–9.

[128] Some might reject this claim, arguing, for example, that someone should be kept alive because continued life is valuable or right even if he wishes to die, or that a denial of consent grounded in what somebody takes to be God's will may be ignored because religion is so much superstition. Various perfectionist or objective-list accounts of human welfare, see, e.g. James Griffin, *Well-Being* (Oxford: Clarendon Press, 1986), 40–72, might (but need not) contribute to similar justifications of paternalistic intervention. My argument rests on the contention, which I shall not defend further here, that these views, as justifications for dishonoring a competent adult's self-regarding higher-order desires, are mistaken. The intrinsic and instrumental value of autonomy, the tension if not outright contradiction in trying to force someone to lead a life he scorns because he judges it differently from the coercing party, and the danger that the power to compel might be abused all point in this direction. I argue below that at least some of these reasons militate against ignoring people's religious or moral opposition to policies maximizing the number of survivors, even if considerations of fairness might overcome that opposition. See below, Sect. 5.4.

privilege actual consent over hypothetical consent, except (in some cases) epistemologically. Indeed, one might well say it does the reverse. Hypothetical consent is, by definition, a perfect expression of someone's autonomous preferences, whereas actual consent, in the non-ideal circumstances of everyday life, is invariably a more or less close approximation. In any case, the decisive moral question (leaving aside any applicable legal restrictions) in deciding whether one may infringe the rights of another is whether the action accords with his will, where his will is a construction of his higher-order preferences, ranked as he would arrange them following adequate rational reflection and having due regard for any dissatisfaction he would feel at infringements of his rights that he did not expressly authorize even when those infringements are intended to serve, and do serve, his interests as he defines them.

As I mentioned, this view of the proper occasions for infringing someone's rights is widely shared by prominent writers on paternalism, whether, like Brock, they view the ultimate ground for intervention as consequentialist, or whether, like Feinberg and VanDeVeer, they see its foundations as deontological. All of them limit their endorsement of actions meeting this test of hypothetical consent to those that would, when performed, benefit the consenting subject or prevent a substantial loss to that person.[129] This limitation might be traced to the conventional boundaries of discussions about paternalism. It certainly owes something to the worry that a broader license for intervention in the name of hypothetical consent might lead to unwarranted governmental restrictions and manipulation.

Be that as it may, the foregoing rationale for acting in another's interest cannot be cabined as representative discussions of paternalism perhaps suggest. It extends to all situations in which a person's highest-order preferences (including his moral convictions) would have approved some action or omission with respect to him, even if, at the time that action is performed, it harms him. There is nothing unnatural in this extension: if autonomy is best respected by acting as somebody's higher-order desires dictate, there is no reason to stop short in cases where those desires do not conduce to that person's self-interest, narrowly construed. Just as the terms of a contract might become onerous, so too hypothetical assent to some policy might prove personally detrimental, even though the policy was prudent or otherwise desired. In both cases, a person must accept the consequences of his actual or hypothetical decisions. Taking personal autonomy seriously means acting as someone desires on balance, bearing in mind that what he immediately wants is not always coincident with what he wills. Just as hypothetical

---

[129] See, e.g. Feinberg, *Harm to Self*, 186–7; VanDeVeer, *Paternalistic Intervention*, 22.

consent may license paternalistic actions that, at the time of their performance, advance someone's good notwithstanding his protests, so too it may
justify actions according to rules that advance someone's good (as he defines
it) even though, at the time of their performance, they work to his actual
disadvantage. The notion of autonomy on which standard accounts of justifiable paternalism rely does not harbor any inherent limitation on rights-
infringing actions (rather than policies for rights-infringing action) that
benefit the person affected, nor, so far as I can see, is there any compelling
independent principle that would so restrict its scope.

My aim in this section is apologetic. I argue that acting in accordance with
rules to which somebody would have consented, in trolley cases and more
mundane situations, is consistent with the high regard we have for autonomy, inasmuch as it respects what is or would be the considered preference
of the person benefitted or harmed by the action. I further argue that this
principle, although it goes beyond what are generally considered prudent
limitations on paternalistic interference, is free from counterintuitive ramifications. Its consequences, even in difficult cases, are readily acceptable. I
later argue, in Section 5.1, that the dangers of altered attitudes and even
errant killings that are attendant on allowing people to kill some to save
more others are not so daunting as to justify not construing or rewriting the
choice-of-evils or necessity defense to homicide to include killing that meets
the criteria I develop over the intervening sections.

Consider, first, a case remote from life-or-death decisions. You discover at
your door a bottle of wine that you often buy for $15. No note is attached,
and you did not order it. You wait a week. Nobody comes for the wine. So
you drink it with a friend one evening. The next day, the person who left the
bottle asks for $5 as reimbursement. Are you morally required to pay? In
discussing a similar case, Paul Menzel assumes that you would have agreed
to buy the wine for $5 if you had been approached. Yet he also thinks it
evident that you are not obligated to pay a penny when asked. That you
would have considered the wine a steal at $5 is irrelevant:

> [A] crucial condition of presuming consent is that obtaining actual consent be either
> impossible or in some sense prohibitively costly. In the rough sense, 'prohibitively
> costly' simply means what the actual individual, with his or her actual values, would
> agree is too high a cost for upgrading from presumed to actual consent.[130]

Menzel believes that articulated consent has greater moral force than presumed consent, even when there is no doubt that an individual would have
consented, because 'people see intrinsic value in making their own explicit
choices.'[131] But both carry considerable moral weight, because conduct

[130] Paul Menzel, *Strong Medicine* (1990), 31 (footnote omitted).
[131] Ibid. 24, 30.

according to either '[b]ring[s] decisions in line with one's values and beliefs.'[132]

Menzel's contention, that presumed consent can legitimate what would otherwise be rights-infringements or can bind a person if the prohibitive-cost condition is met, is plausible.[133] That actual consent is intrinsically more valuable than presumed consent inspires more doubts, unless Menzel merely wishes to note that people prefer making their own choices to having wise choices made for them. If presumed consent is given the meaning I attached to the phrase 'hypothetical consent' above, it should be at no disadvantage morally to its verbalized cousin. Nevertheless, there is no disputing that explicit consent is typically a better indicator of what somebody prefers than whatever other evidence and generalizations provide a basis for inferring consent. And Menzel's contention that presumed consent is at least some-times binding yields the intuitively correct result in the case of the unconscious individual in need of medical treatment. Menzel further contends—less persuasively, as I explain—that his rule also handles the abandoned wine bottle case properly. There, he says, the cost of calling you or attaching a note to the bottle was low, hence the supplier's failure to secure your consent absolves you of all obligation to pay.[134] Menzel would presumably say the same of hypothetical consent to a coin-flip wager featuring an extremely attractive win-loss ratio.

How Menzel would resolve the trolley case is unclear. It would, however, be reasonable to presume that he would regard express advance consent as prohibitively costly, given the slim likelihood that this fatal decision would arise and the trouble of informing whoever might be at the switch of any agreement the workers had made. In that case, if people would have assented to a maximizing rule, the trolley could be switched to kill the smaller group to save a greater number. Menzel's approach should also decree that manda-tory organ transplant schemes are not justified because the prohibitive-cost condition is not satisfied: if people want to run the risks associated with those schemes in exchange for their possible benefits, they may do so if they choose.

Despite these appealing features, Menzel's attempt to delimit the moral

---

[132] Ibid. 31.

[133] Menzel imposes other conditions as well. For advance consent to bind, there must, he says, 'be important advantages for the sort of case at hand in making decisions at a prior point in time,' ibid. 33. He invokes this vague condition to hold people to their earlier health insurance decisions, for controlling health care costs would be impossible if patients could change their minds about the scope of their insurance coverage when in need. See ibid. 32. In addition, a person relying on presumed consent has the burden of showing that it would have been granted. See ibid. 33–4. I shall not discuss these further conditions.

[134] See ibid. 30.

importance of presumed consent in terms of a prohibitive-cost requirement is not entirely successful. One minor flaw is his definition of 'prohibitively costly' by reference to the view of the person whose consent might be presumed.[135] Making the moral propriety of somebody's actions depend upon the affected person's unknown subjective evaluation of the reasonableness of acting without securing explicit consent seems mistaken.[136] If an exceptional individual would not have wanted a doctor to operate on him while he was unconscious because he would have voiced religious or other objections to interference, it hardly seems right to say that the doctor acted wrongly by operating when the overwhelming majority of people would quite sensibly have wanted him to operate. Some objective standard of reasonableness is required.[137]

A larger defect is that intervention is sometimes justified for a person's good even if actual consent is not forthcoming. A person's refusal to consent might be contrary to her own ends through weakness of will or a stubborn failure to recognize what is best given her values and desires. Further, despite her actual resentment of intervention, she might indeed approve it under ideal conditions if the divergence between her actual expressed preference and her good yawns wide. Menzel might, I suppose, insist that actual consent may not be overridden in practice, even if it might be as a theoretical matter. His concern is with the informed consent that patients give medical personnel, and he might think that the perils of permitting health care workers to ignore a patient's expressed wishes exceed the benefits patients might glean from doctors who strive to fulfill their ends by ignoring patients' stated desires. But these practical worries should not be allowed to mask the

[135] Menzel states that defining 'prohibitively costly' by reference to the judgment that would have been made by the person whose consent might be presumed renders 'the whole argument in a sense admittedly circular.' Ibid. 31 n. 24. He adds that he sees no way to avoid circularity and that he is not convinced that it betrays any defect.

[136] Menzel, like VanDeVeer, might only wish to claim that it is only whether somebody's invasive conduct is *justifiable* that should be determined by reference to the person's own view as to whether the prohibitive-cost condition is met, not whether that conduct is *blameworthy*, which depends upon what action was objectively reasonable. See VanDeVeer. *Paternalistic Intervention*, 150–5; but see Douglas N. Husak, 'Paternalism and Autonomy,' *Philosophy & Public Affairs*, 10 (1980), 27. 32–5. This dispute is purely semantic unless VanDeVeer (and Menzel, if he agrees) believes that interventions that are unjustifiable but not blameworthy should be sanctioned in some way. He does not, however, offer any evidence of this belief—for example, by suggesting that, contrary to current practice, doctors not be permitted to recover fees for services provided to unconscious patients if, as might a Jehovah's Witness, they would have refused medical treatment if conscious.

[137] One possibility I mention below is to categorize explicit consent as 'prohibitively costly' if the transaction costs of obtaining consent from somebody exceed the expected net benefits that the person would derive from consenting. This possible test is not self-applying, however. People might count up the costs to themselves differently, because their aversion to risk differs or because their confidence in other people's honesty or ability to calculate benefits is greater or less than that of most other people.

theoretical propriety of intervention in some cases in which the prohibitive-cost condition has not been satisfied.

Another flaw in Menzel's account is that somebody's failure to obtain consent when doing so would not have been prohibitively costly does not seem to deprive him of all right to compensation for any benefits he bestows or to render him liable for all harms he inflicts. Suppose that a wine shop delivered the bottle to your house by mistake, and that the error was not discovered until a week later because the intended recipient was away on holiday. Have you no obligation to pay *anything* for the wine? Or suppose that a friend of yours left it. She found it on sale at a bargain price, and intending to do you a favor, she bought a bottle and brought it by at a time you are usually home. Unfortunately, you went out and she lacked pen and paper, so she simply left the bottle on your porch (carrying it to the opera would have been awkward). She planned to call you later, but forgot. Your mention of the wine a week later jogs her memory. Do you owe your friend nothing for the wine? Would the answer really change if your friend could easily have taken the bottle home with her, but did not bother?

It seems to me that in both cases you do owe compensation, although not necessarily the amount the shop charges or your friend paid. You are morally obligated to provide compensation, moreover, despite its not having been prohibitively costly to request payment beforehand. In my view, in the absence of an independent moral principle requiring some payment for the wine (or over and above what any applicable independent moral principles require),[138] the question is what amount, if any, you would have agreed to pay for it knowing that circumstances would unfold as they did, including any actions you took in reasonable reliance on the fact that you did not pay for the wine when you first found it. This is analogous to the standard that applies to paternalistic intervention: what would ordinarily be rights-invasions are appropriate if someone would reasonably have approved them in those circumstances, knowing the anger or resentment he would feel if his actual consent were not obtained and the setback his interests would suffer if nobody intervened. Thus, if the bottle went into your wine rack and substituted for a purchase you would otherwise have made, you might well owe more than if you reasonably treated the mystery bottle as a windfall and

---

[138] Menzel appears to assume that no moral principle independent of hypothetical consent mandates payment. I am less sure. That people have a duty to repay at least part of any unsolicited benefits they receive at some cost to others, whether through others' mistakes or by their design, seems to me true in some cases, though certainly not in all. If that obligation exists in a given instance, it perforce sets a lower bound to what somebody owes by way of compensation. Moral duties do not vanish just because somebody is blind to them.

enjoyed it more casually than if you had paid for the wine.[139] The question, again, is what payment you would have considered due under the complex circumstances that actually existed.[140]

Of course, as a legal matter you probably would not owe anything. There are obvious benefits to having a rule that obviates determinations of how much somebody would have paid in certain counterfactual situations, that does not allow merchants to press goods on people and demand payment,[141] and that supplies businesses with an incentive to make proper deliveries by making them pay for their errors. But in this case it is hard to see why the existence of that legal rule should alter your moral obligation, any more than the absence of a law penalizing you for failing to save a drowning person at slight risk and cost to yourself frees you from moral responsibility if you stand idly by as a child slips beneath the water.

The importance of reliance on the absence of express consent nevertheless deserves emphasis. If I would have agreed to buy a friend's car but did not actually agree to do so, and if I then purchased a different car, I am not obligated to buy my friend's car when he later hands me the keys. My earlier, hypothetical consent would have been conditioned on my not buying another car before my friend offered to sell me his. The same can be said about the plight of the trolley workers. A worker might have assented to a maximizing rule when he took his job or accepted a particular assignment, but only if he had a better than fifty percent chance of being in the larger group at the time of decision. If he did not assent, and if he accepted solitary posts because he reasonably assumed that no maximizing rule was in effect, it would be wrong to treat him as though he consented to a maximizing rule. He would never have consented *except* on the proviso that job assignments

---

[139] Suppose you guzzled down the wine the moment you spotted the bottle, without making inquiries or waiting for somebody to discover the mistake and ask for the bottle back. The amount you morally owe is, I think, greater than if you waited a reasonable period of time before consuming the apparent windfall, because your action showed insufficient regard for the bottle's owner or intended recipient. This is one example of how an independent moral principle might constrain reliance on hypothetical agreement.

[140] My claim is that if you would have considered yourself obligated to pay under these circumstances, you are so obligated. It is possible, I suppose, that in making this hypothetical determination, somebody would favor Menzel's prohibitive-cost requirement for compensation. If so, then its justification with respect to that person (though not to others) would come from his making this judgment, not from whatever other source Menzel thinks grounds the prohibitive-cost restriction.

[141] Should one pay for goods one keeps that are sent unbidden through the mail, even though the law does not require payment or return? I think not, unless the sender provides compensation for return postage and the time and trouble of sending back the goods. Given the legal background, however, no retailer is likely to provide such compensation. Moreover, even if a retailer promised compensation upon return of the goods, recipients should not have to rely on a mere assurance of payment for the costs they incur, given the practical difficulties of bringing suit for breach of contract. Yet it is hard to imagine an arrangement providing payment up front that retailers would find attractive.

would be random, or at least would be made in a way that antecedently furthered his self-interest.[142]

What these examples suggest is that the consent somebody would have given to some proposal binds him and other agents in the present, provided that the terms on which he would have consented are fully specified and met, *including* whatever provision he would have wanted for decisions he took in the absence of actual consent.[143] This standard does not defer to present values and inclinations completely, rendering the reference to an earlier counterfactual decision otiose. The question in the case of the wine bottle, for example, is what somebody would have agreed to pay for the use to which the bottle was reasonably put, not how much somebody thought the bottle was worth after the wine was served and the experience to which it contributed (an intimate dinner, for example) had been lived. Nor does this standard employ some notion of consent, derived from what a morally or spiritually enlightened person would allegedly agree to, that might not coincide with the preferences the actual person in question would express under the counterfactual circumstances I described. That would be to endorse the hard paternalist position that I deplore, one that yokes people to a vision of their own good they themselves reject. Hypothetical consent is simply the consent that somebody would actually have manifested in a normatively authoritative situation of relevant knowledge and rational choice

[142] Fleshing out the assumptions under which somebody would have consented to an offer explains why the view I propose does not generate the wrong result in the case of the colleague who demands payment after flipping a coin at what she claims was a favorable pay-out rate for you. Suppose the person is a friend. In that case, you probably would not have consented to bet, because you thought the terms unfair and you did not want to take your friend's money. If a stranger proposed the bet, you probably would not have agreed either. You would have thought her mentally unstable or a gambling addict, making it wrong to take advantage of her, or you would not have trusted her. Even if you would have agreed, you would have doubted her word when she came to you later, not having secured your permission in advance. And if you did think she was telling the truth about the bet, you might reasonably suspect that she would not have come to you had the bet gone the other way. In short, you probably would only have agreed to bet if the bet were proposed by a stranger, on terms that were reasonable yet tempting to you, with adequate assurance of fairness in flipping the coin and of payment if you won. You would further have insisted that you not be bound by presumed consent if you relied detrimentally on the fact that you did not make a bet—say, by spending the money you would have bet on lottery tickets at less favorable odds. Some stranger asking for payment would almost certainly be unable to prove that all these conditions were fulfilled. The law sensibly denies her any right to payment.

[143] I ignore the question to what extent, if any, a person should be able to bind himself in the future, either expressly or tacitly, particularly if he intends, or would have wished, to protect against important changes in his values. The starting point for virtually all discussions of this issue is Derek Parfit, *Reasons and Persons* (Oxford: Oxford University Press, 1984), 326–9 (exploring bearing of personal identity on force of moral commitments over time); see also Buchanan, 'Advance Directives and the Personal Identity problem,' 283–302 (discussing need for psychological continuity to preserve personal identity for advance directives); Donald H. Regan, 'Paternalism, Freedom, Identity, and Commitment,' in Rolf Sartorius (ed.), *Paternalism*, 113, 122–34 (discussing implications of changes of identity over time for paternalistic interference).

that never in fact occurred. Thus, the standard I am endorsing merely attempts to explain and guide our intuitive reactions to particular cases by holding people to bargains they would have made, insofar as they would have wanted themselves held to those bargains. It is therefore consonant with, indeed an expression of, the personal autonomy that morality should protect and nurture. Deference to a person's considered higher-order desires, insofar as they can be ascertained, is deference to that person.

The application of this approach to the trolley case is straightforward.[144] If people have a right not to be killed without their consent, it would be wrong to turn the trolley headed for five towards one. If, however, somebody would have agreed to a maximizing rule in preference to this principle and did not act, in the absence of a justified belief that one applied, in a way that would have nullified the benefit he would have sought by consenting to its application, then it is permissible to choose according to a maximizing rule to his detriment in this case. Not to do so would contravene his will, viewed as a construction of his higher-order desires, even if the action turned out to be to his disadvantage.[145]

It is imperative, however, not to overlook the importance of actual, expressed consent as evidence of a person's will, and its absence as evidence of his refusal to consent to some infringement he has a right to rebuff if considered choice and the expression of a preference do not require excessive effort or expense. Menzel's prohibitive-cost requirement may not be a necessary condition for the effectiveness of presumed consent, but it is a useful guide, given a host of practical considerations and anxiety about paternalistic decisionmaking by people we may not trust, for dividing cases

---

[144] One who believes that there is an important difference between hypothetical consensual justifications for suffering actions and hypothetical consensual justifications for duties to perform actions, see supra note 119, should accept the application of the framework I have developed to situations in which some must be killed to spare a larger number of others, even if they reject its application to the case of the wine bottle and other affirmative duties.

[145] Suppose that the worker toward whom the train is redirected could somehow send it back towards the five, say, by radioing commands to it, or that he could prevent its being turned by shooting the person about to switch it toward him. Would his hypothetical consent obligate him to refrain? Perhaps not. In some situations morality might run out, so that actions in defense of one's life defy moral appraisal. See above, nn. 105–6 and accompanying text and below, Section 5.5. Alternatively, even if all actions are subject to moral evaluation, somebody might recognize that he or others could not or would not act as morality demands when their lives are threatened, and thus not agree even hypothetically to conform his conduct to morality's strictures in those situations. In that case, the lone worker might well conclude that pointing the train towards the five or shooting somebody about to take his life so that others would live is morally permissible. Even if self-defense would be morally permissible, however, it does not follow that somebody else would be acting impermissibly if she sought to send the train toward the one, notwithstanding her awareness that he would, quite properly, attempt to save himself even at considerable cost to others. Compare the efforts of an innocent person who stands wrongly condemned to resist state officials bent on enforcing a court order to execute him following a fair trial. Neither deserves blame, yet their actions are at cross-purposes.

in which actual consent should be required from those where it is inessential. If obtaining or furnishing actual consent would not generally be prohibitively costly, in the sense that the net benefits of consent will likely exceed the expected transaction costs of obtaining and giving consent, there is usually no reason to interfere with actual arrangements. For this reason, there appears to be a strong if rebuttable case against compulsory organ transplant schemes for adults using organs taken from live donors. People make medical insurance decisions regularly, and could sign onto plans of this kind if they so desired.[146] Unlike trolley-type cases, which are rarer, less predictable, and harder to register views about beforehand, organ transplants are not operations to which consent may be presumed.

5.3. The Circumstances of Hypothetical Choice

No doubt some will favor Menzel's statement of the conditions under which presumed consent is effective over the view I advance. Intuitions are apt to differ, for example, regarding the existence of a moral obligation to pay for the wine delivered to your home by mistake. But so long as one accepts *either* approach and agrees that the consent a person would have given can serve in lieu of the express consent she never gave, one must address the question of how the counterfactual situation in which consent is given or withheld should be described. What information—about their beliefs, identities, and personal situation—should people be assumed to have when we imagine them facing the choice between consenting and declining?

If the view I have been developing is correct, we should imagine people deciding with full knowledge of their convictions, desires, age, physical attributes, and personal circumstances, including the risks and possible rewards that consent would bring.[147] The purpose of appealing to hypothetical choice is to recognize and give effect to an individual's higher-order preferences. Relying upon the decisions she would have made were she shorn of her individuality would render the appeal nugatory. Just as hard paternalism is rightly condemned because it foists on people a conception of their good that they, on reflection, find unattractive,[148] so too an approach to

---

[146] For further discussion of the unfairness of mandatory organ transplant schemes, see infra text accompanying notes 160–4. I here assume something that is false in the United States today, namely, that voluntary organ transplant schemes are legally permissible.
[147] This appears to be Thomson's answer too. See Thomson, *The Realm of Rights*, 184–7.
[148] Donald VanDeVeer argues, in defending the view that paternalistic interference can be justified only on the basis of a person's own competent, considered beliefs about what makes life meaningful, not what someone else thinks that he *ought* to find valuable or illuminating or pleasurable:

life-saving that brushes aside what concrete individuals would agree to under ideal conditions works an unacceptable abridgment of their autonomy as reasoning beings.

One way of renewing the assault on this view is, of course, to ask why we should assume that people have a pro tanto right not to be killed for any purpose. Given this premise, a critic might say, the conclusion that we must grant robust self-knowledge to those making hypothetical choices follows, as it does in conventional analyses of paternalistic intervention. But whence this premise? In ascertaining whether people have a right not to be killed whenever more lives could be saved by killing, must we not ask what people *without* knowledge of their personal predicaments and without any moral or religious views about the propriety of killing or letting die would decide? And would they not agree that in general it is morally proper, because in these circumstances it is a prudent bet, to permit killing some people whenever more can be kept alive?

This is a formidable challenge. It sets forth the motivation for much broader consequentialist accounts of morality and distributive justice that employ an ideal contractarian framework.[149] It seems to me vulnerable, however, to three distinct objections. The first is that this approach to determining the wrongness of killing appears firmly tied to an ideal contractarian approach to resolving all ethical questions. When that approach is applied to other moral issues or matters of distributive justice, however, it recommends offensive policies and fails to respect the dignity we believe people to have.[150] Exploiting the productive, neglecting the handicapped if they prove to be poor utility producers, harming some people whenever greater gains will flow to others, are all repellant, yet they are arguably unavoidable under certain important consequentialist views unless apparently incompatible distributive constraints are imported from outside. An approach to life-saving that incorporates these deficiencies does not merit assent.

If we are to respect S as an active, autonomous, moral agent with his own conception of the good, we cannot invasively intervene in his choices on the basis of a myopic focus on what constitutes *his own good* even if we happen to possess superior insight on that score (or with regard to means to that end). To allow S to function as an independent moral agent, responsible for his choices and acts, invasive intervention is prohibited except when we have S's valid authorization or there is compelling reason to believe that he would appropriately consent to it. To do otherwise is to treat S as a 'good receptacle' or a 'utility location,' but persons are not just that. They are arbiters of their own well-being, and not merely sentient, computing, devices to be kept in good repair . . . Unlike computers, they originate, adopt, and revise ultimate ends.

Van De Veer, *Paternalistic Intervention*, 112.

[149] See, e.g., Harsanyi, 'Morality and the Theory of Rational Behaviour'; Hare, 'Rawls' Theory of Justice.'

[150] I shall not survey these shortcomings. The literature on utilitarianism and its evident weaknesses is vast. For an argument that it fails as a theory of distributive justice, see Rakowski, *Equal Justice*, 23–39. Additional arguments bearing on its defensibility as a theory of private morality can be found, for example, in Smart and Williams, *Utilitarianism*, and in Sen and Williams (eds.), *Utilitarianism and Beyond*.

The second objection is that, even confined to questions of killing or life-saving, this utilitarian approach seems to support counterintuitive results. For example, it at least appears to require that people lay down their lives or the lives of those they love if more would be kept alive by their doing so, and perhaps to smile on the doctor's cutting up one healthy patient to save five. Two-level or dispositional accounts can go some way toward ameliorating these implications, often by assuming that the hypothetical choosers have certain common human desires that would make their decisions less chilling, such as an overmastering desire to put oneself and family first.[151] But it is questionable how successful this gambit is, particularly if the theory recommends killing innocents who took pains to protect themselves in order to save a greater number of others who chose to run some risk of death—for example, trolley workers who knew that runaway trolleys were possible and often lethal.

The third objection, which is more ethereal but also more fundamental, goes to the aims and origins of moral theory. Although I must assert rather than argue the point, morality seems to me best conceived as stemming from the mutual recognition of people's equality as individual persons, with their differing needs, aspirations, and capacities, rather than from the formal equality of an abstract part of them, such as some unit of desire-intensity. It is an attempt by fully formed human beings to reach an agreement that is fair, given their unequal abilities, disparate desires, and conflicting ambitions and beliefs.[152] The question moral philosophers must answer is what people's moral equality requires of them as an initial matter, and what departures from those requirements people would freely and fairly make. My view is that a Kantian notion of the worth and inviolability of persons forms the base of moral reflection and grounds a right not to be slain for the good of others. The question, then, is whether people would wish to modify this and other background entitlements. Viewed in this light, it would mock their right to fashion their own future to force them to choose without knowing who they are or what they stand to gain.

This reply to partisans of utilitarian approaches is undoubtedly too skeletal to persuade those attracted to them. It merely outlines the long and

---

[151] Richard Hare adopts this strategy, claiming that utility is best advanced if people develop strong propensities to give priority, for example, to those they love, even if, on occasion, acting from these desires will not maximize utility. See R. M. Hare, *Moral Thinking* (Oxford: Clarendon Press, 1981), 135–40. As with most such attempts to square utilitarianism with widespread intuitions, Hare does not consider *degrees* of commitment to friends and family. And he simply *assumes* that utilitarianism prescribes just the amount of loyalty that popular morality condones, without offering a detailed demonstration of the coincidence.

[152] See T. M. Scanlon, 'The Aims and Authority of Moral Theory,' *Oxford Journal of Legal Studies* (1992); T. M. Scanlon, 'Contractualism and Utilitarianism,' in Sen and Williams (eds.), *Utilitarianism and Beyond*. 103.

intricate course that a full response would take. Arguing against utilitarian answers to the specific questions before us would be simpler were there specific proposals, differing in their practical implications from the theory I defend, available for scrutiny. But none exists, to my knowledge. Because I am disinclined to invent opponents with whom to disagree, I shall say little more about possible consequentialist alternatives to the view I present that are anchored in differing notions of an ideal hypothetical contract.

One question about the information available to people choosing hypothetically in the restricted sense I advocate that requires separate consideration is *when* we should imagine people selecting or repudiating a maximizing rule. In the trolley case Thomson sketches, a maximizing rule would have been to every worker's apparent advantage in the morning, before track positions were assigned randomly, but not in the afternoon, when the trolley was racing ahead with lethal abandon. Why should the decision to switch the trolley depend upon the workers' earlier unanimous preferences that the trolley be turned rather than upon the lone worker's almost certain opposition to turning it once he was given the solitary post?

Thomson correctly notes that agreement could only be found in the morning, before jobs were assigned, and that an agreement would only be beneficial to everybody if it controlled the later decision to switch the trolley, despite its then being to the disadvantage of the solo worker that the trolley be turned. Her discussion therefore appears to suggest that *whenever* it would at one time have been to more than one person's advantage to consent to a later course of action, it is permissible for somebody to adopt that course of action later, so far as those people are concerned, provided that any person's later opposition derives entirely from his awareness of who will be harmed by the action.[153]

The final proviso is essential. If a worker would have agreed to a maximizing rule but did not, and if he accepted an assignment with the smaller group because he reasonably thought no maximizing rule was in force, it would be wrong to hold him to what he would have chosen but did not in fact choose. Compare a willingness to buy a friend's car that was premised on your not buying another car in the meantime. What prompts doubts, or at any rate questions, is the generality of Thomson's protasis. Vary her example. Jones

[153] This reading is strengthened by Thomson's remark that what distinguishes her version of the transplant case from the trolley case is that there is nothing in the former analogous to early morning (before track positions were assigned) in the latter. See Thomson, *The Realm of Rights*, 185, 195. She also says that the trolley case belongs to a class of exceptions to the rule against killing 'in which the one who will be killed, and the five who will be saved, are members of a group such that it was to the advantage of all the members that the one (whoever he or she would later turn out to be) would later be killed, and the only thing that has since changed is that it is now clear who the one was going to turn out to be.' Ibid. 195.

took a job with the trolley company. New workers were and still are assigned randomly to different specialities. At that time, it would have made sense for Jones to agree to a maximizing rule. But Jones was not asked and no rule was in place governing life-threatening emergencies. As it happens, Jones was assigned to the corps of beam fitters—workers, Thomson assumes, who invariably labor alone. Jones would now object strenuously to a maximizing rule if he were asked about its implementation. Should he be held to the agreement he would have signed (but did not) when he accepted the job? Has anything changed except that the loser's identity is now known?

Thomson's general principle suggests that Jones should not be heard to complain. In describing the trolley case, however, she supposes that if the lone worker were a beam fitter, it would be impermissible to turn the trolley on him. Thomson's statements therefore appear in tension with one another, *unless* she assumes that workers are not assigned to specialties randomly after joining the trolley company, but rather apply for specific jobs and *not* on the understanding that a maximizing rule applies to all employees (so that beam fitters, for instance, would not extract more favorable compensation for assuming greater risk). Whatever Thomson's position, the question remains: can the morality of aiming the trolley at the lone worker turn on the way jobs are assigned at the start of somebody's career?

Take first the beam fitters who got their jobs directly, rather than by random assignment to specialty jobs. Thomson seems right in applying the general principle that someone may not be killed to save a greater number of others unless he gave or gives his assent.[154] If the probability of confronting a situation in which some could be killed to keep others alive were high, the matter of who dies and who lives would presumably be decided explicitly, so that no resort need be made to this bedrock rule. Beam fitters would likely be paid a risk premium to compensate them for their assent to a maximizing rule because in a well-functioning labor market people would not accept a job that carried an increased risk of death unless they received some consideration.[155] Hence, the knowledgeable person at the switch would not have to ponder the morality of throwing the lever, because the issue would have been decided beforehand.

Only if the risk of death from a rogue trolley were too slight to prompt people to make advance arrangements would a situation arise like the beam fitter case Thomson describes. And there I see no alternative to letting the trolley continue toward the five if people enjoy the right not to be killed that I described above.

---

[154] Or unless, as I explain in Sect. 5.4. fairness requires that his preference yield to others' desires.
[155] I assume that killing in these situations is not a criminal offense.

To be sure, one might imagine some meta-rule at a high level of abstraction requiring that the greater number be saved and leaving it to those who would predictably be hurt by this rule to seek redress, presumably in the form of greater pay or work-related benefits. One might argue that this meta-rule would be favored by most people because, in general, the greater number would be able to compensate the smaller group, if one assumes that risk-aversion is spread fairly uniformly across the work force and that the average income of probable members of the smaller and larger groups is the same. The right result would therefore obtain most often, even if transaction costs blocked the wealth transfers that would occur in a frictionless world.

An obvious problem with this proposal is that normally no compensation would in fact be paid, either because transaction costs were prohibitively high relative to the amount of the transfer or because the risks were so slight that disadvantaged people were not aware that they were hurt by the meta-rule. Its more fundamental flaw, however, is that the imagined agreement could only occur if people abstracted from important features of their personal situations, indeed, from what is alone of relevance in this context, namely, their propensity to find themselves among the damned rather than the saved. To prescind from these features, however, is to forfeit the autonomy of concrete individuals that must, as I argued, be the starting point for determining how we should act in these cases. It is the essential move towards utilitarianism that intuition resists.[156]

What should be done in the remaining case of the beam fitters who are assigned their specialty by lot when they join the trolley company, with no possibility of transfer into this specialty? Notice, first of all, that this question only presses when the risk to which the beam fitters are exposed is so slight that they are unable or do not care to negotiate compensation for the heightened risk they bear. It is therefore of little moment for the affected parties and, derivatively, for social policy. Insofar as the question holds interest, however, its answer seems to me to depend on the temporal proximity of the job assignment to the life-saving decision. If, as Thomson assumes, track positions are assigned randomly each day and everybody has a better than even chance of ending up in the larger group, the bystander at the switch should save the greater number.[157] But as the randomizing event that makes a maximizing rule antecedently beneficial recedes in time, its

---

[156] See text above, accompanying nn. 149–52.

[157] The sole exception to this claim, the motivation for which I set out in Section D, arises if the person at the switch knows that most of the workers oppose switching trolleys to save the larger group, despite the fact that their opposition to switching is contrary to their self-interest. This unlikely situation might occur if all or most of the workers were drawn from some religious sect that opposed killing at all times.

connection to the lives of the people it affects stretches thin, and eventually grows too attenuated to justify applying the rule to them. This seems the temporal analogue of the process by which personal attributes are shaved away to elicit unanimous consent at an overly abstract level. Moving the randomizing event back a week, or a month, does not seem unfair to those facing death. But as the date becomes more remote—perhaps a year or two, certainly once at the start of an adult's life—it seems inappropriate to act towards them in a way that would at some distant time, for a fleeting moment, have been to their advantage.

It is difficult, I admit, to say why this is so. Perhaps we do not think that people would have agreed (would *you* have agreed?) to a maximizing rule upon being assigned to a community or a job, knowing that they would have to live under its shadow their entire life and face certain death if some highly unlikely event occurred. The larger cumulative risk of dying over the course of a lifetime rather than a month or a year might amplify this reluctance. Or perhaps the lapse of time weakens the force of presumed consent more than it does the pull of actual consent. Or maybe both fade in step with, if not necessarily to the same degree as, changes in people's psychological identity.[158] I am by no means sure of the best explanation for this apparent moral fact. Fortunately, the solution to this puzzle will rarely be relevant in deciding how we should act.

5.4. Fairness and Mandatory Participation in Maximizing Schemes

In many situations, a maximizing rule would unquestionably increase everybody's antecedent chance of survival. Authorizing police or other officials to kill or capture terrorists or criminals at the predictable cost of innocent lives, when doing so would likely prevent the taking of yet more lives, would probably enhance everyone's prospect of staying alive because people's proportional chances of becoming casualties of law enforcement officials or becoming terrorist victims seem roughly identical. Likewise, in workplace disasters or other emergencies, such as partially collapsed or burning buildings, workers or citizens generally would have no reason to expect that their

---

[158] Another possible explanation, one might think, rests on an alleged parallel between ignorance of personal characteristics in the circumstances of hypothetical choice and ignorance of the distant future. This is not, however, a reason independent of the possible reasons mentioned in the text. In both cases, the limits to self-knowledge are set by a conception of fairness and by a person's second-order judgments about which hypothetical bargains may morally be enforced. A *separate* reason, of the sort just considered, must inform those second-order judgments.

chances of ending up in the smaller group that might be killed are greater than their chances of joining the larger group of beneficiaries. A maximizing rule would again provide antecedent benefits to all. Military expeditions offer another familiar example when killing some could save more others, if abandoning certain troops to overwhelming enemy fire or sending some to spearhead a dangerous assault constitutes killing. But, as long as the unlucky soldiers are not selected invidiously, the appropriateness of a maximizing rule is widely accepted even among conscripts, given the common aim of achieving victory at the smallest possible loss of life.

Nonetheless, one additional hurdle remains to implementing a maximizing policy in these cases. Some people might refuse to approve a maximizing scheme because they think killing wrong in all circumstances, even if the scheme promises to keep more people alive, possibly including themselves. In fact, opposition of this kind, backed by recognizably moral or religious reasons, seems inevitable in our diverse society. If these reasons formed the basis for opposition to some type of paternalistic intervention designed to promote a person's own good but not the good of others, they would have to be respected. One may not force a life-saving transfusion on a Jehovah's Witness who would rather forgo medical assistance, even if the Witness will survive many years and live what is, on balance, a happy life. Nor can dissent always be quelled by reducing the danger of erroneous killings under the rule or by mitigating the possibility that citizens' respect for life might atrophy.

Opposition might come from other quarters as well. Some people might refuse to participate in a maximizing scheme because they think themselves particularly lucky and prefer to trust fate, even if a maximizing rule would improve their odds of survival. Still others might hold out, if unanimous assent were required, to secure additional compensation from other potential beneficiaries, thereby running the risk that the failure of all to agree would injure them too. May some people be killed to save others in these cases? Or must consent have been unanimous under the relevant counterfactual conditions to license killing?[159]

[159] Thomson never addresses these questions squarely. She mentions the possibility that somebody would prefer to trust Providence or run an irrational risk, but offers cryptic counsel. 'The more firmly held those views are, and the more central to their lives,' she says, 'the more we are going to think [the person at the switch] really must not intervene' by killing some workers in accordance with a maximizing rule that would unquestionably increase their antecedent chance of staying alive. Thomson, *The Realm of Rights*, 182. She then adds: 'But that is just mere possibility. It really can be supposed that the workmen would all consent to [the person's] turning the trolley later, for the reason that his doing so gives them an increased probability of survival.' Ibid. Whether Thomson means that somebody's opposition can rightly be ignored unless it stems from a belief that is sufficiently central to his life is unclear. If that is Thomson's view, one wonders whence the centrality requirement comes. Why is a peripheral belief insufficient if an individual

Some situations are unproblematic. To the extent that one can operate a voluntary maximizing scheme that denies its benefits to people who choose to avoid the risk of being killed, those who think killing wrong or who would rather take their chances could be accommodated. Organ transplant schemes that would kill one person to save two or more other people provide the best example of a potential voluntary arrangement. Even in the hypothetical world Thomson describes, where everyone has an equal chance of needing a transplant that would require killing the donor, it would be inappropriate to force adults to join a scheme maximizing the number kept alive[160] because people could freely weigh the risks, benefits, and morality of the scheme and decide for themselves whether to join. Should they elect to sit out, nobody is harmed but themselves.[161] One might argue, I suppose, that if the odds were favorable, it would be irrational not to join,[162] notwithstanding the fact that a healthy life would often be traded for lives that are more cramped. But even ignoring the costs of compulsion—for instance, widespread anxiety, the use of force in subduing victims who resist, corruption resulting in the unfair selection of victims— it would, I believe, be wrong to force everyone to go along. Unlike mandatory seat belt laws, rules compelling people to surrender an organ or their very lives would require so large a sacrifice that people would wisely not trust their political representatives to decide for them whether participation would be prudent. In addition, people might object to inclusion on religious or moral grounds, and in a state that honors freedom of conscience it would be intolerable to dismiss these beliefs as irrational and unworthy of respect. That is particularly so when, as here, any physical

invokes his rights? Even more confusing are the last two sentences quoted, which seem to suggest something obviously false: that no rational person would put ethical or spiritual considerations before his interest in physical survival, thus permitting us to abstract from possible objections to a maximizing rule. Whatever Thomson's point, the problem of moral or religious opposition must be confronted.

[160] Children present a special problem because they lack the experience and decisionmaking autonomy to decide responsibly. I offer principles for determining what health care minors should receive in Rakowski, *Equal Justice*, 100–6, 180–1, 318–31.

[161] I ignore the problem posed by people who might want to join an organ transplant scheme but who cannot do so because nobody who could provide a tissue match is interested. For thoughts on this issue, see ibid. 182.

[162] The odds of survival are, of course, not the only relevant non-moral factors. People rank different forms of survival differently. Some might wish to live even in a severely debilitated state; others might prefer death under those conditions, particularly if the chance to live in that state would be purchased by incurring the risk of becoming an unwilling donor while in full health. Unless one imagines a world where people share evaluations about how worthwhile assorted lives are, divergent preferences would pose a serious problem to formulating just terms for mandatory inclusion.

harm caused by acting in accordance with those beliefs befalls the believer alone.[163]

This conclusion is even more secure in the world we know, due to the dependence of need or contribution on a host of voluntary decisions. Diet, smoking, employment, pastimes, and many other chosen pursuits affect a person's foreseeable need for transplant organs and the likelihood that his organs will be suitable for transplantation. Requiring everyone to join a single transplant scheme would be unfair to the prudent and a windfall to the reckless.[164] Problems of tissue typing, the difficulty of taking account of age and prognosis in what everyone would agree is a just manner, and the need to coordinate organ transplant schemes with other plans for obtaining and allocating cadaver organs would further complicate the creation of a single arrangement that is fair to all. Of supreme importance, however, is the fact that was decisive even in Thomson's imagined case. The autonomy of those who wish not to risk death or who believe the scheme transgresses their moral or religious beliefs can be respected without harming those who think the wager prudent and morally irreproachable. When this condition holds, it is morally impermissible to compel participation.

Often, however, the condition will not hold. A policy allowing

---

[163] I argue this point at greater length ibid. 344. Thomson's claim that participation may be mandated in a world in which people do not think it appreciably worse to be killed suddenly than to die slowly, or at least not enough worse to make organ transplant schemes irrational, overlooks these considerations favoring individual autonomy in cases in which free-riding can be avoided. See Thomson. *The Realm of Rights*. 185–6. Larry Alexander, in arguing that Thomson's view entails compulsory participation in this imagined world—which he thinks is inappropriate—also pays no attention to these issues. See Alexander, 'Self-Defense, Justification and Excuse,' 58. Frances Kamm equally finds Thomson's conclusion intuitively unsatisfactory. See Kamm, 'Non-Consequentialism, the Person as an End-in-Itself, and the Significance of Status,' 374–6.

[164] Not all differences in people's chances of needing an organ or being called to die for others are within their control. Genetic predispositions to various maladies, for example, are not. If they are detectable, they might encourage some people to join voluntary transplant schemes and drive others away. The injustice of the resulting pattern of participation, like the injustice of different health insurance rates for people who are more likely to need care because of genetic or congenital handicaps, argues for the establishment of a single plan that treats everybody equally.

The contention that disparities in opportunity that afflict people through no fault of their own should be reduced or eliminated through transfers from the naturally lucky to the naturally unfortunate is certainly cogent. Nonetheless, that argument is in my view outweighed by the considerations supporting free choice, particularly if one assumes that people who are born (or raised) unlucky are compensated in other ways—for example, by the provision of health and life insurance at nondiscriminatory rates or subsidies for market purchases. See Rakowski, *Equal Justice*, 73–6, 88–106 (arguing that justice requires compensation for emergent inequalities in people's opportunities, such as those stemming from genetic differences, for which they are not responsible). The argument for mandatory inclusion also falls before the compelling notion that competent adults cannot morally be required to sustain large sacrifices, such as the loss of their lives, to help others for whom they have no special attachment or affection, unless they agree to do so or they would have agreed to do so in the morally significant circumstances of hypothetical choice I describe.

government officials to attack murderous terrorists or criminals even though innocent lives would thereby be placed at risk could not feasibly exempt those who objected to killing. The thought of dissenters wearing some identifying badge that would be visible to possible rescuers in tense emergencies is silly. Even if identification and exception were possible—suppose the person who is always at the switch knows that one of the workers regards all killing, even in the standard trolley case, as an abomination—it seems unfair, at first blush at least, to give the dissenter's view precedence over everybody else's. The dissenter would then exercise his right not to be killed when he was in the smaller group; and when he was in the larger group that could be saved by killing fewer others, he would not stand in the way of others' preference for a maximizing rule, thus saving him here too. He would be hurt only in a case in which the two groups were identical in size (without counting him) and his presence was *not* counted in determining which group should be saved—a rare scenario that would barely detract from his favored situation.

Of course, somebody who opposed killing solely as a matter of principle might want a potential rescuer not to save the larger group by killing others even when he was a member of the larger group. If so, he would not be requesting special treatment. But if those in the smaller group would all have favored a maximizing policy, along with many of those in the larger group, it seems the smaller group should be killed, notwithstanding the dissenter's contrary preference as a member of the larger group. After all, the relevant right is the right of members of the smaller group not to be killed, and their hypothetical consent has extinguished it; the dissenter has no right to bar them from hypothetically surrendering it when he is in the larger group. He might just as well be a bystander. Thus, although the dissenter would not be demanding unfair treatment, he would enjoy a uniquely protected status if he could exercise his right not to be killed when he was in the smaller group yet be saved automatically if he found himself in the larger group. Should his religious or moral opposition to killing entitle him to more favorable treatment than the other people receive?

Begin with an easier case. In Bernard Williams's thought experiment,[165] Pedro and his thugs will murder twenty Indians unless Jim, a foreigner who stumbles onto the scene, shoots one of them. If Jim kills one, the other nineteen will be released, as a sign of respect for the foreign guest. Suppose that one of the Indians abhors killing and says that he believes it wrong for Jim to pull the trigger, even though the alternative is for a vicious man to commit a more terrible wrong. He invokes his alleged right not to be killed

---

[165] See Smart and Williams, *Utilitarianism*, 98–9.

and asks Jim to respect it, despite Pedro's evident intention to disregard it. The other nineteen Indians plead with Jim to kill someone selected at random. What should he do?

Jim has three options, unless he tries to be a hero and points the gun at Pedro. He could stand idle and watch the Indians be slaughtered. He could pick one victim at random from among the twenty and shoot that person himself. Or he could choose a victim randomly from among the nineteen that want him to kill one.[166]

The first course may be excluded. The nineteen prefer both the second and the third options to the first. Further, they apparently have a *right* to see the third option selected over the first, because doing so would significantly advance their interests without harming anybody else, at no cost to Jim (other than any irrational sense of complicity he might feel on slaying one of the Indians). The dissenter opposes both the second and the third options. The third, however, slights no right of his. He might experience moral dissatisfaction upon witnessing what he regards as another's wrongful conduct. But this moral offense, which he would anyway experience if Jim stepped aside and Pedro brandished his gun, hardly empowers him to insist that others die who would rather live and who may live if Jim shoots one. The third course thus dominates the first.

A harder question is whether the third course also dominates the second. Given that a victim should be chosen randomly, should the dissenter be included in the lottery against his will, on the ground that exempting him would lend him an advantage the others lack by ensuring his continued life?

If the dissenter's reason for asserting a right not to be killed in opposing random choice from among all twenty Indians is not as I described, but is motivated by his wanting to live and by his belief that riding free is the surest means to that end, his protest may, I think, be ignored. It would be unfair to exempt him when one must die and all wish to live, and his opposition to participation originates not in moral principle but in a self-interested bargaining strategy he could not honestly wish that all would adopt. On these facts, free-riding need not be permitted because the ethical or economic cost of preventing it is too high. It can be avoided, and should be.

But what if the lone dissenter appeals to some moral or religious principle with evident sincerity, not just as a dodge to keep his head? My view is that Jim ought nevertheless to turn a deaf ear to his pleas. That view is based on three premises: first, that there is no convincing religious reason for not killing in the circumstances described, or, alternatively and perhaps more

---

[166] Jim has many other options too, such as choosing randomly from among nine of the nineteen plus the dissenter. These other options are, however, so intuitively unfair that they may be ignored.

acceptably, that neither government officials nor private citizens of a liberal
state should grant a veto on the implementation of popular, life-enhancing
policies to members of a religious minority who would also physically benefit from those policies; second, that no persuasive moral reason exists for
exempting the dissenting Indian from Jim's random selection of the victim;
third, that in the absence of a sound moral reason, the unfairness of
exempting one person mandates treating everyone alike.

I shall not defend the claim that there is no compelling religious reason for
Jim to refrain from killing. Although traditional Roman Catholic doctrine,
by endorsing the Doctrine of Double Effect with its prohibition on intentional killing, arguably condemns Jim's shooting one Indian,[167] this view is
not, I conjecture, one that most religions would support when the alternative
is that the Indian will be shot anyway and that nineteen others will die too.
Anyone who claims that some divinity forbids killing in this situation also
faces familiar evidentiary problems. In addition, he confronts the difficulty
of showing that divine commands are morally correct, or that sanctions will
be visited on disobedient people (whether or not the commands are morally
irreproachable) that are so severe as to justify or excuse someone's doing the
opposite of what would be morally required in the absence of those sanctions. I am not familiar with a convincing demonstration of the wrongness
of killing that satisfies these conditions.

Setting these points to one side, however, I would further maintain, perhaps less controversially, that whether the members of some religious minority believe that there are convincing theological objections to killing in Jim's
situation should not affect the way a nonbeliever or government official
selects the victim. In a liberal state, while the *fact* of opposition is relevant in
deciding how to proceed, as I explain below, religious *reasons* for opposition
ought, as reasons, to be ignored. Defending this thesis about the character
of public reasons in a liberal community would take me far afield. Here,
I merely note my reliance on it and the difficulty of formulating and
implementing public policy if the presence of religiously inspired opposition
sufficed to circumscribe or overturn that policy.[168]

---

[167] For a helpful analysis of the sometimes conflicting opinions of Roman Catholic moralists on
this question, see Greenawalt, supra note 101, at 6–13, 16–23.

[168] For illuminating discussions of the place of religious principle in grounding arguments
about public policy, see Michael J. Perry, *Love and Power: The Role of Religion and Morality in
American Politics* (1991); James E. Wood Jr. and Dereck Davis (eds.), *The Role of Religion in the
Making of Public Policy* (1991); Kent Greenawalt, *Religious Convictions and Political Choice*
(1987); Robert Audi, 'The Separation of Church and State and the Obligations of Citizen-
ship,' *Philosophy & Public Affairs*, 18 (1989), 259; Paul J. Weithman, 'The Separation of Church
and State: Some Questions for Professor Audi,' *Philosophy & Public Affairs*, 20 (1991), 52;
Robert Audi, 'Religious Commitment and Secular Reason: A Reply to Professor Weithman,'
Philosophy & Public Affairs, 20 (1991), 66; 'Religion and the Ethics of Political Participation,'

A moral objection to Jim's firing would have to be grounded in the wrongness of the act of killing, rather than in the undesirability of the consequences, because the alternative to Jim's killing one is allowing twenty to be killed, and one cannot seriously imagine the victims saying that it is worse to be slain by one unfamiliar executioner rather than another. It is hard to see, however, how killing can be condemned as immoral when it leaves the victim no worse off (he would have been shot anyway), when it benefits others substantially, and when it seems highly unlikely to weaken the public's resistance to inexcusable slaughter or to increase the number of false threats of killing.[169] On the other side, the unfairness of exempting one person is patent. Hence, Jim should, I think, choose from among all twenty.

In fact, while the nineteen would naturally favour that course, because it would inflate their odds of staying alive, the dissenter could not consistently oppose it. Although he would prefer that Jim not shoot anybody, he has, as we saw, no right to insist that Jim refrain from shooting one of the others. In addition, he could hardly think it worse to choose among twenty rather than nineteen, when his objection is to the act of killing rather than to the principle of fairness that underpins random choice. If he asserts a right not to be killed, he does so to no purpose by his own principles, because at least one will be killed in any event. In the interest of fairness, his remonstrations may be disregarded.

It seems more difficult to justify, in the face of moral or religious opposition, the application of a maximizing rule to trolleys, work places, terrorists, and other situations in which everybody's chance of survival would be enhanced by that rule. To be sure, allowing opponents to opt out would lend them an unfair advantage over those who remained subject to the rule, because they lack a right to block its application when it would not harm them and they would stymie its operation when it would injure them. But moral or religious objections seem more forceful here than in Williams's example because those who assert a right not to have their lives sacrificed will not be killed by deliberate human agency anyway if the person who could implement a maximizing policy declines to kill them.

Ethics, 100 (1990), 386 (book review). This debate overlaps with discussions of whether and in what ways a liberal state should strive to be neutral with respect to citizens' competing conceptions of the good life in deciding upon and justifying state action. See, e.g., Peter de Marneffe, 'Liberalism, Liberty, and Neutrality,' *Philosophy and Public Affairs*, 19 (1990), 253 (discussing the views of John Rawls and Ronald Dworkin); Will Kymlicka, 'Liberal Individualism and Liberal Neutrality,' *Ethics*, 99 (1989), 883 (discussing justification for state action in the face of citizens' competing desires); Thomas Nagel, 'Moral Conflict and Political Legitimacy,' *Philosophy & Public Affairs*, 16 (1987), 215.

[169] Samuel Scheffler offers a similar argument. See Scheffler, *The Rejection of Consequentialism*, 108–14.

There are at least three responses to this problem. One is to recognize a right not to be killed that applies in spite of the unfairness of exempting a dissenter, so long as the right is invoked sincerely for some substantial moral or religious reason. If the exercise, or presumed exercise, of such a right wreaks havoc with the implementation of a maximizing policy and frustrates the contrary preferences of a large majority of those persons who would be affected by the policy, that result is simply bad fortune for those who wish the policy to be applied without exception.

The second response is diametrically opposed to the first. It denies the validity, in a liberal community, of moral or religious reasons that might be asserted on behalf of a right not to be killed in situations in which a maximizing policy would definitely enhance everyone's antecedent chance of survival without significantly diminishing their quality of life or causing detrimental side effects, such as enervation of respect for other people that leads to unwarranted injury or killing. One of two consequences might follow. Either people asserting a right to opt out could be ignored altogether if someone affected by a life-saving decision favoured a maximizing policy, because the reasons they invoked are either misplaced or not entitled to consideration if at least some of those affected reject them and if those who reject them would have consented to, and would in the circumstances actually benefit from, a policy of saving the greater number. Or the *preference* of those claiming a right not to be killed for a rule forbidding killing even to keep more people alive could be set against the contrary preference of advocates of a maximizing policy, and the issue could be settled by majority vote.

A third possibility lies between the first two. People might be thought to have a right not to have their lives taken to save more others, but that right might not be so potent as to prevail if a great many other people's preferences are arrayed against it. A person's right to veto the establishment of a maximizing policy would thus overcome a certain amount of opposition, but it could not withstand *all* opposition. Rather, if a sufficiently large majority favoured a maximizing policy, those who opposed it on moral or religious grounds would have to accept the verdict of their peers, as a moral matter and not just as political reality.

All three positions are coherent, and each one might be married to the rest of the theory I am defending. Somebody who believes that numbers always matter when saving lives might dismiss the first option. He might also rule out the second version of the second option except in a modified form. If a maximizing policy lost by a sufficiently small number of votes, he might conclude that the larger number should be saved notwithstanding, because in his judgment the moral force of numbers outweighs the moral reasons that undergird the preference-tabulation rule when only a small majority opposes saving the most lives. Somebody who thinks that numbers are morally irrelevant cannot reduce the range of choice even that much.

The three positions are problematic in different ways. The first is intuitively unattractive to me and, I surmise, to a great many other people. Not only does it countenance unfairness, arguably to the benefit of somebody whose views are badly misguided. It also affronts democratic instincts. Why should one person's opposition to maximizing be permitted to frustrate a plan that hundreds, or thousands, or millions of other people approve because it offers physical benefits to *everybody* touched by it? Indeed, given that in most emergencies in which killing might save lives an agent could not possibly elicit the sincere moral and religious beliefs of members of the smaller group, and given that there is *some* chance that the smaller group would include people who opposed killing for moral or religious reasons, the first position might be construed to block the implementation of maximizing policies in almost every instance in which they would prove beneficial. These consequences are hard to accept.

The major shortcoming of the first version of the second view is that it embodies what some people would regard as a pernicious, and certainly antimajoritarian, strategy for collective decisionmaking. Setting people's views aside entirely so long as at least one other person favors a maximizing rule seems the height of moral hubris. Generalized, an unsympathetic commentator might say, this approach amounts to despotism.

Nevertheless, the assumption on which it is based—that moral and religious objections to maximizing policies are either wrongheaded or inappropriate in a liberal polity—seems to me correct. And even if one rejects this claim, it seems plain that, in the absence of a legal prohibition, an agent ought to do what *she* deems morally proper, and polling those affected by her possible actions seems a poor means for arriving at moral truth, even if it often supplies a salutary spur to reflection. This is not, one might affirm, a prescription for moral despotism, merely a fact about moral agency.

One might rejoin that respect for other people requires that an agent canvass their views (insofar as circumstances permit) and put the matter to a vote. But this is not a rule any of us would accept if our own interests were at stake. Nor is it a rule of general applicability. Few atheists would feel morally impelled to attend religious services if most of those around them worshipped regularly; most gays would not consider themselves obligated to repress their sexuality just because a majority thought homosexual conduct immoral. Moreover, neither group would err morally in refusing to bend to the majority's convictions. So why should a majority's opposition to a maximizing policy[170] bind an agent disposed to save the greater number if he thinks this view, like that of the devout or intolerant heterosexual majority, mistaken? To be sure, in writing legislation a government should probably defer to the joust of preferences, giving each person an equal say, which is what the second version of the second position recommends. But proper public policy and proper private morality are surely two different things.

The third response faces line-drawing problems that neither extreme position encounters. It is hard to justify the selection of a particular number of preferences as weightier than one individual's assertion of a right not to be killed, except by referring to intuitions that will strike many people as infirm. More important, the moral and religious reasons adduced on behalf of the alleged right seem unpersuasive, and the religious reasons are, in any event, out of place in this argument.

Let me repeat that any of the three positions could be adopted consistent with the remainder of the theory I offer. Because I reject the moral and religious reasons on which opposition to a maximizing policy must be founded, I would endorse the second position over the first and third. The difficult question for me is which version of the second position deserves allegiance. This is a question that few, if any, agents will confront, and not only because life-or-death choices are rare. The two versions decree different results only in cases in which the majority explicitly opposes, or would not have given hypothetical consent to, a maximizing rule. In today's liberal democracies, actual or hypothetical opposition is apt to be small unless the *ex ante* advantage of a maximizing rule is doubtful, in which case it would be wrong for an agent to kill anyway. And in societies in which killing in accordance with a maximizing rule would be widely denounced, the law is likely to proscribe killing, which in turn might resolve the matter for private citizens.[171] Moreover, if *everyone* affected by the agent's decision does or would have opposed killing some to save a larger group, the agent's contrary belief that a maximizing convention would be prudent should be irrelevant to his decision. People have, if the foregoing argument is correct, a right not to be killed that must be honored unless invoking that right would be unfair to others or unless that right has been or would be waived. If everyone rejects a maximizing rule, there would be no unfairness in honoring their rights. It would be wrong to disregard them.[172]

---

[170] If only a minority favored it, this second version of the second position would yield the same prescriptions as the first version.

[171] In some cases, morality countenances or commands illegal conduct. It seems doubtful, however, that this is one of them.

[172] We do, of course, think it morally licit or even required to interfere with some accepted practices we deem immoral. Most of us believe wife burning should not be tolerated if we can prevent it, even if women willingly throw themselves on the pyre. Have we not a similar duty to

Nevertheless, we can imagine conflicts between a majority that opposed killing to save lives and a minority that favoured it when a maximizing rule would increase everybody's ex-ante chance of survival, in cases in which at least some of the opponents were numbered among the smaller group that might be killed. I am uncertain how these conflicts should be resolved. My inclination is to respect the majority's assertion of its rights when unfairness is not present.[173] Unlike a majority that would impose its religious views or sexual morality on an unpersuaded minority, the interests of the majority would here be directly and importantly affected by the policy pursued by agents able to save lives. But I cannot boast confidence in the conclusion that the majority's convictions, which I do not share, ought to govern.

In summary, it might be helpful to review why majoritarian principles should prevail here over an asserted right not to have one's life taken in accordance with a rule one considers reprehensible. The reasons are three. First, there is the pull of intuition. It seems wrong that a handful of people whose views most people reject should be able to have their way despite their inability to convince the majority, so long as everybody's antecedent chance of survival would have been increased by the adoption of a maximizing policy that permits killing some to save others. If religious or moral objections to killing permitted someone to veto a maximizing policy, then the danger of contravening a dissenter's will might well prevent such a policy from ever taking effect, however popular it might be. An appeal to majority preferences, in circumstances in which *ex ante* agreement would have benefitted everyone, sidesteps the possible frustration of a rule that all or most would have favored.

But the majoritarian instinct that lies behind this thought is, in this expression, too crude. It is not enough that a majority favors some policy. If that policy would *not* enhance the prospect of survival of some people it would affect, their opposition should suffice to sink it, even if many others

---

employ a maximizing rule when it would be to everyone's antecedent advantage, given that lives are at stake here too? I think not, but confess that I find it difficult to draw lines when the moral belief I reject harms the believer and not other people. (If wives resisted burning, the two cases could easily be distinguished. And this would. I think, typically occur.)

[173] Unfairness *might* obtain in exceptional cases if one accedes to a majority's wishes when they seek to exercise their rights not to be killed. Suppose that fifteen of the twenty Indians Pedro plans to kill invoke their right not to be killed, citing religious reasons. Five want Jim to select a victim randomly so that the rest may walk away with their lives. Should Jim nonetheless choose randomly from among all twenty? Or from among the five? Or consign them all to Pedro's cruelties? In this case, I would include all twenty in the lottery, because the unfairness of exempting anyone when all would gain from Jim's killing one seems to me to outweigh the moral force of the fifteen Indians' misguided insistence that Jim kill no one.

would profit from its adoption.[174] To render the majority's will morally effective, two additional premises are therefore needed. A maximizing policy must, in the circumstances, increase its opponents' chance of survival. And, finally, their reasons for opposing it must, in the case of moral reasons, be invalid or, in the case of religious reasons, be properly excluded as irrelevant (as reasons, though not as individual votes) to policy making in a liberal state. If these conditions are met, fairness requires a democratic solution to the problem, even though some people conscientiously oppose a maximizing policy. Denying veto rights to dissenters is the obverse of treating all those affected as moral equals.

5.5. A Lifeboat Example

Before considering further problems that this qualified defense of maximizing policies encounters, let me illustrate some of its significant limitations by analyzing a somewhat different case. This scene has provoked a wealth of speculation, and thus holds independent interest. But discussing its permutations also aids in elaborating the theory I am commending.

Five men are adrift in the South Atlantic, their ship having broken apart in a violent storm. The scant provisions they managed to carry aboard their small boat are long gone. They have no reason to expect another vessel to happen by soon; perhaps they will never be found. They try to hook fish and snare sea turtles, without success. Nobody, it appears, will live another week unless four of the sailors eat the flesh of the fifth. Yet, another week might suffice for rescue. How may, or should, they act?

Set aside the contention—which may be correct—that morality runs dry in such situations, that an innocent person in imminent danger of dying may do whatever he must to stay alive, even if that means killing other innocent people. Assume that the five are armed and wary and disposed to enforce agreements, or that they are bound together by blood or vows and wish to treat each other fairly. Must they refrain from killing and wait until somebody dies to consume his body? What if waiting might well kill them all, because by the time somebody dies the rest will likely have suffered irreversible tissue damage? May they kill the person most likely to die first now, in the reasonable belief that delay will be fatal? If not, and if some want to draw lots to choose a sacrificial victim, may they force everyone to join in?

---

[174] Those who believe that numbers matter in deciding whom to save would disagree, at least if the numbers are sufficiently uneven. But most who hold this view would agree that people have a right not to be killed when the disparity is not *too* great. For them, my claim would remain true so long as the difference in numbers did not tip the balance.

And if people may not be compelled to participate, must the lucky ones share any leftover flesh with the nonparticipants?

In the absence of consent and assuming that somebody's natural death will not come too late to save the others, it seems to me morally impermissible to kill the weakest member. The sole exception to this result, which might clash with utilitarian solutions, is if some who would otherwise outlive him agree, contrary to their self-interest, to choose a victim by lot and thus to give the weakest person a chance at survival, and the weakest agrees to participate and has his number drawn.[175]

One might venture, however, that if such altruism is lacking, the doomed person may be killed shortly before he is destined to die if doing so would benefit others significantly. After all, he would lose little—a few miserable hours—and they, by hypothesis, would gain noticeably. This approach, however, is not always warranted. If the dying person *cannot* recover, even if one of the others died before him, this prescription seems correct. If the gains are large enough relative to the loss, one could presume general assent to this rule, or at least sufficiently widespread assent to justify, in fairness, taking that person's life. And even if one finds an appeal to presumed consent unavailing, one might agree that at times gains to some can outweigh the loss to another.[176] However, if the person who would die first *can* still be saved if

[175] I again assume that moral rules find purchase here, to the extent of protecting the person who will die first unless he kills somebody else, or that circumstances constrain people from taking others' lives unless all or most agree to that course. I further assume that consent to a rule stipulating that the weakest be killed first is absent. In some cases, such as that of nineteenth-century seamen, that assumption might not hold, because one may forcefully argue that those who undertook lengthy voyages did so on the understanding that the weakest survivor would be killed in this situation. See supra note 118. It is, of course, a separate question whether that convention should have been honored, given the economic duress that drove poor boys and others to sea.

[176] This situation arises frequently in modern hospitals. Suppose that somebody dying from an incurable brain tumor could supply organs to one or more people who will die if they must wait until the person with the brain tumor dies a natural death. If killing him would not deprive him of *too* much time—bearing in mind that it is hard to determine when exactly somebody will die and how much is too much—would it be wrong to take his life if that were the only way of saving another person or several other people, particularly if he has had time to wind up his affairs and the life left to him is of low quality? I am inclined to think that killing him would not be wrong. It would apparently be in everyone's antecedent interest to agree to such a rule. (The same cannot be said of the possible rule Daniel Dinello mentions, which would require a coin-flip to decide whether Smith or Jones should die if both were dying, if each could provide the transplant organ the other needs to live, and if Smith would die two hours after Jones unless Smith were killed first to save Jones. See Daniel Dinello, 'On Killing and Letting Die,' in Steinbock (ed.), *Killing and Letting Die*, 128, 130.)

The main objection to killing in the situation I have described is that the incurable patient has not consented to be killed, and medical insurance policies *could* be written to cover this case. The reply, which some might consider inadequate, is that no mechanism exists for registering consent or objection. Thus, we must appeal to patients' likely antecedent preferences in deciding what to do. Another problem is that this rule takes no account of somebody's responsibility for his condition. This shortcoming could, however, be met by considering this factor in deciding whether or

somebody else were killed, one could not expect him, actually or hypothetically, to surrender his remaining hours if insisting on his right not to be killed
gave him sufficient leverage to extract an offer of a lottery from the others
who, by hypothesis, stood to gain from his (or someone's) immediate demise.
Perhaps he could not get even odds in a draw with the others—the strength
of his hand would turn on myriad facts and his fellows' bargaining
strategies—but he need not give up his ghost to profit others if his advantage
lies elsewhere.

Assume now that the sailors cannot wait until somebody dies naturally if
they are to keep their lives. The case therefore parallels that of the doomed
Indians to this extent: all will die unless one is slain. But it departs from the
Indians' case in one crucial respect: those who are excluded from a random
selection of the victim will not necessarily live if one is killed.[177] Nonparticipants will live only if lottery winners share the dead person's flesh with them
and they are willing to partake of it. These differences ground important
limits to the principle requiring mandatory participation in a survival
lottery.

If the lucky participants have a moral duty to share any flesh they cannot
eat, if they can be counted on to do what they should, and if nonparticipants
will eat what they are given, then it would be unfair to allow some to avoid
the risk of dying by not participating in the lottery. The situation would
resemble that of the twenty Indians in all pertinent respects, and it would be
permissible to force everyone to draw lots. But if there is no moral duty to
share, as there is no moral duty to divide lottery winnings with people who
did not purchase tickets, then I see no reason to compel participation. And
here a moral duty to share appears lacking, because it would usurp the
independent judgment of people who decline to participate. Those who
oppose drawing lots may simply be willing to make a different wager: that
rescuers will spy them before death's grip is firm. Even if there is no chance

when to take life. Of course, if this rule were implemented, procedural checks would be important
to ensure that the patients' prognoses were accurate and that no alternative means were available
for keeping alive possible organ recipients.

[177] I assume that fairness requires that the victim be chosen randomly, given the moral equality
of all who are endangered. As a legal matter, it is unclear whether cannibalism in extremely
exigent circumstances is punishable in the United States as intentional homicide if the victim was
selected fairly. No recent precedent exists. A federal trial court asserted a century and a half ago,
in a case involving an overcrowded lifeboat, that sailors not needed to pilot the boat should be
sacrificed before passengers and that choice from among the passengers should be random. See
United States v. *Holmes*, 26 F. Cas. 360, 367 (E.D. Pa. 1842) (No. 15,383). Whether the judge's
statement was an accurate summary of the law then, and whether it fairly portrays existing law,
are unsettled issues. In *Regina* v. *Dudley & Stephens*, L.R. 14 Q.B.D. 273 (1884), the sailors'
decision to slay the weakened cabin boy without drawing lots resulted in their conviction. See
above, n. 118.

of help arriving in time,[178] they might wish to gamble on the charity of those who win the lottery of lives. And there seems no good reason to curtail rather than enlarge the realm of choice. One can easily imagine a mother electing to participate and offering to share, if she wins, with her children while asking them not to run the risk themselves, or friends doing the same for one another. Why deny people their pick of dice? Unless fairness is to be forfeited, however, the corollary of this choice is that participants have no moral duty—which is not to say that charity is wrong—to cushion people who decline to bet.[179]

People who would rather die than eat human flesh present no problem. They may not be compelled to join in the lottery. They would have nothing to gain by participating, as they would not consume the dead person's flesh if they won. They would have only their remaining days or hours to lose. They would also not be acting unfairly to the others by not wagering their lives because by not participating they would forgo all possible benefit. Hence, neither consent nor fairness could justify their inclusion.

5.6   The Problem of Overlapping Groups

Thus far I have considered groups of people defined primarily by occupation or activity. I have asked whether, if they found themselves in a predicament in which more could be kept alive if some were killed and if they had not entered into an explicit agreement governing a potential rescuer's actions, they would, at some not too distant earlier time, have acceded to a rule permitting killing. What should a potential rescuer do, however, if those who can be saved or killed belong to *different* groups within each of which a maximizing rule separately applies? Suppose, for example, that the trolley will strike five workers unless it is turned on a lone pedestrian who has nothing whatever to do with the trolley company? Or what if a bus's brakes

[178] In an imaginary case Lon Fuller describes, a group of spelunkers becomes trapped in a cave yet retains radio contact with rescue workers and medical advisers. See Lon L. Fuller. 'The Case of the Speluncean Explorers.' *Harvard Law Review*, 62 (1949), 616, 616–18. They know with some accuracy how long it will take help to reach them, and can estimate fairly reliably that nobody will live who does not feed on human flesh. Here it would be irrational to gamble on some miracle breakthrough by the rescuers.

[179] Can charity be morally demanded—rather than a praiseworthy but optional expression of affection or sympathy—yet not rise to the level of a moral *duty*, thus not requiring that everyone who would eat of the dead person's body be included in the lottery, regardless of their wishes? If charity is viewed as an imperfect duty, one that agents are morally required to perform but not on any specific occasion, it would not necessarily mandate an all-inclusive lottery. But the more one conceives morality to require helping precisely those individuals who refuse to risk death to live and who might starve unless aided, the more one will be forced to conclude that fairness forbids people from sitting out. See below, n. 181.

fail and the choice is between running over employees subject to a heightened risk of traffic accidents—road construction workers, for example—and people strolling by on the sidewalk? Should the police wait until the terrorist has his gun to the head of a reporter rather than an ordinary airplane passenger before rushing the plane?

It is no answer to say that those who enter dangerous occupations or engage in perilous leisure activities assume greater risk and that therefore their lives should not be valued as highly as those of bystanders or passersby. For while it is true that they assume *some* risk as part of their job or pastime, the question is whether they also elect to forgo the presumed benefits of a maximizing rule in choosing their livelihood or personal projects. The proper response, I think, is to treat cases of overlapping groups in exactly the same manner as those already discussed. The background rule forbids killing one person to save others. The question in each case, then, is whether the conditions for presumed consent to a maximizing rule are met with respect to those who are imperiled and those who might be killed to save them.

If, for example, pedestrians and road workers are as likely to have errant vehicles bearing down on them that can be turned toward the other group, and if the chance of the pedestrian group's being larger than the workers' group is one in two, it would be in everybody's interest to approve a maximizing rule. If, however, the errant vehicle invariably heads for the road workers and the alternative is always and only to direct it toward the pedestrians, the pedestrians would never consent to a modification of the background rule. The question in each case is whether those who would be killed to save additional others would have favored a maximizing policy. In many situations, determining what rule people would have chosen will be difficult, given the dearth of information available to potential agents and the frequent need for speedy action. If the answer is not obvious and time is short, perhaps a good rule would be not to intervene unless the numbers are lopsided, in which case the policy would likely have been to everyone's antecedent advantage and have won at least majority support. But the theoretically correct course requires a more searching inquiry.

5.7. Ought or May Agents Maximize Lives Saved?

Ought the agent to divert the trolley or activate the ceiling-support machine if hypothetical or actual consent, consistent with the demands of fairness, so dictates? I think so. The reasons I gave in criticism of Thomson's brief remarks on this topic establish a moral imperative, not merely a permission.[180] Turning the trolley, or flipping the switch, is what at least a majority of those in danger would have wanted. Disregarding their will, when complying with it would not exact from the agent a significant sacrifice, manifests disrespect for them as rational creatures entitled to treatment as moral equals. We have, I believe, a duty to confer sizable benefits on others when doing so would cost us little or nothing.[181] Turning the trolley or switching on the machine slips comfortably within this principle's embrace, provided that the agent does not risk legal penalties or other retaliation.

Moreover, if one assumes (which I do not) that the value of lives can be summed for the purpose of deciding whom to keep alive and if it is permissible to kill, then it follows more forcefully that one *ought* to divert the trolley or start the machine.[182] Flipping a coin, or standing idle as events amble by, ensures a worse world, and affronts the reasoned choices of our moral equals.

5.8. Additional Applications

Before detailing the legal implications of my argument and concluding with a few remarks about cases in which no one need be killed to save lives but

---

[180] See above, nn. 102–4 and accompanying text.

[181] Does this claim conflict with my earlier assertion, see supra note 179 and accompanying text, that the survivors of a lifeboat lottery need not share any of the victim's flesh that they cannot themselves consume with those who declined to participate in the lottery? No, for the only condition under which nonparticipants could receive this benefit *fairly* is a condition they deem unacceptable, namely, participation. If they cannot morally be denied this benefit after the lottery, then in fairness they would have to be included in the lottery against their will. And that, in my view, would be a more grievous wrong.

The same result can be reached by viewing the problem from a participant's perspective. If a participant recognized, in advance, a duty to share superfluous flesh with nonparticipants, doing so *would* come at considerable cost to him, because it would increase his chance of death relative to what it would be were nonparticipants included in the survival lottery. Hence, the principle I endorsed would not require that he share. On a more practical level, if everybody recognized a duty to aid nonparticipants, no rational person would participate unless he were unusually altruistic.

[182] Would the government's adoption of a maximizing policy in rescue situations strengthen the argument that citizens have a duty to kill in similar circumstances? I do not see how it could. The government's decision to institute some policy for state officials, without commanding citizens to do likewise, certainly does not oblige citizens to weave that policy into their own lives. The government's decision to engage in affirmative-action hiring for racial minorities or to subsidize domestic industries, for example, does not obligate private employers to use the same hiring criteria or supply consumers with a moral imperative to buy local manufactures. People must decide for themselves whether the course their government pursues is right and whether they ought to embrace it; the bare fact that the government follows that course says nothing about its merits or its proper scope. What effect the government's adoption of maximizing policies should have on individuals' conduct, moreover, seems (at least for the moment) academic, because the official actions of virtually all existing governments fall well short of unambiguously endorsing maximization.

different numbers of people can be saved, let me strengthen the case for appealing to hypothetical consent and fairness by describing the consequences of my view in several situations not yet considered. Unlike Costa's gloss on the 'ends not means' principle and Kamm's Principle of (Im)Permissible Harm, the notion of hypothetical consent I have outlined dictates the same approach to all versions of the trolley case, whether in its simplest incarnation or its loop variants or versions in which bystanders can be pushed onto the track or killed in rock slides or explosions if necessary to halt the train. The same is true of the various permutations of the hospital case: it matters not at all that the single patient's death would come from the ceiling-support machine's exhaust, from therapeutic treatment given to the five, or from movement of the weight atop the ceiling. In all these cases, distinctions among the way in which somebody's body is used to prevent the death of other people, and among the closeness of the causal connections between that action and the deaths of some people and the rescue of more numerous others, are morally irrelevant. Approaches that give prominence to these factors overlook the moral equality of persons, and fail to focus sufficiently on the fact that in every case, either some must be killed to save others, or through inaction more will die. Respect for our fellows as responsible, reasoning creatures forbids our taking their lives for purposes for which they are unwilling to die, in circumstances in which they can refuse endorsement without reneging on their agreements and without unfairness. The decisive question is always whether they (or a majority of those who might be killed) would be killed pursuant to a policy they would have approved beforehand, from which dissenters could not be excepted without treating the others unfairly, and which would antecedently have improved the dissenters' chances of staying alive.

   In some cases, ascertaining whether these conditions have been met will be difficult. This seems particularly likely when one must decide whether to kill people who lack important characteristics of those who might be saved. Suppose, for example, that the person beside the trolley tracks who might be knocked beneath the train to save five workers is not a worker himself but a neighbor out for a stroll. Or suppose that the possible victim in the next hospital room is not another patient but a visitor, or a nurse, or somebody delivering supplies. Although the proper prescription depends upon the facts of a given case, it would, I think, ordinarily be impermissible to push a non-worker onto the trolley tracks or to explode the train beside him because in most instances he would have had little or no chance of ending up in a group that would have benefitted statistically from a maximizing rule. The identity of the person in the adjacent hospital room does not seem similarly relevant,

290 ERIC RAKOWSKI

however, because that person might just as likely have found himself in the more crowded room.

As indicated,[183] I do not think it matters that the threat to the larger group was created intentionally by a wicked mind rather than accidentally or naturally. Whether the trolley's brakes fail through sabotage, poor maintenance, or unforeseeable mechanical malfunction, the person sitting at the switch should turn the train to save the greater number if he can reasonably predict that turning the train would antecedently have been the course preferred by those whose lives are at stake. Nor does it matter that the evil person forcing the choice has the power to prevent harm altogether, so long as he is certain enough to fulfill his threat. In making that determination, one would have to consider the possibility that a policy of ignoring threats would save the most lives in the long run and assess, as best one could, the likelihood that the evildoer will perform the threatened deed. But a desire not to become the instrument of another person's condemned will is not an adequate reason to refrain from doing what those with much more to lose—people whose lives might end—would have wanted one to do.

McCloskey's famous case poses a more troubling decision.[184] In a more realistic variation of McCloskey's example, a Southern sheriff some time ago has in custody a black man accused of some serious crime. The man is innocent, and the sheriff believes him to be innocent. A crazed mob thinks otherwise. The crowd has seized five black men who happen to live nearby, and threatens to lynch them unless the prisoner is released into its hands to suffer a cruel death in place of the five. The sheriff reasonably expects the shouting throng to kill the five unless he complies with their demand. If he declines to hand over his prisoner, the sheriff can protect him indefinitely. What should he do?

This example often serves as a springboard for criticizing utilitarianism. Critics assume that handing over the man in custody would be unequivocally wrong; but utilitarianism, they contend, requires that the sheriff surrender him. Ancillary considerations, such as detrimental effects on the administration of justice and the prospect of more vigilante action, are supposedly too weak to permit utilitarians to prescribe the intuitively proper outcome.

---

[183] See above, nn. 99–101 and accompanying text.

[184] See H. J. McCloskey, 'A Note on Utilitarian Punishment,' *Mind*, 72 (1963), 599. For an argument that under certain circumstances, the sheriff should send an innocent person to his death, see Smart's contribution to Smart and Williams, *Utilitarianism*, 69–72. Considering a case in which the judge must frame an innocent man to save five innocent men from a mob, Richard McCormick argues that the judge must refrain from an unjust act because of its detrimental long-term effects. See Richard McCormick, 'Ambiguity in Moral Choice,' in R. McCormick and P. Ramsey (eds.), *Doing Evil to Achieve Good* (1978), 7, 33. McCormick's subsequent discussion of this case, however, leaves his reasons for opposing the sacrifice of the one man less clear. See Richard McCormick, 'A Commentary on the Commentaries,' in ibid. 193.

Would the same criticism apply to an appeal to the hypothetical consent of the six black men?

It is hard to know without more facts. Did the one stand as great a chance as the five of being picked up and lynched in similar circumstances? If so, would turning over a prisoner in this case really further the interests of blacks and other members of that community in the long run? One can, I suppose, imagine circumstances in which, by consulting the antecedent advantage of the black men facing death and speculating about what policy they would have favored, the sheriff ought to bow to the mob's will. But it is difficult to believe that, in those circumstances, the better course is to ignore the crowd's shouts, wash one's hands, and thereby cause more innocent people to die. Taking one's cue from what those affected would have wanted rules out an absolute bar on appeasing the crowd. But an absolute prohibition has no firm moral foundation, whatever its initial appeal.

Finally, consider Michael Tooley's Diabolical Machine.[185] The machine contains two innocent children. Its design ensures that one child will be killed and one will be released unharmed. You cannot free both. You can, however, push a button that will redirect the machine's lethal force, causing it to kill the child that would have been released and freeing the child that would have been killed. You do not know which child will die if you refrain from acting. Would it be morally permissible to push the button? Tooley contends that it would be. He thinks that flipping a coin to decide whether to push the button would be best, because it would give each child an equal chance of surviving. But if no coin is available, it seems to him a matter of indifference what one does.[186]

Tooley offers his example to cast doubt on the claim that it is intrinsically more wrong to kill somebody than to let someone die. Tooley's argument might seem to threaten my view as well, insofar as that view incorporates some version of that claim in holding that we may not kill somebody unless he expressly consents, even if in consequence we must let more people die, unless killing him is consistent with a rule he would have endorsed beforehand, or unless fairness requires his sacrifice. For pushing the button appears, at least at first sight, to override somebody's right not to be killed, even if that person's identity is unknown to the agent. It thus seems impermissible. Yet pushing the button does not, as Tooley says, seem morally outrageous.[187]

---

[185] See Michael Tooley, *Abortion and Infanticide* (Oxford: Oxford University Press, 1983), 189–90, 206–11.

[186] See ibid. 189–90.

[187] Not everyone would agree, I am sure. Judith Thomson, for example, presumably would not. She recently stated that it would be morally impermissible to redirect a trolley headed toward one

The Diabolical Machine grounds no serious objection to the view I propose. Except in highly unusual cases, of which this is one, it would plainly be
wrong to kill one person to prevent another person from dying. A doctor
may not remove a heart from a healthy patient to save one near death. She
may not kill one patient even to save several dying patients, so long as the
one does not or did not consent to becoming a donor. The best explanation
of this moral fact, I have suggested, is that people have a right not to be
killed. Although that right can be waived or trumped by considerations of
fairness, in these circumstances it ordinarily would not be relinquished,
it cannot be presumed to have been surrendered, and it may be exercised
without unfairness to others.[188]

The Diabolical Machine does not, in my view, furnish a reason to doubt
the existence of that right. Nor does it cast suspicion on the claim that a
person's right not to be killed morally overrides whatever right other people
have not to be allowed to die. We see no immediate obstacle to pushing the
button because, in contrast to the more typical case of the two patients, we
cannot think of any good reason the children might have for objecting. No
convention or rule makes whatever events put one child in the death chair
and destined the other for freedom the controlling factors for deciding which
one lives. We think it might be permissible to flip a coin, or at least that it
would not be gravely wrong to do so, because the children would almost
certainly be indifferent to what we do. Suppose that a roulette wheel were
spun and that where the ball stopped would determine which child died.
Suppose that, while it was whirling rapidly, we gave the wheel an additional
push. There is a fifty-fifty chance that we changed the outcome. But while
doing something that kills somebody every second time would generally be
impermissible, even if it also saves a life every second time, adding impetus
to the wheel can hardly be thought wicked. Unless they wished their anxiety
to come to as speedy an end as possible, the children would not mind.
Tooley's example therefore exposes no deficiency in the proposed analysis.

5.9. Legal Implications

Even if one ought to kill if certain conditions are met, it is a separate
question whether the law should permit, or even require, people to kill in

---

person so that it strikes another person instead. See Thomson, 'Self-Defense,' 309. Thomson does
not, however, defend her conclusion or address Tooley's example explicitly. For an argument that
Thomson's conclusion is incompatible with her appeal to antecedent advantage in at least some
cases, see Alexander, 'Self-Defense, Justification, and Excuse,' 58.

[188] See above, Sect. 5.4.

those situations. One reason this question is hard is that situations satisfying the conditions set forth above do not come clearly labeled for the benefit of agents, judges, and juries. If they did, governments might (if they thought it right not to respect conscientious dissents from official policy) require killing in just those situations in which the conditions were met and punish it in all other cases except, suitably qualified, unprovoked self-defense and euthanasia. In fact, however, reasonable people would in some cases almost certainly disagree over whether all the affected individuals would antecedently have approved killing some to save more others or whether a majority would have and fairness requires that the majority's preferences prevail. Punishing people whose judgment reasonably diverged from government officials' opinions would be highhanded. Absolving from blame any killer who asserted that his action cleared the relevant hurdles, however, would only invite ill-conceived slaughter. As Samuel Scheffler observes, '[t]he world has known all too many people whose zeal for killing has not been matched by any great talent for accurately predicting the consequences of their actions, and all too many killers whose judgements about what ends are valuable have been deranged, biased, self-serving, or otherwise misguided.'[189] If killing is to be permitted or required in situations in which morality appears to allow or command it, we cannot exempt from punishment all killers proclaiming pureness of heart, irrespective of the feebleness of their judgment.

Would it suffice to exempt from punishment for murder or manslaughter anyone who killed, in the apparently sincere and demonstrably reasonable (if mistaken) belief that killing would maximize the number of people kept alive consistent with the constraints described above? The law in most American jurisdictions might be interpreted as accepting this approach, although the absence of recorded cases and explicit statutory commands in most states renders a more definite statement impossible. The Model Penal Code and many state criminal codes allow a person charged with a crime to defend his action by showing that he reasonably believed it necessary to avoid a greater evil than he brought about.[190] So long as the defendant is able to produce sufficient evidence to support his claim, the burden is on the prosecution to prove, beyond a reasonable doubt, that the defendant's belief was unreasonable and that the other elements of the offense were present.[191] The

---

[189] Scheffler, *The Rejection of Consequentialism*, 110. Similarly, Tim Scanlon thinks that mistrust of others' judgment, coupled with an irrational belief in one's own good fortune, lies behind laws forbidding killing even to save more numerous others. That same mistrust, Scanlon thinks, explains our proclivity to condemn people who refused to save others because they thought (perhaps rightly) the world would be better off with those people dead. See T. M. Scanlon, 'Rights, Goals, and Fairness,' in Stuart Hampshire (ed.), *Public and Private Morality* (Cambridge: Cambridge University Press, 1978), 93, 108–11.

[190] See Model Penal Code, §3.02 (Proposed Official Draft 1962).

[191] See ibid., §§1.12(2), 3.01.

Model Penal Code does not, however, specifically identify killing some people as a lesser evil than allowing a larger number of other people to die. Nor does any state statute. To be sure, the Commentary to the Model Penal Code asserts that taking life to increase the number of people remaining alive should be regarded as justifiable under the necessity or choice-of-evils defense.[192] But in the absence of decided cases, it is unclear whether states that have enacted provisions tracking the Model Penal Code would interpret them as the Commentary counsels. Some states, moreover, have rejected the Model Penal Code's approach, either by increasing the burden on a defendant entering a choice-of-evils defense[193] or by precluding him from raising the defense to a charge of intentional homicide.[194]

Should political communities hearken to the Model Penal Code's Commentary and permit killing if the conditions outlined above are met and if a defendant can satisfy the evidentiary requirements set by the generally applicable choice-of-evils defense? I believe that they should. If the preceding argument is correct, killing some people to save a larger number of other people is, ignoring contrary legal requirements, morally imperative in certain instances. The law should not impede the performance of this moral duty. It should, moreover, provide explicitly that killing in those instances is protected conduct, in order to safeguard defendants from the possibly discordant moral beliefs of some judges or jurors who would otherwise be left to give shape to the nebulous choice-of-evils defense as their consciences direct.

To be sure, allowing defendants to invoke the choice-of-evils defense might encourage unjustified killing because those inclined to take others' lives might believe that they will be able to escape punishment for conduct they know is wrongful. This risk, however, seems slight, given the necessity of showing that one's conduct was reasonable to shield oneself from conviction. And the fear that recognizing the defense in exceptional murder cases would have a noticeable detrimental effect on the respect people accord innocent life seems fatuous.

One might, of course, argue more forcefully that it would be best not to extend, either legislatively or by judicial decision, the choice-of-evils defense

---

[192] See Model Penal Code and Commentaries, §3.02 cmt., 14–16 (1985). There seems little doubt that the Commentary's approach to weighing evils is consequentialist and that it assumes the value of lives can be added to determine which outcome is less bad, without assigning any special weight to the arguable inherent wrongness of intentionally taking innocent life. See Greenawalt, 'Natural Law and Political Choice,' 5–6.

[193] Some states require that the defendant show that the threatened harm *clearly* outweighed the harm caused by the defendant. See Paul H. Robinson, 2 Criminal Law Defenses §125(g) (1984). Others require that the defendant show by a preponderance of the evidence that the evil averted was greater than the evil caused. See ibid., §124(c) (Supp. 1988).

[194] See e.g., Sanford H. Kadish et al., Criminal Law and its Processes (1983), 785 n. 5 (collecting examples of states limiting the choice-of-evils defense).

of killing, so as to enhance the deterrent effect of laws proscribing murder and manslaughter, but instead to trust prosecutors not to seek indictments in cases in which the killer plausibly attempted to save lives on balance. But for the same reasons that a general necessity defense warrants codification,[195] its extension to cases of justified killing should be rendered explicit too. The existence of a choice-of-evils defense would not, in any case, eliminate prosecutorial discretion. Government officials would still have to decide whether to go forward with a case whenever one person takes another's life. If the evidence strongly supports a defendant's claimed justification under the principles elaborated above, prosecutors plainly should not initiate proceedings. This will typically be so if a killer deflected an existing threat toward a smaller group with the evident intention of keeping alive as many people as he could; there is generally less reason to mistrust the motives of people who divert dangers that they did not create than to question the motives of people who bring new perils into being. The distinction between diverting and originating harm thus has considerable practical utility, even if it is not always an accurate or illuminating guide to distinguish between justified and unjustified killing. Because abuse of discretion is possible and the stakes are so high, however, prosecutors ought to be checked by a legal standard of justification to which a defendant can appeal in court.

The arguable flaw in this approach is that, by making the choice of the lesser evil an affirmative *defense* to intentional homicide, it establishes a disincentive to kill even when killing is morally justified. For even if the killer's judgment is sound and he can show that he ought to have killed, he still faces at least the *possibility* of prosecution and the anxiety and expense of defending himself. If the evidence for the correctness of his view is less plain, the risk dilates. If he does nothing, however, he need not fear prosecution, at least under current law, for in no jurisdiction is *failure* to kill a criminal offense. Admittedly, the law could be changed to make failure to kill punishable if the conditions for applying a maximizing rule were met. But then agents who found themselves in perilous emergencies would face possible prosecutions whether they acted or refrained from acting. That seems to place unwarranted pressure on people who are unlucky enough to

---

[195] Kent Greenawalt notes:

That very few cases actually raise the [necessity] defense does show that most appealing claims of justification are handled in some informal way; yet, despite its limited practical significance, the defense fills important offices. It serves most plainly as a safeguard against prosecutorial abuse. Even when prosecutorial policy is enlightened, actors who are genuinely justified should have legal confirmation that they have acted appropriately, rather than having to conceive themselves as depending on a prosecutor's grace. Moreover, when claimed justifying facts are in doubt, or the crime is very serious, or the balance of relevant values is controversial, formal adjudication may be preferable to prosecutorial judgment of whether or not a possibly justified actor should be punished.

Kent Greenawalt, *Conflicts of Law and Morality*, (1989), 287 (footnote omitted).

confront these tense and trying choices. In addition, the law would show an inconsistent face if it penalized people for failing to kill when more could thereby be kept alive, but not for failing to save if identical results would ensue.[196] There, too, the law could be amended to impose duties to assist.[197] But even if this change were made, panicked agents would still have to walk the tightrope.

Fining or incarcerating those who failed to kill in accordance with a maximizing rule would be inappropriate for still other reasons. The first is the unusual and frantic circumstances of choice. Situations in which killing might save lives consistent with the requirements I have defended are rare, decisions are frequently hurried, and ascertaining the presence of the pre-conditions for justified killing is often difficult. While the wise use of prosecutorial discretion would allow for these factors, it might be best to forestall the misuse of that discretion, whether willful or unintentional, by not criminalizing failure to kill under any circumstances. Further, some people might reject the moral principles on which a maximizing rule is prem-ised, and to a society that considers it improper to visit criminal penalties on citizens who conscientiously object to killing enemy soldiers in combat, criminal penalties for failure to kill innocent fellow citizens would be even more offensive. Sometimes, of course, we think it permissible to punish people for what they, in good conscience, do or refuse to do. But it seems unlikely that we would benefit in the future from penalizing those who conscientiously decided not to kill some people to save others, because it is highly improbable that they would ever again face such a choice. In addition, the threat of punishment, discounted by the slim odds that any omission would be discovered and prosecuted, would probably prove an ineffectual spur to action if someone's moral convictions stood opposed. For these reasons, it seems best to refrain altogether from penalizing failure to kill.

---

[196] Under the law of the overwhelming majority of states, '[g]enerally one has no legal duty to aid another person in peril, even when that aid can be rendered without danger or inconvenience to himself.' Wayne R. LaFave and Austin W. Scott Jr., *Criminal Law*, 2nd edn. (1986), §3 3(a) (footnote omitted).

[197] That change seems overdue. Although Anglo-American criminal and civil legal regimes have long tolerated bad Samaritans, most continental European countries have for many years penal-ized people who failed to rescue others in serious need when rescue was easy. See Joel Feinberg, *Harm to Others*, 126–7. Feinberg argues forcefully that failure to prevent grave harm to another should be punishable if helping would clearly not have imposed an unreasonable risk, cost, or inconvenience on the rescuer. See ibid. 127–86.

5.10. Saving without Killing

Rescuers forced to choose between groups of different sizes because they are unable to save both frequently need not kill some people to save the rest. Think of rescue helicopters that can save one of two sets of swamped sailors, but not both. For those who believe that the value of lives can be summed for the purpose of choosing survivors, these choices are uncomplicated. In the absence of special duties, obligations, or permissions, and assuming that the people who might be saved are equally guiltless, rescuers ought in their view to save the larger group straightaway. Most people's intuitions approve this advice. The view that numbers are morally irrelevant, which I and others hold,[198] might be thought to founder on this intuitive conviction, for it apparently requires that we choose survivors randomly—say, by flipping a coin—even when groups differ vastly in size.

In fact, however, its implications are not as unpalatable as appearances suggest. The hypothetical consent approach has the merit of reconciling the view that numbers are morally irrelevant with our intuitive convictions in life-saving cases. In the vast majority of situations in which rescuers must choose between groups of different sizes, most imperiled individuals would antecedently have favoured a rule requiring that the more numerous group be saved, as that rule would have increased their odds of surviving the calamity. And those who would have balked would ordinarily have had their chance of surviving improved by the introduction of a maximizing rule. Think of people trapped in different parts of burning buildings, or miners caught in separate tunnels following a cave-in, or the overboard passengers of a sinking ship. By appealing to what would have been to their unanimous advantage beforehand and what, in the absence of unusual moral or religious beliefs, a majority would have preferred, one may retain the view that the value of people's lives cannot be added for purposes of moral decisionmaking without endorsing a counterintuitive approach to these cases.[199]

---

[198] I defend this view at length in Rakowski, *Equal Justice*, 277–309. The first sustained presentation and defense of the claim that numbers do not matter is John Taurek's article 'Should the Numbers Count?' Judith Thomson espouses this view as well. See *The Realm of Rights*, 166–7. It nevertheless remains a minority position.

[199] In *Equal Justice*, I stopped short of endorsing direct reliance on what people would reasonably have preferred in an ideal setting for choice. Instead, I argued that prospective rescuers are obligated to intend to save the larger group if all those affected would have favored that course, because forming that intention would confer a significant benefit on other people at no cost to themselves. I further maintained, however, that if they neglected to form that intention, they should in most instances choose survivors randomly. See Rakowski, *Equal Justice* 304–9. That view now seems to me mistaken. The prior formation of an intention to save the larger group is not a morally necessary precondition for departing from a random choice of survivors.

ERIC RAKOWSKI

In some situations, however, the view I propose parts company from one that always requires that the larger group be saved. John Taurek provides an example.[200] A volcano erupts on a small island inhabited by poor villagers with no means of escape. We own a boat and can save some of them before they are engulfed by the lava and smoke. Lamentably, we cannot save them all. The villagers are divided between the northern end of the island, where most of them live, and the southern end, where a minority lives. They did not choose their residences knowing that the volcano might erupt and that, if it did, our policy would be to save the larger group wherever it happened to be. Everyone thought the volcano extinct. What should we do?

Those who believe that the value of lives can be summed morally would steer automatically for the island's northern end, as more people could be saved there. If Taurek and I were skippering the craft and knew nobody on the island, we would flip a coin. None of the islanders is to blame for her plight or her proximity to one end of the island or the other. Because we care about them equally as individuals, we would give each the same chance of survival. When somebody loses his life, he loses what is often most previous to him. That others perish alongside him does not compound his loss, nor does the loss experienced by any other individual wax beyond that which he or another suffers. What matters morally is not the vanishing of some valuable object, of which we as moral agents are caretakers. What matters are the losses that particular individuals suffer, people with whom we can identify and whose plight we can imagine, and nobody (save the universe poetically conceived) suffers the sum of those losses. Treating those in danger as moral equals requires that we accord them the same chance of coming away with their lives, unless a different rule would have been to the advantage of all and most would have welcomed its adoption.

This is not the place, however, to offer an extended argument for this view. My point is merely that the approach defended in this Article goes a long way to acquitting the thesis that numbers are morally irrelevant in the court of intuition. That approach is in no way undermined if one rejects the thesis that numbers are morally inconsequential and adheres to the common view that they wield some moral weight.

6. CONCLUSION

Killing some people to save others from death is wrong, unless the killing accords with a rule that everyone killed accepted overtly or would reasonably

---

[200] See Taurek, 'Should the Numbers Count?', 310–16.

have found beneficial to adopt, or unless, although some or all of the victims opposed killing on religious or moral grounds, their deaths were brought about in accordance with a rule that would antecedently have advanced their self-interest and was or would have been favored by a larger number of those people who were also covered by the policy. Determining when these conditions are met might at times be difficult. Life-saving choices are frequently pressured and unexpected; rescuers often lack pertinent information. If the preceding argument is correct, however, this difficult determination may not be shirked. For unless these preconditions are met, killing somebody to save others is morally intolerable. It is intolerable because it takes from someone what he probably values most, without his consent, indeed without even the possibility of his having benefited, and for the sake of somebody else who, as his moral peer, is entitled to no preference. To conform killing to a less demanding standard is to blink our moral equality and the value of human life.

9

THE SURVIVAL LOTTERY

JOHN HARRIS

Let's suppose that organ transplant procedures have been perfected; in such circumstances if two dying patients could be saved by organ transplants then, if surgeons have the requisite organs in stock and no other needy patients, but they notwithstanding allow their patients to die, we would be inclined to say, and be justified in saying, that the patients died because the doctors refused to save them. But if there are no spare organs in stock and none otherwise available, the doctors have no choice, they cannot save their patients and so must let them die. In this case we would be disinclined to say that the doctors are in any sense the cause of their patients' deaths.

But let's further suppose that the two dying patients, Y and Z are not happy about being left to die. They might argue that it is not strictly true that there are no organs which could be used to save them. Y needs a new heart and Z new lungs. They point out that if just one healthy person were to be killed his organs could be removed and both of them be saved. We and the doctors would probably be alike in thinking that such a step, while technically possible, would be out of the question. We would not say that the doctors were killing their patients if they refused to prey upon the healthy to save the sick. And because this sort of surgical Robin Hoodery is out of the question we can tell Y and Z that they cannot be saved and that when they die, they will have died of natural causes and not of the neglect of their doctors. Y and Z do not, however, agree; they insist that if the doctors fail to kill a healthy man and use his organs to save them, then the doctors will be responsible for their deaths.

The rejection of Y's and Z's plea for life is based on the view that we must not kill even if by doing so we could save life, that there is a moral difference between killing and letting die. On this view, to kill someone, B let's say, so that Y and Z might live is ruled out because we have a strict obligation not to kill but a duty of some lesser kind to save life. The dying Y and Z may be

From John Harris, 'The Survival Lottery', first pub. in *Philosophy*, 50/191 (Jan. 1975); this version from Harris, *Violence and Responsibility* (London: Routledge & Kegan Paul, 1980).

excused for not being over-much impressed by this view. They accept that it is wrong to kill the innocent and are prepared to agree to an absolute prohibition against so doing. They do not agree, however, that B is more innocent than they are. Y and Z might go on to point out that the currently acknowledged right of the innocent not to be killed even where their deaths might give life to others, is just a decision to prefer the lives of the fortunate to those of the unfortunate. B is innocent in the sense that he has done nothing to deserve death, but Y and Z are also innocent in this sense. Why should they be the ones to die, simply because they are so unlucky as to have diseased organs? Why, they might argue, should their living or dying be left to chance when in so many other areas of human life we believe that we have an obligation to ensure the survival of the maximum number of lives possible?

Y and Z argue that, if a doctor refuses to treat a patient with the result that the patient dies, he has killed that patient as sure as shooting; in exactly the same way, if the doctors refuse Y and Z the transplants that they need, then their refusal will kill Y and Z, again as sure as shooting. The doctors, and indeed the society which supports their inaction, cannot defend themselves by arguing that they are neither expected, nor required by law or convention, to kill so that lives may be saved (indeed quite the reverse), since this is just an appeal to custom or authority. A man who does his own moral thinking must decide whether, in these circumstances, he ought to save two lives at the cost of one or one life at the cost of two. The fact that so called 'third parties' have never before been brought into such calculations, have never before been thought of as being involved, is not an argument against their now becoming so.

There are, of course, good arguments against allowing doctors simply to haul passers-by off the streets whenever they have a couple of patients in need of new organs. And the harmful side-effects of such a practice in terms of terror and distress to the victims, the witnesses and society generally, would give us further reasons for dismissing the idea; Y and Z realise this and have a proposal, which they will shortly produce, which would largely meet objections to placing such power in the hands of doctors and eliminate at least some of the harmful side-effects.

KILLING THE INNOCENT

In the unlikely event of their feeling obliged to reply to the reproaches of Y and Z, the doctors might make the following argument: they might maintain that a man is only responsible for the death of someone whose life he might have saved if, in all the circumstances of the case, he ought to have saved the man by the means available. This is why a doctor might be a murderer if he simply refused or neglected to treat a patient who would die without treatment, but not if he could only save the patient by doing something he ought in no circumstances to do—kill the innocent. Y and Z readily agree that a man ought not to do what he ought not to do, but they point out that if the doctors, and for that matter society at large, ought on balance to kill one man if two can thereby be saved, then failure to do so will involve responsibility for the consequent deaths. The fact that Y's and Z's proposal involves killing the innocent cannot be a reason for refusing to consider their proposals, for this would just be a refusal to face the question at issue and so avoid having to make a decision as to what ought to be done in circumstances like these. It is Y's and Z's claim that failure to adopt their plan will also involve killing the innocent, rather more of the innocent than the proposed alternative.

THE SURVIVAL LOTTERY

To back up this last point, to remove the arbitrariness of permitting doctors to select their donors from among the chance passers-by outside hospitals, and the tremendous power this would place in doctors' hands, to mitigate worries about side-effects and lastly to appease those who wonder why poor old B should be singled out for sacrifice, Y and Z put forward the following scheme. They propose that everyone be given a sort of lottery number. Whenever doctors have two or more dying patients who could be saved by transplants, and no suitable organs have come to hand through 'natural' deaths, they can ask a central computer to supply a suitable donor. The computer will then pick the number of a suitable donor at random and he will be killed so that the lives of two or more others may be saved. No doubt if the scheme were ever to be implemented a suitable euphemism for 'killed' would be employed. Perhaps we would begin to talk about citizens being called upon to 'give life' to others. With the refinement of transplant procedures such a scheme could offer the chance of saving large numbers of lives that are now lost. Indeed, even taking into account the loss of the lives of donors, the numbers of untimely deaths each year might be dramatically reduced, so much so that everyone's chance of living to a ripe old age might be increased. If this were to be the consequence of the adoption of such a scheme—and it might well be—it could not be dismissed lightly.

Suppose, for example, that inter-planetary travel revealed a world of people like ourselves, but who organised their society according to this scheme. No one was considered to have an absolute right to life or freedom from interference, but everything was always done to ensure that as many people as possible would enjoy long and happy lives. In such a world a man who attempted to escape when his number was up or who resisted on the grounds that no one had a right to take his life, might well be regarded as a murderer. We might or might not prefer to live in such a world, but the morality of its inhabitants would surely be one that we could respect. It would not be obviously more barbaric or cruel or immoral than our own.

A FATAL EXEMPTION

Y and Z are willing to concede one exception to the universal application of their scheme. They realise that it would be unfair to allow people who have brought their misfortune on themselves to benefit from the lottery. There would clearly be something unjust about killing the abstemious B so that W, whose heavy smoking has given him lung cancer, and X, whose drinking has destroyed his liver, should be preserved to over indulge again.

SECURITY

What objections could be made to the lottery scheme? A first straw at which to clutch would be the desire for security. Under such a scheme we would never know when we would hear *them* knocking at the door. Every post might bring a sentence of death, every sound in the night might be the sound of boots on the stairs. But, as we have seen, the chances of actually being called upon to make the ultimate sacrifice might be slimmer than is the present risk of being killed on the roads, and most of us do not lie trembling abed, appalled at the prospect of being dispatched on the morrow. The truth is that lives might well be more secure under such a scheme.

INDIVIDUALITY

If we respect individuality and see every human being as unique in his own way, we might want to reject a society in which it appeared that individuals were seen merely as interchangeable units in a structure, the value of which lies in its having as many healthy units as possible. But of course Y and Z would want to know why A's individuality was more worthy of respect than theirs.

PLAYING GOD

Another plausible objection is the natural reluctance to play God with man's lives, the feeling that it is wrong to make any attempt to re-allot the life opportunities that fate has determined, the feeling that the deaths of Y and Z would be 'natural', whereas the death of anyone killed to save them would have been perpetrated by men. But if we are able to change things, then to elect not to do so is also to determine what will happen in the world. We would be playing God quite as much if we left Y and Z to their fate as we would if we killed B.

Of course if Y alone could be saved by the killing of B we would be reluctant to play God, but this is not because it's wrong to play God, but wrong to do so *to no purpose*. In the present example we do have a reason to re-allot the life opportunities that fate has determined—we can thereby save an extra life.

Professor Anscombe has attacked the moral importance of saving more lives rather than fewer.[1]

If there are a lot of people stranded on a rock, and one person on another, and someone goes with a boat to rescue the single one, what cause so far have any of the others for complaint? They are not injured unless help that was owing to them was withheld. There was one boat that could have helped them: but it was not left idle; no, it went to save that other one. What is the accusation that each of them can make? What wrong can he claim has been done him? None whatever: unless the preference signalises some ignoble contempt.

Professor Anscombe insists that a man 'doesn't act badly if he uses his resources to save X ... *for no bad reason*, and is not affected by the consideration that he could save a larger number of people'.[2]

Professor Anscombe's view is certainly eccentric for it robs us of a perspective from which to criticise wasteful social policies, at least those which are wasteful of lives. But there are two alternative and equally catastrophic assumptions behind Professor Anscombe's position. I cannot improve upon Jonathan Glover's[3] ingenious exposure of these assumptions:[4]

Underlying this is the unstated belief that the time at which someone's life is in jeopardy is relevant to the moral importance of saving it. This curious assumption is a necessary feature of the position as we can see from consideration of some more people stranded on the rocks.

Suppose there are two rocks and on Monday the lifeboatman hears that A and B

---

[1] G. E. M. Anscombe, 'Who is Wronged?', *Oxford Review* (Trinity, 1967), 16.

[2] Ibid. 17.

[3] Jonathan Glover, *Causing Death and Saving Lives* (Harmondsworth: Penguin: 1977).

[4] I have constructed this quotation from an earlier draft of Glover's book and from the final version, but see ibid. 208, 209.

are stranded one on each rock. He has only time to go to one rock before both are submerged by the tide. Neither rock is harder to reach than the other. He knows nothing about the identity of A and B, only that they are different people. Here we might all agree that it is morally indifferent which rock he goes to. Now suppose a third person, C, is stranded on one of the two rocks on Tuesday. We may all agree that it is of some moral importance that the lifeboatman should rescue him. But, according to Professor Anscombe's view, if C had instead been stranded with either A or B on Monday, the prospect of saving him as well as one of the others need not have been considered of any moral importance at all. This will appeal to all those who think that saving lives consecutively is more important than saving lives simultaneously. (The alternative assumption is that the rightness of saving a life has nothing to do with any value placed on the life which is saved.)

POSITIVE AND NEGATIVE ACTIONS AGAIN

Neither does the alleged moral difference between killing and letting die afford a respectable way of rejecting the claims of Y and Z. For if we really want to counter proponents of the lottery, if we really want to answer Y and Z and not just put them off, we cannot do so by saying that the lottery involves killing and object to it for that reason, because to do so would, as we have seen, just beg the question as to whether the failure to save as many people as possible might not also amount to killing. To put this point another way: the view that there is a moral difference between killing and letting die cannot be used in support of the alleged moral difference between killing B and letting Y and Z die because it presupposes such a difference.

LAST-DOOR ARGUMENTS

An argument that has sometimes been used to support the doctrine that there is a moral difference between killing and letting die is that to kill someone is, as it were, to close the *last*[5] door on his opportunities for life, whereas any failure to prevent his death merely closes *one* door—not necessarily the last—on his life chances. On this view, to kill someone is surely and certainly to kill him, whereas to let him die is to act so that his death will *probably* result. But it is a question of fact in each case whether positive actions are a sure, or less ambitiously, a more probable, method of securing death than are negative actions. To draw again on an earlier example, it is a question of fact whether or not my bedridden granny will more probably die if I bring her poisoned food than if I bring her no food at all. I may

---

[5] See P. J. FitzGerald, 'Acting and Refraining', *Analysis*, 27/4 (Mar. 1967).

miscalculate the dose and she may gain nourishment from the food in which it is concealed thus prolonging her life, whereas if I bring her no food at all she may be rescued, or manna may fall from Heaven.

So, in each case it will be a question of fact whether the last door has indeed been closed upon the life of a particular person. There is nothing in the difference between positive and negative acts which makes the one inevitably or of itself a more certain method of bringing about death than the other.

SELF DEFENCE

To opt for the society which Y and Z propose would be, then, to adopt a society in which saintliness would be mandatory. Each of us would have to recognise a binding obligation to give up our own life for others when called upon to do so. In such a society anyone who reneged upon this duty would be a murderer. The most promising objection to such a society and indeed to any principle which required us to kill B in order to save Y and Z, is I suspect, that we are committed to the right of self defence. If I can kill B and save Y and Z then he can kill me to save P and Q, and it is only if I am prepared to agree to this that I will opt for the lottery or be prepared to agree to a man's being killed if doing so would save the lives of more than one other man.

Of course, there is something paradoxical about basing objections to the lottery scheme on the right of self defence since, *ex hypothesi*, each person would have a better chance of living to a ripe old age if the lottery scheme were to be implemented. Nonetheless, the feeling that no man should be required to lay down his life for others, makes many people shy away from such a scheme even though it might be rational to accept it on prudential grounds, and perhaps even mandatory on utilitarian grounds. Again, of course, Y and Z would reply that the right of self defence must extend to them as much as to anyone else. And while it is true that they can only live if another man is killed, they would claim that it is also true that if they are left to die, then someone who lives on does so literally over their dead bodies.

SIDE-EFFECTS

It might be argued that the institution of the survival lottery has not gone far to mitigate the harmful side-effects in terms of terror and distress to victims, witnesses and society generally, that would be occasioned by doctors simply snatching passers-by off the streets and disorganising them for the benefit of the unfortunate. Donors would, after all, still have to be procured, and this process, however it was carried out, would still be likely to prove distressing to all concerned. The lottery scheme would eliminate the arbitrariness of leaving the life and death decisions to the doctors, and remove the possibility of such terrible power falling into the hands of any individuals, but the terror and distress would remain. The effect of having to apprehend presumably unwilling victims would give us pause.

Perhaps only a long period of education or propaganda could remove our abhorrence. What this abhorrence reveals about the rights and wrongs of the situation is, however, more difficult to assess. We might be inclined to say that only monsters could ignore the promptings of conscience so far as to operate the lottery scheme. But the promptings of conscience are not necessarily the most reliable guide. In the present case Y and Z would argue that such promptings are mere squeamishness, an over nice self-indulgence that costs lives. Death, Y and Z would remind us, is a distressing experience whenever and to whomever it occurs, so the later it occurs the better. Fewer victims and witnesses will be distressed as part of the side-effects of the lottery scheme than would suffer as part of the side-effects of not instituting it.

COMMON DECENCY

One form of absolutist argument perhaps remains. This involves taking an Orwellian stand of some principle of common decency. The argument would then be that even to enter into the sort of 'macabre' calculations that Y and Z propose, displays a blunted sensibility, a corrupted and vitiated mind. Forms of this argument have been advanced recently by Noam Chomsky,[6] Stuart Hampshire,[7] Bernard Williams[8] and Jonathan Bennett.[9] The indefatigable Y and Z would, of course, deny that their calculations are in any sense 'macabre', but on the contrary are the most humane course available in the circumstances. Moreover, they would claim that the Orwellian stand on decency is the product of a closed mind and not susceptible to rational argument. Any reasoned defence of such a principle would

---

[6] Noam Chomsky, *American Power and the New Mandarins* (Harmondsworth: Penguin, 1969), 11.
[7] Stuart Hampshire, *Morality and Pessimism* (Cambridge: Cambridge University Press, 1972).
[8] Bernard Williams, 'A Critique of Utilitarianism', in J. J. C. Smart and Bernard Williams, *Utilitarianism: For and Against* (Cambridge: Cambridge University Press, 1973).
[9] Jonathan Bennett, 'The Conscience of Huckleberry Finn', *Philosophy*, 49/188 (Apr. 1974).

have to appeal to notions like respect of human life (as Hampshire's argument in fact does) and these Y and Z could of course make comfortable to their own position.

RIGHTS

A particularly tenacious form of objection to the survival lottery is that we have no *right* so much as to assault A, even if we could thereby save any number of lives. Well, we may well not have such a right, but so much the worse for us. I am concerned not so much with what rights people happen to have, but with what we ought to do. It may be that we ought not to respect rights if the cost of doing so is this high or, perhaps, that we ought to revise our system of rights.

   J. G. Hanink[10] has set out an objection of this form in some detail. Hanink accuses Y and Z of falling for an outrageously sophistical argument, only to fall for it himself. I pointed out that Y and Z can say that they did not intentionally seek A's death, only his heart and lungs, and if A could live without these that would be fine with Y and Z. Hanink's point is that since the organs in question are *vital* organs, the link between their removal and death is conceptual, not contingent, and so in removing them Y and Z must intentionally seek A's death. But then Hanink offers us the following case. Jones, Smith and Robinson are confined to close quarters with one another on a ship. Jones has a highly contagious disease which will kill Smith and Robinson but not Jones himself. If Smith and Robinson expel Jones he will die, but they will escape infection; if they don't, they will die and he won't. Hanink argues, 'Smith and Robinson cannot kill Jones in self defence. *For Jones does not violate any right of theirs intentionally or otherwise.*'[11] But, the absence in Smith and Robinson of Jones's bacteria is a *vital absence*, just as the presence in A of a heart and lungs is a vital presence. Can one really say that one intentionally acts so as to communicate a deadly contagion but does not intend the consequent death?

   Hanink's real difficulty is that he does not see Jones knowingly infecting Smith and Robinson with a deadly disease as something he is *doing* to them.

   If Smith and Robinson cannot throw Jones off the boat in self defence, can they refuse to allow him on board knowing that they will die if they do

[10] J. G. Hanink, 'On the Survival Lottery', *Philosophy*, 51/196 (Apr. 1976), 223–5.
[11] Ibid. 225. And again 'intention' proves far too supple a notion to be of help.

and that he will if they don't? Jones has, after all, no *right* to come aboard.[12] Can thirty people on a lifeboat refuse to let one more aboard if he will sink the boat but now throw someone off for the same reason? Sure, they must choose the one to be ejected fairly, but that is what the survival lottery is for.

These are hard choices and hard cases, but I don't think a normative moral theory which sacrifices the lives of many to preserve the rights of one, can be too confident of a knockdown victory over its rivals.

CHOICE OF VICTIMS

Lastly, a more limited objection to the survival lottery might be made, not to the idea of killing to save lives, but to the involvement of 'third parties'. Why, so the objection goes, should we not give Z's heart to Y or Y's lungs to Z, the same number of lives being thereby preserved and no one else's life set at risk?

Y's and Z's reply to this objection differs from their previous line of argument. To amend their plan so that the involvement of so called 'third parties' is ruled out would, Y and Z claim, violate their right to equal concern and respect with the rest of society. They argue that such a proposal would amount to treating the unfortunate, who need new organs if they are to survive, as a class within society whose lives are considered to be of less value than those of its more fortunate members. What possible justification could there be for singling out one group of people whom we would be justified in using as donors but not another?

The idea in the mind of those who would propose such a step must be something like the following: since Y and Z cannot survive, since they are going to die in any event, there is no harm in putting their names into the lottery, for the chances of their dying cannot thereby be increased and will, in fact, almost certainly be reduced. But this is just to ignore everything that Y and Z have been saying. For if their lottery scheme is adopted they are not going to die in any event, their chances of dying are no greater and no less than any other participant in the lottery whose number may come up.[13] This ground for confining selection of donors to the unfortunate therefore disappears, as does any which discriminates against Y and Z as members of a class whose lives are less worthy of respect than those of the rest of society.

---

[12] In an otherwise sensitive treatment of this sort of problem Onora Nell seems to fall for something like the Hanink line; see 'Lifeboat Earth', *Philosophy & Public Affairs*, 4/3 (Spring 1975), esp. 281.

[13] This is not strictly true of course since there is always some risk in surgical operations but, assuming as we have, that transplant procedures have been perfected, the risk would be small compared with the alternatives and can be disregarded for our present purposes.

It might be argued more plausibly that the dying who cannot themselves be saved by transplants or by any other means at all, should be the priority selection group for the computer programme. But how far off must death be for a man to be classified as 'dying'? Those so classified might argue that their last few days or weeks of life are as valuable to them—if not more valuable—than the possibly longer span remaining to others. The problem of narrowing down the class of possible donors without discriminating unfairly against some sub-class of society is, I suspect, insoluble.

Such is the case for the survival lottery. There seem to be good reasons for utilitarians to be in favour of it, and absolutists cannot object to it on the ground that it involves killing the innocent, for it is Y's and Z's case that any alternative must also involve killing the innocent. If the absolutist wishes to maintain his objection he must point to some morally relevant difference between positive and negative killing. The most likely candidate for something which might make this moral difference is 'intention'. An absolutist might argue that Y and Z intend the death of A whereas no one wishes to kill Y and Z. But Y and Z can reply that the death of A is no part of their plan, they merely wish to use a couple of his organs and if he cannot live without them . . . *tant pis*!

A fit, either of exaltation or of depression (to which those such as Y and Z whose philosophical deliberations are of the life and death variety are prone) has led Y and Z to underestimate some of the difficulties faced by their version of the survival lottery.

A FATAL EXEMPTION RE-VISITED

Conscious of the injustice of allowing people who have brought their illness on themselves to benefit from the lottery at the expense of the prudent who have led 'healthy' lives, Y and Z were prepared to exempt such people from the otherwise universal application of the lottery. The unfairness of killing the abstemious B so that W (whose heavy smoking has given him cancer) and X (whose drinking has destroyed his liver) should be preserved to over-indulge again, weighed heavily with Y and Z. But the exemption they consequently proposed brings grave problems in its wake.

First, the difficulty of deciding whether or how far someone was responsible for their illness is overwhelming. The connection between various items of diet and diseases of various organs has been established and new connections are suggested almost daily. In addition to the sometimes fatal consequences of alcohol and tobacco, sugar, eggs, milk, butter, cheese and meat have all been cited as possible causes of disease. In addition to factors of diet, how heavy we are, how much exercise we take and of what type, where we live, the sorts of job we do—in short, the sorts of lives we lead—may all plausibly be shown to contribute to our state of health. Even if there were cases where we could be confident that a person had in no way contributed to their illness, could we acquire this confidence in time to save them? The meticulous investigation of the life and work of each citizen would, even if theoretically possible, be hopelessly time-consuming.

In the face of this there are two courses we might take. We could try to regulate every aspect of the lives of everyone, so that all unhealthy or risky practices were eliminated. This, even if it were possible and acceptable, would probably be self-defeating, since depression can also be fatal. Alternatively, we might decide that a certain amount of injustice was a price worth paying for the saving of large numbers of lives, and push ahead with the survival lottery despite the impossibility of exempting the careless. This raises a further difficulty over which the exalted or depressed Y and Z have been somewhat cavalier.

WOULD THE SURVIVAL LOTTERY SAVE LIVES?

One feature of the survival lottery as proposed by Y and Z makes its implementation less than attractive. This feature is the tendency of the lottery to lead to a gradual deterioration of the health of any society which operates it. This happens in two ways. The first is caused by the fact that since diseased organs are no use for transplantation, the computer would select only healthy donors, thus discriminating unfairly against the healthy (a point to which we will return) and also, and more crucially, gradually leading to a society in which those with healthy organs, and perhaps healthy living patterns, were weeded out. This would be re-enforced by the second way in which the lottery would operate to undermine the health of society, namely by removing disincentives to imprudent action.[14] For why should I curtail my smoking and drinking because they are unhealthy practices when my diseased organs can and will always be replaced. And since they are likely to be replaced from people who do not have the same bad habits as I do (indeed from people who do not have any bad, i.e. unhealthy habits) the survival lottery will gradually lead to a society depopulated of the prudent and populated by the imprudent. And thus to a society in which eventually it would be difficult to find suitable donors and thus both to a situation in which the

[14] For an interesting discussion of this question, see Peter Singer, 'Utility and the Survival Lottery', *Philosophy*, 52 (1977).

lottery would cease to save many lives and also to one in which the healthy would live under virtual sentence of death.

Perhaps the last nail in the coffin of a society-wide lottery would be our fears as to its misuse. The lottery would be a powerful weapon in the hands of someone prepared and able to misuse it. Could we ever feel certain that the lottery could be made safe from unscrupulous computer programmers?

CHOICE OF VICTIMS AGAIN

Y and Z, it will be remembered, were distressed at the prospect of the lottery being confined to themselves and others like them. When it was asked why Z's heart should not simply be given to Y or Y's lungs to Z thus saving the same number of lives, Y and Z replied that this would discriminate unfairly against the dying. But we can now see that a society-wide lottery would discriminate unfairly against the healthy. If this was merely the price that had to be paid for saving large numbers of lives it would have been a price well worth paying and one indeed that we often do have to pay already. Since wherever we have to choose between rescuing two different groups of people in circumstances in which we cannot rescue both, we choose to rescue the more numerous group. Indeed to believe that one should always save more lives rather than fewer, is always to discriminate against minorities.[15] Thus the principles of saving lives and of fairness are 'lexically' ordered in that we prefer to save lives and try to do so fairly, but where we have to choose between the principles, we choose to save lives.

Thus, if we have to choose between a society-wide lottery and one confined to the dying, where each lottery would save the same numbers of lives but where one was fairer than the other, we would have a reason to choose the fairer. But where both a society-wide lottery and one confined to the dying each involve discrimination in the selection of victims and neither offers a gain in the numbers of lives saved, then we have no reason gratuitously to swap one group of victims for another.

Moreover, because of the deteriorating effect that a society-wide lottery would have on the general health of the community, we have a good reason to confine the lottery to the dying. So Y's and Z's arguments against confining the choice of victims to the dying fail.

---

[15] There has been a vigorous debate on this point; see John M. Taurek, 'Should the Numbers Count?', *Philosophy & Public Affairs*, 6/4 (Summer 1977), and Derek Parfit, 'Innumerate Ethics', *Philosophy & Public Affairs*, 7/4 (Summer 1978).

A Modest Proposal

We are left, then, with a more modest proposal, that in the event of the perfection of transplant procedures a survival lottery be instituted confined to the dying. Whenever two or more patients could be saved by the sacrifice of one then either straws could be drawn, or more fairly, a nation-wide scheme would be introduced to maximise the advantage. This could be a voluntary scheme and ought to prove attractive to the dying. For, in any group of three or more dying people where the sacrifice of one would save the other two and where all would die if the sacrifice was not made, then to fail to sacrifice one for two is to kill two people. So long as the choice of who to sacrifice is made fairly there would seem to be overwhelming reasons in favour of a survival lottery confined to the dying.

So we have to tell Y and Z that their original scheme was sound in principle but self-defeating in practice. But that a more limited version of the survival lottery, one confined to the dying, is both viable and imperative.

I say sound in principle because it is in a sense an unhappy[16] accident that only sound organs can be transplanted and that health is in large part contingent upon lifestyle. If, for example, a wonder drug were to be discovered that would cure any disease but that its only source was minced human brain and moreover that one brain would supply two or more doses, then so long as it did not matter whether or not the brains used were themselves diseased or what age they were, we could re-introduce the society-wide survival lottery. And all the arguments of Y and Z could then be re-introduced in all their pristine cogency.

THE RE-CONDITIONING LOTTERY

Alternatively and for good measure, if a process were to be discovered whereby we could extract human organs and re-condition them, then again the society-wide lottery could be resurrected. I am imagining circumstances which would allow for the extraction and re-conditioning of living human organs however far gone they were, but which do not allow for the survival of the donor. Donors would not have to be healthy, nor would they have to have tissue types compatible with the eventual recipients of their organs. Here all citizens could be in the lottery each time the lottery runs, including those who are about to benefit from the lottery and those who have recently done so. There would be no progressive deterioration in the health of a

---

[16] 'Unhappy' for the argument.

society which introduced it, nor would such a lottery discriminate unfairly against either the healthy or the sick.

Incentives to lead healthy lives and thus avoid a gradual deterioration in the health of society would be built in to this lottery. The imprudent as a class would not prey upon the healthy and all would have a reason to minimise their chance of being selected by the lottery, by minimising the number of times the lottery would have to be called upon to rescue the dying.

The arguments against confining this scheme to the dying would be those originally conceived by Y and Z. For these were only defeated by the discovery that the unconfined original lottery led both to injustice to the healthy and to a gradual sickening of society.

To be sure, it would discriminate unfairly against the victims, those picked as donors by the computer. But if it is bad luck to be a victim it is also bad luck to be dying of disease. What we should try to do is minimise the bad luck where we cannot eradicate it.

The re-conditioning lottery, however, allows for a less impartial alternative, but one more frugal of lives. If the gradual deterioration of the health of a society which operated it is an argument against the original survival lottery, then the gradual amelioration of the health of society should count in favour of a scheme such as that above, but which selects donors only from among the unhealthy *and* also the imprudent. This scheme would have the double advantage of gradually weeding out the unhealthy and replacing them with the fit, but also of re-enforcing healthy patterns of living. People would have the most powerful of incentives to adopt healthy ways of life and thus avoid placing themselves within the priority selection group for the health-promoting lottery. Lives immediately at risk would be saved *and* the general health of the community gradually improved.

But at what cost? First and foremost certainly at a cost to justice. The health-promoting lottery would re-introduce unfair discrimination against the unhealthy and imprudent. Second, and not far behind in importance, at a tremendous cost in terms of freedom. The pervasive inspection and control over the lives of all in the community which would be required for effective implementation of the health-promoting lottery coupled with the consequent disaffection and hostility of all those who would resent such controls, would prove formidable arguments against it.

In the face of such costs the gains might seem less attractive. The extra lives saved by the health-promoting lottery would not, of course, be those of people immediately at risk but rather of those of people who will not fall ill in the future thanks to the general improvement in health. We are inclined to give less weight to lives which will be saved in an uncertain future than to those in real and present danger.

But if we end this chapter preferring the magisterial justice of a completely impartial re-conditioning lottery to the rigours of its more frugal alternative, we should be aware that the cost of our preference is the lives of a number, perhaps a large number of once but future people.[17]

---

[17] Even those who feel they must reject the survival lottery at all costs in any of its versions, should be grateful for what they will see as a counter-example both to utilitarianism and to Rawls's theory of justice. The ways in which the survival lottery should be mandatory for utilitarians have already been considered. Rawlsians would accept it for a number of reasons: because it is rational in the Rawlsian sense; because it is fair; because, at the level of legislation, it improves the position of the least advantaged (the dying). It would, in short, clearly be chosen by people in the initial position.

PART IV

ALLOCATION OF SCARCE RESOURCES AND QUALITY OF LIFE

10

HEALTH-CARE NEEDS AND DISTRIBUTIVE JUSTICE

NORMAN DANIELS

1. WHY A THEORY OF HEALTH-CARE NEEDS?

A theory of health-care needs should serve two central purposes. First, it should illuminate the sense in which we—at least many of us—think health care is 'special,' that it should be treated differently from other social goods. Specifically, even in societies in which people tolerate (and glorify) significant and pervasive inequalities in the distribution of most social goods, many feel there are special reasons of justice for distributing health care more equally. Some societies even have institutions for doing so. To be sure, others argue it is perverse to single out health care in this way, or that if we have reasons for doing so, they are rooted in charity, not justice. But in any case, a theory of health-care needs should show their connection to other central notions in an acceptable theory of justice. It should help us see what kind of social good health-care is by properly relating it to social goods whose importance is similar and for which we may have a clearer grasp of appropriate distributive principles.

Second, such a theory should provide a basis for distinguishing the more from the less important among the many kinds of things health care does for us. It should tell us which health-care services are 'more special' than others. Thus, a broad category of health-services functions to improve quality of life, not to extend or save it. Some of these services restore or compensate for diminished capacities and functions; others improve life quality in other

From Norman Daniels, 'Health-Care Needs and Distributive Justice,' in his *Justice and Justification* (Cambridge: Cambridge University Press, 1996).

Research for this paper was supported by Grant Number HS03097 from the National Center for Health Services Research, OASH, and by a Tufts Sabbatical Leave. I am also indebted to the Commonwealth Fund, which sponsored a seminar on this material at Brown University. Earlier drafts benefited from presentations to the Hastings Center Institute project on Ethics and Health Policy (funded by the Kaiser Foundation), a NCHSR staff seminar, and colloquia at Tufts, NYU Medical Center, University of Michigan, and University of Georgia. Helpful comments were provided by Ronald Bayer, Hugo Bedau, Richard Brandt, Dan Brock, Arthur Caplan, Josh Cohen, Allen Gibbard, Ruth Macklin, Carola Mone, John Rawls, Daniel Wikler, and the Editors of *Philosophy & Public Affairs*.

ways. We do draw distinctions about the urgency and importance of such services. Our theory of health-care needs should provide a basis for a reasonable set of such distinctions. If we can assume some scarcity of health-care resources,[1] and if we cannot (or should not) rely just on market mechanisms to allocate these resources, then we need such a theory to guide macro-allocation decisions about priorities among health-care needs.

In short, a theory of health-care needs must come to grips with two widely held judgments: that there is something especially important about health care, and that some kinds of health care are more important than others. The philosophical task is to assess, explain, and justify or modify these distinctions we make about the importance of different wants, interests, or needs. After considering a preliminary objection to the claim that we need a theory of health-care needs (Section 2), I shall offer an account of basic needs in general (Section 3) and health-care needs in particular (Section 4). These needs are important to maintaining normal species functioning, and in turn, such normal functioning is an important determinant of the range of opportunity open to an individual. This connection to opportunity helps clarify the kind of social good health care is and provides the basis for subsuming health-care institutions under principles of distributive justice (Section 5 and 6).

2. A PRELIMINARY OBJECTION

Before turning to the theory, I would like to address one objection to the project as a whole, for there is reason to think that talk about health-care needs and their priorities both is avoidable and undesirable. The objection, which challenges the assumption that we cannot rely on medical markets even where there is adequate income redistribution, can be put as follows: Suppose we could agree on a theory of distributive justice that gives us a notion of a *fair income share*. Then individuals could protect themselves against the risk of needing health care by voluntary insurance schemes. Each person would be responsible for buying insurance at a level of protection he or she desires. No one (except children and the congenitally handicapped) has a *claim* on social resources to meet health-care needs unless he is prudent enough to buy the relevant insurance (which does not preclude charity). Resource allocation to meet demand, expressed through varying insurance packages, can be accommodated by the medical market, provided appropriate

---

[1] The objection that health-care resources are scarce only because we waste money on frivolous things presupposes distinctions which a theory of needs should illuminate.

competitive conditions obtain. In this way there is protection against expensive but rare needs for health care, for which relatively inexpensive insurance can be bought; so too, common but inexpensive services can either be risk shared through insurance or paid out of pocket without great sacrifice, if preferred. But expensive and potentially common 'needs'—for example, to be provided with artificial hearts or to be cryogenically preserved—would not become a drain on social resources since individuals who want protection against the risks of facing them would have to buy expensive insurance out of their own fair shares. This way of meeting health needs does not create a bottomless pit into which we are forced to drain all available social resources.[2]

Sometimes needs-based theories are criticized because they give us too small a claim on social resources, providing only a floor on deprivation.[3] In contrast, the objection we face here warns against granting precedence to the satisfaction of needs because we then allow too great a claim on social resources. I postpone until Section 6 considering how a need-based theory can avoid this problem. Similarly, I shall not here defend the assumption that medical markets fail to be acceptable allocative mechanisms.[4] Instead, I would like to suggest that the insurance scheme fails to obviate the need for a theory of health-care needs.

The key assumption underlying this scheme is that the prudent citizen will be able to buy a *reasonable* health-care insurance package from his fair share. Such a package can meet the health-care needs it is *reasonable for people to want to be protected against*. However, if some fair shares turn out to be inadequate to pay the premium for such a package, then there is something unacceptable about them. Intuitively, they are not fair to those people. But we can describe such a benefit package, and thus determine minimum constraints on a fair share, only if we already use a notion of basic or reasonable health-care needs, the ones it is rational for a prudent person to insure

[2] I paraphrase Charles Fried, *Right and Wrong* (Cambridge, Mass.: Harvard University Press, 1978), 126 ff. See my comments on Fried's proposal in 'Rights to Health Care: Programmatic Worries,' *Journal of Medicine and Philosophy*, 4/2 (June 1979), 174–91. I ignore here an issue of paternalism which Fried may have wanted to pursue but which is better raised when fair shares are clearly large enough to purchase a reasonable insurance package: Should the premium purchase be compulsory?

[3] Needs-based theories cut two ways. Egalitarians use them to criticize the failure of inegalitarian systems to meet basic human needs. Inegalitarians use them to justify providing only minimally for basic needs while allowing significant inequalities above the floor. Here I resist the temptation to respond to the inegalitarian by expanding the category of needs to consume such inequalities.

[4] Arrow's classic paper traces the anomalies of the medical market to the uncertainties in it. My analysis has a bearing on the further moral issue, whether health care ought to be marketed even in an ideal market. Cf. Kenneth Arrow, 'Uncertainty and the Welfare Economics of Medical Care,' *American Economic Review*, 53 (1963), 941–73.

against. So the 'fair share plus insurance' approach only *appears* to avoid talk about health-care needs. Either it must smuggle such a theory in when it arrives at constraints on fair shares, or else it is open to the objection the shares are not fair.

There is another way in which a theory of health-care needs is implicit in the insurance-scheme market approach: the approach puts health-care needs on a par with other wants and preferences and allows them to compete for resources with no constraints other than market mechanisms operating.[5] But such a stance, far from avoiding the need to develop a theory of needs, already is a view of health-care needs. It sees them as one kind of preference among many, with no special claim on social resources except that which derives from strength of preference. To be sure, where strength of preference is high, needs may be met, but strength may vary in ways that fail to reflect the importance we ought (and usually do) ascribe to health care. Such a market view needs justification, and it is not a justification simply to point to the *existence* of such a market.

3. NEEDS AND PREFERENCES

Not all Preferences are Created Equal

Before turning to health-care needs in particular, it is worth noting that the concept of needs has been in philosophical disrepute, and with some good reason. The concept seems both too weak and too strong to get us very far toward a theory of distributive justice. Too many things become needs, and too few. And finding a middle ground seems to involve many of the issues of distributive justice one might hope to resolve by appeal to a clear notion of needs.

It is easy to see why too many things appear to be needs. Without abuse of language, we refer to the means necessary to reach any of our goals as needs. To reawaken memories of Miller's, the neighborhood delicatessen of my childhood, I need only the smell of sour pickles in a barrel. To paint my son's swing set, I need a clean brush.[6] The problem of the importance of

---

[5] The presence of people with preferences for more-than-reasonable coverage may result in inflationary pressures on the premium for 'reasonable' insurance packages. So interference in the market is likely to be necessary to protect the adequacy of fair shares.

[6] For emphasis, we often refer to things we simply desire or want as things we need. Sometimes we invoke a distinction between noun and verb uses of 'need,' so that not everything we say we need counts as a *need*. Any distinction we might draw between noun and verb uses depends on our purposes and the context and would still have to be explained by the kind of analysis I undertake above.

needs seems to reduce to the problem of the importance or urgency of preferences or wants in general (leaving aside the fact that not all the things we need are expressed as preferences).

But just as not all preferences are on a par—some are more important than others—so too not all the things we say we need are. It is possible to pick out various things we say we need, including needs for health care, which play a special role in a variety of moral contexts. Taking a cue from T. M. Scanlon's discussion in 'Preference and Urgency,' we should distinguish *subjective* and *objective* criteria of well-being.[7] We need *some* such criterion to assess the importance of competing claims on resources in a variety of moral contexts. A *subjective* criterion uses the relevant individual's own assessment of how well-off he is with and without the claimed benefit to determine the importance of his preference or claim. An *objective* criterion invokes a measure of importance independent of the individual's own assessment, for example, independent of the *strength* of his preference.

In contexts of distributive justice and other moral contexts, we do *in fact* appeal to some *objective* criteria of well-being. We refuse to rely solely on subjective ones. If I appeal to my friend's duty of beneficence in requesting $100, I will most likely get a quite different reaction if I tell him I need the money to get a root canal than if I tell him I need the money to go to the Brooklyn neighborhood of my childhood to smell pickles in a barrel. Indeed, it is not likely to matter in his assessment of *obligations* that I strongly *prefer* to go to Brooklyn. Nor is it likely to matter if I insist I feel a great *need* to reawaken memories of my childhood—I am overcome by nostalgia. (He might give me the money for either purpose, but if he gives it so I can smell pickles, we would probably say he is not doing it out of any duty at all, that he feels no obligation.) Similarly, if my appeal was directed to some (even utopian) social welfare agency rather than my friend, it would adopt objective criteria in assessing the importance of the request independent of my own strength of preference.

The issue as Scanlon has drawn it, between subjective and objective standards of well-being, is not just a claim about the *epistemic* status of our criteria of well-being. He is surely right that we do not rely on subjective standards of well-being: we do not just accept an individual's assessment of his well-being as the *relevant* measure of his well-being in important moral contexts. But the issue here is not just that such a measure is *subjective* and we use an *objective* measure. Nor is the issue that we may be skeptical about the feasibility of developing an objective interpersonal measure of satisfaction, and so we use another measure. Suppose we had an intersubjectively

[7] T. M. Scanlon, 'Preference and Urgency,' *Journal of Philosophy*, 77/19 (Nov. 1975), 655–69.

acceptable way of determining individual levels of well-being, where well-being is viewed as the level of satisfaction of the individual's *full range of preferences*. That is, suppose we had some deep social-utility function that enabled us to compare different persons' levels of satisfaction, given the full range of their preferences and the social goods they have available. Such a scale would be the wrong scale to use in a broad range of moral contexts involving justice and the design of social institutions—at least it is not just an improvement on the scale we do in fact use. We would continue to use a far narrower scale of well-being, one that *does not include the full range of kinds of preferences* people have. So the real issue behind Scanlon's insightful discussion is the choice between objective *truncated* or selective scales of well-being and either objective or subjective *full-range* or 'satisfaction' scales of well-being.[8] I shall return shortly to consider why the truncated scale *ought to be* (and not just *is*) the measure used in issues of social justice.

One indication that we appeal to an objective, truncated standard is that I might say the root canal, but not the smell of pickles in a barrel, is something I *really* need (assuming the dentist is right). It is a *need* and not just a desire. The implication is that some of the things we claim to need fall into special categories which give them a weightier moral claim in contexts involving the distribution of resources (depending, of course, on how well-off we already are within those categories of need).[9] Our task is to characterize the relevant categories of needs in a way that *explains* two central properties these special needs have. First, these needs are *objectively ascribable*: we can ascribe them to a person even if he does not realize he has them and even if he denies he has them because his preferences run contrary to the ascribed needs. Second, and of greater interest to us, these needs are *objectively important*: we attach a special weight to claims based on them in a variety of moral contexts, and we do so independently of the weight attached to these and competing claims by the relevant individuals. So our philosophical task is to characterize the class of things we need which has these properties and to do so in such a way that we explain why such importance is attached to them.

---

[8] The difference might not be in the *extent* but in the *content* of the scale. An objective full-range satisfaction scale might be constructed so that some categories of (key) preferences are lexically primary to others; preferences not included on a truncated scale never enter the full-range scale except to break ties among those equally well-off on key preferences. Such a scale may avoid my worries, but it needs a rationale for its ranking. The objection raised here to full-range satisfaction measures applies, I believe, with equal force to happiness or enjoyment measures of the sort Richard Brandt defends in *A Theory of the Good and the Right*. (Oxford: Oxford University Press, 1979), ch. 14.

[9] See Scanlon, 'Preference and Urgency,' 660.

Needs and Species-typical Functioning

One plausible suggestion for distinguishing the relevant needs from all the things we can come to need is David Braybrooke's distinction between 'course-of-life needs' and 'adventitious needs.' *Course-of-life needs* are those needs which people 'have all through their lives or at certain stages of life through which all must pass.' *Adventitious needs* are the things we need because of the particular contingent projects (which may be long-term ones) on which we embark. Human course-of-life needs would include food, shelter, clothing, exercise, rest, companionship, a mate (in one's prime), and so on. Such needs are not themselves deficiencies, for example, when they are anticipated. But a deficiency with respect to them 'endangers the normal functioning of the subject of need *considered as a member of a natural species*.'[10] A related suggestion can be found in McCloskey's discussion of the human and personal needs we appeal to in political argument. He argues that needs 'relate to what it would be detrimental to us to lack, *where the detrimental is explained by reference to our natures as men and specific persons*.'[11]

The suggestion here is that the needs which interest us are those things we need in order to achieve or maintain species-typical normal functioning. Do such needs have the two properties noted earlier? Clearly they are objectively ascribable, assuming we can come up with the appropriate notion of species-typical functioning. (So, incidentally, are adventitious needs, assuming we can determine the relevant goals by reference to which the adventitious needs become determinate.) Are these needs objectively important in the appropriate way? In a broad range of contexts we do treat them as such—a claim I shall not trouble to argue. What is of interest is to see *why* being in such a need category gives them their special importance.

A tempting first answer might be this: whatever our specific chosen goals

---

[10] David Braybrooke, 'Let Needs Diminish that Preferences may Prosper,' in *Studies in Moral Philosophy*, American Philosophical Quarterly Monograph Series, no. 1 (Oxford: Blackwell, 1968), 90 (my emphasis). Personal medical services do not count as course-of-life needs on the criterion that we need them all through our lives or at certain (developmental) stages, but they do count as course-of-life needs in that deficiency with respect to them may endanger normal functioning.

[11] McCloskey, unlike Braybrooke, is committed to distinguishing a narrower noun use of 'need' from the verb use. See J. H. McCloskey, 'Human Needs, Rights, and Political Values,' *American Philosophical Quarterly*, 13/1 (Jan. 1976), 2–3 (my emphasis). McCloskey's proposal is less clear to me than Braybrooke's: presumably our natures include species-typical functioning but something more as well. Moreover, McCloskey is more insistent than Braybrooke in leaving room for *individual natures*, though Braybrooke at least leaves room for something like this when he refers to the needs that we may have by virtue of individual temperament. The hard problem that faces McCloskey is distinguishing between things we need *to develop our individual natures* and things we come to need in the process of what he calls 'self-making,' the carrying out of projects one chooses, perhaps in accordance with one's nature but not just by way of developing it.

or tasks, our ability to achieve them (and consequently our happiness) will
be diminished if we fall short of normal species functioning. So, whatever
our specific goals, we need these course-of-life needs, and therein lies their
objective importance. We need them whatever else we need. For example, it
is sometimes said that whatever our chosen goals or tasks, we need our
health, and so appropriate health care. But this claim is not strictly speaking
true. For many of us, some of our goals, perhaps even those we feel most
important to us, are not necessarily undermined by failing health or disability. Moreover, we can often adjust our goals—and presumably our levels
of satisfaction—to fit better with our dysfunction or disability. Coping in
this way does not necessarily diminish happiness or satisfaction in life.

Still, there is a clue here to a more plausible account: impairments of
normal species functioning reduce the range of opportunity we have within
which to construct life plans and conceptions of the good we have a reasonable expectation of finding satisfying or happiness producing. Moreover, if
persons have a high-order interest in preserving the opportunity to revise
their conceptions of the good through time, then they will have a pressing
interest in maintaining normal species functioning by establishing
institutions—such as health-care systems—which do just that. So the kinds
of needs Braybrooke and McCloskey pick out by reference to normal species functioning are objectively important because they meet this high-order
interest persons have in maintaining a normal range of opportunities. I shall
try to refine this admittedly vague answer, but first I want to characterize
health-care needs more specifically and show that they fit within this more
general framework.

4. HEALTH-CARE NEEDS

Disease and Health

To specify a notion of health-care needs, we need clear notions of health and
disease. I shall begin with a narrow, if not uncontroversial, 'biomedical'
model of disease and health. The basic idea is that health is the absence of
disease, and diseases (I here include deformities and, disabilities that result
from trauma) are *deviations from the natural functional organization of a
typical member of a species.*[12] The task of characterizing this natural

[12] The account here draws on a fine series of articles by Christopher Boorse; see 'On the
Distinction between Disease and Illness,' *Philosophy & Public Affairs*, 5/1 (Fall 1975), 49–68;
'Health as a Theoretical Concept,' *Philosophy of Science*, 44 (1977), 542–73. See also Ruth Mack-
lin, 'Mental Health and Mental Illness: Some Problems of Definition and Concept Formation,'
Philosophy of Science, 39/3 (Sept. 1972), 341–65.

functional organization falls to the biomedical sciences, which must include evolutionary theory since claims about the design of the species and its fitness to meeting biological goals underlie at least some of the relevant functional ascriptions. The task is the same for man and beast with two complications. For humans we require an account of the species-typical functions that permit us to pursue biological goals as social animals. So there must be a way of characterizing the species-typical apparatus under-lying such functions as the acquisition of knowledge; linguistic communica-tion and social cooperation. Moreover, adding mental disease and health into the picture complicates the issue further, most particularly because we have a less well-developed theory of species-typical mental functions and functional organization. The 'biomedical' model clearly presupposes we can, in theory, supply the missing account and that a reasonable part of what we now take to be psychopathology would show up as diseases.[13]

The biomedical model has two controversial features. First, the deviations that play a role in the definition of disease are from species-typical func-tional organization. In contrast, some treat health as an idealized level of fully developed functioning, as in the WHO definition.[14] Others insist that the notion of disease is strictly normative and that diseases are deviations from socially preferred functional norms.[15] Still, the WHO definition seems to conflate notions of health with those of general well-being, satisfaction, or happiness, overmedicalizing the domain of social philosophy. And, his-torical arguments which show that 'deviant' functioning—for example, 'Drapetomania' (the running-away disease of slaves) or masturbation—have been medicalized and viewed as diseases do not establish the strongly nor-mative thesis that deviance from social norms of functioning constitutes disease. So I shall accept the first feature of the model, noting, of course, that the model does not exclude normative judgments *about* diseases, for example, about which are undesirable or which excuse us from normally criticizable behavior and justify our entering a 'sick role.' These judgments circumscribe the normative notion of illness or sickness, not the theoretic-ally more basic notion of disease (which thus admittedly departs from looser ordinary usage).[16]

[13] Boorse, 'What a Theory of Mental Health should Be,' 77.

[14] 'Health is a state of complete physical, mental, and social well-being, and not merely the absence of disease or infirmity.' From the Preamble to the Constitution of the World Health Organization. Adopted by the International Health Conference held in New York, 19 June–22 July 1946, and signed on 22 July 1946. *Off. Rec. Wld. Health Org.* 2, no. 100. See Daniel Callahan, 'The WHO Definition of "Health,"' *Hastings Center Studies*, 1/3 (1973), 77–88.

[15] See H. Tristram Engelhardt Jr., 'The Disease of Masturbation: Values and the Concept of Disease,' *Bulletin of the History of Medicine*, 48/2 (Summer 1974), 234–48.

[16] Boorse's critique of strongly normative views of disease is persuasive independently of some problematic features of his own account.

Second, pure forms of the biomedical model also involve a deeper claim, namely that species-normal functional organization can itself be characterized without invoking normative or value judgments. Here the debate turns on hard issues in the philosophy of biology.[17] Fortunately, these need not detain us since my discussion does not turn on so strong a claim. It is enough for my purposes if the line between disease and the absence of disease is, for the general run of cases, *uncontroversial* and ascertainable through publicly acceptable methods, for example, primarily those of the biomedical sciences. It will not matter if there is some relativization of what counts as a disease category to some features of social roles in a given society, and thus to some normative judgments, provided the core of the notion of species-normal functioning is left intact. The model would still, I presume, count infertility as a disease, even though some or many individuals might prefer to be infertile and seek medical treatment to render themselves so. Similarly, unwanted pregnancy is not a disease. Again, dysfunctional noses are diseases, since noses have normal species functions and anatomy. If the dysfunction or deformity is serious, it might warrant treatment as an illness. But deviation of nasal anatomy from individual or social conceptions of beauty does not constitute disease.[18]

Thus the modified biomedical model still allows me to draw a fairly sharp line between uses of health-care services to prevent and treat diseases and uses to meet other social goals. The importance of such other goals may be different and may rest on other bases, for example, in the induced infertility or unwanted pregnancy cases. My intention is to show which principles of justice are relevant to distributing health-care services where we can take as fixed, primarily by nature, a generally uncontroversial baseline of species-normal functional organization. If important moral considerations enter at yet another level, to determine what counts as health and what disease, then the principles I discuss and these others must be reconciled, a task the

---

[17] For example, we need an account of functional ascriptions in biology (see Boorse, 'Wright on Functions,' *Philosophical Review*, 85/1 (Jan. 1976), 70–86). More specifically, we need to be able to distinguish genetic variations from disease, and we must specify the range of environments taken as 'natural' for the purpose of revealing dysfunction. The latter is critical to the second feature of the biomedical model: for example, what range of social roles and environments is included in the natural range? If we allow too much of the social environment, then racially discriminatory environments might make being of the wrong race a disease; if we disallow all socially created environments, then we seem not to be able to call dyslexia a disease (disability).

[18] Anyone who doubts the appropriateness of treating some physiognomic deformities as serious diseases with strong claims on surgical resources should look at Frances C. MacGreggor's *After Plastic Surgery: Adaptation and Adjustment* (New York: Praeger, 1979). Even where there is no disease or deformity, there is nothing in the analysis I offer that precludes individuals or society from deciding to use health-care technology to make physiognomy conform to some standard of beauty. But such uses of health technology will not be justifiable as the fulfillment of health-care *needs*.

biomedical model makes unnecessary at this stage and which I want to avoid here in any case. Of course, a complete theory, which I do not pursue, would presumably have to establish priorities among principles governing the meeting of health-care needs and principles for using health-care services to meet other social or individual goals, for example the termination of unwanted pregnancy or the upgrading of the beauty of the population.[19]

Though I have deliberately selected a rather narrow model of disease and health, at least by comparison to some fashionable construals, *health-care needs* emerge as a broad and diverse set. Health-care needs will be those things we need in order to maintain, restore, or provide functional equivalents (where possible) to normal species functioning. They can be divided into:

1. adequate nutrition, shelter
2. sanitary, safe, unpolluted living and working conditions
3. exercise, rest, and other features of healthy life-styles
4. preventive, curative, and rehabilitative personal medical services
5. nonmedical personal (and social) support services

Of course, we do not tend to think of all these things as included among health-care needs, partly because we tend to think narrowly about personal medical services when we think about health care. But the list is not constructed to conform to our ordinary notion of health care but to point out a functional relation between quite diverse goods and services and the various institutions responsible for delivering them.

Disease and Opportunity

The *normal opportunity range* for a given society will be the array of 'life plans' reasonable persons in it are likely to construct for themselves. The range is thus relative to key features of the society—its stage of historical development, its level of material wealth and technological development, and even important cultural facts about it. Facts about social organization, including the conception of justice regulating its basic institutions, will of course determine how that total normal range is distributed in the

---

[19] My account has the following bearing on the debate about Medicaid-funded abortions. Nontherapeutic abortions do not count as health-care needs, so *if* Medicaid has as its only function the meeting of the health-care needs of the poor, then we cannot argue for funding the abortions just like any other procedure. Their justifications will be different. But if Medicaid should serve other important goals, like ensuring that poor and well-off women can equally well control their bodies, then there is justification for funding abortions. There is also the worry that not funding them will contribute to other health problems induced by illegal abortions.

population. Nevertheless, that issue of distribution aside, normal species-typical functioning provides us with one clear parameter relevant to defining the normal opportunity range. Consequently, impairment of normal functioning through disease constitutes a fundamental restriction on individual opportunity relative to the normal opportunity range.

There are two important points to note about the normal opportunity range. Obviously some diseases constitute more serious curtailments of opportunity than others relative to a given range. But because normal ranges are society relative, the same disease in two societies may impair opportunity differently and so have its importance assessed differently. Thus the social importance of particular diseases is a notion we plausibly ought to relativize between societies, assuming for the moment that impairment of opportunity is a relevant consideration. Within a society, however, the normal opportunity range abstracts from important individual differences in what might be called *effective opportunity*. From the perspective of an individual with a particular conception of the good (life plan or utility function), one who has developed certain skills and capacities needed to carry out chosen projects, *effective* opportunity range will be a subspace of the normal range. A college teacher whose career and recreational skills rely little on certain kinds of manual dexterity might find his effective opportunity diminished little compared to what a skilled laborer might find if disease impaired that dexterity. By appealing to the normal range I abstract from these differences in effective range, just as I avoid appeals directly to a person's conception of the good when I seek a measure for the social importance (for claims of justice) of health-care needs.[20]

What emerges here is the suggestion that we use impairment of the normal opportunity range as a fairly crude measure of the relative importance of health-care needs at the macro level. In general, it will be more important to prevent, cure, or compensate for those disease conditions which involve a greater curtailment of normal opportunity range. Of course, impairment of normal species functioning has another distinct effect. It can diminish satisfaction or happiness for an individual, as judged by that individual's conception of the good. Such effects are important at the micro level—for example, to individual decision making about health-care utilization. But I am here seeking the appropriate framework within which to apply principles of justice to health care at the macro level. So we shall have to look further at considerations that weigh against appeals to satisfaction at the macro level.

---

[20] One issue here is to avoid 'hijacking' by past preferences which themselves define the effective range. Of course, effective range may be important in microallocation decisions.

5. TOWARD A DISTRIBUTIVE THEORY

Satisfaction and Narrower Measures of Well-Being

So far my discussion has been primarily descriptive, not normative. As Scanlon suggests, we do not in fact use a full-range satisfaction criterion of well-being when we assess the importance or urgency of individual claims on our resources. Rather, we treat as important only a narrow range of kinds of preferences. More specifically, preferences that bear on the fulfillment of certain kinds of needs are important components of this truncated scale of well-being. In a broad range of moral contexts, we give precedence to claims based on such needs, including health-care needs, over claims based on other kinds of preferences. The Braybrooke and McCloskey suggestion gives us a general characterization of this class of needs: deficiency with regard to them threatens normal species functioning. More specifically, we can characterize health-care needs as things we need to maintain, restore, or compensate for the loss of normal species functioning. Since serious impairments of normal functioning diminish our capacities and abilities, they impair individual opportunity range relative to the range normal for our society. If we suppose people have an interest in maintaining a fair and roughly equal opportunity range, we can give at least a plausible *explanation* why they think health-care needs are special and important (which is not to say we actually do distribute them accordingly).

In what follows, I shall urge a normative claim: we ought to subsume health care under a principle of justice guaranteeing fair equality of opportunity. Actually, since I cannot here defend such a general principle without going too deeply into the general theory of distributive justice, I shall urge a weaker claim: *if* an acceptable theory of justice includes a principle providing for fair equality of opportunity, then health-care institutions should be among those governed by it. Indeed, I shall sketch briefly how one general theory, Rawls' theory of justice as fairness, might be extended in this way to provide a distributive theory for health care. *But my account does not presuppose the acceptability of Rawls' theory.* If a rule or ideal code utilitarianism, or some other theory, establishes a fair equality of opportunity principle, my account will probably be compatible with it (though some of the argument that follows may not be).

In order to introduce some issues relevant to extending Rawls' theory, I want to consider an issue we have thus far left hanging. *Should* we, for purposes of justice, use the objective, truncated scale of well-being we happen to use rather than a full-range satisfaction scale? Clearly, this too is a general question that takes us beyond the scope of this essay. Moreover, it is unlikely that we could establish conclusively a case against the satisfaction scale by considering the health care context alone. For example, a utilitarian proponent of a satisfaction or enjoyment scale might claim that the general tendencies of different diseases to diminish satisfaction provides, at worst, a rough equivalent to the 'impairment of opportunity' criterion I am proposing.[21] Still, it is worth suggesting some of the considerations that weight against the use of a satisfaction scale.

We can begin by pointing to a special case where our moral judgment would incline us against using a satisfaction scale, namely the case of 'social hijacking' by persons with expensive tastes.[22] Suppose we judge how well-off someone is by reference to the full range of individual preferences in a satisfaction scale. Suppose further that moderate people adjust their tastes and preferences so that they have a reasonable chance of being satisfied with their share of social goods. Other more extravagant people form exotic and expensive tastes, even though they have comparable shares to the moderates, and, because their preferences are very strong, they are desperately unhappy when these tastes are not satisfied. Assume we can agree intersubjectively that the extravagant are less satisfied. Then if we are interested in maximizing—or even equalizing—satisfaction, extravagants seem to have a greater claim on further distributions of social resources than moderates. But something seems clearly unjust if we deny the moderates equal claims on further distributions just because they have been modest in forming their tastes. With regard to tastes and preferences that *could have been otherwise* had the extravagants chosen differently, it seems reasonable to hold them *responsible* for their own low level of satisfaction.[23]

A more general division of responsibility is suggested by this hijacking case. Rawls urges that we hold *society* responsible for guaranteeing the individual a fair share of basic liberties, opportunity, and all purpose means, like income and wealth, needed for pursuing individual conceptions of the good. But the *individual* is responsible for choosing his ends in such a way that he has a reasonable chance of satisfying them under such just arrangements.[24]

---

[21] Presumably, he must also claim that we improve satisfaction more by treating and preventing disease than by finding ways to encourage people to adjust to their conditions by reordering their preference curves.

[22] I draw on Rawls' unpublished lecture, 'Responsibility for Ends,' in the following three paragraphs.

[23] Here again the utilitarian proponent of the satisfaction scale may issue a typical promissory note, assuring us that maximizing satisfaction overall requires institutional arrangements that act to minimize social hijacking.

[24] The division presupposes, as Rawls points out in response to Scanlon, that people have the ability and know they have the responsibility to adjust their desires in view of their fair shares of (primary) social goods. See Scanlon, 'Preference and Urgency,', 665–6.

Consequently, the special features of an individual's conception of the good—here his extravagant tastes and resulting dissatisfaction—do not give rise to any special claims of justice on social resources. This suggestion about a division of responsibility is really a claim about the *scope* of theories of justice: just arrangements are supposed to guarantee individuals a reasonable share of certain basic social goods which constitute the relevant—truncated—scale of well-being for purposes of justice. The immediate object of justice is not, then, happiness or the satisfaction of desires, though just institutions provide individuals with an acceptable framework within which they can seek happiness and pursue their interests. But individuals remain responsible for the choice of their ends, so there is no injustice in not having sufficient means to reach extravagant ends.

Obviously, a full defense of this claim about the scope of justice and the social division of responsibility, and thus about the reasons for using a truncated scale of well-being, cannot rest on isolated intuitions about cases like the hijacking one. In Rawls' case, a full argument involves the claim that adopting a satisfaction scale commits us to an unacceptable view of persons as mere 'containers' for satisfaction, one that departs significantly from our moral practice.[25] Because I cannot pursue these issues here, beyond suggesting there are problems with a satisfaction scale, I am content to show there is a systematic, plausible alternative to using a satisfaction scale (and ultimately to utilitarianism) whose acceptability depends on more general issues. Consequently I stick with my weaker, conditional claim above.

Rawls' argument for a truncated scale is, of course, for a specific scale, one composed of his primary social goods. But my talk about a truncated scale has focused on talk about certain basic needs, in particular, things we need to maintain species-typical normal functioning. Health-care needs are paradigmatic among these. The task that remains is to fit the two scales together. My analysis of the relation between disease and normal opportunity range provides the key to doing that.

---

[25] Satisfaction scales leave us no basis for not wanting to *be* whatever person, construed as a set of preferences, has higher satisfaction. To borrow Bernard Williams' term, they leave us with no basis for insisting on the *integrity* of persons. See Rawls, 'Responsibility for Ends.' The view that issues here turn in a fundamental way on the nature of persons is pursued in Derek Parfit, 'Later Selves and Moral Principles,' in Alan Montefiore (ed.), *Philosophy and Personal Relations* (London: Routledge & Kegan Paul, 1973); Rawls, 'Independence of Moral Theory,' *Proceedings and Addresses of the American Philosophical Association* 48 (1974–5), 5–22; and Daniels, 'Moral Theory and the Plasticity of Persons,' *Monist*, 62/3 (July 1979), 265–87.

Extending Rawls' Theory to Health Care

Rawls' *index of primary social goods*—his truncated scale of well-being used in the contract—includes five types of social goods: (a) a set of basic liberties; (b) freedom of movement and choice of occupations against a background of diverse opportunities; (c) powers and prerogatives of office; (d) income and wealth; (e) the social bases of self-respect. Actually, Rawls uses two simplifying assumptions when using the index to assess how well-off (representative) individuals are. First, income and wealth are used as approximations to the whole index. Thus the two principles of justice[26] require basic structures to maximize the long-term expectations of the least advantaged, estimated by their income and wealth, given fixed background institutions that guarantee equal basic liberties and fair equality of opportunity. More importantly for our purposes, the theory is *idealized* to apply to individuals who are 'normal, active and fully cooperating members of society over the course of a complete life.'[27] There is no distributive theory for health care because no one is sick.

This simplification seems to put Rawls' index at odds with the thrust of my earlier discussion, for the truncated scale of well-being we in fact use includes needs for health care. The primary goods seem to be *too truncated* a scale, once we drop the idealizing assumption. People with equal indices will not be equally well-off once we allow them to differ in health-care needs. Moreover, we cannot simply dismiss these needs as irrelevant to questions of justice, as we did certain tastes and preferences. But if we simply build another entry into the index, we raise special issues about how to arrive at an approximate weighting of the index items.[28] Similarly, if we treat health-care services as a specially important primary social good, we abandon the useful generality of the notion of a primary social good. Moreover, we risk generating a long list of such goods, one to meet each important need.[29] Finally, as I argued earlier in answer to Fried's proposal about insurance schemes, we cannot just finesse the question whether there are special issues of justice in the distribution of health care by assuming fair shares of primary goods will be used in part to buy decent health-care insurance. A constraint on the adequacy of those shares is that they permit one to buy reasonable

---

[26] See *A Theory of Justice* (Cambridge, Mass.: Harvard University Press, 1971), 302.

[27] Rawls, 'Responsibility for Ends.'

[28] Some weighting problems will have to be faced anyway; see my 'Rights to Health Care' for further discussion. Also see Kenneth Arrow, 'Some Ordinalist Utilitarian Notes on Rawls's Theory of Justice,' *Journal of Philosophy* 70/9 (1973), 245–63. Also see Joshua Cohen, 'Studies in Political Philosophy,' Ph.D. diss., Harvard University, 1978, pt. III and apps.

[29] See Ronald Greene, 'Health Care and Justice in Contract Theory Perspective,' in Robert Veatch and Roy Branson (eds.), *Ethics and Health Policy* (Cambridge, Mass.: Ballinger, 1976).

protection—so we must already know what justice requires by way of reasonable health care.

The most promising strategy for extending Rawls' theory without tampering with useful assumptions about the index of primary goods simply includes health-care institutions among the background institutions involved in providing for fair equality of opportunity.[30] Once we note the special connection of normal species functioning to the opportunity range open to an individual, this strategy seems the natural way to extend Rawls' view that *the subject* of theories of social justice are the *basic institutions* which provide a framework of liberties and opportunities within which individuals can use fair income shares to pursue their own conceptions of the good. Insofar as meeting health-care needs has an important effect on the distribution of health, and more to the point, on the distribution of opportunity, the health-care institutions are plausibly included on the list of basic institutions a fair equality of opportunity principle should regulate.[31]

Including health-care institutions among those which are to protect fair equality of opportunity is compatible with the central intuitions behind wanting to guarantee such opportunity in the first place. Rawls is primarily concerned with *the opportunity to pursue careers*—jobs and offices—that have various benefits attached to them. So equality of opportunity is *strategically* important: a person's well-being will be measured for the most part by the primary goods that accompany placement in such jobs and offices.[32] Rawls argues it is not enough simply to eliminate formal or legal barriers to persons seeking such jobs—for example, race, class, ethnic, or sex barriers. Rather, positive steps should be taken to enhance the opportunity of those disadvantaged by such social factors as family background.[33] The point is that none of us *deserves* the advantages conferred by accidents of birth—

[30] The primary social goods themselves remain general and abstract properties of social arrangements—basic liberties, opportunities, and certain all-purpose exchangeable means (income and wealth). We can still simplify matters in using the index by looking solely at income and wealth—assuming a background of equal basic liberties and fair equality of opportunity. Health care is not a primary social good—neither are food, clothing, shelter, or other basic needs. The presumption is that the latter will be adequately provided for from fair shares of income and wealth. The special importance and unequal distribution of health-care needs, like educational needs, are acknowledged by their connection to other institutions that provide for fair equality of opportunity. But opportunity, not health care or education, is the primary social good.

[31] Here I shift emphasis from Rawls when he remarks that health is a *natural* as opposed to *social* primary good because its possession is less influenced by basic institutions. See *A Theory of Justice*, 62. Moreover, it seems to follow that where health care is generally inefficacious—say, in earlier centuries—it loses its status as a special concern of justice and the 'caring' it offers may more properly be viewed as a concern of charity.

[32] The ways in which disease affects normal opportunity range are more extensive than the ways in which it affects opportunity to pursue careers, a point I return to later.

[33] Of course, the effects of family background cannot all be eliminated. See *A Theory of Justice*, 74.

either the genetic or social advantages. These advantages from the 'natural lottery' are morally arbitrary, and to let them determine individual opportunity—and reward and success in life—is to confer arbitrariness on the outcomes. So positive steps, for example, through the educational system, are to be taken to provide fair equality of opportunity.[34]

But if it is important to use resources to counter the advantages in opportunity some get in the natural lottery, it is equally important to use resources to counter the natural disadvantages induced by disease (and since class-differentiated social conditions contribute significantly to the etiology of disease, we are reminded disease is not just a product of the natural component of the lottery). But this does not mean we are committed to the futile goal of eliminating all natural differences between persons. Health care has as its goal normal functioning and so concentrates on a specific class of obvious disadvantages and tries to eliminate them. That is its *limited* contribution to guaranteeing fair equality of opportunity.

The approach taken here allows us to draw some interesting parallels between education and health care, for both are strategically important con-tributors to fair equality of opportunity. Both address needs which are not equally distributed between individuals. Various social factors, such as race, class, and family background, may produce special learning needs; so too may natural factors, such as the broad class of learning disabilities. To the extent that education is aimed at providing fair equality of opportunity, special provision must be made to meet these special needs. Here educational needs, like health-care needs, differ from other basic needs, such as the need for food and clothing, which are more equally distributed between persons. The combination of unequal distribution and the great strategic importance of the opportunity to have health care and education puts these needs in a separate category from those basic needs we can expect people to purchase from their fair income shares.

It is worth noting another point of fit between my analysis and Rawls' theory. In Rawls' contract situation, a 'thick' veil of ignorance is imposed on contractors choosing basic principles of justice: they do not know their abilities, talents, place in society, or historical period. In selecting principles to govern health-care resource-allocation decisions, we need a thinner veil, for we must know about some features of the society, for example, its resource limitations. Still, using the normal opportunity range and not just

[34] Rawls allows individual differences in talents and abilities to remain relevant to issues of job placement, for example, through their effects on productivity. So fair equality of opportunity does not mean that individual differences no longer confer advantages. Advantages are constrained by the difference principle. See my 'Merit and Meritocracy,' *Philosophy & Public Affairs*, 7/3 (Spring 1978), 206–23.

the effective range as the baseline has the effect of imposing a plausibly thinned veil. It reflects basic facts about the society but keeps facts about individuals' particular ends from unduly influencing social decisions. Ultimately, defense of a veil depends on the theory of the person underlying the account. The intuition here is that persons are not defined by a particular set of interests but are free to revise their life plans. Consequently, they have an interest in maintaining conditions under which they can revise such plans, which makes the normal range a plausible reference point.

Subsuming health-care institutions under the opportunity principle can be viewed as a way of keeping the system as close as possible to the original idealization under which Rawls' theory was constructed, namely, that we are concerned with normal, fully functioning persons with a complete life-span. An important set of institutions can thus be viewed as a first defense of the idealization: they act to minimize the likelihood of departures from the normality assumption. Included here are institutions which provide for public health, environmental cleanliness, preventive personal medical services, occupational health and safety, food and drug protection, nutritional education, and educational and incentive measures to promote individual responsibility for healthy life-styles. A second layer of institutions corrects departures from the idealization. It includes those which deliver personal medical and rehabilitative services that restore normal functioning. A third layer attempts, where feasible, to maintain persons in a way that is as close as possible to the idealization. Institutions involved with more extended medical and social support services for the (moderately) chronically ill and disabled and the frail elderly would fit here. Finally, a fourth layer involves health care and related social services for those who can in no way be brought closer to the idealization. Terminal care and care for the seriously mentally and physically disabled fit here, but they raise serious issues which may not just be issues of justice. Indeed, by the time we get to the fourth layer moral virtues other than justice become prominent.

6. WORRIES AND QUALIFICATIONS

I would like to address two kinds of worries that arise in response to the approach to equality of opportunity that I have been sketching, though no doubt there are others.[35] One is that the account cannot be *exhaustive* of

---

[35] For example, appeals to equality of opportunity have historically played a conservative, deceptive role, blinding people to the injustice of class and race inequalities in rewards. Historically, appeals to the ideal of equal opportunity have implicitly justified strong competitive individual relations. More concretely, we often find institutions, like the United States educational

distributive issues in health care—the connection to opportunity is but one consideration among many. A second worry is that the appeal to opportunity is not a *useable* one—it commits us to too much or fails to tell us what we are committed to. Both worries emphasize the degree to which my account is programmatic.

One way to put the first worry is that my account makes the 'specialness' of health care rest on quite abstract considerations. After all, when we reflect on the importance of health-care needs, many other factors than their effects on opportunity come to mind. Some might say health care in a direct and simple way reduces pain and suffering—and no fancy analysis of opportunity is needed to show why people value reducing them. Still, much health care affects quality of life in other ways, so the benefit of reducing pain and suffering is not general enough for our purposes. Moreover, some suffering, for example, some emotional suffering, though a cause for concern, does not obviously become a concern of justice. Others may point to psychological or cultural bases for our viewing health care as special, for example, disease reminds us of the fragility of life and the limits of human existence. But even if this point is relevant to sociological or psychological explanations of the importance some of us attribute to some kinds of health care, I have been attempting a different kind of analysis, one that can be used to justify and not just explain the importance attached to health care. So I have abstracted a central *function* of health care, the maintenance of species-typical function, and noted its central *effect* on opportunity. As a result, we are in a better position to frame distributive principles that account for the special way we treat health care because we can now say what kind of a social good health care is, namely one that maintains normal opportunity range. My analysis, while not exhaustive, focuses on that general benefit which is most relevant from the point of view of distributive justice.

Still, this qualification does not settle the first worry, which can be raised in another way. Within the confines of Rawls' theory, fair equality of opportunity—and Rawls' principle guaranteeing it—is concerned solely with access to jobs and offices. In contrast, my notion of normal opportunity range is far broader. To be sure, the narrower notion, whatever its problems, is far clearer than the broader one. But if we stick with the narrower one, we immediately import a strong age bias into our distributive theory. The opportunity of the elderly to enter jobs or offices is not impaired by

system, praised as embodying (at least approximately) that ideal, whereas there is strong evidence the system functions primarily to replicate class inequalities. See my 'IQ, Heritability and Human nature' in R. S. Cohen (ed.), *Proceedings of the Philosophy of Science Association*, 1974 (Dordrecht: Reidel, 1976); and, with J. Cronin, A. Krock, and R. Webber, 'Race, Class and Intelligence: A Critical Look at the IQ Controversy,' *International Journal of Mental Health*, 3/4 (1976), 46–123; and S. Bowles and H. Gintis, *Schooling in Capitalist America* (New York: Basic Books, 1976).

disease since they are beyond, as the crass phrase goes, their 'productive' years. Thus fair equality of opportunity narrowly construed seems open to one of the standard objections raised against 'productivity' measures of the value of life.[36]

There are two ways to respond to this problem while still adhering to the narrower construal of opportunity. One is to admit that equality of opportunity is only one among several considerations that bear on the justice of health-care distribution. Still, even on this view, it is an important consideration with broad implications for health-care delivery. Fleshing out this response would require showing how the opportunity principle fits with these other considerations. A stronger response is to claim that the domain of basic considerations of *justice* regarding health care is exhausted by the equal opportunity principle. Other moral considerations may bear on distribution, but claims of justice will be based on the narrowly construed opportunity principle. This response bites the bullet about the age effect.

If we turn to the broader construal of equality of opportunity, using the notion of normal opportunity range, the problem reemerges, as do the weaker and stronger responses, but there may be more flexibility. The problem reemerges because it might seem that the young will always suffer greater impairment of opportunity than the elderly if health-care needs are not met. But a further alternative suggests itself: it may be possible to make the normal opportunity range relative to age. On this view, for each age (stage of life) there is a normal opportunity range, but it reflects basic facts about the life cycle and a society's responses to it. Consequently, diseases may have different effects on the young and elderly and their importance will be assessed differently.[37] This approach may avoid the most serious objections about age bias. It still leaves open the weak claim that the opportunity principle is only one consideration among many or the stronger claim that it circumscribes the scope of basic claims of justice. The stronger claim may seem more plausible since the opportunity principle has broader scope on this construal. But employing the broader construal brings with it other serious problems: do arguments which establish the priority of fair equality of opportunity on the narrow construal with its competitive aspect extend to

---

[36] See E. J. Mishan, 'Evaluation of Life and Limb: A Theoretical Approach,' *Journal of Political Economy*, 79/4 (1971), 687–705; Jan Paul Acton, 'Measuring the Monetary Value of Life Saving Programs,' *Law and Contemporary Problems*, 40/4 (Autumn 1976), 46–72; Michael Bayles, 'The Price of Life,' *Ethics*, 89/1 (Oct. 1978), 20–34.

[37] It would be interesting to know if this age-relativized opportunity range yields results similar to that achieved by the Rawlsian device of a veil. If people who do not know their age are asked to design a system of health-care delivery for the society they will be in, they would presumably budget their resources in a fashion that takes the special features of each stage of the life cycle into account and gives each stage a reasonable claim on resources.

the broader notion? These issues and alternatives require more careful discussion than they can be given here.

The second worry, about what commitments the appeal to equal opportunity generates, also has several sources. Certain 'hard' cases raise the issue sharply. What does asking for the restoration of normal opportunity range mean for the terminally ill, on whom we lavish exotic life-prolonging technology, or for the severely mentally retarded? We are not required to pour all our resources into the worst cases, for that would undermine our ability to protect the opportunity of many others. But I am not sure what the approach requires here, if it delivers an answer at all. Similarly, the approach provides little help with another sort of hard case, the resource-allocation decisions in which we must choose between services which remove serious impairments of opportunity for a few people and those which remove significant but less serious impairments from many. But these shortcomings are not special to the approach I sketch: distributive theories generally founder on such cases. It seems reasonable to test my approach first in the cases where we have a better understanding of what kind of health care is owed. In any case, I do not rule out here the strong response sketched earlier to the worry about exhaustiveness, namely that our problem with at least the first kind of hard case derives from the fact that it takes us beyond the domain of justice into other considerations of right.

The second worry also has more fundamental sources. Suppose supplying a car to everyone who cannot afford one would do more to remove individual impairments of normal opportunity range than supplying certain health-care services to those who need them. does the opportunity approach commit us now to supply cars instead of treatments?[38] The example is an instance of a far more general problem, namely, that socioeconomic (and other) inequalities affect opportunity (broadly or narrowly construed), not just the health-care and educational needs we have picked out as strategically important. But my approach does not require me to deny that certain inequalities in wealth and income may conflict with fair equality of opportunity and that guaranteeing fair equality of opportunity may thus constrain acceptable inequalities in these goods. Rather, my approach rests on the calculation that certain institutions meet needs which quite generally have a central impact on opportunity range and which should therefore be governed directly by the opportunity principle.

Finally, the second worry can be traced to the fear that health-care needs

---

[38] Using medical technology to enhance normal capacities or functions—say strength or vision—makes the problem easier: the burden of proof is on proposals that give priority to altering the normal opportunity range rather than protecting individuals whose normal range is compromised.

are so *expansive* (and expensive), given the advance of technology, that they create a bottomless pit. Fried, for example, argues that recognizing individual right claims to the satisfaction of health-care needs would force society to forgo realizing other social goals. He cautions we would end up worshipping the opportunity to pursue our goals but having to forgo the pursuit. Here we have the other form of the social hijacking argument, hijacking by needs rather than preferences.[39]

Two points can be offered in response to Fried's version of the second worry. First, the narrow model I have given of health-care needs excludes some of the kinds of cases Fried uses to demonstrate the threat of the bottomless pit. Thus Fried's example of retarding the effects of normal aging does not emerge as a *need* on my analysis, since normal aging does not involve a departure from normal species functioning. Such uses of health-care technology may be thought important in a particular society. Then, arguments about the relative merits of this use of scarce resources may be advanced. But such arguments would not rest on claims about basic health-care needs and thus may have different justificatory force. Still, technology does expand the ways (and costs) we have of meeting genuine health-care needs. So my account of needs at best reduces but does not eliminate Fried's worry.

Second, there is a difference between Fried's account of individual rights and entitlements and the one I am assuming here (which is quite Rawlsian). Fried is worried that if we posit a fundamental individual right to have needs satisfied, no other social goals will be able to override the right claims to all health care needs.[40] But no such fundamental right is *directly* posited on the view I have sketched. Rather, the particular rights and entitlements of individuals to have certain needs met are specified only *indirectly*, as a result of the basic health-care institutions acting in accord with the general principle governing opportunity. Deciding which needs are to be met and what resources are to be devoted to doing so requires careful moral judgment. The various institutions which affect opportunity must be weighed against each other. Similarly, the resources required to provide for fair equality of opportunity must be weighed against what is needed to provide for other important social institutions. Clearly, health-care institutions capable of protecting opportunity can be maintained only in societies whose productive capacities they do not undermine. The bugaboo of the bottomless pit is less threatening in the context of such a theory. The price paid is that we are less

---

[39] See Fried, *Right and Wrong*, ch. 5. The problem also worries Braybrooke, 'Let Needs Diminish.'

[40] It is not clear to me how much Fried's side-constraints resemble Nozick's.

clear—in general and abstracting from the application of the theory to a given society—just what the individual claim comes to. The price is worth paying.

These worries emphasize the sense in which my account is sketchy and programmatic. It is worth a reminder that my account is incomplete in other ways. I have not argued that opportunity-based considerations are the only ones that should bear on the design of health-care systems. Other important social goals—some protected by right claims or other claims of need—may require the use of health-care technology. I have not considered when, if ever, these needs or rights take precedence over other wants and preferences or over some health-care needs.[41] Similarly, there is the question whether the demand for equality in health care extends beyond some decent adequate minimum—which we may suppose is defined by reference to fair equality of opportunity. Should those health-care services not considered basic be allowed to operate on a market basis? Should we insist on equality even here? These issues are not addressed by my analysis.[42]

Finally, my account is incomplete because I have concentrated on social obligations to maintain and restore health and have ignored individual responsibility to do so. But there is substantial evidence that individuals can do much to avoid incurring risks to their health—by avoiding smoking, excess alcohol, and certain foods, and by getting adequate exercise and rest. Now, nothing in my approach is incompatible with encouraging people to adopt healthy life-styles. The harder issue, however, is deciding how to distribute the burdens that result when people 'voluntarily' incur extra risks and swell the costs of health care by doing so (by over 10 percent, on some estimates). After all, the consequences of such behavior cannot be easily dismissed as the arbitrary outcome of the natural lottery. Should smokers be forced to pay higher insurance premiums of special health-care taxes? I do not believe my account forces us to ignore the source of health-care risks in assigning such burdens. But at this point little more can be said because much here depends on very specific details of social history. In the United States, government subsidies of the tobacco industry, the legality of cigarette advertising, the legality of smoking in public places, and special subculture pressures on key groups (for example, teenagers) all undermine the view that we have clear-cut cases of informed, individual decision making for which individuals must be held fully accountable.

[41] See n. 19 above.

[42] Except where conditions of extensive scarcity leave basic health-care needs unmet and so no room for less important uses of health-care services, or except where the existence of a market-based health-care system threatens the ability of the basic system to deliver its important product.

7. APPLICATIONS

The account of health-care needs sketched here has a number of implications of interest to health planners. Here I can only note some of them and set aside the many difficulties that face drawing implications from ideal theory for nonideal settings.[43]

Access

My account is compatible with (but does not imply) a multitiered health-care system. The basic tier would include health-care services that meet important health-care needs, defined by reference to their effects on opportunity. Other tiers would include services that meet less important health-care needs or other preferences. However the upper tiers are to be financed—through cost sharing, at full price, at 'zero' price[44]—there should be no obstacles, financial, racial, sexual, or geographical to *initial access* to the system as a whole.

The equality of initial access derives from basic facts about the sociology and epistemology of the determination of health-care needs.[45] The 'felt needs' of patients are (unreliable) initial indicators of real health-care needs. Financial and geographical barriers to initial access—say to primary care—compel people to make their own determinations of the importance of their symptoms. Of course, every system requires some patient self-assessment, but financial and geographical barriers impose different burdens in such assessment on particular groups. Indeed, where sociological barriers exist to people utilizing services, positive steps are needed (in the schools, at work, in neighborhoods) to make sure unmet needs are detected.

It is sometimes argued that the difficult access problems are ones deriving from geographical barriers and the maldistribution of physicians within specialities. In the United States, it is often argued that achieving more equitable distribution of health-care providers would unduly constrain physician liberties. It is important to see that no fundamental liberties need be violated.

---

[43] I discuss these difficulties in 'Conflicting Objectives and the Priorities Problem,' in Peter Brown, Conrad Johnson, and Paul Vernier (eds.), *Income Support: Conceptual and Policy Issues* (Totowa, NJ: Rowman & Littlefield, 1981). *My Just Health Care* (Cambridge: Cambridge University Press, 1985) develops some applications in detail.

[44] The strongest objections to such mixed systems is that the upper tier competes for resources with the lower tiers. See Claudine McCreadie, 'Rawlsian Justice and the Financing of the National Health Service,' *Journal of Social Policy*, 5/2 (1976), 113–31.

[45] See Avedis Donabedian, *Aspects of Medical Care Administration* (Cambridge, Mass.: Harvard University Press, 1973).

Suppose that the basic tier of a health-care system is redistributively financed through a national health insurance scheme that eliminates financial barriers, that no alternative insurance for the basic tier is allowed, and that there is central planning of resource allocation to guarantee needs are met. To achieve a more equitable distribution of physicians, planners *license those eligible for reimbursement* in a given health-planning region according to some reasonable formula involving physician-patient ratios.[46] Additional providers might practice in an area, but they would be without benefit of third-party payments for all services in the basic tier (or for other tiers if the national insurance scheme is more comprehensive). Most providers would follow the reimbursement dollar and practice where they are most needed.

Far from violating basic liberties, the scheme merely puts physicians in the same relation to market constraints on job availability that face most other workers and professionals. A college professor cannot simply decide there are people to be taught in Scarsdale or Chevy Chase or Shaker Heights; he must accept what jobs are available within universities, wherever they are. Of course, he is 'free' to ignore the market, but then he may not be able to teach. Similarly, managers and many types of workers face the need to locate themselves where there is need for their skills. So the physician's sacrifice of liberty under the scheme (or variants on it, including a National Health Service) is merely the imposition of a burden already faced by much of the working population. Indeed, the scheme does not change in principle the forces that already motivate physicians; it merely shifts where it is profitable for some physicians to practice. The appearance that there is an enshrined liberty under attack is the legacy of an historical accident, one more visible in the United States than elsewhere, namely, that physicians have been more independent of institutional settings for the delivery of their skills than many other workers, and even than physicians in other countries. But this too shall pass.

Resource Allocation

My account of health-care needs and their connection to fair equality of opportunity has a number of implications for resource-allocation issues. I have already noted that we get an important distinction between the use of health-care services to meet health-care needs and their use to meet other

---

[46] I ignore the crudeness of such measures. For fuller discussion of these manpower distribution issues see my 'What is the Obligation of the Medical Profession in the Distribution of Health Care?', *Social Science and Medicine*, 15F (1981), 129–35.

wants and preferences. The tie of health-care needs to opportunity makes the former use special and important in a way not true of the latter. Moreover, we get a crude criterion—impact on normal opportunity range—for distinguishing the importance of different health-care needs, though I have also noted how far short this falls of being a solution to many hard allocation questions. Three further implications are worth noting here.

There has been much debate about whether the United States' health-care system overemphasizes acute therapeutic services as opposed to preventive and public health measures. Sometimes the argument focuses on the relative-efficacy and cost of preventive, as opposed to acute, services. My account suggests there is also an important issue of distributive justice here. Suppose a system is heavily weighted toward acute interventions, yet it provides equal access to its services. Thus anyone with severe respiratory ailments—black lung, brown lung, asbestosis, emphysema, and so on—is given adequate and comprehensive services as needed. Does the system meet the demands of equity? Not if they are determined by the approach of fair equality of opportunity. The point is that people are differentially at risk of contracting such diseases because of work and living conditions. Efficacy aside, preventive measures have distinct distributive implications from acute measures. The opportunity approach requires we attend to both.

My account points to another allocational inequity. One important function of health-care services, here personal medical services, is to restore handicapping dysfunctions, for example, of vision, mobility, and so on. The medical goal is to cure the diseased organ or limb where possible. Where cure is impossible, we try to make function as normal as possible, through corrective lenses or prosthesis and rehabilitative therapy. But where restoration of function is beyond the ability of medicine per se, we begin to enter another area of services, nonmedical social support (we move from (4) to (5) on the list of health-care needs in Section 4). Such support services provide the blind person with the closest he can get to the functional equivalent of vision—for example, he is taught how to navigate, provided with a seeing-eye dog, taught braille, and so on. From the point of view of their impact on opportunity, medical services and social support services that meet health-care needs have the same rationale and are equally important. Yet, for various reasons, probably having to do with the profitability and glamor of personal medical service and careers in them as compared to services for the handicapped, our society has taken only slow and halting steps to meet the health-care needs of those with permanent disabilities. These are matters of justice, not charity; we are not facing conditions of scarcity so severe that these steps to provide equality of opportunity must be forgone in favor of more pressing needs. The point also has implications for the problem of long-term care for the frail elderly, but I cannot develop them here.

A final implication of the account raises a different set of issues, namely, how to reconcile the demands of justice with certain traditional views of a physician's obligation to his patients. The traditional view is that the physician's direct responsibility is to the well-being of his patients, that (with their consent) he is to do everything in his power to preserve their lives and well-being. One effect of leaving all resource-allocation decisions in this way to the micro-level decisions of physicians and patients, especially where third-party payment schemes mean little or no rationing by price, is that cost-ineffective utilization results. In the current cost-conscious climate, there is pressure to make physicians see themselves as responsible for introducing economic considerations into their utilization decisions. But the issue raised here goes beyond cost-effectiveness. My account suggests that there are important resource-allocation priorities that derive from considerations of justice. In a context of moderate scarcity, this suggests it is not possible for physicians to see as their ideal the maximization of the quality of care they deliver regardless of cost: pursuing that ideal upsets resource-allocation priorities determined by the opportunity principle. Considerations of justice challenge the traditional (perhaps mythical) view that physicians can act as the unrestrained agents of their patients. The remaining task, which I pursue elsewhere, is to show at what level the constraints should be imposed so as to disturb as little as possible of what is valuable about the traditional view of physician responsibility.[47]

These remarks on applications are frustratingly brief, and fuller development of them is required if we are to assess the practical import of the account I offer. Nevertheless, I think the account offers enough that is attractive at the theoretical level to warrant further development of its practical implications.

[47] See Avedis Donabedian, 'The Quality of Medical Care: A Concept in Search of a Definition,' *Journal of Family Practice*, 9/2 (1979), 277–84; and Daniels, 'Cost-Effectiveness and Patient Welfare,' in Marc Basson (ed.), *Ethics, Humanism and Medicine*, ii (New York: Aldon Liss, 1981).

11

EQUALITY OR PRIORITY?

DEREK PARFIT

In his article 'Equality', Nagel imagines that he has two children, one healthy and happy, the other suffering from a painful handicap. He could either move to a city where the second child could receive special treatment, or move to a suburb where the first child would flourish. Nagel writes:

This is a difficult choice on any view. To make it a test for the value of equality, I want to suppose that the case has the following feature: the gain to the first child of moving to the suburb is substantially greater than the gain to the second child of moving to the city.

He then comments:

If one chose to move to the city, it would be an egalitarian decision. It is more urgent to benefit the second child, even though the benefit we can give him is less than the benefit we can give to the first child. This urgency is not necessarily decisive. It may be outweighed by other considerations, for equality is not the only value. But it is a factor, and it depends on the worse off position of the second child.[1]

My aim, in this lecture, is to discuss this kind of egalitarian reasoning.

Nagel's decision turns on the relative importance of two facts: he could give one child a greater benefit, but the other child is worse off.

There are countless cases of this kind. In these cases, when we are choosing between two acts or policies, one relevant fact is how great the resulting benefits would be. For Utilitarians, that is all that matters. On their view, we should always aim for the greatest sum of benefits. But, for Egalitarians, it also matters how well off the beneficiaries would be. We should sometimes choose a smaller sum of benefits, for the sake of a better distribution.

From Derek Parfit, *Equality or Priority?* the Lindley Lecture, University of Kansas, 21 Nov. 1991 (Lawrence: University of Kansas, Department of Philosophy, 1995).

This article owes much to the ideas of Brian Barry, David Brink, Jerry Cohen, Ronald Dworkin, James Griffin, Shelly Kagan, Dennis McKerlie, David Miller, Thomas Nagel, Richard Norman, Robert Nozick, Ingmar Persson, Janet Radcliffe Richards, Joseph Raz, Thomas Scanlon, and Larry Temkin.

[1] Thomas Nagel, *Mortal Questions* (Cambridge: Cambridge University Press, 1979), 123. See also Nagel's *Equality and Partiality* (New York: Oxford University Press, 1991).

How can we make a distribution better? Some say: by aiming for equality between different people. Others say: by giving priority to those who are worse off. As we shall see, these are different ideas.

Should we accept these ideas? Does equality matter? If so, when and why? What kind of priority, if any, should we give to those who are worse off?

These are difficult questions, but their subject matter is, in a way, simple. It is enough to consider different possible states of affairs, or outcomes, each involving the same set of people. We imagine that we know how well off, in these outcomes, these people would be. We then ask whether either outcome would be better, or would be the outcome that we ought to bring about. This subject we can call *the ethics of distribution*.

Some writers reject this subject. For example, Nozick claims that we should not ask what would be the best distribution, since that question wrongly assumes that there is something to be distributed. Most goods, Nozick argues, are not up for distribution, or redistribution.[2] They are goods to which particular people already have entitlements, or special claims. To decide what justice demands, we cannot look merely at the abstract pattern: at how well off, in the different outcomes, different people would be. We must know these people's histories, and how each situation came about. Others make similar claims about merit, or desert. To be just, these writers claim, we must give everyone their due, and people's dues depend entirely on the differences between them, and on what they have done. As before, it is these other facts which are morally decisive.

These objections we can here set aside. We can assume that, in the cases we are considering, there are no such differences between people. No one deserves to be better off than anyone else; nor does anyone have entitlements, or special claims. Since there are *some* cases of this kind, we have a subject. If we can reach conclusions, we can then consider how widely these apply. Like Rawls and others, I believe that, at the fundamental level, most cases are of this kind. But that can be argued later.[3]

There are many ways in which, in one of two outcomes, people can be worse off. They may be poorer, or less happy, or have fewer opportunities, or worse health, or shorter lives. Though the difference between these cases often matters, I shall be discussing some general claims, which apply to them all.

To ask my questions, we need only two assumptions. First, some people can be worse off than others, in ways that are morally relevant. Second,

---

[2] Robert Nozick, *Anarchy, State, and Utopia* (New York: Basic Books, 1974). 149–50.

[3] Since acts may differ morally from omissions, we can also assume that each of the possible outcomes would result from the same kind of act. And, since it may make a difference whether any outcome would be a continuation of the status quo, we should assume that this would not be so.

these differences can be matters of degree. For example, A could be much worse off than B, who is slightly worse off than C.

In describing my examples, I shall use figures. One description might be:

(1) A is at 20   B is at 10
(2) A is at 25   B is at 9

Though such figures suggest precision, that is misleading. Such differences are, I believe, even in reality imprecise. These figures merely show that the choice between these outcomes makes much more difference to A, but that, in both outcomes, B would be much worse off. That is what Nagel assumes about his two imagined children.

One point about my figures is important. Each extra unit is a roughly equal benefit, however well off the person is who receives it. If someone rises from 99 to 100, this person benefits as much as someone else who rises from 9 to 10. Without this assumption we cannot make sense of some of our questions. We cannot ask, for example, whether some benefit would matter more if it came to someone who was worse off. Consider Nagel's claim that, in his example, it would be more urgent to benefit the handicapped child. Nagel tells us to assume that, compared with the healthy child, the handicapped child would benefit *less*. Without this assumption, as he notes, his example would not test the value of equality. Nagel's conclusion is egalitarian because he believes that it is the *lesser* benefit which *matters more*.

For each extra unit to be an equal benefit, however well off the recipient is, these units cannot be thought of as equal quantities of resources. The same increase in resources usually brings greater benefits to those who are worse off. But these benefits need not be thought of in narrowly Utilitarian terms: as involving only happiness and the relief of suffering, or the fulfilment of desire. These benefits might include improvements in health, or length of life, or education, or other substantive goods.[4]

I

What do Egalitarians believe? The obvious answer is: they believe in equality. On this definition, most of us are Egalitarians, since most of us believe in some kind of equality. We believe in political equality, or equality before the

[4] For two such broader accounts of well-being, see Amartya Sen, 'Capability and Well-Being', and Thomas Scanlon. 'Value Desire, and the Quality of Life', both in Martha Nussbaum and Amartya Sen (eds.), *The Quality of Life* (Oxford: Oxford University Press, 1993), and Amartya Sen, *Inequality Reexamined* (Oxford: Oxford University Press, 1992), ch. 3.

law, or we believe that everyone has equal rights, or that everyone's interests should be given equal weight.[5]

Though these kinds of equality are of great importance, they are not my subject. I am concerned with people's being *equally well off*. To count as Egalitarians, in my sense, this is the kind of equality in which we must believe.

There are two main ways in which we can believe in equality. We may believe that inequality is *bad*. On such a view, when we should aim for equality, that is because we shall thereby make the outcome better. We can then be called *Teleological*—or, for short *Telic*—Egalitarians. Our view may instead be *Deontological* or, for short, *Deontic*. We may believe we should aim for equality, not to make the outcome better, but for some other moral reason. We may believe, for example, that people have rights to equal shares. (We might of course have beliefs of both kinds. We might believe we should aim for equality both because this will make the outcome better, and for other reasons. But such a view does not need a separate discussion. It is enough to consider its components.)[6]

We can first consider Telic Egalitarians. These accept

The Principle of Equality: It is in itself bad if some people are worse off than others.[7]

In a fuller statement of this principle, we would need to assess the relative badness of different patterns of inequality. But we can here ignore these complications.[8]

Suppose next that the people in some community could all be either (1) equally well off, or (2) equally badly off. The Principle of Equality does not tell us that (2) would be worse. This principle is about the badness of inequality; and, though it would be clearly worse if everyone were equally worse off, our ground for thinking this cannot be egalitarian.

To explain why (2) would be worse, we might appeal to

The Principle of Utility: It is in itself better if people are better off.

When people would be on average better off, or would receive a greater net sum of benefits, we can say, for short, that there would be more *utility*. (But, as I have said, these benefits need not be thought of in narrowly utilitarian terms.)

[5] See Sen, *Inequality Reexamined*, ch. 1.

[6] On these definitions, we are Egalitarians if, in any area, we believe we should aim for equality. If we had that belief in only some small area, we would not naturally be called 'Egalitarians'. In that respect my definitions are misleading.

[7] We might add, 'through no fault or choice of theirs'.

[8] They are well discussed in Larry Temkin's *Inequality* (New York: Oxford University Press, 1993).

If we cared only about equality, we would be *Pure* Egalitarians. If we cared only about utility, we would be Pure Utilitarians—or what are normally just called Utilitarians. But most of us accept a *pluralist* view: one that appeals to more than one principle or value. On what I shall call the *Pluralist Egalitarian View*, we believe that it would be better both if there was more equality, and if there was more utility. In deciding which of two outcomes would be better, we give weight to both these values.

These values may conflict. One of two outcomes may be in one way worse, because there would be more inequality, but in another way better, because there would be more utility, or a greater sum of benefits. We must then decide which of these two facts would be more important. Consider, for example, the following possible states of affairs:

(1) Everyone at 150
(2) Half at 199   Half at 200
(3) Half at 101   Half at 200

For Pure Egalitarians, (1) is the best of these three outcomes, since it contains less inequality than both (2) and (3). For Utilitarians, (1) is the worst of these outcomes, since it contains less utility than both (2) and (3). (In a move from (1) to (3), the benefits to the half who gained would be slightly greater than the losses to the half who lost.) For most Pluralist Egalitarians, (1) would be neither the best nor the worst of these outcomes. (1) would be all-things-considered worse than (2), since it would be *much* worse in terms of utility, and only *slightly* better in terms of equality. Similarly, (1) would be all-things-considered better than (3), since it would be much better in terms of equality, and only slightly worse in terms of utility.

In many cases the Pluralist View is harder to apply. Compare

(1) Everyone at 150

with

(4) Half at *N*   Half at 200.

If we are Pluralist Egalitarians, for which values of *N* would we believe (1) to be worse than (4)? For some range of values—such as 120 to 150—we may find this question hard to answer. And this case is unusually simple. Patterns of inequality can be much harder to assess.

As such cases show, if we give weight to both equality and utility, we have no principled way to assess their relative importance. To defend a particular decision, we can only claim that it seems right. (Rawls therefore calls this view *intuitionist*.)

I have said that, for Telic Egalitarians, inequality is bad. That seems to me the heart of this view. But I shall keep the familiar claim that, on this view, equality has value. It would be pedantic to claim instead that *in*equality has *dis*value.

We should next distinguish two kinds of value. If we claim that equality has value, we may only mean that it has good effects. Equality has many kinds of good effect, and inequality many kinds of bad effect. If people are unequal, for example, that can produce conflict, or envy, or put some people in the power of others. If we value equality because we are concerned with such effects, we believe that equality has *instrumental* value: we think it good as a means. But I am concerned with a different idea. For true Egalitarians, equality has *intrinsic* value. As Nagel claims, it 'is in itself good'.

This distinction, as we shall see, is theoretically important. And it makes a practical difference. If we believe that, besides having bad effects, inequality is in itself bad, we shall think it to be worse. And we shall think it bad even when it has no bad effects.

Nagel sometimes blurs this distinction. He mentions two kinds of argument 'for the intrinsic value of equality'[9]; but neither seems to deserve this description.

The first kind of argument is *individualistic*, since it appeals to what is good or bad for individuals. Nagel's example is the claim that, when there is inequality, this weakens the self-respect of those people who are worse off. But what is claimed to be bad here is not inequality itself, but only one of its effects. Nor, to judge this effect bad, need we be egalitarians. Other effects we may think bad only because our conception of well-being is in part egalitarian. Thus we may think it bad for people if they are servile or too deferential, even if this does not frustrate their desires, or affect their experienced well-being. But though such a view is, in one way, egalitarian, it too does not claim that equality has intrinsic value. As before, it claims only that inequality has bad effects.

Nagel's second type of argument is *communitarian*. According to this argument, he writes.

equality is good for society taken as a whole. It is a condition of the right kind of relations among its members, and of the formation in them of healthy fraternal attitudes, desires, and sympathies.

For this to be a different type of argument, it must claim that such relations are not merely good for people, but have intrinsic value. This, however, would still not be the claim that *equality* has intrinsic value. What would be

---

[9] *Mortal Questions*, 108. Cf. David Miller, 'Arguments for Equality', *Midwest Studies in Philosophy*, vii (Minneapolis: University of Minnesota Press, 1982).

claimed to be good would still not be equality itself, but only some of its effects.[10]

The difference can be shown like this. Consider what I shall call *the Divided World*. This contains two groups of people, each unaware of the other's existence. Perhaps the Atlantic has not yet been crossed. Consider next two possible states of this world:

(1) Half at 100   Half at 200
(2) Half at 140   Half at 140

Of these two states, (1) is in one way better than (2), since people are on average better off. But we may believe that, all things considered, (1) is worse than (2). How could we explain this view?

If we are Telic Egalitarians, our explanation would be this. While it is good that, in (1), people are on average better off, it is bad that some people are worse off than others. The badness of this inequality morally outweighs the extra benefits.

In making such a claim, we could not appeal to inequality's effects. Since the two halves of the world's population are quite unconnected, the inequality in (1) has no bad effects on the worse-off group. Nor does the equality in (2) produce desirable fraternal relations between the two groups. If we are to claim that (1) is worse because of its inequality, we must claim that this inequality is in itself bad.

Suppose we decide that, in this example, (1) is *not* worse than (2). Would this show that, in our view, inequality is *not* in itself bad?

This would depend on our answer to another question. What should be the *scope* of an egalitarian view? Who are the people who, ideally, should be equally well off?

The simplest answer would be: everyone who ever lives. And, on the Telic View, this seems the natural answer. If it is in itself bad if some people are worse off than others, why should it matter where or when these people live? On such a view, it is in itself bad if there are or have been, even in unrelated communities, and in different centuries, people who are not equally well off. Thus it is bad if Inca peasants, or Stone Age hunter-gatherers, were worse off than we are now.

We may reject this view. We may believe that, if two groups of people are quite unrelated, it is in no way bad if they are not equally well off. This might be why, in my example, we deny that (1) is worse than (2).

If that is our reaction, might we still believe that, when it holds between

---

[10] There are some other possibilities. As Kagan and Brink suggest, equality might be intrinsically good, neither by itself, nor because of its effects, but because it was an essential part of some larger good. Cf. Miller, 'Arguments for Equality'.

related groups, inequality is in itself bad? This seems unlikely. Why is it only in these cases that we object to inequality? Why would it make a difference if these groups were not aware of each other's existence? The obvious answer is that, in such cases, inequality cannot have its usual bad effects. It would be coherent to claim that inequality is in itself bad, but only when it holds between related groups. But, though coherent, this view does not seem plausible, since it would involve a strange coincidence.

We might claim, more plausibly, that inequality is in itself bad, but only when it holds within one *community*. But that would suggest that our real view is that such inequality involves social injustice. And we may then be *Deontic* Egalitarians.

II

Let us now consider this second kind of view. Deontic Egalitarians believe that, though we should sometimes aim for equality, that is *not* because we shall thereby make the outcome better, but is always for some other reason. On such a view, it is not in itself good if people are equally well off, or bad if they are not.

Such a view typically appeals to claims about justice. More exactly, it appeals to claims about *comparative* justice. Whether people are unjustly treated, in this comparative sense, depends on whether they are treated *differently* from other people. Thus it may be unfair if, in a distribution of resources, some people are denied their share. Fairness may require that, if such goods are given to some, they should be given to all.

Another kind of justice is concerned with treating people as they deserve. This kind of justice is *non-comparative*. Whether people are unjustly treated, in this sense, depends only on facts about *them*. It is irrelevant whether others are treated differently. Thus, if we treated no one as they deserved, this treatment would be unjust in the non-comparative sense. But, if we treated everyone equally unjustly, there would be no comparative injustice.[11]

It is sometimes hard to distinguish these two kinds of justice, and there are difficult questions about the relation between them.[12] One point should be mentioned here. Non-comparative justice may tell us to produce equality. Perhaps, if everyone were equally deserving, we should make everyone equally well off. But such equality would be merely the effect of giving

---

[11] Cf. Joel Feinberg, 'Noncomparative Justice', *Philosophical Review*, 83 (July 1974).
[12] Cf. Philip Montague, 'Comparative and Non-Comparative Justice', *Philosophical Quarterly*, 30 (Apr. 1980).

people what they deserved. Only comparative justice makes equality our aim.

When I said that, in my examples, no one deserves to be better off than others, I did not mean that everyone is equally deserving. I meant that, in these cases, we are considering benefits that no one deserves. So it is only comparative justice with which we shall be concerned.

There is another relevant distinction. In some cases, justice is *purely procedural*. It requires only that we act in a certain way. For example, when some good cannot be divided, we may be required to conduct a fair lottery, which gives everyone an equal chance to receive this good. In other cases, justice is in part *substantive*. Here too, justice may require a certain kind of procedure; but there is a separate criterion of what the outcome ought to be. One example would be the claim that people should be given equal shares.

There is an intermediate case. Justice may require a certain outcome, but only because this avoids a procedural flaw. One such flaw is partiality. Suppose that we have to distribute certain publicly owned goods. If we could easily divide these goods, others might be rightly suspicious if we gave to different people unequal shares. That might involve favouritism, or wrongful discrimination.[13] We may thus believe that, to avoid these flaws, we should distribute these goods equally. The same conclusion might be reached in a slightly different way. We may think that, in such a case, equality is the *default:* that we need some moral reason if we are to justify giving to some people more than we give to others.

How does this view differ from a view that requires equality for substantive reasons? One difference is this. Suppose that we have manifestly tried to distribute equally, but our procedure has innocently failed. If we aimed for equality only to avoid the taint of partiality or discrimination, there would be no case for correcting the result.[14]

We can now redescribe my two kinds of Egalitarian. On the Telic View, inequality is bad; on the Deontic View, it is unjust.

It may be objected that, when inequality is unjust, it is, for that reason, bad. But this does not undermine this way of drawing our distinction. On the Deontic View, injustice is a special kind of badness, one that necessarily involves wrong-doing. When we claim that inequality is unjust, our objection is not really to the inequality itself. What is unjust, and therefore bad, is not strictly the state of affairs, but the way in which it was produced.

There is one kind of case which most clearly separates our two kinds of

---

[13] See Robert Goodin, 'Egalitarianism, Fetishistic and Otherwise', *Ethics*, 98 (Oct. 1987), and 'Epiphenomenal Egalitarianism', *Social Research*, 52 (Spring 1985).

[14] Cf. the distinctions drawn in Lawrence Sager and Lewis Kornhauser, 'Just Lotteries', in *Social Science Information*, 27 (London: Sage, 1988)

view. These are cases where some inequality cannot be avoided. For Deontic Egalitarians, if nothing can be done, there can be no injustice. In Rawls's words, if some situation 'is unalterable . . . the question of justice does not arise.'[15]

Consider, for example, the inequality in our natural endowments. Some of us are born more talented or healthier than others, or are more fortunate in other ways. If we are Deontic Egalitarians, we shall not believe that such inequality is in itself bad. We might agree that, if we *could* distribute talents, it would be unjust or unfair to distribute them unequally. But, except when there are bad effects, we shall see nothing to regret in the inequalities produced by the random shuffling of our genes.

Many Telic Egalitarians take a different view. They believe that, even when such inequality is unavoidable, it is in itself bad.[16]

III

It is worth developing here some remarks of Rawls. As I have said, Rawls assumes that injustice essentially involves wrongdoing. When he discusses the inequality of our inherited talents, he writes:

The natural distribution is neither just nor unjust . . . These are simply natural facts. What is just and unjust is the way that institutions deal with these facts.

This may suggest a purely deontic view. But Rawls continues:

Aristocratic and caste societies are unjust because . . . the basic structure of these societies incorporates the arbitrariness found in nature. But there is no necessity for men to resign themselves to these contingencies.[17]

This use of the word *resign* seems to assume that natural inequality *is* bad. And Rawls elsewhere writes that, in a society governed by his principles, we need no longer 'view it as a *misfortune* that some are by nature better endowed than others'. These remarks suggest that Rawls is in part a Telic Egalitarian. An objection to natural inequality is, I believe, one of the foundations of his theory, and one of its driving forces. If Rawls denies that such inequality is unjust, that may only be because he wishes to preserve the

---

[15] John Rawls, *A Theory of Justice* (Cambridge, Mass.: Harvard University Press, 1971), 291.

[16] There is now a complication. Those who take this second view do not merely think that such inequality is bad. They often speak of natural injustice. On their view, it is unjust or unfair that some people are born less able, or less healthy, than others. Similarly, it is unfair if nature bestows on some richer resources. Talk of unfairness here is sometimes claimed to make no sense. I believe that it does make sense. But, even on this view, our distinction stands. For Telic Egalitarians, it is the state of affairs which is bad, or unjust; but Deontic Egalitarians are concerned only with what we ought to do.

[17] *A Theory of Justice*, 102.

analytic link between injustice and wrong-doing. And, given the substance of his theory, that may be merely a terminological decision.

Rawls's objection to natural inequality is not so much that it is bad, but that it is morally arbitrary. This objection, as Rawls suggests, can be reapplied at several points in one natural line of thought.

We can start with external goods. In some cases, we enjoy resources whose availability, or discovery, is in no sense due to us. Such resources simply appear, like manna falling from the sky. There will be inequality if such manna falls unequally on different people. Let us call these *windfall* cases.

In such cases, the inequality is entirely due to differences in the bounty of nature. Such differences are, in the clearest sense, morally arbitrary. If some people receive less than others, that is merely their bad luck. Since such inequalities have this arbitrary cause, we may conclude that they are bad. Or we may conclude that we ought to redress these inequalities, by a redistribution of resources.

Consider next cases in which we are not merely passive. We do some work, either in discovering resources, or in converting them for use. We plant seeds, prospect and mine, or fish the sea; we till the soil, and manufacture goods.

Suppose that we all work equally hard, and with equal skill. In such cases, the human input is the same. But there may still be inequality between us, which results from differences in the natural input. These might be differences in mineral wealth, or in the climate, or in the fruitfulness of the soil, or sea. Because of such variations, some of us may soon become much better off than others. These are cases of *productive luck*.[18]

Some of these cases hardly differ from pure windfalls. Perhaps we merely have to shake our trees, or stroll over to where the fruit fell. And all these cases may seem relevantly similar. Since we all work equally hard, and with equal skill, the inequality is again due to differences in the bounty of nature, which we believe to be morally arbitrary. Can the other element, the equal human input, make this fact irrelevant? Can it justify the resulting inequality? We may decide that it cannot, and that such inequality also calls for redistribution.

Now consider inequality of a third kind. In these cases, there are no differences either in external resources, or in the efforts people make. The inequality is entirely due to differences in people's native talents. These are cases of *genetic luck*.[19]

---

[18] They include environmental or circumstantial luck. Cf. Brian Barry, *Theories of Justice* (London: Harvester, 1989), 239.

[19] Some object that it cannot be luck that we have the genes we do, since we could not have had other genes. But this use of 'luck' does not imply that things could have been otherwise. Something is 'luck', in this sense, if it is not something for which we ourselves are responsible. (Cf. Thomas Nagel, 'Moral luck', in *Mortal Questions* (Cambridge: Cambridge University Press, 1979).)

We may decide that such genetic differences are, in the relevant respect, like differences in nature's bounty. As Rawls says, they are not deserved. Our native talents are inner resources, which, like manna, merely fell upon us.

In some of these cases, people receive greater rewards simply for *having* certain natural endowments. These are like pure windfalls. But, in most of these cases, people develop and use the talents with which they were born. We must ask again whether this infusion of effort cancels out the arbitrariness of genetic luck. Can it justify the resulting inequalities?

This may be the most important question in this whole debate. Many people answer Yes. But, like Rawls and Nagel, we may answer No. We may conclude that these inequalities should also be redressed.

Consider next a fourth kind of case. The natural input is the same, and we all have equal talents. But inequality results from differences in how hard we work. These are cases of *differential effort*.

We must here note one complication. There are two uncontroversial ways in which, when people work harder, they should sometimes be paid more. They may work for a longer time, or in a more unpleasant way. In such cases, overtime or hardship pay may be mere compensation, which does not create real inequality. These are not the cases that I have in mind. I am thinking of people who enjoy working hard, and who, because they do, become much better off than others.

Of those who appeal to the arbitrariness of the natural lottery, many stop here. Differences in effort seem to them to justify such inequality. But we may press on. Such differences involve two elements: the ability to make an effort, and the decision to try. We may decide that the first is merely another native talent, which cannot justify inequality.

This leaves only inequalities that are the result of choice. To most Egalitarians, these inequalities are of no concern. That is why some writers argue for equality, not of well-being, but of *opportunity* for well-being.[20] But some of us may still press on. We may decide that it is bad if some people are worse off than others, even when this is merely because these people do not enjoy working hard, or because, for some other reason, they make choices that leave them worse off. These may seem to be merely other kinds of bad luck.

The line of thought that I have just sketched raises many questions. I shall make only three brief comments.

First, to some people this reasoning may seem a *reductio*. If these people find the last step absurd, they may be led to reject the others. But that would be too swift, since there could be grounds for stopping earlier.

---

[20] Cf. C. A. Cohen, 'On the Currency of Egalitarian Justice' *Ethics*, 99 (1989) and R. Arneson, 'Equality and Equality of Opportunity for Welfare', *Philosophical Studies*, 56 (1989).

Second, we should state more clearly what such reasoning might show. The reasoning appeals to the claim that certain kinds of inequality have a morally arbitrary cause. Such a claim might show that such inequality is *not* justified. But it may not show that such inequality is *un*justified, and ought to be redressed. These are quite different conclusions.

If such inequality is not justified, people have no positive claim to their advantages, or to the resources which they now control. But this conclusion only clears the decks. It means that, *if* there is a moral reason for redistribution, those who are better off can have no principled objection. It would be a further claim that there *is* such a reason, and that the aim of such redistribution should be to produce equality.[21]

The difference can be shown like this. Utilitarians would also claim that, if some distribution of resources has an arbitrary natural cause, it is not justified. Since that is so, they would claim, there can be no objection to redistribution. But, on their view, the best distribution is the one that would maximize the sum of benefits. Such a distribution would not be morally arbitrary. But it may not be an equal distribution.

Third, Rawls regards Utilitarians as his main opponents. At the level of theory, he may be right. But the questions I have been discussing are, in practice, more important. If nature gave to some of us more resources, have we a moral claim to keep these resources, and the wealth they bring? If we happen to be born with greater talents, and in consequence produce more, have we a claim to greater rewards? In practical terms, Rawls's main opponents are those who answer Yes to such questions. Egalitarians and Utilitarians both answer No. Both agree that such inequalities are *not* justified. In this disagreement, Rawls, Mill, and Sidgwick are on the same side.

IV

I have distinguished two kinds of Egalitarian view. On the Telic View, we believe that inequality is in itself bad, or unfair. On the Deontic View, our concern about equality is only a concern about what we should do.

Why does this distinction matter? It has theoretical implications. As we shall later see, these views can be defended or attacked in different ways. There are also practical implications, some of which I shall mention now.

Each view has many versions. That is especially true of the Deontic View, which is really a group of views. Telic and Deontic Views might, in practice,

[21] Cf. Nozick, *Anarchy, State and Utopia*, 216, and Nagel, *Mortal Questions*, 119.

coincide. It might be true that, whenever the first view claims that some kind of inequality is bad, the second claims that we should prevent it, if we can. But when we look at the versions of these views that are in fact advanced, and found plausible, we find that they often conflict.

The Telic View is likely to have wider scope. As I have said, if we think it in itself bad if some people are worse off than others, we may think this bad whoever these people are. It may seem to make no difference where these people live: whether they are in the same or different communities. We may also think it irrelevant what the respects are in which some people are worse off than others: whether they have less income, or worse health, or are less fortunate in other ways. *Any* inequality, if undeserved and unchosen, we may think bad. Nor, third, will it seem to make a difference how such inequality arose. That is implied by the very notion of intrinsic badness. If some state is in itself bad, it is irrelevant how it came about.

If we are Deontic Egalitarians, our view may have none of these features.

Though there are many versions of the Deontic View, one large group are broadly contractarian. Such views often appeal to the ideas of reciprocity, or mutual benefit. On some views of this kind, when goods are co-operatively produced, and no one has special claims, all the contributors should get equal shares. There are here two restrictions. First, what is shared are only the fruits of co-operation. Nothing is said about other goods, such as those that come from nature. Second, the distribution covers only those who produce these goods. Those who cannot contribute, such as the handicapped, or children, or future generations, have no claims.[22]

Other views of this type are less restrictive. They may cover all the members of the same community, and all types of good. But they still exclude outsiders. It is irrelevant that those other people may be far worse off.

On such views, if there is inequality between people in different communities, this need not be anyone's concern. Since the greatest inequalities are on this global scale, this restriction has immense importance. (Here is one way to make this point. If Egalitarians oppose inequality only within particular communities, their view may, on a global scale, call for *less* redistribution than a Utilitarian view.)

Consider next the question of causation. The Telic View naturally applies to all cases. On this view, we always have a reason to prevent or reduce inequality, if we can.

If we are Deontic Egalitarians, we might think the same. But that is less likely. Since our view is not about the goodness of outcomes, it may cover

---

[22] See, for example, David Gauthier, *Morals by Agreement* (Oxford: Oxford University Press, 1980), 18 and 268.

only inequalities that result from acts, or only those that are intentionally produced. And it may tell us to be concerned only with the inequalities that we ourselves produce.

Here is one example. In a highly restricted way, Gauthier is a Deontic Egalitarian. Thus he writes that 'If there were a distributor of natural assets . . . we might reasonably suppose that in so far as possible shares should be equal.'[23] But, when assets are distributed by nature, Gauthier has no objection to inequality. He sees no ground to undo the effects of the natural lottery.

On such a view, when we are responsible for some distribution, we ought to distribute equally. But, when we are not responsible, inequality is not unjust. In such cases, there is nothing morally amiss. We have no reason to remove such inequality, by redistribution.

Is this a defensible position? Suppose we are about to distribute some resources. We agree that we ought to give people equal shares. A gust of wind snatches these resources from our hands, and distributes them unequally. Have we then no reason to redistribute?

It makes a difference here why we believe that we ought to distribute equally. Suppose, first, that our concern is with procedural justice. We believe that we should distribute equally because that is the only way to avoid partiality. Or we believe that equality is the default: what we should aim for when we cannot justify distributing unequally. When there is natural inequality, neither belief applies. Nature is not discriminatory; nor is she an agent, who must justify what she does. On such a view, *if* we distribute, we should distribute equally. But we have no ground for thinking that we *should* distribute. If the distributor is Nature, there has been no partiality. Nothing needs to be undone.

Suppose, next, that we are concerned with substantive justice. Our aim is not merely to avoid procedural flaws, since we have a separate criterion for what the result should be. On such a view, we might believe that, wherever possible, we should intervene, to produce the right result. But, as before, that belief need not be part of such a view. As in the case of procedural justice, we might believe only that, *if* we distribute, we should distribute equally. When inequality arises naturally, our view may not apply.

Things are different on the Telic View, according to which such inequality is in itself bad, or unjust. On this view, we have a reason to redistribute. The onus of the argument shifts. If people oppose redistribution, they must provide contrary reasons.

It is worth mentioning some of these reasons. Some would claim that, even if *we* should distribute equally, once there has been a natural distribution, it is wrong to intervene. Such a claim may seem to assume that what is natural is right, or that the status quo is privileged—assumptions that are now hard to defend. But there are other ways in which people might defend such claims. They might appeal to the difference between acts and omissions, or between negative and positive duties, or something of the kind.[24]

In some cases, such a view is plausible. Suppose that some natural process threatens to kill many people. We could save them if we intervened, and killed one person as a means to save the many. Many believe that, even though the deaths of many would be a worse outcome than the death of one, we ought not to intervene in such a way. We should allow this natural process to bring about the worse of these two outcomes.

Could we apply such a view to inequality? If some natural process has distributed resources in an unequal way, could it be similarly claimed that, though such inequality makes the outcome worse, we ought not to intervene? That seems less plausible. In the case of killing, our objection might appeal to the special features of this act, our relation to the person killed, her right not to be injured, or to the fact that her death is used as a means. There seem to be no such features when we correct a natural distribution. If the wind blows more manna into the laps of certain people, and we conceded that, as an outcome, this is worse, there seems no ground for a constraint against redistribution. If we remove and redistribute these people's extra manna, so that everyone has equal shares, we do not injure these people, or use them as a means.

It may next be claimed that, once a natural distribution has occurred, people acquire entitlements. In pure windfall cases, such a claim seems far-fetched. The fact that the manna fell on you does not make it *yours*. But similar claims are widely made. Thus it may be said that you staked out a valid claim to the ground on which the manna fell, and that this makes it yours. Or it may be said that, once you interact with the manna—or mix your labour with it—it becomes yours.

Such claims may have some force if they are made within some existing institutional scheme, or agreement. But we are here discussing a more fundamental question. What should our institutions, or agreements, be? If such claims are not convincing, as answers to that question, we may conclude that, in pure windfall cases, we ought to redistribute. It may then be harder to defend such claims in cases of productive luck. If we reject such claims

[24] Cf. Nagel, *Equality and Partiality*, 99–102, and Thomas Pogge's discussion of Nozick, in his *Realizing Rawls* (Ithaca, NY: Cornell University Press, 1989), ch. 1.

here, it may then be harder to defend them in cases of genetic luck, and so on down the series.

For those who hold a Deontic View, there is no need even to make these claims. On such a view, since natural inequality is not in itself bad, there is no argument *for* redistribution; so there need not be an argument against. This, for conservatives, is a stronger position.

V

Let us now consider two objections to the Telic View.

On the widest version of this view, any inequality is bad. It is bad, for example, that some people are sighted and others are blind. We would therefore have a reason, if we could, to take single eyes from some of the sighted and give them to the blind. That may seem a horrific conclusion.

If Egalitarians wish to avoid this conclusion, they might claim that their view applies only to inequality in resources. But, as Nozick says, such a restriction may be hard to explain. If natural inequality is in itself bad, why is that not true of the inequality between the sighted and the blind?

Should we be horrified by this conclusion? To set aside some irrelevant complications, let us purify the example. Suppose that, after some genetic change, people are henceforth born as twins, one of whom is always blind. And suppose that, as a universal policy, operations are performed after every birth, in which one eye from the sighted twin is transplanted into its blind sibling. That would be a forcible redistribution, since new-born babies cannot give consent. But I am inclined to believe that such a policy would be justified.

Some of us may disagree. We may believe that people have rights to keep the organs with which they were born. But that belief would not give us grounds to reject the Telic View. Egalitarians could agree that the State should not redistribute organs. Since they do not believe equality to be the only value, they could think that, in this example, some other principle has greater weight. Their belief is only that, if we all had one eye, that would be *in one way* better than if half of us had two eyes and the other half had none. Far from being moustrous, that belief is clearly true. If we all had one eye, that would be much better for all of the people who would otherwise be blind.[25]

A second objection is more serious. If inequality is bad, its disappearance

---

[25] Cf. Nozick, *Anarchy, State and Utopia*, 206 (though Nozick's target here is not the Principle of Equality but Rawls's Difference Principle).

must be in one way a change for the better, *however this change occurs*. Suppose that those who are better off suffer some misfortune, so that they become as badly off as everyone else. Since these events would remove the inequality, they must be in one way welcome, on the Telic View, even though they would be worse for some people, and better for no one. This implication seems to many to be quite absurd. I call this *the Levelling Down Objection*.[26]

Consider first those Egalitarians who regret the inequalities in our natural endowments. On their view, it would be in one way better if we removed the eyes of the sighted, not to give them to the blind, but simply to make the sighted blind. That would be in one way better even if it was in *no* way better for the blind. This we may find impossible to believe. Egalitarians would avoid this form of the objection if what they think bad is only inequality in resources. But they must admit that, on their view, it would be in one way better if, in some natural disaster those who are better off lost all of their extra resources, in a way that benefitted no one. That conclusion may seem almost as implausible.

It is worth repeating that, to criticize Egalitarians by appealing to the Levelling Down Objection, it is not enough to claim that it would be *wrong* to produce equality by levelling down. As we have seen, since they are pluralists, Telic Egalitarians could accept that claim. Our objection must be that, if we achieve equality by levelling down, there is *nothing* good about what we have done. And we must claim that, if some natural disaster makes everyone equally badly off, that is not in any way good news. These claims do contradict the Telic Egalitarian View, even in its pluralist form.

I shall return to the Levelling Down Objection. The point to notice now is that, on a Deontic view, we can avoid all forms of this objection. If we are Deontic Egalitarians, we do not believe that inequality is bad, so we are not forced to admit that, on our view, it would be in one way better if inequality were removed by levelling down. We can believe that we have a reason to remove inequality only *when*, and only *because*, our way of doing so benefits the people who are worse off. Or we might believe that, when some people are worse off than others, through no fault or choice of theirs, they have a special claim to be raised up to the level of the others, but they have no claim that others be brought down to their level.

---

[26] Such an objection is suggested, for example, in Joseph Raz, *The Morality of Freedom* (Oxford: Oxford University Press, 1986), ch. 9, and Larry Temkin, *Inequality*, 247–8.

VI

There are, then, several differences between the Telic and Deontic Views. Though these views might coincide, they are likely to have different scope, and different implications. And, as we have just seen, they can be challenged in different ways. If we are Egalitarians, it is thus important to decide which kind of view we hold.

If we are impressed by the Levelling Down Objection, we may be tempted by the Deontic View. But, if we give up the Telic View, we may find it harder to justify some of our beliefs. If inequality is not in itself bad, we may find it harder to explain, for example, why we should redistribute resources.

Some of our beliefs would also have to go. Reconsider the Divided World, in which the two possible states are these:

(1) Half at 100   Half at 200
(2) Half at 140   Half at 140

In outcome (1) there is inequality. But, since the two groups are unaware of each other's existence, this inequality was not deliberately produced, or maintained. Since this inequality does not involve wrong-doing, there is no injustice. On the Deontic View, there is nothing more to say. On this view, we cannot claim that (1) is worse than (2). If we believe that (1) is worse, and because of the inequality, we must accept the Telic form of the Egalitarian View. We must claim that the inequality in (1) is in itself bad.

We might, however, give a different explanation. Rather than believing in equality, we might be especially concerned about those people who are worse off. That could be our reason for preferring (2).

Let us now consider this alternative.

VII

In discussing his imaged case, Nagel writes:

If one chose to move to the city, it would be an egalitarian decision. It is more urgent to benefit the second child ... This urgency is not necessarily decisive. It may be outweighed by other considerations, for equality is not the only value. But it is a factor, and it depends on the worse off position of the second child. An improvement in his situation is more important than an equal or somewhat greater improvement in the situation of the first child.[27]

---

[27] Nagel, *Mortal Questions*, 124.

This passage contains the idea that equality has value. But it gives more prominence to another idea. Nagel believes it is more important to benefit the child who is worse off. That idea can lead us to a quite different view.

Consider first those people who are badly off: those who are suffering, or destitute, or those whose fundamental needs have not been met. It is widely claimed that we should give priority to helping such people. This would be claimed even by Utilitarians, since, if people are badly off, they are likely to be easier to help.

I am concerned with a different view. On this view, it is more urgent to help these people even if they are *harder* to help. While Utilitarians claim that we should give these people priority when, and because, we can help them *more*, this view claims that we should give them priority, even when we can help them *less*. That is what makes this a distinctive view.

Some apply this view only to the two groups of the well off and the badly off.[28] But I shall consider a more general version of this view, which can be applied to everyone. On what I shall call

> *The Priority View:* Benefiting people matters more the worse off these people are.

For Utilitarians, the moral importance of each benefit depends only on how great this benefit would be. For *Prioritarians*, it also depends on how well off the person is to whom this benefit comes. We should not give equal weight to equal benefits, whoever receives them. Benefits to the worse off should be given more weight.[29]

Like the Egalitarian Pluralist View, this view is, in Rawls's sense, intuitionist. It does not tell us how much priority we should give to those who are worse off. On this view, benefits to the worse off could be morally outweighed by sufficient benefits to the better off. To decide what would be sufficient, we must simply use our judgement.

Like the belief in equality, the Priority View can take either Telic or Deontic forms. It can be a view about which outcomes would be better, or a view that is only about what we ought to do. But, for most of my discussion, this difference does not matter.

---

[28] Cf. H. Frankfurt, *The Importance of what we Care About* (Cambridge: Cambridge University Press, 1988), ch. 11, and Joseph Raz, *The Morality of Freedom*, ch. 9.

[29] Several other writers have suggested such a view. See, for example, Thomas Scanlon, 'Nozick on Rights, Liberty, and Property', *Philosophy & Public Affairs*, 6/1 (Fall 1976), 6 to 10; Joseph Raz, *The Morality of Freedom*; Harry Frankfurt, 'Equality as a Moral Ideal', in *The Importance of what we Care About*; David Wiggins, 'Claims of Need', in his *Needs, Values, Truth* (Oxford: Blackwell, 1987); Dennis McKerlie, 'Egalitarianism', *Dialogue*, 23 (1984); and 'Equality and Priority', *Philosophy & Public Affairs*.

VIII

Let us now look more closely at this view. To whom should we give priority? Here are three answers:

(1) those who are worse off in their lives as a whole,
(2) those who are worse off at the time,
(3) those who have needs that are morally more urgent.

(1) and (2) frequently diverge. One of two people may be worse off now, even though she has earlier been, and will later be, much better off.

(2) and (3), in contrast, usually coincide. If one of two people has more urgent needs, she is likely to be worse off at the time. But, on some views about the urgency of needs, that is not always true. Compare A, who is disabled, with the less fortunate but able-bodied B. A's need for a wheelchair may be claimed to be more urgent than any of B's needs, even though A's other advantages make her, on the whole, better off.[30]

The choice between (1) and (2) is the choice of what Nagel calls *units* for distributive principles: the items to which we apply these principles.[31] Nagel takes these units to be 'individual persons, individual human lives'. And he writes, 'what makes a system egalitarian is the priority it gives to the claims of those whose overall life prospects put them at the bottom.' Rawls and many others take the same view.

If lives are the relevant units, this increases the difference between giving priority to those who are worse off, and giving priority to meeting more urgent needs.

Nagel sometimes favours the second of these. Thus he claims that an egalitarian view 'establishes an order of priority among needs and gives preference to the most urgent'. And he writes:

An arrangement must be acceptable first from the point of view of everyone's most basic claims, then from the point of view of everyone's next most basic claims, etc. . . . [T]he principles grant to each person the same claim to have his most urgent needs satisfied prior to the less urgent needs of anyone else.[32]

This implies that we should give priority to needs rather than persons. The more urgent needs of someone who, on the whole, is better off, take priority over the less urgent needs of someone who is worse off.

---

[30] Cf. Frankfurt, *The Importance of what we Care About*, 149.

[31] Nagel, *Mortal Questions*, 111. I have claimed elsewhere that, on what I take to be the truth about personal identity, there is an argument for taking these units to be people at particular times, and that, on that view, our distributive principles move us towards Negative Utilitarianism. (*Reasons and Persons* (Oxford: Oxford University Press, 1984), sect. 117, and 'Comments', *Ethics* (July 1986), 869–72.)

[32] *Mortal Questions*, 117 and 121.

Nagel seems to have overlooked this implication. Thus he also writes, 'Priority is given to individuals who, *taking their lives as a whole, have more urgent needs*'.[33] This claim conflates the distinction I have drawn. X's needs may *now* be more urgent than Y's, even though, in most of her life, X has been, and will later be, much better off than Y. If we should give priority to more urgent needs, we should help X. If we should give priority to those who are worse off in their lives as a whole, we should help Y.

Which answer should we give? Suppose that we could support one of two programs. The first would provide treatment for a painful illness that occasionally afflicts the rich. The second would benefit an equal number of the poor, by subsidising sports grounds, or seaside holidays. Which of these should have priority?

For this case to be relevant, it must be true that, even without the treatment, the rich would on the whole be better off. And it must be true that our decision would make *less difference* to them: that it would give them lesser benefits. We can thus suppose that the treatment in question would not bring much relief to this painful illness. Since the benefits to both groups would be hedonistic, they can be roughly estimated by an appeal to people's preferences. Let us suppose that everyone involved would prefer a seaside holiday, or a new sports ground, to the relief of this amount of suffering.

Suppose we believe that, even in such a case, the relief of suffering should take priority. And suppose we take a similar view about other urgent needs, such as those produced by disability. We then have a view which is not, in any way, egalitarian. We think it more important to give *lesser* benefits to people who, in the relevant sense, are *better off*.

Such a view is not, I think, absurd. But, because it is so different, I shall ignore it here. I shall assume that, on the Priority View, we should give priority, not to meeting special needs, but to benefiting those people who are worse off. And I shall assume that, in my examples, there is no difference between those who would be worse off at the time, and those who would be worse off in their lives as a whole.

IX

What is the relation between the Priority View and Egalitarianism?

On the Priority View, it is morally more important to benefit the people who are worse off. But this claim, by itself, does not define a different view, since it would be made by all Egalitarians. If we believe that we should aim

[33] *Mortal Questions*, 121.

for equality, we shall think it more important to benefit those who are worse off. Such benefits reduce inequality. If that is why we give such benefits priority, we do not hold the Priority View. On this view, as I define it here, we do *not* believe in equality. We give priority to the worse off, not because this will reduce inequality, but for other reasons. That is what makes this a distinctive view.

As before, we may hold a mixed view. We may give priority to the worse off, partly because this will reduce inequality, and partly for other reasons. But such a view does not need a separate discussion. It is enough to consider the pure version of the Priority View.

How does this view differ from an Egalitarian view?

One difference is purely structural. As we have seen, equality cannot plausibly be our only value. If we are Egalitarians, we must hold some more complicated view. Thus, on the Telic form of the Pluralist View, the belief that inequality is bad is combined with the belief that benefits are good. The Priority View, in contrast, can be held as a complete moral view. This view contains the idea that benefits are good. It merely adds that benefits matter more the worse off the people are who receive them. Unlike the Principle of Equality, which might be combined with the Principle of Utility, the Priority View can replace that principle. It can be regarded as the only principle we need.

The chief difference can be introduced like this. I have said that, on the Priority View, we do not believe in equality. We do not think it in itself bad, or unjust, that some people are worse off than others. This claim can be misunderstood. We do of course think it bad that some people are worse off. But what is bad is not that these people are worse off than *others*. It is rather that they are worse off than *they* might have been.

Consider next the central claim of the Priority View: benefits to the worse off matter more. The same ambiguity can lead one astray. On this view, if I am worse off than you, benefits to me are more important. Is this *because* I am worse off than you? In one sense, yes. But this has nothing to do with my relation to you.

It may help to use this analogy. People at higher altitudes find it harder to breathe. Is this because they are higher up than other people? In one sense, yes. But they would find it just as hard to breathe even if there were no other people who were lower down. In the same way, on the Priority View, benefits to the worse off matter more, but that is only because these people are at a lower *absolute* level. It is irrelevant that these people are worse off *than others*. Benefits to them would matter just as much even if there *were* no others who were better off.

The chief difference is, then, this. Egalitarians are concerned with *relativities*: with how each person's level compares with the level of other people. On the Priority View, we are concerned only with people's absolute levels.[34]

This is a fundamental structural difference. Because of this difference, there are several ways in which these views have different implications.

One example concerns scope. Telic Egalitarians may, I have said, give their view wide scope. They may believe that inequality is bad even when it holds between people who have no connections with each other. But this can seem a dubious view. Why is it bad if, in some far off land, and quite unknown to me, there are other people who are better off than me?

On the Priority View, there is no ground for such doubts. This view naturally has universal scope. And that is true of both its telic and deontic forms. If it is more important to benefit one of two people, because this person is worse off, it is irrelevant whether these people are in the same community, or are aware of each other's existence. The greater urgency of benefiting this person does not depend on her *relation* to the other person. It depends only on her lower absolute level.

There are other ways in which, given the structural difference between these views, they are likely to have different implications. I cannot discuss these here. But I have described the kind of case in which these views most deeply disagree. These are the cases which raise the Levelling Down Objection. Egalitarians face this objection because they believe that inequality is in itself bad. If we accept the Priority View, we avoid this objection. We are more concerned for people the worse off these people are. But, as we have just seen, it makes no difference to our concern whether there are other people who are better off. On this view, when inequality is not bad for people, it simply does not matter. If the better off suffer some misfortune, so that they become as badly off as anyone else, we do not think this in any way a change for the better.

---

[34] Raz puts the difference well. He writes:

what makes us care about various inequalities is not the inequality but the concern identified by the underlying principle. It is the hunger of the hungry, the need of the needy, the suffering of the ill, and so on. The fact that they are worse off in the relevant respect than their neighbours is relevant. But it is relevant not as an independent evil of inequality. Its relevance is in showing that their hunger is greater, their need more pressing, their suffering more hurtful, and therefore our concern for the hungry, the needy, the suffering, and not our concern for equality, makes us give them priority. (*The Morality of Freedom*, 240)

When we are comparing benefits to different people, it is easy to confuse concern with relative and absolute levels. On the Priority View, if one of two people is worse off, benefits to this person matter more. They matter more, as I have said, because this person is at a lower absolute level. But in calling this a *lower* level, I cannot help describing the *relation* between these levels. (This is why I sometimes say: benefits to people matter more the worse off *these people* are.)

X

I have explained the sense in which, on the Priority View, we do not believe in equality. Though we give priority to benefiting those who are worse off, that is not because such benefits reduce inequality.

It may be objected that, on the Priority View, we shall often aim for equality. But that is not enough to make us Egalitarians. In the same way, Utilitarians often aim for equality, because inequality has bad effects. But Utilitarians are not Egalitarians, since they regard equality as a mere means.

It is worth pursuing this analogy. There is an important Utilitarian reason to aim for equality, not of well-being, but of resources. This reason appeals to *diminishing marginal utility*, or the claim that, if resources go to people who are better off, they will benefit these people less. Utilitarians therefore argue that, whenever we transfer resources to those who are worse off, we shall produce greater benefits, and shall thereby make the outcome better.

On the telic version of the Priority View, we appeal to a similar claim. We believe that, if benefits go to people who are better off, these benefits matter less. Just as *resources* have diminishing marginal *utility*, so *utility* has diminishing marginal *moral importance*. Given the similarity between these claims, there is a second similar argument in favour of equality: this time, not of resources, but of well-being. On this argument, whenever we transfer resources to people who are worse off, the resulting benefits will not merely be, in themselves, greater. They will also, on the moral scale, matter more. There are thus *two* ways in which the outcome will be better.

The Utilitarian argument in favour of equality of resources is, as Nagel says, a 'non-egalitarian instrumental argument'. It treats such equality as good, not in itself, but only because it increases the size of the resulting benefits. A similar claim applies to the Priority View. Here too, equality is good only because it increases the moral value of these benefits.[35]

There are, however, two differences. First, diminishing marginal utility is not a universal law. In some cases, if resources went to the people who were

---

[35] We might go even further. In some Utilitarian arguments, equality plays an essential causal role. It really is a means, because it has various good effects. But, in the argument that appeals to diminishing marginal utility, this may not be so. Suppose that, as Utilitarians, we set out to redistribute resources whenever this would increase the sum of benefits. We might not even notice that, if we carry this process to its limit, equality of resources will be the result. And, even when we do notice this, we may regard equality, not as a means, but as a by-product. If we decide to aim for equality, this may be like aiming at a target merely to ensure that our arrow passes through some point en route.

better off, they would give these people *greater* benefits.[36] Utilitarians would then believe that we should transfer resources to these people. That would increase inequality.

The law of diminishing moral goodness is, in contrast, quite secure. As a moral claim, it always holds. On the Priority View, benefits to the worse off always matter more. This argument for equality is thus more securely grounded. But this does not make it different in kind. Like the Utilitarian argument, it still treats equality as a mere means.

A second difference goes deeper. Since diminishing marginal utility is an empirical generalization, the Utilitarian argument for equality is, in a way, coincidental. It merely happens to be true that, if people are better off, resources give them smaller benefits.

On the Priority View, there is no coincidence. It does not merely happen to be true that, if people are worse off, benefits to them matter more. On this view, these benefits matter more *because* these people are worse off. This is a fact, not about the size of these benefits, but about their distribution. And, in telling us to give priority to such benefits, this view has what Nagel calls 'a built-in bias towards equality'.

On the definition with which I began, the Priority View is not Egalitarian. On this view, though we ought to give priority to the worse off, that is not because we shall be reducing inequality. We do not believe that inequality is, in itself, either bad or unjust. But, since this view has a built-in bias towards equality, it could be called Egalitarian in a second, looser sense. We might say that, if we take this view, we are *Non-Relational Egalitarians*.

XI

Though equality and priority are different ideas, the distinction is often overlooked, with unfortunate results.

It is worth suggesting why this distinction has been overlooked. First, especially in earlier centuries, Egalitarians were often fighting battles in which this distinction did not arise. They were demanding legal or political equality, or attacking arbitrary privileges, or differences in status. These are not the kinds of good to which our distinction applies. And it is here that the demand for equality is most plausible.

---

[36] See, for example, Amartya Sen, *On Economic Inequality* (Oxford: Oxford University Press, 1973), 15–23. Sen has argued that this may be true of those who are crippled. While this would seldom be true of those with physical disabilities, it seems plausible for those who have certain kinds of mental illness, or impairment. If such people gain less from each unit of resources, utilitarians must claim that they should get *fewer* resources. On Sen's proposed *Weak Equity Axiom*, they should either get more, or at least no fewer.

Second, when Egalitarians considered other kinds of good, they often assumed that, if equality were achieved, this would either increase the sum of these goods, or would at least not reduce this sum. If they thought of benefits in utilitarian terms, they may have assumed that the redistribution of resources would increase the resulting benefits. If instead they were concerned only with resources, they may have regarded these as a fixed sum, which would not be altered by redistribution. In either of these cases, equality and priority cannot conflict.

Third, even when a move to equality might reduce the total sum of benefits, Egalitarians often assumed that such a move would at least bring *some* benefits to the people who were worse off. In such cases, equality and priority could not deeply conflict. Egalitarians overlooked the cases where equality could not be achieved except by levelling down.

I shall now mention certain recent statements of Egalitarian views. In the case of some views, though they are presented as being about equality, that fact is superficial. These views could be restated as views about priority, and they would then become more plausible. But other views are essentially about equality, and cannot be restated in this way.

We can start by asking which kind of view Nagel holds. In his review of Nozick's book, Nagel seemed to conflate equality and priority. He wrote:

To defend equality as a good in itself, one would have to argue that improvements in the lot of people lower on the scale of well-being took priority over greater improvements to those higher on the scale.[37]

In his article 'Equality', Nagel does argue this. And, after claiming that it is more urgent to benefit the child who is worse off, he writes:

This urgency is not necessarily decisive. It may be outweighed by other considerations, for equality is not the only value.[38]

This suggests that, to the question 'Why is it more urgent to benefit this child?', Nagel would answer, 'Because this would reduce the inequality between these two children'. But I doubt that this is really Nagel's view. Would it be just as urgent to benefit the handicapped child, even if he had no sibling who was better off? I suspect that, on Nagel's view, it would. Nagel is thus one writer who sometimes uses the language of equality, when he is really appealing to the Priority View.[39]

Consider next a remark of Dworkin's:

It is perhaps the final evil of a genuinely unequal distribution of resources that some

---

[37] Jeffrey Paul (ed.), *Reading Nozick* (Oxford: Blackwell, 1981), 203.

[38] *Mortal Questions*, 124.

[39] Similar remarks apply to sect. 117 of my *Reasons and Persons*. Nagel returns to the choices between these views in his later *Equality and Partiality*, chs. 7 and 8.

people have reason for regret just in the fact that they have been cheated of the chances others have had to make something valuable of their lives.[40]

Why does Dworkin write 'the chances *others* have had'? That suggests that there would be no evil if *no one* had such chances. That seems wrong. The real evil seems to be that these people were cheated of the chances that *they* could have had. The argument for an equal distribution is not to give people *equal* chances to make something valuable of their lives. That could be achieved by levelling down. The argument is rather that, while an unequal distribution gives good chances only to some people, the same resources, if shared out, would give them to everyone.[41]

We can now turn to the idea of distribution according to need. Several writers argue that, when we are moved by this idea, our aim is to achieve equality. Thus Raphael writes:

If the man with greater needs is given more than the man with lesser needs, the intended result is that each of them should have (or at least approach) the same level of satisfaction; the inequality of nature is corrected.[42]

Others make similar claims. Thus, when discussing the giving of extra resources to meet the needs of the ill, or handicapped, Norman writes, 'the underlying idea is one of equality. The aim is that everybody should, as far as possible, have an equally worthwhile life.'[43] As before, if this is the aim, it could be as well achieved by levelling down. This cannot be what Norman means. He could avoid this implication by omitting the word 'equally'. He could simply say, 'the aim is that everybody should, as far as possible, have a worthwhile life.' With this revision, Norman could no longer claim that equality is the underlying idea. But that, I believe, would strengthen his argument. Distribution according to need is more naturally interpreted as a form of the Priority View.[44]

Some ideas, however, cannot be reinterpreted in this way. For example, Cohen suggests that 'the right reading of egalitarianism' is that 'its purpose is to eliminate involuntary disadvantage'.[45] He means by this comparative

---

[40] 'What is Equality? Part 1: Equality of Welfare', *Philosophy & Public Affairs*, 10/3 (Summer 1981), 219.
[41] Cf. Frankfurt, *The Importance of what we Care About*, 147–8. It may of course be unfair if these people were cheated of such chances, while others had them. I am not claiming that Dworkin's claim can be fully phrased in terms of priority. But equality is not the only issue, or, it seems, the most important.
[42] D. D. Raphael, *Justice and Liberty* (London: Athlone Press, 1980). 10. Cf. 49.
[43] Richard Norman, *Free and Equal* (Oxford: Oxford University Press, 1987), 80.
[44] See, however, the excellent discussion in David Miller, 'Social Justice and the Principle of Need', in Michael Freeman and David Robertson (eds.), *The Frontiers of Political Theory* (Brighton: Harvester Press, 1980).
[45] 916.

disadvantage: being worse off than others. That is an essentially relational idea. Only equality could eliminate such disadvantage. Cohen's view could not be re-expressed in the language of priority. Remember next the view that it is in itself bad, or unfair, that some people are born abler or healthier than others, or that through the differences in the natural distribution of resources, some people are worse off than others. That view is essentially about inequality. There are many other cases. For example, Ake writes:

Justice in a society as a whole ought to be understood as a complete equality of the overall level of benefits and burdens of each member of that society.

The various maxims of distributive justice, Ake claims, can all be interpreted as having as their aim 'to restore a situation of complete equality to the greatest degree possible'.[46]

It is sometimes claimed that, though Egalitarians may seem committed to the intrinsic value of equality, that is not really so, and that no Egalitarian would believe that there was any case for levelling down.[47] But, while that is true of some Egalitarians, it is not true of all. For example, Ake writes:

What about the case of someone who suddenly comes into good fortune, perhaps entirely by his or her own efforts? Should additional burdens . . . be imposed on that person in order to restore equality and safeguard justice? . . . Why wouldn't it be just to impose any kind of additional burden whatsoever on him in order to restore the equality? The answer is that, strictly speaking, it would be . . . [48]

Ake concedes that, on his view, it would be just to level down, by imposing burdens on this person. He merely believes that the claim of justice would here be overridden, just as the claims of efficiency, or happiness, can be overridden. Levelling down would be in one way good, or be something that we would have a moral reason to do. Similarly, Temkin writes:

I, for one, believe that inequality is bad. But do I *really* think that there is some respect in which a world where only some are blind is worse than one where all are? Yes. Does this mean I think it would be better if we blinded everybody? No. Equality is not all that matters.[49]

Several other writers make such claims.[50]

[46] Christopher Ake, 'Justice as Equality', *Philosophy & Public Affairs* (Fall 1975) 71 and 77.

[47] See, for example, Robert Young. 'Envy and Inequality', *Journal of Philosophy* (Nov. 1992). (But Young may only be claiming that, in the terms I introduce below, there are no Strong Egalitarians.)

[48] 'Justice as Equality', 73.

[49] *Inequality*, 282.

[50] See, for example, Amartya Sen, *Inequality Reexamined*, 92–3.

DEREK PARFIT

XII

Since some writers are unmoved by the Levelling Down Objection, let us now reconsider what that objection claims. The objection appeals to cases where, if some inequality were removed, that would be worse for some people and better for no one. As I have said, these are the cases which raise the deepest disagreement between our two kinds of view.

On the Priority View, we do not object to inequality except when it is bad for people. We shall see nothing good in the removal of inequality, when this would benefit no one. Telic Egalitarians disagree. On their view, inequality is *in itself* bad. This implies that inequality is bad *whether or not it is bad for people*.

My last claim assumes that inequality is not in itself bad for people. Is this assumption justified? If we are worse off than other people, is that in itself bad for us?

Inequality may, of course, have bad effects. For example, if I am worse off than other people, this may put me in their power, or make me envious, or undermine my self-respect. But such effects are irrelevant here. We are concerned with the mere fact that I am worse off than other people. To isolate this fact, we can suppose that I am not aware of these people, and that their existence has no other effect on me. In such a case, though the inequality has no effects, it remains true that I am worse off than these other people. Is that bad for me?

This question is easily misunderstood. It is, of course, in one sense bad for me that I am worse off than these people. It would be better for me if I was not worse-off than them, *because I was as well-off as they actually are*. If that were true, I would be better off. But this is not the relevant comparison. Clearly, it is bad for me that *I am not* that well off. But is it bad for me that *they are*?

It may help to rephrase our question. We should not ask, 'Is it bad for me that I am worse off than other people?' This suggests that the relevant alternative is my being better off. Rather we should ask, 'Is it bad for me that, unknown to me, there are other people who are better off than me? Would it be better for me if there were no such people? Would it be better for me if these people had never existed, or were as badly off as me?'

The answer depends on our view about what is in or against people's interests, and there are several theories here. But I shall simply claim that, on all the plausible versions of these theories, the answer is No. The mere fact of inequality is not, in itself, bad for the people who are worse off. Such inequalities may be naturally unfair. And it would of course be better for these people if they themselves were better off. But it would not be better for them if, without any effects on them, the other people were just as badly off.[51]

We can now return to my earlier claim. For Telic Egalitarians, inequality is in itself bad. If that is so, it must be bad even when it is not bad for people. For these Egalitarians, inequality is bad *even when it is bad for no one*.

That may seem enough reason to reject this view. We may think that nothing can be bad if it is bad for no one. But, before we assess this objection, we must distinguish two versions of this view. Consider these alternatives:

(1) Everyone at some level
(2) Some at this level   Others better off

In outcome (1) everyone is equally well off. In outcome (2), some people are better off. In (2) there is inequality, but this outcome is worse for no one. For Telic Egalitarians, the inequality in (2) is bad. Could this make (2), all things considered, a worse outcome than (1)?

Some Egalitarians answer Yes. These people do not believe that inequality would always make outcomes, all things considered, worse. On their view, the loss of equality could be morally outweighed by a sufficient increase in the sum of benefits. But inequality is a great evil. It *can* make an outcome worse, even when this outcome would be better for everyone. Those who hold this view I shall call *Strong Egalitarians*.

Others hold a different view. Since they believe that inequality is bad, they agree that outcome (2) is in one way worse. But they do not think it worse on balance, or all things considered. In a move from (1) to (2), some people would become better off. For these Egalitarians, the loss of equality would be morally outweighed by the benefits to these people. On their view, (2) would be, on balance, better than (1). Those who hold this view I shall call *Moderates*.

This version of Egalitarianism is often overlooked, or dismissed. People typically produce the standard objection to Strong Egalitarianism: the appeal to cases where a move to inequality would be bad for no one. They then either ignore the Moderate view, or treat it as not worth considering. They assume that, if we claim that the badness of the inequality would always be outweighed by the extra benefits, our view must be trivial.[52]

This, I believe, is a mistake. Our view would indeed be trivial if we held

---

[51] For a contrary view, which would need a further discussion, see John Broome, *Weighing Goods* (Oxford: Blackwell, 1991), ch. 9.

[52] See, for example, Antony Flew, *The Politics of Procrustes* (Buffalo: Prometheus, 1981), 26; McKerlie, 'Egalitarianism', 232. See also Nozick, *Anarchy, State, and Utopia*, 211.

that any loss of equality, however great, could be outweighed by any gain in utility, however small. But that is not what Moderates claim. They claim only that, in *this* kind of case, those in which greater inequality would be worse for no one, the badness of the inequality would in fact be outweighed by the extra benefits. This claim can be subdivided into a pair of claims. One is a view about the relative importance of equality and utility. The other, which has been overlooked, is a claim about the structure of these cases. If there is greater inequality, in a way that is worse for no one, the inequality must come from benefits to certain people. And there cannot be a *great* loss of equality unless these benefits are also great. These gains and losses would roughly march in step.

In the simplest cases, this is obvious. Consider these alternatives:

(1) All at 100
(2) Half at 100   Half at 101
(3) Half at 100   Half at 110
(4) Half at 100   Half at 200

In a move from (1) to (2), there would be a small gain in utility but only a small loss in equality. In a move from (1) to (3) the loss in equality would be greater, but so would be the gain in utility. As we move lower down the list, both gains and losses would steadily grow. In more complicated cases, the point still holds. If one of two outcomes involves more inequality, but is worse for no one, the better-off must gain. There can be much more inequality only if the better-off gain a great deal. But there would then be much more utility.[53]

Since these gains and losses roughly march in step, there is room for Moderates to hold a significant position. Moderates claim that, in all such cases, the gain in utility would outweigh the loss in equality. That is consistent with the claim that, in other kinds of case, that may not be so. Moderates can claim that *some* gains in utility, even if *great*, would *not* outweigh some losses in equality. Consider, for example, these alternatives:

(1) All at 100
(4) Half at 100   Half at 200
(5) Half at 70   Half at 200

[53] Shelly Kagan has suggested a possible counter-example: one in which a very few people became much better off than everyone else. The gain in utility would here be very small; and, on certain views, the loss of equality would be great. On Temkin's account, that would be true of views which take the badness of inequality to depend on how much worse off people are than the best-off person. On other views, however, which I find more plausible, the loss of equality would not be great. That would be true of views which appeal to how much worse off people are than the average person, or than everyone who is better off than them.

Moderates believe that, compared with (1), (4) is better. But they might claim that (5) is worse. This would not be a trivial claim. In a move from (1) to (5), the worse-off would lose, but the better-off would gain more than three times as much. Compared with (1), (5) would involve a great gain in utility. But, for these Moderates, this gain would be too small to outweigh the loss of equality. They would here choose a smaller sum of benefits, for the sake of a more equal distribution. That is why, though Moderate, they are true Egalitarians.

Return now to the Levelling Down Objection. Strong Egalitarians believe that, in some cases, a move towards inequality, even though it would be worse for no-one, would make the outcome worse. This may seen incredible. We may claim that one of two outcomes *cannot* be worse if it would be worse for no one. To challenge Strong Egalitarians, it would be enough to defend this claim.

To challenge Moderates, this claim may not be enough. Moderates believe that, if the outcome with greater inequality would be worse for no one, it would *not* be a worse outcome. But their claim is only that it would not be worse on balance, or all-things-considered. They must agree that, on their view, this outcome would be *in one way* worse. On their view, inequality is *bad*, even when it is bad for no one. To reject their view, we must claim that even this cannot be true.

In the space remaining, I can make only a few remarks about this disagreement. It is widely assumed that, if an outcome is worse for no one, it cannot be in any way worse. This we can call *the Person-affecting Claim*.

This claim might be defended by an appeal to some view about the nature of morality, or moral reasoning. Some, for example, argue as follows. It is not hard to see how an outcome can be worse for particular people. But it can seem puzzling how an outcome can be simply worse—worse, period. What is meant by this impersonal use of 'worse'? Some suggest that this use of 'worse' can be explained, or constructed, out of the concept 'worse for'. There are other lines of thought which may lead to the Person-affecting Claim, such as a contractualist view about moral reasoning.[54]

Egalitarians might respond by defending a different meta-ethical view. Or they might argue that this claim has unacceptable implications, since it conflicts too sharply with some of our beliefs.

Temkin responds in the second way. The Person-affecting Claim, he argues, is incompatible with many of our ideals.[55]

---

[54] Such as the view advanced in Thomas Scanlon's 'Contractualism and Utilitarianism', in Amartya Sen and Bernard Williams (eds.), *Utilitarianism and Beyond* (Cambridge: Cambridge University Press, 1982).

[55] *Inequality*, ch. 9.

Temkin's best example seems to me his appeal to what he calls 'proportional justice'. Would it not be bad, he asks, if 'the evilest mass murderers fare better than the most benign saints?' But this might not be bad for any of these people.

It may be bad that the saints fare worse than the murderers. But this comparative element is too close to the question at issue: whether inequality is bad. So we should forget the saints. Is it bad that the murderers fare as well as they do? Would it be better if they fared worse?

We might think this better if it would give the murderers the punishment that they deserve. Note that, in thinking this, we are not merely claiming that they ought to be punished. We may think that, if they are not punished, perhaps because they cannot be caught, this would be bad. The badness here may not involve any further wrong-doing. And we may think this bad even if their punishment would do no one any good—perhaps because, as in Kant's example, our community is about to dissolve.

If we accept this retributive view, we must reject the Person-affecting Claim. We believe that, if people are not punished as they deserve, this would be bad, even if it would be bad for no one. And, if that is true, the same could be true of the badness of inequality.

Even if we reject the retributive view, as I do, this analogy may still be useful. Consider the claim that it would have been better if Hitler, unknown to others, had suffered for what he did. If we reject this claim, what would our reason be? Would it be enough to say, 'How could this have been better? It would not have been better for him.' This remark may seem to us inadequate. We may reject retribution, not because it is good for no one, but because we do not believe in the kind of free will that it seems to require. Perhaps we believe that, to deserve to suffer for what we do, we would have to be responsible for our own characters, in a way that seems to us to make no sense.

If that is why we reject retribution, this analogy may still, in a somewhat curious way, tell against the Person-affecting Claim. We believe that, in one sense, retribution could have been good, even when it is good for no one. Or rather, what makes this impossible is not the truth of the Person-affecting Claim, but the incoherence of the required kind of free will. We might imagine coming to believe that this kind of freedom is not incoherent. We may agree that, in that case, we could not reject retribution *merely* by claiming that it is good for no one. If that objection would not be sufficient, why should it be sufficient as an objection to Egalitarianism?

Fully to assess the Person-affecting Claim, we would need to discuss meta-ethics, or the nature of morality and moral reasoning. Since I cannot do that here, I shall merely express an opinion.[56] The, Person affecting Claim has, I think, less force than, and cannot be used to strengthen, the Levelling Down Objection.

XIII

I shall now summarise what I have claimed.

I began by discussing the view that it is in itself bad, or unfair, if some people are worse off than others through no fault or choice of theirs. This, the Telic Egalitarian view, can seem very plausible. But it faces the Levelling Down Objection. This objection seems to me to have great force, but is not, I think, decisive.

Suppose we began by being Telic Egalitarians, but are convinced by this objection. Suppose that we cannot believe that, if inequality were removed in a way that is bad for some people, and better for no one, that change would be in any way good. If we are to salvage something of our view, we then have two alternatives.

We might become Deontic Egalitarians. We might believe that, though we should sometimes aim for equality, that is not because we would thereby make the outcome better. We must then explain our view in some other way. And the resulting view may have a narrower scope. For example, it may apply only to goods of certain kinds, such as those that are co-operatively produced, and it may apply only to inequality between certain people, such as members of the same community.

We may also have to abandon some of our beliefs. Reconsider the Divided World:

(1) Half at 100   Half at 200
(2) Half at 140   Half at 140

On the Deontic View, we cannot claim that it would be better if the situation changed from (1) to (2). Our view is only about what people ought to do, and makes no comparisons between states of affairs.

Our alternative is to move to the Priority View. We could then keep our view about the Divided World. It is true that, in a change from (1) to (2), the better off would lose more than the worse off would gain. That is why, in utilitarian terms, (2) is worse than (1). But, on the Priority View, though the better off would lose more, the gain to the worse off counts for more.

---

[56] Another objection to the Person-affecting View comes from what I have called *the Non-Identity Problem* (in my *Reasons and Persons*, ch. 16).

Benefits to the worse off do more to make the outcome better. We could claim that this is why (1) is worse than (2).

The Priority View often coincides with the belief in equality. But, as I have suggested, they are quite different kinds of view. They can be attacked or defended in different ways. The same is true of Telic and Deontic views. So, in trying to decide what we believe, the first step is to draw these distinctions. Taxonomy is unexciting, but it needs to be done.

Appendix: Rawls's View

How do the distinctions I have drawn apply to Rawls's theory?

Rawls's Difference Principle seems to be an extreme version of the Priority View: one which gives *absolute* priority to benefiting those who are worse off. There are, however, three qualifications. We should apply the Difference Principle (1) only to the basic structure of society, (2) only in conjunction with Rawls's other principles, which require equal liberty and equality of opportunity, and (3) we do not apply this principle to individuals, but only to the representative member of the worst-off group.

Instead of claiming that the worst-off group should be as well off as possible, Rawls states his view in a less direct way. He makes claims about when inequality is unjust. On his view, whether some pattern of inequality is unjust depends on its effects upon the worst-off group. What these effects are depends on what alternatives were possible. Let us say that inequality *harms* the worst-off group when it is true that, without this inequality, this group could have been better off. Inequality *benefits* this group when it is true that, in every possible alternative without this inequality, they would have been even worse off.

Rawls often claims

(A) Inequality is not unjust if it benefits the worst-off group.

Egalitarians might accept this claim. They might say, 'Even in such cases, inequality is bad. But it is not unjust. Such inequality is, all things considered, justified by the fact that it benefits the worst off.' They might add that this inequality is, in a way, naturally unfair. It would then be a case of what Barry calls justified unfairness.

Rawls's arguments do not suggest that such inequality is, in itself, bad. He seems to accept claim (A) in the spirit of the Priority View. On his Difference Principle, since we should give absolute priority to the worst-off group, if inequality benefits this group, it is straightforwardly morally required. There is no moral balancing to be done—no intrinsic badness needing to be outweighed.

Rawls just as often claims

(B) Inequality is unjust if it harms the worst-off group.

Egalitarians might make this claim. But, here again, it could be fully explained on the absolute version of the Priority View. On this view, if the worst-off group could have been made better off, this is what should have been done. What is unjust is that the required priority has not been given to these people.

I have suggested that Rawls's view could be regarded as one version of the Priority View. What would show that it *cannot* be so regarded?

That might be shown by Rawls's answer to a further question. On his view, inequality is *not* unjust if it benefits the worst-off group, and it *is* unjust if it harms this group. What if inequality neither benefits nor harms this group? Would it then be unjust?

Suppose that, in some case, the only possible alternatives are these:

(1) Everyone at some level
(2) Some at this level   Others better off

If we choose (2), there would be inequality, and this would not benefit those who are worst-off. But there is no way in which the gains to the better off could be shared by both groups. The benefits to the better off are, for some reason, not transferable. Since that is so, though the inequality in (2) would not benefit the worst-off group, it would not be worse for them.

In such cases, on the Priority View, we *must* favour (2). The benefits to the better off are unequivocally good. The fact that they increase inequality is, for us, of no concern. But, if we are Egalitarians, we might oppose (2). We might claim that the inequality in (2) is bad, or unjust.

Would Rawls agree? If he would, this *would* show that he does not hold a version of the Priority View.

It is clear that, on Rawls's view, inequality is not unjust *if* it benefits the worst-off group. Does he mean if and only if? Is inequality unjust if it does *not* benefit this group?

The answer may seem to be Yes. Rawls's Second Principle merely reads 'Social and economic inequalities are to be arranged so that they are . . . to the greatest benefit of the least advantaged'. This is compatible with either answer. But his General Conception reads. 'All social primary goods . . . are to be distributed equally unless an unequal distribution . . . is to the advantage of the least favored'. Similarly, Rawls writes, 'Injustice, then, is simply inequalities that are not to the benefit of all.' And he often makes such claims.[57] This suggest that he accepts.

(C) Inequality is unjust, unless it benefits the worst-off group.

But Rawls may not intend (C). When he makes these claims, he may be assuming that the levels of the different groups are what he calls *close-knit*. This is true when any

---

[57] Cf. Rawls, *A Theory of Justice*: 'The inequality in expectation is permissible only if lowering it would make the working class even . . . worse off.' (78) 'No one is to benefit from these contingencies except in ways that redound to the well-being of others.' (100) 'Those who have been favoured by nature . . . may gain from their good fortune only on terms that improve the situation of those who have lost out.' (101) 'The more fortunate are to benefit only in ways that help those who have lost out.' (179) 'Inequalities are permissible when they maximize, or at least contribute to, the long-term expectations of the least fortunate group in society.' (151)

change in the level of one group would change the levels of the other groups.[58] When levels are close-knit, if inequality does *not* benefit the worst-off group, it must *harm* that group. In such cases, (C) coincides with

(D) Inequality is unjust only if it harms the worst-off group.

In the passages to which I have referred, this may be all that Rawls means.

In one section of his book, Rawls directly addresses my question. He considers a case in which the alternatives are these:

(1) Two people are both at some level
(2) One is at this level   The other is better off

On Rawls's Difference Principle, which of these outcomes should we choose?

Rawls gives three answers. The Difference Principle, he writes, 'is a strongly egalitarian conception in the sense that unless there is a distribution that makes both persons better off . . . an equal distribution is to be preferred'. (76) On this first answer, outcome (2) is *worse* than outcome (1). This remark *does* commit Rawls to a version of claim (C). It tells us to avoid inequality unless it benefits those who are worst-off.

Rawls's second answer is implied by the indifference map with which he illustrates this case:[59]

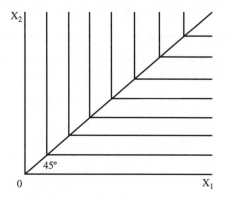

This shows (2) to be *as good as* (1). On this map, (1) would be some point on the 45 degree diagonal, and (2) would be on the horizontal line passing through this point. Since this is an *indifference* map, all points on this line are equally good. As Rawls writes, 'No matter how much either person's situation is improved, there is no gain from the standpoint of the difference principle unless the other gains also'. No *gain*

---

[58] As Rawls writes: 'It is impossible to raise or lower the expectation of any representative man without raising or lowering the expectation of every other representative man'. (80) Though he knows that this is not always true, and he claims that his principles apply even when it is not true, he writes, at one point, 'close-knitness is assumed in order to simplify the statement of the Difference Principle.' Perhaps it was assumed in all of the passages quoted above.

[59] Rawls, *A Theory of Justice*, fig. 5 on p. 76.

from the standpoint of this principle; but also, as the indifference map implies, no *loss*. Later in this section, however, Rawls writes, 'the difference principle is compatible with the principle of efficiency'. (79) This implies that (2) is *better* than (1). Compared with (1), (2) is better for someone, and worse for no one.

Given the further assumptions that Rawls makes, and the use to which he puts his principles, this inconsistency is not in practice damaging. But, for the purposes of theory, it is worth asking which of these three answers is Rawls's true view. If he accepts the first or second answer, he cannot hold a version of the Priority View. And this would affect the arguments that could be given for or against his view.

I believe that the third answer, though less often supported in his text, is Rawls's true view. He would accept, not (C), but (D). On his view, inequality is unjust only if it worsens the position of those who are worse off. That is what is implied by the Lexical version of his Difference Principle. On that principle, if we cannot make other groups better off, we should, if we can, make the *best*-off group even better off. We should, that is, *increase* inequality, in a way that does not benefit any of the people who are worse off.

More important, this is the view to which we are led by Rawls's main arguments. From the standpoint of the Original Position, we would clearly favour giving benefits to the better off, when this would not worsen the position of those who are worse off. For all we know, we might *be* the people who are better off. On Rawls's assumptions, we would not limit the gains to ourselves if we *were* in this position for the sake of limiting other people's gains if we were not. Describing the motivation of his parties, Rawls writes: 'Nor do they try to gain relative to one another . . . They strive for as high an absolute score as possible. They do not wish a high or a low score for their opponents, nor do they seek to maximize or minimize the difference between their successes and those of others.' (144)

As these last remarks suggest, Rawls's view is not merely compatible with the Priority View. Given his main argument, it *must* be, in its content, a version of this view, since it must be concerned with absolute not relative levels. On the Difference Principle, we should make the worst-off group as well off as possible. It is quite irrelevant whether, in so doing, we reduce or increase inequality. This means that, on my definition, Rawls is at most a Non-Relational Egalitarian.

Rawls's view is not, however, *merely* a version of the Priority View. If it were, it would be implausibly extreme. If we are not egalitarians, and are not concerned with whether some people are worse off *than others*, it is hard to see why we should give *absolute* priority to benefiting people who are worse off. And that view seems too extreme even when, as in Rawls's case, it applies only to the basic structure of society, and only to the representative member of the worst-off group. If we are not concerned with relative levels, why should the smallest benefit to the representative worst-off person count for infinitely more than much greater benefits to other representative people?

To explain this feature of Rawls's view, we should, I believe, reintroduce the moral importance of equality. An objection to natural inequality is, I have suggested, one of the foundations of Rawls's theory. And Rawls himself claims that, in an account of justice, equal division is the natural first step, and provides the benchmark by reference to which we can defend our final principles.

As Barry notes, this suggests a different way to defend Rawls's Difference Principle.[60] First we argue for equality, by appealing to the arbitrariness of the natural lottery. Then we allow departures from equality provided that these are not worse for those who are worst-off. This explains why, in Rawls's phrase, the worst-off have the *veto*, so that benefits to them should have absolute priority.

[60] See Barry, *Theories of Justice*, ch. VI.

12

QUALITY OF LIFE MEASURES IN HEALTH CARE AND MEDICAL ETHICS

DAN BROCK

INTRODUCTION

There has been considerable philosophical work during the last two decades, especially in the United States but not limited to there, in a relatively new field called medical ethics. My aim in this paper is to explore what illumination that body of work might offer to our understanding of the quality of life. If one looks only to the medical ethics literature explicitly addressing the notion of the quality of life, there are few sustained analyses of it and of its role in various medical and health care contexts. Consequently, it is necessary to look more broadly to issues and areas of research that often do not explicitly address the quality of life, but that nevertheless have an important bearing on it. I believe there are two main areas of work in medical ethics that fit this criterion. The first is work on ethical frameworks for medical treatment decision-making in a clinical context, including accounts of informed consent and life-sustaining treatment decisions. The second is the development of valuational measures of outcomes of health care treatments and programmes; these outcome measures are designed to guide health policy and so must be able to be applied to substantial numbers of people, including across or even between whole societies. The two main parts of this paper will address these two main bodies of work. Before doing so, however, several preliminary issues need to be briefly addressed.

I have mentioned that the literature that I will be summarizing and drawing on often does not explicitly address the concept of the 'quality of life', but instead uses other notions that are either closely related or roughly equivalent in the context. Sometimes a notion of 'health' is employed, particularly in its broader interpretations, as exemplified in the World Health Organization definition of 'health' as a state of complete physical, mental,

From Dan Brock, 'Quality of Life Measures in Health Care and Medical Ethics', in Martha C. Nussbaum and Amartya Sen (eds.), *The Quality of Life* (Oxford: Clarendon Press, 1993).

and social well-being.[1] The notion of patient 'well-being', independent of its use within a definition of health, is also often employed for evaluation of outcomes in health care. Another conceptual framework commonly employed for evaluating health care outcomes is the assessment of the benefits and burdens of that care for the patient (and sometimes for others as well). Still another common conceptual framework often employed looks to the effects of health care on patients' interests, with a best interests standard particularly prominent for patients whose preferences cannot be determined. These and other conceptual schemes are not fully interchangeable in health care, much less in broader contexts. Nevertheless, they all have in common their use in evaluating health care outcomes for patients and their employment as at least part of a comprehensive account of a good life for persons. I shall freely draw here on each of these conceptual frameworks, and others, though indicating where differences between them become important.

The 'quality of life' can be given a number of more or less broad interpretations, depending on the scope of the evaluative factors concerning a person's life that it is taken to include. Medicine and health care often affect a person's life in only some limited areas or respects. Nevertheless, my concern will be with the broadest conception of, in Derek Parfit's words, 'what makes a life go best', and I shall try to show that medicine and health care may affect and illuminate more aspects of that question than might at first be thought.[2] No concept is entirely apt or widely accepted in either philosophical or common usage for this broad role, but I shall use the concept of a 'good life' to refer to the quality of life of persons in its broadest interpretation.

It is common in much philosophical work on theories of the good for persons or of a good life to distinguish three broad kinds of theory. While this classification misses some distinctions important for my purposes here, it provides a natural starting point. These three alternative theories I will call the hedonist, preference satisfaction, and ideal theories of a good life.[3] Much of the philosophical work on these theories has been in the service of developing an account of 'utility', broadly construed for employment in consequentialist moral theories.[4] What is common to hedonist theories, as I will

---

[1] Lester Breslow, 'A Quantitative Approach to the World Health Organization Definition of Health: Physical, Mental and Social Well-Being', *International Journal of Epidemiology*, 1 (1972), 347–55.

[2] Derek Parfit, *Reasons and Persons* (Oxford: Oxford University Press, 1984); cf. esp. app. I.

[3] See T. M. Scanlon's discussion in this volume of these alternative theories. What I call preference satisfaction and ideal theories he calls desire and substantive good theories.

[4] Some time ago I discussed these as alternative interpretations of utility (Dan W. Brock, 'Recent Work in Utilitarianism', *American Philosophical Quarterly*, 10 (1973), 241–76). The most subtle and detailed recent discussion of these alternative theories is James Griffin, *Well-Being* (Oxford: Oxford University Press, 1986), chs. 1–4.

understand them here, is that they take the ultimate good for persons to be the undergoing of certain kinds of conscious experience. The particular kinds of conscious experience are variously characterized as pleasure, happiness, or the satisfaction or enjoyment that typically accompanies the successful pursuit of our desires. Particular states of the person that do not make reference to conscious experience, such as having diseased or healthy lungs, and particular activities, such as studying philosophy or playing tennis, are part of a good life on this view only to the extent that they produce the valuable conscious experience.

Preference satisfaction theories take a good life to consist in the satisfaction of people's desires or preferences. I here understand desires or preferences as taking states of affairs as their objects: for example, my desire to be in Boston on Tuesday is satisfied just when the state of affairs of my being in Boston on Tuesday obtains. This is to be distinguished from any feelings of satisfaction, understood as a conscious experience of mine, that I may experience if I am in Boston on Tuesday. The difference is clearest in cases in which my desire is satisfied, but I either do not or could not know that it is and so receive no satisfaction from getting what I desire: for example, my desire that my children should have long and fulfilling lives, a state of affairs that will only fully obtain after my death. For preference satisfaction theories of a good life to be at all plausible, they must allow for some correcting or 'laundering' of a person's actual preferences.[5] The most obvious example is the need to correct for misinformed preferences: for example, my desire to eat the sandwich before me not knowing that its ingredients are bad and will make me ill. Other corrections of preferences have also been supported by proponents of the preference satisfaction theory that are compatible with its underlying idea that ultimately what is good for persons is that they should get what they most want or prefer.

The third kind of theory holds that at least part of a good life consists neither of any conscious experience of a broadly hedonist sort nor of the satisfaction of the person's corrected preferences or desires, but instead consists of the realization of specific, explicitly normative ideals.[6] For example, many have held that one component of a good life consists in being a self-determined or autonomous agent, and that this is part of a good life for a

---

[5] Virtually all discussions of desire or preference satisfaction theories of the good contain some provision for correcting preferences. One of the better treatments, with extensive references to the literature, is Robert Goodin, 'Laundering Preferences', in Jon Elster and Aanund Hylland (eds.), *Foundations of Social Choice Theory* (Cambridge: Cambridge University Press, 1986), 75–101.

[6] What I call ideal theories are what Parfit (*Reasons and Persons*) calls 'objective list' theories. I prefer the label 'ideal theories', because what is usually distinctive about this kind of theory is its proposal of specific, normative ideals of the person.

person even if he or she is no happier as a result and has no desire to be autonomous. Ideal theories will differ both in the specific ideals the theories endorse and in the place they give to happiness and preference satisfaction in their full account of the good for persons. There is a strong tendency in much of the philosophical literature to seek a simple, comprehensive theory, such as the hedonist or preference satisfaction theories: proponents of ideal theories commonly acknowledge a plurality of component ideals that place constraints on and/or supplement the extent to which happiness and/or preference satisfaction serves a person's good. The account I will develop of quality of life judgements in health care strongly suggests that it is a mistake to let the attractions of a simple, unified theory of a good life force a choice between the hedonist and preference satisfaction theories. Instead, these quality-of-life judgments suggest the importance of giving independent place to the considerations singled out by each of the three main alternative theories, as ideal theories do, in any adequate overall account of the quality of life or of a good life for persons. The quality of life judgements made in medicine and health care also help some to fill in the content of a theory of a good life.

A major issue concerning ethical judgements generally, and judgements concerning a good life in particular, is the sense and extent to which such judgements are objective or subjective. A number of different senses have been given to the notions of 'objectivity' and 'subjectivity' in these contexts, and other essays in this volume take up some of these general theoretical issues and will develop some of these alternative senses.[7] I will not attempt an extended analysis of this general theoretical issue here. Nevertheless, one sense in which what constitutes a good life for a particular person is believed to be subjective or objective mirrors the distinction between hedonist and preference satisfaction theories on the one hand, and ideal theories on the other. Hedonist and preference theories are both subjective in the sense that both hold that what is good for a particular person depends on what in fact makes that person happy or what that person in fact (with appropriate corrections) desires. (This is compatible, of course, with acknowledging that what will make a particular person happy or satisfy his or her preferences is an 'objective matter of fact', even if often an extremely difficult one to determine.)

Ideal theories are objective, or at least contain objective components, in the sense that they hold a good life for a person is, at least in part, objectively

---

[7] See Hilary Putnam, 'Objectivity and the Science–Ethics Distinction', Ruth Anna Putnam, 'Commentary on Michael Walzer', and Michael Walzer, 'Objectivity and Social Meaning', all in Nussbaum and Sen (eds.), *The Quality of Life*.

determined by the correct or justified ideals of the good life, and does not in those respects depend either on what makes that person happy or on what that person's (even corrected) preferences happen to be. The question of whether accounts of a good life are objective or subjective is, then, an explicitly normative issue about what is the correct or most justified substantive theory of a good life. This sense of the objective-subjective dispute has been a central concern in the debates in medical ethics and health care about the quality of life. Interestingly, I believe that medicine and health care provide some of the most persuasive instances for both the objective *and* the subjective components of a good life, and so point the way towards a theory that incorporates hedonist, preference, and ideal components.

Haavi Morreim has distinguished a different sense in which quality of life judgements in medicine are either objective or subjective.[8] In her account, objective quality of life judgements are made on the basis of intersubjectively observable, material facts about a person (facts concerning his or her body, mind, functional capabilities, and environment), together with a socially shared evaluation of those facts, specifically of how those facts determine the person's quality of life. Subjective quality of life judgements also appeal to material facts about a person and his or her condition (though these may also include facts about the person's private psychological states), together with *that person's* value judgements about how those facts affect his or her quality of life. According to this account, the essential issue that determines whether a quality of life judgement is objective or subjective is whether the evaluative judgements concerning a particular individual's quality of life are and must be shared by some wider group or are, instead, only the individual's own. Since there are many possible wider social groups, one respect in which one could make sense of degrees of this kind of objectivity is in terms of the size, breadth, or nature of the wider social group; important variants include an individual's community or larger society, and a maximally wide group might be all humans or rational agents. It should be obvious that my and Morreim's senses of the objective-subjective distinction are independent: the individual whose quality of life is in question might hold any of the three substantive theories of the good for persons distinguished above, as might any wider social group.

A full conception of a good life for a person that does not reduce to a single property like happiness or preference satisfaction must assign a weight to the various components that contribute to that life's being good, though there may not be full comparability between different components and so in

---

[8] E. Haavi Moreim, 'Computing the Quality of Life', in G. J. Agich and C. E. Begley (eds.), *The Price of Health* (Dordrecht: Reidel, 1986), 45–69.

turn only partial comparability between different possible life courses for a person. Amartya Sen has suggested in several places the formal device of understanding these different components as independent vectors, each of which contributes to an overall assessment of the degree to which a person has a good life.[9] There are several benefits to an analysis of what constitutes a good life into a number of independent vectors. First, it allows us to accept part of what proponents of each of the three traditional theories of a good life have wanted to insist on, namely the theoretical independence of those components. The three components of happiness, preference satisfaction, and ideals of a good life can each be represented by their individual vectors, or subdivided further into distinct vectors within each component, having independent weight within an overall account of a good life. Second, the vector approach quite naturally yields the possibility of two senses of partial comparability of the quality of different lives. For a single individual, alternative possible lives may be only partially commensurable if one alternative life provides a greater value on one vector, but a lesser value on another vector, than another possible life. But for two different persons it is important that at least partial comparability between their lives may be possible, contrary to the dogma about the impossibility of interpersonal comparisons of utility, by comparing common vectors or by comparing different changes in common vectors making up a good life for each. Medicine and health care provide strong grounds for insisting on these independent vectors and, perhaps more important, also suggest a content and structure to the ideals along the lines proposed by Sen in his work on agency and capabilities, which drew on settings largely outside of health care.

We also need to distinguish between the relative importance of a particular feature or condition, say as represented by a specific vector, in its contribution to a person having a good life, compared with what I shall call its broader moral importance. A simple example will suffice. One condition that may plausibly contribute to a person's quality of life or good life is his or her physical mobility. It may be possible to specify roughly a normal level of physical mobility for persons of a similar age at a particular historical stage and in a particular society, and then to specify roughly levels of mobility say 25 per cent below and 25 per cent above the norm, such that the effect on a

---

[9] Sen's main discussion of the 'vector view' applied to the notion of utility is in 'Plural Utility', *Proceedings of the Aristotelian Society*, 81 (1980), 193–218. I am much indebted to Sen's subtle discussion in a number of places of distinctions of importance to conceptions of the quality of life and of a good life. Besides his essay in this volume ['Capability and Well-Being', in Nussbaum and Sen (eds.), *The Quality of Life*], see esp. *Commodities and Capabilities* (Amsterdam: Elsevier Science Publishers, 1985), 'Well-Being, Agency and Freedom: The Dewey Lectures', *Journal of Philosophy*, 82 (1985), 169–221, and *The Standard of Living* (Cambridge: Cambridge University Press, 1987).

person's quality of life in moving from 25 per cent below the norm up to the norm is quantitatively roughly the same as moving from the norm to 25 per cent above it. While the degree or importance of the two changes in a person's quality of life or good life may be roughly the same, it can none the less be consistently held that these two comparable effects on the person's quality of life have different *moral* importance or priority. It might be held, for example, that on grounds of equality of opportunity bringing a person's mobility from 25 per cent below the norm up to the norm has greater moral priority than increasing his mobility from the norm to 25 per cent above it. The general point is that aspects of a person's quality of life may play a role not only in judgements about his quality of life or about how good a life he has, but also in other distinct moral and political judgements, or in the application of independent moral principles such as a principle of equal opportunity. This is, of course, a thoroughly familiar point in moral and political philosophy generally, and concerning consequentialist moralities in particular, against which it is often objected that they ignore the moral importance of whether the good is fairly or justly distributed. In the present context its importance is in reminding us to distinguish judgements concerning the improvement or reduction of people's quality of life from other independent moral evaluations of those same changes so as not to confuse needlessly the nature of quality of life judgements in health care.

ETHICAL FRAMEWORKS FOR HEALTH CARE TREATMENT DECISION-MAKING

The first broad area of work within medical ethics bearing on the concept of the quality of life concerns the aims of medicine and the account of medical treatment decision-making appropriate to those aims. It may be helpful to begin with a natural objection to thinking that these issues in medical ethics will illuminate any broad notion of the good life. On the contrary, as Leon Kass has argued, medicine's proper end is the much narrower one of health, or the healthy human being, and other goals such as happiness and gratifying patient desires are false goals for medicine.[10] Kass understands health to be a naturalistically defined property of individual biological organisms, organisms which must be understood as organic wholes, and whose parts

have specific functions that define their nature as parts: the bone marrow for making red blood cells; the lungs for exchange of oxygen and carbon dioxide; the heart for pumping the blood. Even at a biochemical level, every molecule can be characterized

[10] Leon Kass, *Toward a More Natural Science* (New York: Free Press, 1985).

in terms of its function. The parts, both macroscopic and microscopic, contribute to the maintenance and functioning of the other parts, and make possible the maintenance and functioning of the whole.[11]

What constitutes well-functioning varies with the particular biological species in question, but Kass is at pains to argue that 'health is a natural standard or norm—not a moral norm, not a "value" as opposed to a "fact", not an obligation—a state of being that reveals itself in activity as a standard of bodily excellence or fitness'.[12]

Kass's work constitutes one of the more ambitious attempts to justify two common-sense beliefs about the 'objectivity' of medicine: that the aim of medicine is and should be the patient's health, and that health is a biologically determined, objective matter of fact. If so, then physicians, with their impressive body of scientific knowledge concerning human biological functioning and the impact of therapeutic interventions on diseases and their natural courses, would seem to be the proper judges of whether we are healthy and, if we are not, what therapeutic interventions will be likely to make us more so. This hardly begins to do justice to the subtlety of Kass's view—though it is a view that I believe to be fundamentally mistaken—but it does bring out why one might think medicine, properly aimed only at human health defined in terms of biological functioning, has little to teach us regarding broader social issues about the quality of life. I believe it is fair to say that the main body of work in medical ethics within the last two decades has rejected Kass's view that the sole proper aim of medicine is health, defined in naturalistic, biological terms, and the ethical framework for medical treatment decision-making that it would seem to imply. We need to see how the alternative, broader view of the aims of medicine that should guide medical treatment decision-making bears on an understanding of the quality of life.

It has become a commonplace, at least in the developed countries, that medicine has achieved the capacity commonly to offer to patients suffering from particular diseases a number of alternative treatments, and to extend patients' lives in circumstances in which the benefit to the patient of doing so is increasingly problematic. In the United States this has led to patients pursuing various means of gaining control over decisions about their treat-

---

[11] *Toward a More Natural Science*, 171.

[12] Ibid. 173. For a more philosophically sophisticated analysis of the concept of health that also construes it in functional terms as a natural, biological norm not involving value judgements, see Christopher Boorse, 'On the Distinction between Disease and Illness', *Philosophy and Public Affairs*, 5 (1975), 49–68, and 'Health as a Theoretical Concept', *Philosophy of Science*, 44 (1977). One of the most useful collections of papers on concepts of health is Arthur L. Caplan *et al.* (eds.), *Concepts of Health and Disease: Interdisciplinary Perspectives* (Reading, Mass.: Addison-Wesley, 1981).

ment. In the case of competent patients, a broad consensus has developed that such patients have the right to decide about their care in a process of shared decision-making with their physicians and to reject any proffered treatment. In the case of incompetent patients, an analogous consensus has been developing that an incompetent patient's surrogate, seeking to decide as the patient would have decided in the circumstances if competent, is likewise entitled to decide about the patient's care with the patient's physician and to reject any care the patient would not have wanted—though the consensus concerning incompetent patients is less broad and more ringed with qualifications. Each consensus is reflected in a large medical ethics literature, a growing body of legal decisions, legal mechanisms such as Living Wills and Durable Powers of Attorney for Health Care, whose purpose is to ensure patients' control over their care, pronouncements and studies of authoritative bodies and commissions, policies of health care institutions, and the practice of health care professionals.[13]

The common view is now that health care decision-making should be a process of shared decision-making between patient (or the patient's surrogate in the case of an incompetent patient) and physician.[14] Each is seen as indispensable to sound decision-making. The physician brings his or her training, knowledge, and expertise to bear for the diagnosis of the patient's condition, the estimation of the patient's prognosis with different alternative

[13] I make no attempt here to provide any more than a few representative references to this very large literature. Probably the single best source for the medical ethics literature in this area is the Hastings Center Report *Guidelines on the Termination of Treatment and the Care of the Dying* (Briarcliff Manor, NY: Hastings Center, 1987). In the medical literature, see Sidney H. Wanzer *et al.*, 'The Physicians' Responsibility toward Hopelessly Ill Patients', *New England Journal of Medicine*, 310 (Apr. 1984), 955–9, and John E. Ruark *et al.*, 'Initiating and Withdrawing Life Support', *New England Journal of Medicine*, 318 (Jan. 1988), 25–30. For a good review of most of the principal legal decisions in the United States concerning life-sustaining treatment, see George Annas and Leonard Glantz, 'The Right of Elderly Patients to Refuse Life-Sustaining Treatment', *Milbank Quarterly*, 64 (1986), suppl. 2: 95–162. The most influential treatment of these issues by a governmental body in the United States is the report of the President's Commission for the Study of Ethical Problems in Medicine and Biomedical and Behavioral Research, *Deciding to Forgo Life-SustainingTreatment* (Washington, DC: US Government Printing Office, 1983). See also the recent report by the Hastings Center *Guidelines on the Termination of Treatment and the Care of the Dying*. For discussion of Living Wills and Durable Powers of Attorney, see Robert Steinbrook and Bernard Lo, 'Decision Making for Incompetent Patients by Designated Proxy: California's New Law', *New England Journal of Medicine*, 310 (1984), 1598–1601, and Lawrence Schneiderman and John Arras, 'Counseling Patients to Counsel Physicians on Future Care in the Event of Patients' Incompetence', *Annals of Internal Medicine*, 102 (1985), 693–8. An application to clinical practice of the consensus that patients should have rights to decide about their care is Albert R. Jonsen, Mark Siegler, and William J. Winslade, *Clinical Ethics* (New York: Macmillan, 1982).

[14] An influential statement of the shared decision-making view is another report of the President's Commission for the Study of Ethical Problem in Medicine and Biomedical and Behavioral Research, *Making Health Care Decisions* (Washington, DC: US Government Printing Office, 1982). A sensitive discussion of the difficulties of achieving shared decision-making in clinical practice is Jay Katz, *The Silent World of Doctor and Patient* (New York: Free Press, 1984).

treatments, including the alternative of no treatment, and a recommendation regarding treatment. The patient brings the knowledge of his or her
aims, ends, and values that are likely to be affected by different courses of
treatment, and this enables a comparative evaluation of different possible
outcomes to be made. As alternative treatments have multiplied and become
possible in circumstances promising increasingly marginal or questionable
benefits, both physicians and patients are called upon to make increasingly
difficult judgements about the effects of treatment on patients' quality of
life. It is worth noting that proponents of shared decision-making need not
reject the functional account of health as a biological norm defended by
Kass and others. What they can reject is the claim that the only proper goal
of medicine is health. Instead, medicine's goal should be to provide treatment that best enables patients to pursue successfully their overall aims and
ends, or life plans. It is the relative value of health, and of different aspects
of health, as compared with other ends, that varies for different persons and
circumstances.

Most patients' decisions about life-sustaining treatment will be based on
their judgement of the benefits and burdens of the proposed treatment and
the life it sustains, though in some instances patients may give significant
weight to other factors such as religious obligations, the emotional burdens
and financial costs for their families, and so forth. Except for patients who
hold a form of vitalism according to which human life should or must be
sustained at all costs and whatever its quality, these decisions by competent
patients must inevitably involve an assessment of their expected quality of
life if life-sustaining treatment is employed, though, as I shall note shortly,
of only a very restricted sort.

Some have rejected the acceptability of quality of life judgements in the
case of incompetent patients unable to decide for themselves, for whom
others must therefore make treatment decisions.[15] One version of the objection is that no one should decide for another whether that other's quality of
life is such that it is not worth continuing it. More specifically, the objection
is that it is unacceptable to judge that the quality of another person's life is
so poor that it is not worth the cost and effort to others to sustain that
person's life. This objection, however, is not to making quality of life judgements in this context generally, but only to concluding that a person's life is
not worth sustaining because its poor quality makes it not of value, but
instead a burden, to *others*. The sound point that this objection confusingly
makes is that quality of life judgements concerning a particular person

---

[15] e.g. Paul Ramsey, *Ethics at the Edge of Life* (New Haven, Conn.: Yale University Press, 1978),
206–7.

should address how the conditions of a person's life affect its quality or value to *that person*, and not its value to others. Moreover, persons might judge their quality of life to be low and nevertheless value their lives as precious. In economic and policy analysis one version of the so-called human capital method of valuing human life, which values a person's life at a given point in time by his or her expected future earnings minus personal consumption, in effect values a person's life in terms of its economic value to others.[16] But there is no reason to reject the soundness of any evaluation by one person of another's quality of life simply because some might draw a further unjustified conclusion that if its quality is sufficiently low to make it on balance a burden to others, it ought not to be sustained.

The quality of life judgement appropriate to life-sustaining treatment decisions, whether made by a competent patient or an incompetent patient's surrogate, should thus assess how the conditions of the patient's life affect the value of that life to that patient. Nevertheless, even properly focused in this way, the role of quality of life judgements in decisions about whether to withhold or withdraw life-sustaining treatment is extremely limited. This quality of life judgement focuses only on which side of a *single threshold* a person's quality of life lies. The threshold question is: 'Is the quality of the patient's life so poor that for that person continued life is worse than no further life at all?' Or, in the language of benefits and burdens commonly employed in this context: 'Is the patient's quality of life so poor that the use of life-sustaining treatment is unduly burdensome, that is, such that the burdens to the patient of the treatment and/or the life that it sustains are sufficiently great and the benefits to the patient of the life that is sustained sufficiently limited, to make continued life on balance no longer a benefit or good to the patient?'[17] The only discrimination in quality of life required here is whether the quality of the life is on balance sufficiently poor to make it worse than non-existence to the person whose life it is.

Some have objected that this judgement is incoherent since, though it is possible to compare the quality of two lives, or of a single person's life under different conditions, it is not possible to make the quality of life comparison needed here because one of the alternatives to be compared is non-existence. If a person no longer exists, there is no life that could possibly have any

---

[16] I have discussed some of the ethical implications of different measures for valuing lives found in the economic and policy literature (Dan W. Brock, 'The Value of Prolonging Human Life', *Philosophical Studies*, 50 (1986), 401–28).

[17] It has been argued that this is the proper understanding of the distinction between 'ordinary' and 'extraordinary' treatment. That is, extraordinary treatment is treatment that for the patient in question and in the circumstances that obtain is unduly burdensome. Cf. President's Commission, *Deciding to Forgo Life-Sustaining Treatment*, 82–9.

quality so as to enter into a comparison with the quality of the life sustained by treatment. This objection does correctly point out that the judgement in question cannot involve a comparison of the quality of two alternative periods of life, though it could compare two possible lives, one that ends at that time and another that continues longer. However, it does not follow that there is no sense to the question of whether the best life possible for a person with some form of life-sustaining treatment is of sufficiently poor quality, or sufficiently burdensome, to be worse for that person than no further life at all. Perhaps the most plausible example is the case of a patient suffering from an advanced stage of invariably fatal cancer, who is virtually certain to die within a matter of days whatever is done, and whose life will be filled in those remaining days with great and unrelievable pain and suffering. (With the appropriate use of presently available measures of pain relief, it is in fact only very rarely the case that great pain and suffering in such cases cannot be substantially relieved.) The burden of those remaining days may then be found by the patient to be virtually unbearable, while the life sustained provides nothing of value or benefit to the patient. This judgement addresses the quality of the life sustained and appears to be a sensible judgement. It is just the judgement that patients or their surrogates commonly understand themselves to be making when they decide whether to employ or continue life-sustaining treatment.

Alternatively, the objection to someone ever making such a judgement for another may not be based on any putative incoherence of such judgements, but may express instead a concern about the difficulty of ever reliably deciding how *another* would in such circumstances decide, due perhaps to the diversity and unpredictability of people's actual decisions for themselves. Moreover, if the difficulty of reliably making such judgements for others is in fact this great, then we might well have a related practical concern that the interests of others, which may be in conflict with those of the patient, may consciously or unconsciously infect judgements about what is best for the patient.

Despite these difficulties, there have been attempts to formulate some general substantive standards to determine when an incompetent patient's quality of life is so poor that withholding or withdrawing further life-sustaining treatment is justified. Nicholas Rango, for example, has proposed standards for nursing home patients with dementia.[18] He emphasizes the importance of being clear about the purposes for which care is provided and distinguishes three forms of care: (1) palliative care aimed at relieving physical

---

[18] Nicholas Rango, 'The Nursing Home Resident with Dementia', *Annals of Internal Medicine*, 102 (1985), 835–41.

pain and psychological distress; (2) rehabilitative care aimed at identifying and treating 'excess disabilities, the gap between actual level of physical, psychological or social functioning and potential functioning capacity',[19] and (3) medical care aimed at reducing the risk of mortality or morbidity. He emphasizes the importance of therapeutic caution because a seriously demented patient will not be able to understand the purposes of painful or invasive interventions, and so presumably cannot choose to undergo and bear burdensome treatment for the sake of promised benefits.[20] Rango proposes two conditions, either of which is sufficient to justify forgoing further treatment of a chronic medical condition or a superimposed acute illness: (a) when the patient is burdened by great suffering despite palliative and rehabilitative efforts; (b) when the dementia progresses 'to a stuporous state of consciousness in which the person lives with a negligible awareness of self, other, and the world'.[21] Even within the relatively narrow focus of life-sustaining treatment decisions for demented patients, Rango's proposal can be seen to include three different kinds of components of quality of life assessments. The first, covered by treatment aim (1) and patient conditions (a) and (b), concerns the quality of the patient's conscious experience. The second, covered especially by treatment aim (2) and patient condition (b), concerns the patient's broad functional capacities. The third, covered especially by patient condition (b) and by the patient's ability to understand the purpose of treatment and in turn to choose to undergo it, concerns the centrality to quality of life of the capacity to exercise choice in forming and pursuing an integrated and coherent life plan. I shall argue below that each of these three kinds of condition is an essential component of an adequate account of the quality of life.

At the other end of life, the debate in the United States about treatment for critically ill new-born infants has also focused on the role of quality of life considerations in determining when life-sustaining treatment is a benefit for the infant. One influential attempt to bring quality of life considerations into these decisions is the proposal of the moral theologian, Richard McCormick, that a new-born infant's life is a value that must be preserved only if the infant has the potential for a 'meaningful life'.[22] A meaningful life is one that contains some potential for human relationships: anencephalic

[19] Ibid. 836, quoting E. M. Brody.
[20] The importance of this factor was stressed in a widely publicized legal decision concerning the use of painful chemotherapy for a man suffering from cancer who had been severely retarded from birth (*Superintendent of Belchertown State School v. Saikewicz* (1977) 370 N.E. 2D 417).
[21] Rango, 'The Nursing Home Resident with Dementia', 838.
[22] Richard J. McCormack SJ, 'To Save or Let Die: The Dilemma of Modern Medicine', *Journal of the American Medical Association*, 229 (1974), 172–6.

new-borns, for example, wholly lack this potential, while those with Down's syndrome or spina bifida (to cite two of the most discussed kinds of case) normally do not. Nancy Rhoden has developed a more detailed proposal along similar lines regarding life-sustaining treatment for new-born infants:

aggressive treatment is not mandatory if an infant: (1) is in the process of dying; (2) will never be conscious; (3) will suffer unremitting pain; (4) can only live with major, highly restrictive technology which is not intended to be temporary (e.g., artificial ventilation); (5) cannot live past infancy (i.e., a few years); or (6) lacks potential for human interaction as a result of profound retardation.[23]

Rhoden's proposal is typical of those accepting the use of quality of life considerations in decisions about life-sustaining treatment for new-born infants in its focus on the infant's at least minimal capacity for positive conscious experience (conditions 2 and 3): the infant's capacities for physical, mental, and social functioning (conditions 2, 3, 4, and 6), and the infant's capacities to live far enough into childhood to begin a life that can be viewed and experienced 'from the inside' by the child as a life lived in a biographical, not biological, sense (conditions 1 and 4; I will say more about this special feature of infant 'life years' below in discussing the relevance of mortality data to good lives). However, the very limited, single-threshold character of the quality of life assessments required in decisions as to whether to forgo or to employ life-sustaining treatment, whether for adults or new-born infants, takes us only a little way in understanding quality of life assessments in health care treatment decision-making.

It is necessary, consequently, to broaden the focus from life-sustaining treatment decisions to medical treatment decisions generally. Here, as noted earlier, there is a widespread consensus that competent patients are entitled, in a process of shared decision-making with their physicians, to decide about their treatment and to refuse any proffered or recommended treatment. In the United States, the doctrine of informed consent, both in medical ethics and in the law, requires that treatment should not be given to a competent patient without that patient's informed and voluntary consent.[24] What does this doctrine, which lodges decision-making authority with the patient,

[23] Nancy K. Rhoden, 'Treatment Dilemmas for Imperiled Newborns: Why Quality of Life Counts', *Southern California Law Review*, 58 (1985), 1283–1347. Another sensitive discussion of the need for quality of life judgments in treatments decisions for imperilled new-born babies is John Arras, 'Toward an Ethic of Ambiguity', *Hastings Center Report*, 14 (Apr. 1984), 25–33.

[24] The most comprehensive treatment of the informed consent doctrine is Ruth R. Faden and Tom L. Beauchamp, *A History and Theory of Informed Consent* (New York: Oxford University Press, 1986). See also President's Commission, *Making Health Care Decisions*. The exceptions to the legal requirement of informed consent are discussed in Alan Meisel, 'The "Exceptions" to the Informed Consent Doctrine: Striking a Balance between Competing Values in Medical Decision-Making', *Wisconsin Law Review* (1979), 413–88.

imply about the nature of judgements concerning the patient's quality of life? An argument that it presupposes the normatively subjective, preference satisfaction account of a good life might, in rough outline, go as follows.

Each of the requirements of the informed consent doctrine can be understood as designed to provide reasonable assurance that the patient has chosen the treatment alternative most in accord with his or her own settled preferences and values. If the patient's decision is not informed—specifically, if the patient is not provided in understandable form with information regarding his or her diagnosis, the prognosis when different treatment alternatives (including the alternative of no treatment) are pursued, including the expected risks and benefits, with their attendant probabilities, of treatment alternatives—then the patient will lack the information needed to select the alternative most in accord with his or her settled preferences. If the patient's decision is not voluntary, but is instead forced, coerced, or manipulated by another, then it is likely not to be in accordance with the patient's settled preferences, but instead will forward another's interests, or another's view of what is best for the patient. If the patient is not competent to make the choice in question, then he or she will lack the ability to use the information provided to deliberate about the alternatives and to select the one most in accord with his or her settled preferences. When all three requirements are satisfied—the decision is informed and voluntary, and the patient competent—others can be reasonably assured that the patient's choice fits the patient's own conception of a good life, as reflected in his or her settled preferences.[25] Viewed in this way, the informed consent doctrine may appear to be grounded in a preference satisfaction account of the good or the quality of life, and so not to require any more complex vector account of the sort suggested earlier. Even in this very crude form, however, this argument can be seen to be unsound if one asks what values the informed consent doctrine and the account of shared decision-making in

---

[25] When patients' settled preferences are not in accord with their values, then their informed and voluntary choices may not reflect their conception of their good. One of the clearest examples is the patient who is addicted to morphine, hates his addiction and tries unsuccessfully to resist it, but in the end is overpowered by his desire for the morphine and takes it. This in essence is Harry Frankfurt's example in his classic paper 'Freedom of the Will and the Concept of a Person', *Journal of Philosophy*, 68 (1971), 5–20. Frankfurt's analysis is in terms of first- and second-order desires, but can also be put in terms of the desires a person in fact has as opposed to the desires the person values and wants to have. When these are in conflict his informed and voluntary choice may not reflect the values that define his own conception of his good. There is a sense in which his choice in these conditions is involuntary, so it would be possible to extend the informed consent doctrine's requirement of voluntariness to include this sense. Alternatively, it might be possible to interpret the requirement of competence in a way that makes the morphine addict incompetent to decide whether to continue using morphine.

medicine are usually thought to promote, and what values support their acceptance.

The most natural and obvious first answer has already implicitly been given: the informed consent doctrine in health-care treatment decision-making is designed, when its three requirements are satisfied, to serve and promote the patient's well-being, as defined by the patient's settled, unco-erced, and informed preferences. If this were the only value at stake, or at least clearly the dominant value, then it would be plausible to argue that the informed consent doctrine rests, at least implicitly, on a preference satisfac-tion account of the good life. However, it is not the only value at stake. Usually regarded as at least of roughly commensurate importance is respect-ing the patient's self-determination or autonomy.[26] The interest in self-determination I understand to be the interest of persons, broadly stated, in forming, revising over time, and pursuing in their choices and actions their own conception of a good life; more narrowly stated for my specific pur-poses here, it is people's interest in making significant decisions affecting their lives, such as decisions about their medical care, for themselves and according to their own values. Sometimes this is formulated as the right to self-determination.

Whether interest or right, however, the greater the moral weight accorded to individual self-determination as one of the values underlying and sup-porting the informed consent doctrine, the weaker the basis for inferring that the doctrine presupposes the normatively subjective, preference satisfaction account of the good life. This is because the greater the moral weight accorded to individual self-determination, the more self-determination can explain the requirement of informed consent, even assuming the patient chooses in a manner sharply contrary to his or her own well-being. More-over, there is substantial reason to suppose that the doctrine does in fact largely rest on respect for patients' self-determination. In the celebrated 1914 legal case of *Schloendorf* v. *Society of New York Hospitals*, usually cited as the first important enunciation of the legal requirement of consent for med-ical care, Justice Cardozo held that: 'Every human being of adult years and sound mind has a right to determine what shall be done to his own body; and a surgeon who performs an operation without his patient's consent commits an assault, for which he is liable in damages.'[27] I shall make no attempt here to trace the development of the legal doctrine of informed

[26] This account of the principal values underlying the informed consent doctrine as patient well-being and self-determination is common to many analyses of that doctrine; cf. President's Commission, *Making Health Care Decisions*. I have employed it in Dan W. Brock, 'Informed Consent', in Tom Regan and Donald VanDeVeer (eds.), *Health Care Ethics* (Philadelphia: Temple University Press, 1987).

[27] *Schloendorf* v. *Society of New York Hospitals*, 1914.

consent since *Schloendorff*, but it is probably fair to say that no other subsequent case has been as influential or as often cited in that development. And the later cases, in one form or another, repeatedly appeal to a right to self-determination to support that developing doctrine.[28] Nearly half a century later, for example, in the important 1960 case of *Natanson* v. *Kline* the Kansas Supreme Court made an equally ringing appeal to self-determination:

Anglo-American law starts with the premise of thorough-going self-determination. It follows that each man is considered to be master of his own body, and he may, if he be of sound mind, expressly prohibit the performance of life-saving surgery, or other medical treatment. A doctor might well believe that an operation or form of treatment is desirable or necessary but the law does not permit him to substitute his own judgment for that of the patient by any form of artifice or deception.[29]

The philosophical tradition regarding the problem of paternalism is equally bound up in a commitment to the importance of individual self-determination or autonomy. Here, the *locus classicus* is John Stuart Mill's renowned assertion of the 'one very simple principle' that

the sole end for which mankind are warranted, individually or collectively, in interfering with the liberty of action of any of their number is self-protection. That the only purpose for which power can be rightfully exercised over any member of a civilized community, against his will, is to prevent harm to others. His own good, either physical or moral, is not a sufficient warrant. He cannot rightfully be compelled to do or forbear because it will be better for him to do so, because it will make him happier, because, in the opinions of others, to do so would be wise or even right.[30]

The voluminous subsequent philosophical literature on paternalism certainly suggests that this principle is not as simple as Mill supposed, but it also makes clear that, even for one like Mill who in other contexts was an avowed utilitarian, the case for non-interference with individual self-determination and liberty of action does not rest on any claim that doing so cannot be for a person's 'good', understood in a normatively subjective interpretation. Quite to the contrary, Mill and the many who have followed him have been at pains to insist that such interference is not justified even when it would truly be for the good of the one interfered with.[31] The result is

[28] Cf. Faden and Beauchamp, *A History and Theory of Informed Consent*, ch. 4.

[29] *Natanson* v. *Kline*, 1960.

[30] J. S. Mill, *On Liberty* (1859; Indiana: Bobbs-Merrill, 1956).

[31] The most detailed recent account of justified paternalism in the spirit of Mill's position is Donald VanDeVeer, *Paternalistic Intervention* (Princeton: Princeton University Press, 1986). The most sophisticated development of a Millian position on paternalism in criminal law is Joel Feinberg, *Harm to Self* (New York: Oxford University Press, 1986). I have explored some of the issues between rights-based and consequentialist accounts of paternalism in Dan W. Brock, 'Paternalism and Promoting the Good', in Rolf Sartorius (ed.), *Paternalism* (Minneapolis: University of Minnesota Press, 1983), and 'Paternalism and Autonomy', *Ethics*, 98 (1988), 550–65.

that it is not possible to draw any firm conclusion from the doctrine of informed consent in medicine that patients' well-being or quality of life is understood according to a normatively subjective interpretation. Individual self-determination can serve as the foundation for the informed consent doctrine and can make that doctrine compatible with any of the three main alternative accounts of the good or quality of life that I have distinguished.

What is the relation between these two values of patient self-determination and well-being, commonly taken as underlying the informed consent doctrine, and the broad concept of a good life? The conventional view, I believe, is that the patient's well-being is roughly equivalent to the patient's good and that individual self-determination is a value independent of the patient's well-being or good. Respecting the patient's right to self-determination, then, at least sometimes justifies respecting treatment choices that are contrary to the patient's well-being or good.[32] Respecting self-determination is commonly held to be what is required by recognizing the individual as a person, capable of forming a conception of the good life for him or herself. If personal self-determination is a fundamental value—fundamental in that it is what is involved in respecting persons—however, then I suggest that our broadest conception of a good life should be capable of encompassing it rather than setting it off as separate from and in potential conflict with a person's well-being or good, as in the conventional account of informed consent. What we need is a distinction between a good life for a person in the broadest sense and a person's personal well-being, such that only personal well-being is independent of and potentially in conflict with individual self-determination.

We should think of being self-determined as central to—a central part of—having a good life in the broadest sense. It is in the exercise of self-determination that we maintain some control over, and take responsibility for, our lives and for what we will become. This is not to deny, of course, that there are always substantial limits and constraints within which we must exercise this judgement and choice. But it is to say that showing respect for people through respecting their self-determination acknowledges the fundamental place of self-determination in a good life. I take this to be essentially what Rawls intends by his claim that people have a highest-order

<hr>

[32] This conventional view is reflected in the independent ethical principles of beneficence and autonomy in Tom L. Beauchamp and James F. Childress, *Principles of Biomedical Ethics* (New York: Oxford University Press, 1979). This book has probably been the account of moral principles most influential with people in medicine and health care without philosophical training in ethics.

interest in autonomy and what Sen means by his notion of agency freedom.[33] We do not want this broad conception of a good life, however, to prevent our making sense of persons freely and knowingly choosing to sacrifice their own personal well-being for the sake of other persons. To cite an extreme case, a parent might knowingly and freely choose not to pursue expensive life-sustaining treatment such as a heart transplant in order to preserve financial resources for his children's education. Given his love and sense of responsibility for his children, he would judge his life to be worse if he had the transplant at the expense of his children's education, though certainly his health and his personal well-being would be improved. We might say here that he values his personal well-being in these circumstances less than the well-being of his children. In its requirement that such a choice be respected, the informed consent doctrine implicitly accepts that the best life for a person is a life of self-determination or choice, even if the exercise of that self-determination or choice results in a lessened state of personal well-being. Precisely how to make this distinction between the good life, as opposed to the personal well-being, of an individual raises difficulties that I cannot pursue here. The rough idea is that personal well-being makes essential reference to the states of consciousness, activities, and capacities for functioning of the person in question (I will pursue this further in the next section of this paper), and it is these that are worsened when the parent pursues his conception of a good life in sacrificing his personal well-being for that of his child.[34]

---

[33] Cf. John Rawls, 'Kantian Constructivism in Moral Theory', *Journal of Philosophy*, 77 (1980), 515–72, and Amartya Sen, *Commodities and Capabilities* (Amsterdam: Elsevier, 1985) and 'Well-Being, Agency and Freedom: The Dewey Lecture', *Journal of Philosophy*, 82 (1985), 169–221.

[34] If personal well-being is understood in this way, it suggests that satisfaction of a person's non-personal desires that make no such reference to him do not increase the person's well-being. Consider a loyal fan of the Boston Red Sox baseball team, who wants the Red Sox to win the pennant. On the last day of the season, tied for first place with the New York Yankees, the Red Sox beat the Yankees and win the pennant. Suppose the fan is travelling in a remote area of Alaska on the day of the big game and a week later, before getting out of the wilderness area and learning of the Red Sox victory, he is killed by a rock slide. Was his personal well-being increased at all simply because the state of affairs he desired—the Red Sox victory—obtained? I believe the answer should be no.

The harder question is whether, in our broader sense of a good life, he had a better life even unbeknownst to him. And was the quality of his life any better? Certainly his life *as experienced by him* was no better and not of higher quality. Even in our broad sense of a good life, his life may seem not to have gone better, but perhaps that is only because this is a relatively unimportant desire. Suppose instead, to adapt an example of Parfit's (*Reasons and Persons*), a person devotes fifty years of his life to saving Venice and then, confident that it is safe, goes on vacation to the Alaskan wilderness. While he is there a flood destroys Venice, but, like the Red Sox fan, he never learns of it because a week after the flood and before getting out of the wilderness he is killed by a rock slide. Parfit notes that it is plausible to say of the destruction of Venice both that it has made the person's life go less well because he had invested his life in this goal and his life's work is now in vain, but also that it cannot lower the quality of his life if it does not affect the quality of his

Medical treatment decisions must often be made for patients who are not themselves competent to make them. There has been considerable discussion both in medical ethics and in the law regarding appropriate ethical standards for such decisions.[35] Since quality of life considerations are virtually always relevant to these decisions, the ethical frameworks developed for these decisions must employ, either explicitly or implicitly, a conception of the quality of life of patients. There is considerable consensus that if the patient in question, while still competent, formulated and left an explicit advance directive clearly and unambiguously specifying his or her wishes regarding treatment in the circumstances now obtaining, then those wishes should be followed, at least within very broad limits, by those treating the patient. At the present time in the United States, most states have adopted legislation giving the force of law to one or another form of so-called Living Will, which allows people to give binding instructions about their treatment should they become incompetent and unable to decide for themselves. Several other states have more recently enacted legislation permitting people to draw up a Durable Power of Attorney for Health Care, which combines the giving of instructions about the person's wishes regarding treatment with the designation of who is to act as surrogate decision-maker, and so to interpret those instructions, should one become incompetent to make the decisions oneself.

In the usual case in which an incompetent patient has left no formal advance directive, two principles for the guidance of those who must decide about treatment for the patient have been supported—the *substituted judgement* principle and the *best interests* principle. The substituted judgement principle requires the surrogate to decide as the patient would have decided if competent and in the circumstances that currently obtain. The best interests principle requires the surrogate to make the treatment decision that best serves the patient's interests. This has the appearance of a dispute between what I earlier called normatively subjective and normatively objective accounts of a good life, since the only point of the best interests principle as an alternative to substituted judgement might seem to be that it employs a normatively objective standard of the person's good that does not depend on his or her particular subjective preferences and values. However, this appearance is misleading. These two principles of surrogate decision-

experience. This suggests a point where a broad notion of a good life may diverge from the notion of the quality of life. Since I believe that medicine and medical ethics have little illumination to offer on this point, I set it aside here and shall in the body of the paper continue to use the broad notion of a good life largely interchangeably with the quality of life.

[35] Allen Buchanan and I have discussed ethical issues in decision-making for incompetent persons in our paper 'Deciding for Others', *Milbank Quarterly*, 64 (1986), suppl. 2: 17–94, and in our book *Deciding for Others* (Cambridge: Cambridge University Press, 1989).

making are properly understood, in my view, not as competing alternative principles to be used for the same cases, but instead as an ordered pair of principles to cover all cases of surrogate decision-making for incompetent patients in which an advance directive does not exist, with each of the two principles to apply in a different subset of these cases. (This is not to say that these two principles are always in fact understood in medical ethics, the law, or health care practice as applying to distinct groups of cases; the treatment of these two principles is rife with confusion.)

The two groups of cases are differentiated with regard to the information available or obtainable concerning the patient's general preferences and values that has some bearing on the treatment choice at hand. The two principles are an ordered pair in the sense that when sufficient information is available about the relevant preferences and values of the patient to permit a reasonably well-grounded application of the substituted judgement principle, then surrogate decision-makers for the patient are to use that information and that principle to infer what the patient's decision would have been in the circumstances if he or she were competent.[36] In the absence of such information, and only then, surrogate decision-makers for the patient are to select the alternative that is in the best interests of the patient, which is usually interpreted to mean the alternative that most reasonable and informed persons would select in the circumstances. Thus, these two principles are not competing principles for application in the same cases, but alternative principles to be applied in different cases.

Nevertheless, it might seem that the best interests standard remains a normatively objective account when it is employed. However, this need not be so. If the best interests standard is understood as appealing to what most informed and reasonable persons would choose in the circumstances, it employs the normatively subjective preference standard. And it applies the choice of most persons to the patient in question because in the absence of any information to establish that the patient's relevant preferences and values are different than most people's, the most reasonable presumption is that the patient is like most others in the relevant respects and would choose like those others. Thus, the best interests standard, like the two other standards of choice for incompetent patients—the advance directive and substituted judgement standards—can be understood as requiring the selection of

---

[36] Rebecca Dresser has developed a Parfitian challenge to the substituted judgement principle as well as to the authority of advance directives in cases in which the conditions creating the patient's incompetence also reduce or eliminate the psychological continuity and connectedness necessary for personal identity to be maintained. Cf. Rebecca Dresser, 'Life, Death, and Incompetent Patients: Conceptual Infirmities and Hidden Values in the Law,' *Arizona Law Review*, 28 (1986), 373–405. Cf. also Allen Buchanan, 'Advance Directives and the Personal Identity Problem', *Philosophy and Public Affairs*, 17 (1988), 277–302.

the alternative the patient would most likely have selected, with the variations in the standards suited to the different levels of information about the patient that is available. Just as with the informed consent doctrine that applies to competent patients, so these three principles—advance directives, substituted judgement, and best interests—guiding surrogate choice for incompetent patients can all be understood as supported and justified by the values of patient well-being *and* self-determination. Thus, each of these three principles implicitly employs an account of a good life that is a life of choice and self-determination concerning one's aims, values, and life plan.

Before leaving the ethical frameworks that have been developed in the medical ethics, legal, and medical literatures for treatment decision-making for competent and incompetent patients, I want to make explicit an indeterminacy in these frameworks concerning the nature of the ethical theory they presuppose. I have noted that it is common to base these ethical frameworks on two central values in a good life: patient well-being and self-determination. What is commonly left unclear, however, is the foundational status of the ethical value of individual self-determination in the underlying ethical theory supporting these decision-making frameworks. Self-determination might be held to have only derivative or instrumental value within a broadly consequentialist moral theory. Specifically, it might be held to be instrumentally valuable for the fundamental value of happiness or preference satisfaction within normatively subjective theories of a good life of a hedonist or preference satisfaction sort. If, as seems true at least for many social conditions and historical periods, most people have a relatively strong desire to make significant decisions about their lives for themselves, then it is at least a plausible presumption that their doing so will generally promote their happiness or the satisfaction of their desires. If self-determination is only valuable at bottom in so far as it leads to happiness or preference satisfaction, then it will not be part of an ideal of the person that is objective in the sense of its value not being entirely dependent on happiness or satisfaction. Since on most plausible theories of the good, happiness and desire satisfaction are significant *part* of a good life, and since self-determination does commonly make a significant contribution to people's happiness or desire satisfaction, self-determination will commonly have significant instrumental value on any plausible theory of a good life.[37]

As a result, to single out self-determination as one of the two principal values underlying the informed consent doctrine in medical ethics as it

[37] Thomas Scanlon argues in this volume ['Value, Desire and Quality of Life', in Nussbaum and Sen (eds.), *The Quality of Life*] that desire satisfaction is not itself a basic part of individual well-being, but is dependent on hedonistic or ideal (what he calls substantive good) reasons for its support.

applies both to competent and incompetent patients is not to make clear at a foundational level of ethical theory whether self-determination is held to have only instrumental value, or also significant non-instrumental value as an important component of an objective ideal of the person. The vast majority of ethical discussions of informed consent and health care treatment decision-making simply do not either explicitly address this foundational question of ethical theory or even implicitly presuppose a particular position on it. From a practical perspective, this foundational indeterminacy has the value of allowing proponents of incompatible ethical theories, for example consequentialists and rights-based theorists, to agree on the fundamental importance of self-determination and choice in a good life.

There is one final difficulty to be noted in attempting to infer the account of a good life at the level of basic ethical theory from the ethical frameworks for treatment decision-making advocated for and employed in medical practice. There is a general difficulty in inferring the underlying values or ethical principles that support social practices. A social practice like that of informed consent and shared decision-making in medicine must guide over time a very great number of treatment decisions carried out in a wide variety of circumstances by many and diverse patients, family members, and health care professionals. A well-structured practice must take account of and appropriately minimize the potential in all involved parties for well-intentioned misuse or ill-intentioned abuse of their roles. Institutional constraints may thus be justified, though on some particular occasions they will produce undesirable results, because in the long run their overall results are better than those of any feasible alternatives. For example, even if we appeal only to the value of patient well-being and leave aside any independent value of self-determination, a strong right of patients to refuse any treatment might be justified if most of the time people are themselves the best judges of what health care treatment will best promote their happiness or satisfy their enduring preferences and values. Alternatively, that same strong right to refuse treatment might be justified within a normatively objective ideal theory of a good life for persons because, though individuals can be mistaken about their own good when they pursue their happiness or seek to satisfy their desires, no reliable alternative social and legal practice is feasible that will produce better results in the long run, even judged by that ideal theory of a good life. The imperfections and limitations of people and institutions may lead supporters of quite different accounts of a good life to support roughly the same institutions in practice. In a more general form, this is a thoroughly familiar point in moral philosophy where defenders of fundamentally different moral theories, such as consequentialists and rights theorists, may converge on the institutions justified by their quite different theories. Without explicitly uncovering the justificatory rationales for specific social institutions accepted by particular persons, we cannot confidently infer the ethical principles or judgements, and specifically the conception of a good life, that they presuppose.

HEALTH POLICY MEASURES OF THE QUALITY OF LIFE

I want now to shift attention from the account of the quality of life presupposed by ethical frameworks for medical treatment decision-making to more explicit measures used to assess health levels and the quality of life as it is affected by health and disease within larger population groups. Early measurement attempts focused on morbidity and mortality rates in different populations and societies. These yield only extremely crude comparisons, since they often employ only such statistics as life expectancy, infant mortality, and reported rates of specific diseases in a population. Nevertheless, they will show gross differences between countries, especially between economically developed and underdeveloped countries, and between different historical periods, in both length and quality of life as it is affected by disease. Major changes in these measures during this century, as is well known, have been due principally to public health measures such as improved water supplies, sewage treatment, and other sanitation programmes and to the effects of economic development in improving nutrition, housing, and education; improvements in the quality of and access to medical care have been less important. In recent decades, health policy researchers have developed a variety of measures that go substantially beyond crude morbidity and mortality measures. Before shifting our attention to them, however, it is worth underlining the importance of mortality measures to the broad concept of a good life.

When quality and quantity of life are distinguished, both are relevant to the degree to which a person has a good life. People whose lives are of high quality, by whatever measure of quality, but whose lives are cut short well before reaching the normal life span in their society, have had lives that have gone substantially less well, because of their premature death, than reasonably might have been expected. People typically develop, at least by adolescence, more or less articulated and detailed plans for their lives; commonly, the further into the future those plans stretch, the less detailed, more general, and more open-ended they are. Our life plans undergo continuous revision, both minor and substantial, over the course of our lives, but at any point in time within a life people's plans for their lives will be based in part on assumptions about what they can reasonably expect in the way of a normal life span.[38] When their lives are cut short prematurely by illness and disease they lose not just the experiences, happiness, and satisfactions that they would otherwise have had in those lost years, but they often lose as well the opportunity to complete long-term projects and to achieve and live out the full shape, coherence, and conclusion that they had planned for their lives. It is this rounding out and completion of a life plan and a life that helps enable many elderly people, when near death, to feel that they have lived a full and complete life and so to accept their approaching death with equanimity and dignity. The loss from premature death is thus not simply the loss of a unit of a good thing, so many desired and expected-to-be-happy life-years, but the cutting short of the as yet incompletely realized life plan that gave meaning and coherence to the person's life.

The importance of life plans for a good life suggests at least two other ways in which different mortality rates within societies affect the opportunities of their members to attain good lives. Citizens of economically underdeveloped countries typically have shorter life expectancies than do citizens of the developed countries. Thus, even those who reach a normal life span will have less time to develop and enjoy a richly complex and satisfying life than will those who reach a normal, but significantly longer, life span in the developed countries. Mortality data indicate that citizens of underdeveloped countries typically have less good lives as a result of inadequate health care *both* because of their shorter life expectancies *and* because of their increased risk of not living to even the normal life span in their own society.

One final relation between mortality data and the importance of life plans in a good life concerns infant and extremely early childhood mortality. It is common to view such early mortality as particularly tragic, both because of the greater amount of expected life-years lost to the individual and because the life was cut short just as it was getting started. The loss is often deep for the parents, in part because of the hopes and plans for the infant's future that *they* had for the infant. But the death of an infant or extremely young child before he or she has developed the capacity to form desires, hopes, and plans for the future cuts that life short—'life' understood as a connected plan or unfolding biography with a beginning, middle, and end—before it has begun; the infant is alive, but does not yet have a life in this biographical

[38] Two of the more important discussions of life plans and of how they can give structure and coherence to life are Charles Fried, *An Anatomy of Values* (Cambridge, Mass.: Harvard University Press, 1970), ch. 10, and John Rawls, *A Theory of Justice* (Cambridge, Mass.: Harvard University Press, 1971), ch. 7.

sense.[39] From the perspective of this biographical sense of having a life as lived from the 'inside', premature death in later childhood, adolescence, or early adulthood commonly makes a life that has got started go badly, whereas infant death does not make a life go badly, but instead prevents it from getting started.

There is a voluminous medical and health policy literature focused on the evaluation of people's quality of life as it is affected by various disease states and/or treatments to ameliorate or cure those diseases.[40] The dominant

[39] The notion of a biographical life is employed in the medical ethics literature by James Rachels, *The End of Life* (Oxford: Oxford University Press, 1986), 5–6; by Peter Singer and Helga Kuhse, *Should this Baby Live*? (Oxford: Oxford University Press, 1985), 129–39; and by Daniel Callahan, *Setting Limits* (New York: Simon & Schuster, 1987). It is also implicit in Michael Tooley's account (*Abortion and Infanticide* (Oxford: Oxford University Press, 1983)) of the right to life.

[40] Among the useful papers consulted for this third section on health policy measures of quality of life, and not cited in other notes, are: John P. Anderson, 'Classifying Function for Health Outcome and Quality-of-Life Evaluation', *Medical Care*, 24 (1986), 454–71; Robert L. Berg, 'Neglected Aspects of the Quality of Life', *Health Services Research*, 21 (1986), 391–5; Marilyn Bergner *et al.*, 'The Sickness Impact Profile: Conceptual Formulation and Methodology for the Development of a Health Status Measure', *International Journal of Health Services*, 6 (1976), 393–415; K. C. Calman, 'Quality of Life in Cancer Patients: An Hypothesis', *Journal of Medical Ethics*, 10 (1984), 124–7; Carl Cohen, 'On the Quality of Life: Some Philosophical Reflections', *Circulation*, 66 (1982), suppl. 3: 29–33; Alan Cribb, 'Quality of Life: A Response to K. C. Calman', *Journal of Medical Ethics*, 11 (1985), 142–5; 'Assessment of Quality of Life in Clinical Trials', Editorial, *Acta Medica Scandia*, 220 (1986), 1–3; Mathew Edlund and Lawrence Tancredi, 'Quality of Life: An Ideological Critique', *Perspectives in Biology and Medicine*, 28 (1985), 591–607; John C. Flanagan, 'Measurement of Quality of Life: Current State of the Art', *Archives of Physical Rehabilitation Medicine*, 63 (1982), 56–9; Friedhelm Gehrmann, '"Valid" Empirical Measurement of Quality of Life', *Social Indicators Research*, 5 (1978), 73–109; Robert Gillingham and William S. Reece, 'Analytical Problems in the Measurement of the Quality of Life', *Social Indicators Research*, 7 (1980), 91–101; A. W. Grogono, 'Index for Measuring Health', *Lancet* (1971), 2: 1024–6; Gordon H. Guyatt *et al.*, 'Measuring Disease-Specific Quality of Life in Clinical Trials', *Canadian Medical Association Journal*, 1314 (1986), 889–95; Sonya Hunt and James McEwen, 'The Development of a Subjective Health Indicator', *Sociology of Health and Illness*, 2 (1980), 203–31; Sidney Katz *et al.*, 'Studies of Illness in the Aged. The Index of ADL: A Standardized Measure of Biological and Psychosocial Function', *Journal of the American Medical Association*, 185 (1963), 914–19; Frederic J. Klotkem, 'Philosophic Considerations of Quality of Life for the Disabled', *Archives of Physical Rehabilitation Medicine*, 63 (1982), 59–63; Donald S. Kornfeld *et al.*, 'Psychological and Behavioral Responses after Coronary Artery Bypass Surgery', *Circulation*, 66 (1982), suppl. 3: 24–8; Mathew Liang *et al.*, 'In Search of a More Perfect Mouse-trap (Health Status of Quality of Life Instrument)', *Journal of Rheumatology*, 9 (1982), 775–9; Jackob Najman and Sol Levine, 'Evaluating the Impact of Medical Care and Technologies on the Quality of Life: A Review and Critique', *Social Science and Medicine*, 15F (1981), 107–15; Robert Pearlman and James Speer, 'Quality of Life Considerations in Geriatric Care', *Journal of the American Geriatrics Society*, 31 (1983), 113–20; Cary A. Presant, 'Quality of Life in Cancer Patients', *American Journal of Clinical Oncology*, 7 (1984), 571–3; 'The 1984 Report of the Joint National Committee on Detection, Evaluation, and Treatment of High Blood Pressure', *Archives of Internal Medicine*, 144 (1984), 1045–57; R. Jolene Starr *et al.*, 'Quality of Life and Resuscitation Decisions in Elderly Patients', *Journal of General Internal Medicine*, 1 (1986), 373–9; Daniel F. Sullivan, 'Conceptual Problems in Developing an Index of Health', *Vital and Health Statistics*, 2 (1966), 1–18; David C. Thomasma, 'Ethical Judgment of Quality of Life in the Care of the Aged', *Journal of the American Geriatrics Society*, 32 (1984), 525–7; 'Quality of Life, Treatment

conception of the appropriate aims of medicine focuses on medicine as an intervention aimed at preventing, ameliorating, or curing disease and its associated effects of suffering and disability, and thereby restoring, or preventing the loss of, normal function or of life. Whether the norm be that of the particular individual, or that typical in the particular society or species, the aim of raising people's function to *above* the norm is not commonly accepted as an aim of medicine of equal importance to restoring function *up to* the norm. Problematic though the distinction may be, quality of life measures in medicine, and health care consequently tend to focus on individuals' or patients' *dysfunction* and its relation to some such norm. At a deep level, medicine views bodily parts and organs, individual human bodies, and people from a functional perspective. Both health policy analysts and other social scientists have done considerable work constructing and employing measures of health and quality of life for use with large and relatively diverse populations. Sometimes these measures explicitly address only part of an overall evaluation of people's quality of life, while in other instances they address something like overall quality of life as it is affected by disease. A closely related body of work focuses somewhat more narrowly on an evaluation of the effect on quality of life of specific modes of treatment for specific disease states. This research is more clinically oriented, though the breadth of impact on quality of life researchers seek to measure does vary to some extent, depending often on the usual breadth of impact on the person of the disease being treated. Generally speaking, the population-wide measures tend to be less sensitive to individual differences as regards both the manner and the degree to which a particular factor affects people's quality of life. It will be helpful to have before us a few representative examples of the evaluative frameworks employed.[41]

The Sickness Impact Profile (SIP) was developed by Marilyn Bergner and colleagues to measure the impact of a wide variety of forms of ill health on the quality of people's lives.[42] Table 1 enumerates the items measured.

A second example of an evaluative framework is the Quality of Life Index

Decisions, and Medical Ethics', *Clinics in Geriatric Medicine*, 2 (1986), 17–27; George W. Torrance, 'Social Preferences for Health States: An Empirical Evaluation of Three Measurement Techniques', *Socio-Economic Planning Sciences*, 10: 129–36; 'Toward a Utility Theory Foundation for Health Status Index Models', *Health Services Research*, 10 (1976), 129–36.

[41] An example of a broad quality of life measure not focused on health care and disease can be found in the Swedish Level of Living Surveys discussed by Robert Erikson in this volume ['Description of Inequality: The Swedish Approach to Welfare Research', in Nussbaum and Sen (eds.), *The Quality of Life*].

[42] Marilyn Bergner, 'The Sickness Impact Profile: Development and Final Revision of a Health Status Measure', *Medical Care*, 19 (1981), 787–805.

TABLE I. *Sickness impact profile categories and selected items*

Dimension	Category	Items describing behaviour related to:	Selected items
Independent categories	SR	Sleep and rest	I sit during much of the day
			I sleep or nap during the day
	E	Eating	I am eating no food at all, nutrition is taken through tubes or intravenous fluids
			I am eating special or different food
	W	Work	I am not working at all
			I often act irritable towards my work associates
	HM	Home managmeent	I am not doing any of the maintenance or repair work around the house that I usually do
			I am not doing heavy work around the house
	RP	Recreation and pastimes	I am going out for entertainment less
			I am not doing any of my usual physical recreation or activities
I. Physical	A	Ambulation	I walk shorter distances or stop to rest often
			I do not walk at all
	M	Mobility	I stay within one room
			I stay away from home only for brief periods of time
	BCM	Body care and movement	I do not bath myself at all, but am bathed by someone else
			I am very clumsy in my body movements
II. Psychosocial	SI	Social interaction	I am doing fewer social activities with groups of people
			I isolate myself as much as I can from the rest of the family
	AB	Alertness behaviour	I have difficulty reasoning and solving problems, e.g. making plans, making decisions, learning new things
			I sometimes behave as if I were confused or disoriented in place or time, e.g., where I am, who is around, directions, what day it is

Dimension	Category	Items describing behaviour related to:	Selected items
	EB	Emotional behaviour	I laugh or cry suddenly I act irritable and impatient with myself, e.g. talk badly about myself, swear at myself, blame myself for things that happen
	C	Communication	I am having trouble writing or typing I do not speak clearly when I am under stress

(QLI) developed by Walter O. Spitzer and colleagues to measure the quality of life of cancer patients (see Figure 1).[43]

A third prominent measure developed by Milton Chen, S. Fanshel and others is the Health Status Index (HSI), which measures levels of function along certain dimensions (see Table 2).[44]

It would be a mistake, of course, to attempt to infer precise and comprehensive philosophical theories of the quality of life or of a good life from measures such as these. The people who develop them are commonly social scientists and health care researchers who are often not philosophically sophisticated or concerned with the issues that divide competing philosophical accounts of a good life. The practical and theoretical difficulties in constructing valid measures that are feasible for large and varied populations require compromises with and simplifications of—or simply passing over—issues of philosophical importance. Nevertheless, several features of these measures are significant in showing the complexity of the quality of life measures employed in health care and, I believe, of any adequate account of the quality of life or of a good life.

First, the principal emphasis in each of the three measures of quality of life is on function, and functions of the 'whole person' as opposed to body parts and organ systems. In each case the functions are broadly characterized so as to be relevant not simply to a relatively limited and narrow class of life plans, but to virtually any life plan common in modern societies. Following

[43] Walter O. Spitzer *et al.*, 'Measuring the Quality of Life of Cancer Patients: A Concise QL-Index for Use by Physicians', *Journal of Chronic Disease*, 34 (1981), 585–97.

[44] Milton M. Chen, J. W. Bush, and Donald L. Patrick, 'Social Indicators for Health Planning and Policy Analysis', *Policy Sciences*, 6 (1975), 71–89.

Study No. _____

Age _____

Sex M₁ F₂ (Ring appropriate letter) _____

Primary Problem or Diagnosis _____

Secondary Problem or Diagnosis, or complication (if appropriate) _____

Scorer's Speciality _____

Scoring Form

Score each Reading 2, 1 or 0 according to your most recent assessment of the patient.

ACTIVITY

During the last week, the patient

- has been working or studying full time, or nearly so, in usual occupation: or managing own household, or participating in unpaid or voluntary activities, whether retired or not 2

- has been working or studying in usual occupation or managing own household or participating in unpaid or voluntary activities, but requiring major assistance or a significant reduction in hours worked or a sheltered situation or was on sick leave 1

- has not been working or studying in any capacity and not managing own household 0

DAILY LIVING

During the last week, the patient

- has been self-reliant in eating, washing, toiletting, and dressing: using public transport or driving own car 2

- has been requiring assistance (another person or special equipment) for daily activities and transport but performing light tasks 1

- has not been managing personal care or light tasks and/or not leaving own home or institution at all 0

HEALTH

During the last week, the patient
- has been appearing to feel well or reporting feeling 'great' most of the time 2
- has been lacking energy or not feeling entirely 'up to par' more than just occasionally 1
- has been feeling very ill or 'lousy', seeming weak and washed out most of the time, or was unconscious 0

☐

SUPPORT

During the last week
- the patient has been having good relationships with others and receiving strong support from at least one family member and/or friend 2
- support received or perceived has been limited from family and friends and/or by the patient's condition 1
- support from family and friends occurred infrequently or only when absolutely necessary or patient was unconscious 0

☐

OUTLOOK

During the last week the patient
- has usually been appearing calm and positive in outlook, accepting and in control of personal circumstances, including surroundings 2
- has sometimes been troubled because not fully in control of personal circumstances or has been having periods of obvious anxiety or depression 1
- has been seriously confused or very frightened or consistently anxious and depressed or unconscious 0

☐

QL INDEX TOTAL ☐☐

How confident are you that your scoring of the preceding dimensions is accurate? Please ring the appropriate category.

Absolutely Confident	Very Confident	Quite Confident	Not Very Confident	Very Doubtful	Not at all Confident
1	2	3	4	5	6

☐

Figure 1 Quality of Life Index: format of the final version adopted

TABLE 2 *Scales and definitions for the classification of function levels*

Scale	Step	Definition
Mobility scale		
5	Travelled freely	Used public transportation or drove alone. For below 6 age group, travelled as usual for age.
4	Travelled with difficulty	(a) Went outside alone, but had trouble getting around community freely, or (b) required assistance to use public transportation or automobile.
3	In house	(a) All day, because of illness or condition, or (b) needed human assistance to go outside.
2	In hospital	Not only general hospital, but also nursing home, extended care facility, sanatorium, or similar institution.
1	In special unit	For some part of the day in a restricted area of the hospital such as intensive care, operating room, recovery room, isolation ward, or similar unit.
0	Death	
Physical activity scale		
4	Walked freely	With no limitations of any kind.
3	Walked with limitations	(a) With cane, crutches, or mechanical aid, or (b) limited in lifting, stooping, or using stairs or inclines, or (c) limited in speed or distance by general physical condition.
2	Moved independently in wheelchair	Propelled self alone in wheelchair.
1	In bed or chair	For most or all of the day.
0	Death	
Social activity scale		
5	Performed major and other activities	*Major* means specifically: play for below 6, school for 6–17, and work or maintain household for adults. *Other* means all activities not classified as major, such as athletics, clubs, shopping, church, hobbies, civic projects, or games as appropriate for age.
4	Performed major but limited in other activities	Played, went to school, worked, or kept house but limited in other activities as defined above.
3	Performed major activity with limitation	Limited in the amount or kind of major activity performed, for instance, needed special rest periods, special school, or special working aids.
2	Did not perform major activity but performed self-care activities	Did not play, go to school, work or keep house, but dressed, bathed, and fed self.

Scale	Step	Definition
1	Required assistance with self-care activities	Required human help with one or more of the following—dressing, bathing, or eating—and did not perform major or other activities. For below 6 age group, means assistance not usually required for age.
0	Death	

the lead of Rawls's notion of 'primary goods', I shall call these 'primary functions'.[45] In the SIP, the categories of sleep and rest, and eating are necessary for biological function. The categories of work, home management, and recreation and pastimes are central activities common in virtually all lives, though the relative importance they have in a particular life can be adjusted for by making the measure relative to what had been the individual's normal level of activity in each of these areas prior to sickness. The two broad groups of functions, physical and psychosocial, are each broken down into several distinct components. For each primary function, the SIP measures the impact of sickness by eliciting information concerning whether activities typical in the exercise of that function continue to be performed, or have become limited. Even for primary functions, about which it is plausible to claim that they have a place in virtually any life, the different functions can have a different *relative* value or importance within different lives, and the SIP makes no attempt to measure those differences. The QLI likewise addresses a person's levels of activity in daily living, specifically measuring the presence of related behaviours in the relevant areas. In measuring health and outlook, the primary concern is with subjective feeling states of the person, though here too there is concern with relevant behaviour. The category of support addresses both the social behaviour of the individual and the availability of people in the individual's environment to provide such relationships. This category illustrates the important point that most primary functional capacities require both behavioural capacities in the individual and relevant resources in the individual's external environment. The HSI addresses three broad categories of primary function—mobility, physical activity, and social activity—with evidence of current functional capacity found in current levels of activity. It is noteworthy that even this index, which focuses explicitly on the health status of individuals, does not measure the presence or absence of disease, as one might expect given common understandings of 'health' as the absence of disease; like the SIP and QLI, it too measures levels of very broad primary functions.

[45] Rawls, *A Theory of Justice*, 62, 90–5.

A second important feature of these measures shows up explicitly only in the first two—SIP and QLI—and is best displayed in the 'outlook' category of the QLI, though it is also at least partly captured in the 'emotional behaviour' category of the SIP. Both these categories can be understood as attempts to capture people's subjective response to their objective physical condition and level of function, or, in short, their level of happiness or satisfaction with their lives, though the actual measures are far too crude to measure happiness with much sensitivity. The important point is that the use of these categories represents a recognition that *part* of what makes a good life is that the person in question is happy or pleased with how it is going; that is, subjectively experiences it as going well, as fulfilling his or her major aims, and as satisfying. This subjective happiness component is not unrelated, of course, to how well the person's life is going as measured by the level of the other objective primary functions. How happy we are with our lives is significantly determined by how well our lives are in fact going in other objective respects. Nevertheless, medicine provides many examples that show it is a mistake to assume that the subjective happiness component correlates closely and invariably with other objective functional measures. In one study, for example, researchers found a substantial relation between different objective function variables and also between different subjective response or outlook variables, but only a very limited relation between objective and subjective variables.[46] These data reinforce the importance of including both objective function and subjective response categories in a full conception of the quality of life, since neither is a reliable surrogate for the other. Given this at least partial independence between happiness and function variables, what is their relative weight in an overall assessment of a good life? Here, too, medicine brings out forcefully that there can be no uniform answer to this question. In the face of seriously debilitating injuries, one patient will adjust her aspirations and expectations to her newly limited functional capacities and place great value on achieving happiness despite these limitations. Faced with similar debilitating injuries, another patient will assign little value to adjusting to the disabilities in order to achieve happiness in spite of them, stating that she 'does not want to become the kind of person who is happy in that debilitated and dependent state'.[47]

There are other important qualifications of the generally positive relation between this happiness component of a good life and both the other primary

[46] Roger W. Evans, 'The Quality of Life of Patients with End Stage Renal Disease', *New England Journal of Medicine*, 312 (1985), 553–9.

[47] The main character in the popular play and subsequent film *Whose Life is it Anyway?*, having become paralysed from the neck down, displayed this attitude of not wanting to become a person who had adjusted to his condition.

function components and the overall assessment of how good a life it is. These qualifications are not all special to health care and the quality of life, but some are perhaps more evident and important in the area of health care than elsewhere. The first qualification concerns people's adjustments to limitations of the other primary functions. Sometimes the limitation in function, or potential limitation, is due to congenital abnormalities or other handicaps present from birth. For example, an American television programme recently reported on a follow-up of some of the children, now young adults, born to pregnant women who had taken the drug Thalidomide in the late 1950s.[48] The people reported on had suffered no brain damage but had been born with serious physical deformities, including lacking some or any arms and legs. While this placed many impairments in the way of carrying out primary functions such as eating, working, home management, physical mobility, and ambulation in the manner of normal adults, these people had made remarkable adjustments to compensate for their physical limitations: one was able to perform all the normal functions of eating using his foot in place of missing arms and hands; another made his living as an artist painting with a brush held between his teeth; another without legs was able to drive in a specially equipped car; and a mother of three without legs had adapted so as to be able to perform virtually all the normal tasks of managing a family and home.

These were cases where physical limitations that commonly restrict and impair people's primary functional capacities and overall quality of life had been so well compensated for as to enable them to perform the *same* primary functions, though in different ways, as well as normal, unimpaired persons do. While a few life plans possible for others remained impossible for them because of their limitations (for example, being professional athletes), their essentially unimpaired level of primary functions as a result of the compensations they had made left them with choice from among a sufficiently wide array of life plans that it is probably a mistake to believe that their quality of life had been lowered much or at all by their impairments. These cases illustrate that even serious physical limitations do not always lower quality of life if the disabled persons have been able or helped sufficiently to compensate for their disabilities so that their level of primary functional capacity remains essentially unimpaired; in such cases it becomes problematic even to characterize those affected as disabled.

In other cases, compensating for functional disabilities, particularly when they arise later in life, may require adjustments involving substantial changes in the kind of work performed, social and recreational activities pursued,

[48] *60 Minutes*, CBS television network programme, 21 Feb. 1988.

and so forth. When these disabilities significantly restrict the activities that had been and would otherwise have been available to and pursued by the person, they will, all other things being equal, constitute reductions in the person's quality of life. If they do so, however, it will be because they significantly restrict the choices, or what Norman Daniels has called the normal opportunity range, available to the persons, and not because the compensating paths chosen need be, once entered on, any less desirable or satisfying.[49] The *opportunity for choice* from among a reasonable array of life plans is an important and independent component of quality of life: it is insufficient to measure only the quality of the life plan the disabled person now pursues and his or her satisfaction with it. Adjustments to impairments that leave primary functions undiminished or that redirect one's life plan into areas where function will be better—both central aims of rehabilitative medicine—can, however, enhance quality of life even in the face of a diminished opportunity range.

In his theory of just health care Daniels uses the notion of an *age-adjusted* normal opportunity range, which is important for the relation between opportunity and quality of life or a good life. Some impairments in primary functions occur as common features of even the normal aging process, for example, limitations in previous levels of physical activity. Choosing to adjust the nature and level of our planned activities to such impairments in function is usually considered a healthy adjustment to the aging process. This adjustment can substantially diminish the reduction in the person's quality of life from the limitations of normal aging. Nevertheless, even under the best of circumstances, the normal aging process (especially, say, beyond the age of 80), does produce limitations in primary functions that will reduce quality of life. Thus, while quality of life must always be measured against normal, primary functional capacities for humans, it can be diminished by reductions both in individual function below the age-adjusted norm and by reductions in normal function for humans as they age.

I have suggested above that adjustments in chosen pursuits as a result of impairments in primary, or previously pursued individual, functions can compensate substantially (fully, in the effects on happiness) for impaired function, but will often not compensate fully for significant reductions in the range of *opportunities* available for choice, and so will not leave quality of life undiminished. In some cases, however, a patient's response and adjustment to the limitations of illness or injury may be so complete, as regards his commitment to and happiness from the new chosen life path, that there is

---

[49] Norman Daniels, *Just Health Care* (Cambridge: Cambridge University Press, 1985), chs. 2 and 3.

reason to hold that his quality of life is as high as before, particularly as he gets further away in time from the onset of the limiting illness or injury and as the new life becomes more securely and authentically the person's own. An undiminished or even increased level of happiness and satisfaction, together with an increased commitment to the new life, often seem the primary relevant factors when they are present. But we must also distinguish different *reasons* why the affective or subjective component of quality of life, which I have lumped under the notion of happiness, may remain undiminished, since this is important for an evaluation of the effect on quality of life.

A person's happiness is to some significant extent a function of the *degree* to which his or her major aims are being at least reasonably successfully pursued. Serious illness or injury resulting in serious functional impairment often requires a major revaluation of one's plan of life and its major aims and expectations. Over time, such revaluations can result in undiminished or even increased levels of happiness, despite decreased function, because the person's aspirations and expectations have likewise been revised and reduced. The common cases in medicine in which, following serious illness, people come to be satisfied with much less in the way of hopes and accomplishments illustrate clearly the incompleteness of happiness as a full account of the quality of life. To be satisfied or happy with getting much less from life, because one has come to expect much less, is still to get *less* from life or to have a less good life. (The converse of this effect is when rising levels of affluence and of other objective primary functions in periods of economic development lead to even more rapidly rising aspirations and expectations, and in turn to an *increasing gap* between accomplishments and expectations.) Moreover, whether the relation of the person's choices to his aspirations and expectations reflects his exercise of self-determination in response to changed circumstances is important in an overall assessment of his quality of life and shows another aspect of the importance of self-determination to quality of life.

Illness and injury resulting in serious limitations of primary functions often strike individuals without warning and seemingly at random, and are then seen by them and others as a piece of bad luck or misfortune. Every life is ended by death, and few people reach death after a normal life span without some serious illness and attendant decline in function. This is simply an inevitable part of the human condition. Individual character strengths and social support services enable people unfortunately impaired by disease or injury to adjust their aims and expectations realistically to their adversity, and then to get on with their lives, instead of responding to their misfortune with despair and self-pity. Circumstances beyond individuals' control may have dealt them a cruel blow, but they can retain dignity as self-determining agents capable of responsible choice in directing and retaining control over their lives within the limits that their new circumstances permit. We generally admire people who make the best of their lot in this way, and achieve happiness and accomplishment despite what seems a cruel fate. This reduction in aims and expectations, with its resultant reduction in the gap between accomplishments and aims, and the in turn resultant increase in happiness, is an outcome of the continued exercise of self-determination. It constitutes an increase in the happiness and self-determination components of quality of life though, of course, only in response to an earlier decrease in the person's level of primary functions.

Other ways of reducing this gap between accomplishments and expectations bypass the person's self-determination and are more problematic as regards their desirability and their effect on a person's quality of life. Jon Elster has written, for example, outside of the medical context, of different kinds of non-autonomous preferences and preference change.[50] Precisely characterizing the difference between what Elster calls non-autonomous preferences and what I have called the exercise of self-determination in adjusting to the impact of illness and injury raises deep and difficult issues that I cannot pursue here. Nevertheless, I believe that response to illness through the exercise of self-determined choice, in the service of protecting or restoring quality of life, is one of the most important practical examples of the significance for overall assessments of the quality of life of *how* to achieve the reasonable accord between aims and accomplishments that happiness requires.

CONCLUSION

Let us tie together some of the main themes in accounts of the quality of life or of a good life suggested by the literature in medical ethics and health policy. While that literature provides little in the way of well-developed, philosophically sophisticated accounts of the quality of life or of a good life, it is a rich body of analysis, data, and experience on which philosophical accounts of a good life can draw. I have presented here at least the main outlines of a general account of a good life suggested by that work. The account will be a complex one which, among the main philosophical theories distinguished earlier, probably most comfortably fits within ideal theories.

---

[50] Jon Elster, 'Sour Grapes: Utilitarianism and the Genesis of Wants', in Amartya Sen and Bernard Williams (eds.), *Utilitarianism and Beyond* (Cambridge: Cambridge University Press, 1982).

I have suggested that we can employ Sen's construction of a plurality of independent vectors, each of which is an independent component of a full assessment of the degree to which a person has a good life.

The ethical frameworks for medical treatment decision-making bring out the centrality of a person's capacity as a valuing agent, or what I have called self-determination in a good life. The capacity for and exercise of self-determination can be taken to be a—or I believe *the*—fundamental ideal of the person within medical ethics. The exercise of self-determination in constructing a relatively full human life will require in an individual four broad types of primary functions: biological, including, for example, well-functioning organs; physical, including, for example, ambulation; social, including, for example, capacities to communicate; mental, including, for example, a variety of reasoning and emotional capabilities. There are no sharp boundaries between these broad types of primary function, and for different purposes they can be specified in more or less detail and in a variety of different bundles. The idea is to pick out human functions that are necessary for, or at least valuable in, the pursuit of nearly all relatively full and complete human life plans. These different functions can be represented on different vectors and they will be normatively objective components of a good life, though their relative weight within any particular life may be subjectively determined.

There are in turn what we can call agent-specific functions, again specifiable at varying levels of generality or detail, which are necessary for a person to pursue successfully the particular purposes and life plan he or she has chosen: examples are functional capacities to do highly abstract reasoning of the sort required in mathematics or philosophy and the physical dexterity needed for success as a musician, surgeon, or athlete. Once again, these functions can be represented on independent vectors, though their place in the good life for a particular person is determined on more normatively subjective grounds depending on the particular life plan chosen. The relative weight assigned to agent-specific functions and, to a substantially lesser degree, to primary functions, will ultimately be determined by the valuations of the self-determining agent, together with factual determinations of what functions are necessary in the pursuit of different specific life plans. The centrality of the valuing and choosing agent in this account of a good life gives both primary and, to a lesser extent, agent-specific functional capacities a central place in the good life because of their necessary role in making possible a significant range of opportunities and alternatives for choice.

At a more agent-specific level still are the particular desires pursued by people on particular occasions in the course of pursuing their valued aims and activities. Different desires and the degree to which they can be successfully satisfied can also be represented using the vector approach. It bears repeating that the level of a person's primary functional capacities, agent-specific functional capacities, and satisfaction of specific desires will all depend both on properties of the agent and on features of his or her environment that affect those functional capacities and desire pursuits. The inclusion of primary functions, agent-specific functions, and the satisfaction of specific desires all within an account of the good life allows us to recognize both its normatively objective and normatively subjective components. Analogously, these various components show why we can expect partial, but only partial, interpersonal comparability of the quality of life or of good lives—comparability will require interpersonal overlapping of similarly weighted primary functions, agent-specific functions, and specific desires. The importance of functional capacities at these different levels of generality reflects the centrality of personal choice in a good life and the necessity for a choice of alternatives and opportunities.

Finally, there will be the hedonic or happiness component of a good life, that aspect which represents a person's subjective, conscious response in terms of enjoyments and satisfactions to the life he or she has chosen and the activities and achievements it contains. These may be representable on a single vector or on a number of distinct vectors if the person has distinct and incommensurable satisfactions and enjoyments. Happiness will usually be only partially dependent on the person's relative success in satisfying his or her desires and broader aims and projects. Once again, it is the valuations of the specific person in question that will determine the relative weight the happiness vector receives in the overall account of a good life for that person.

Needless to say, in drawing together these features of an account of the quality of life or of a good life from the medical ethics and health policy literatures, I have done no more than sketch a few of the barest bones of a full account of a good life. However, even these few bones suggest the need for more complex accounts of the quality of life than are often employed in programmes designed to improve the quality of life of real people.

PART V

FUTURE GENERATIONS

13

FUTURE PEOPLE, DISABILITY, AND SCREENING

JONATHAN GLOVER

Our interests may conflict with those of future generations. For instance, if we use fuel resources in ways that most benefit ourselves, future people may go short. This raises the question of justice between generations. How should our actions be constrained by fairness to people not yet born? There are two crude but popular views about social decision making. According to one, all that matters is that issues be decided democratically. The other is that economic decisions should be left to the market. Both majorities and market forces can generate notoriously unjust outcomes. Future generations provide a dramatic illustration of this, since those yet unborn have no vote and no purchasing power.

But the principles of justice that should guide our relations to future generations are not obvious. We have limited knowledge of what their circumstances and needs will be. We do not know how many of the generations stretching into the future should be considered, and to what extent, if at all, those farther off should be given less weight. Other problems are created by the effects of our actions on both the size and the composition of future generations. Different economic and social policies will affect such variables as where people live, which will affect which people meet one another, and so in turn will determine which people are born. Justice is made more complicated when different people, and different numbers of people, will exist to feel the impact of the policies under consideration.

Both political and everyday decisions unintentionally affect who is born. For instance, the man my grandmother first loved was killed in the First World War. If he had lived, my maternal grandparents would almost certainly not have married, and so my mother would not have been born, nor would I, nor my children, nor their descendants. Our existence is one minute consequence of the First World War. More trivial factors affected our

From Jonathan Glover, 'Future People, Disability, and Screening,' in J. Fishkin and P. Laslett (eds.), *Justice between Age Groups and Generations* (New Haven: Yale University Press, 1992), ch. 6.

existence, too: for instance, my grandfather's decision to learn marine engineering in Newcastle rather than in Belfast. Had he made the other choice, he
would not have met and married my grandmother and our fate would have
been nonexistence.

We also affect who is born by deliberate choice. For those not wanting to
have children, contraception has enlarged the options beyond the rather
bleak alternatives of chastity and abortion. With the development of more
advanced reproductive technologies, the present generation has new powers
of prediction and intervention. One issue raised by those powers is the topic
of this chapter: should we aim for the birth of 'normal' babies rather than
those with disabilities?

Many people will think that this question need not detain us for more
than a moment: the answer is yes. Surely everyone agrees that it is better if a
baby is born without a disability? Although I have a lot of sympathy with
this brisk response, the question is not so easily disposed of. It raises some of
the most abstract issues in ethics. To a surprising extent, those abstract issues
make a difference to social policy.

Our own decisions affect the likelihood of a disabled child being born. A
simple case is the decision to smoke in pregnancy. Another is the decision to
abort a fetus after exposure to rubella in pregnancy or when prenatal tests
have detected some disorder. Others arise as a result of in vitro fertilization
(IVF): the egg, having been fertilized in the laboratory, has to be transferred
to the womb. If several eggs have been fertilized, tests may show that some
are normal and some have a disorder. Deciding which egg to transfer will
determine the kind of person to be born. Also relevant are decisions about
the genetic screening of potential donors of semen or eggs.

'Gene therapy' can also lead to such decisions. When disorders are caused
by the absence of a gene or the presence of a 'wrong' gene, it is attractive to
think of inserting or deleting genes in embryos as required. In our present
state of medical development, this procedure carries a serious risk of
unwanted side effects. It is much safer to conduct genetic testing before
implanting a fertilized egg than to try to delete or insert genes. But the day
may come when this sort of gene therapy can be performed without harmful
side effects. Choosing between a normal baby and one with a disability will
become a genuine possibility.

One kind of intervention against disability is uncontroversially right. This
is any treatment that does not prevent the existence of the person with the
disability but aims to alleviate or cure the disability. (The mirror image is
that it is uncontroversially wrong to give a disability to someone who otherwise would be normal, for instance, by smoking during pregnancy.) What is
controversial is to eliminate or prevent the disability by eliminating or

preventing the existence of the person who has the disability. This controversial policy is the basis of screening programs.

TWO CASES OF DISABILITY

A Girl

In 1987, there was a debate in Britain about lowering the time limit for
abortion. The proposed lower limit would have excluded some cases where
prenatal tests reveal severe disability. As part of the debate, two parents
wrote to the *Guardian*:

In December 1986 our newly-born daughter was diagnosed to be suffering from
a genetically caused disease called Dystrophic epidermolysis Bullosa (EB). This is a
disease in which the skin of the sufferer is lacking in certain essential fibres. As a
result, any contact with her skin caused large blisters to form, which subsequently
burst leaving raw open skin that only healed slowly and left terrible scarring. As EB is
a genetically caused disease it is incurable and the form that our daughter suffered
from usually causes death within the first six months of life. In our daughter's case the
condition extended to her digestive and respiratory tracts and as a result of such
internal blistering and scarring she died after a painful and short life at the age of only
12 weeks.

Following our daughter's death we were told that if we wanted any more children
there was a one-in-four probability that any child we conceived would be affected by
the disease but that it was possible to detect the disease ante-natally. In May 1987 we
decided to restart our family only because we knew that such a test was available and
that should we conceive an affected child the pregnancy could be terminated, such a
decision is not taken lightly or easily . . .

If the time limit for abortions was to be reduced below about 22–24 weeks such
testing would be of no value as the results would not be available in time for the
pregnancy to be terminated.

We have had to watch our first child die slowly and painfully and we could not
contemplate having another child if there was a risk that it too would have to die in the
same way.

Anyone will feel sympathy with the determination of these parents that
any future child of theirs should be spared the life their daughter had. Given
that determination, their only hope of having their own biological children
depends on abortion being available after the test results. This is part of the
case for such abortion being legal. But to those who believe that abortion is
murder, or something close to it, the case may seem insufficient. To avoid
going into this familiar debate, it is worth thinking about the position if the
birth of a child with such a disability could be avoided by means other than
abortion.

Suppose there is a large-scale IVE program, using donated semen or eggs, to help infertile couples have children. Should donors be screened to exclude carriers of EB? Some of us believe that it is better not to bring into the world babies who will have only a few painful months of life. Those of us who think this have a reason to screen the donors. We have a reason, in the case of EB and similar disorders, for choosing to bring into the world a normal child rather than one with a severe disability.

A Woman

The same issue of the *Guardian* included another contribution to the debate:

Thank God this 'abnormal' fetus was conceived in 1947. I was born with spina bifida. My parents were told I would die within three days (wrong!) wouldn't walk (wrong!) and would be ineducable (wrong!). Yes, they were devastated but they picked themselves up and got on with the job of being responsible parents who wanted their children to achieve their potential. I attended normal schools from the age of seven, have a degree and two post graduate professional qualifications. I worked for many years as a Probation Officer and now as an Independent Guardian ad Litem (court social worker). I have a husband and two small children.

Yes, life can be difficult sometimes (isn't it for everyone?). Yes it cost money to get me where I am now (but a nuclear weapon would cost a damned sight more and probably cause more damage.) . . .

Years ago we kept 'the handicapped' in institutions, out of sight, out of mind. Now, we can destroy them before we need to look at them or think of them. But we the handicapped are still here, still playing a part in society. Funnily enough, not only do many of us contribute to society, we even enjoy being alive.

Many of us who face daily the problems of being disabled, are amongst those pressing for stricter abortion laws because we know life is good and believe in protecting the weak from the strong.

Let us together build a caring society which has room for all its members no matter what race or disability.

Spina bifida can be screened for prenatally and is widely accepted as one of the conditions that justify abortion. But this letter raises an extremely difficult question for those who support such a policy. As the writer says, she is playing her part in society and enjoying being alive. Is anyone in a position to make the Godlike judgment: 'It would have been better if you had been aborted'?

Again, to avoid the complications of the abortion debate, suppose that donors of eggs and sperm can be screened in an effort to prevent conception of children with spina bifida. (For most forms of spina bifida this would not be possible, but one rare form is genetic and such screening might one day be effective.) The objection to abortion as murder falls away. But the other difficult question remains. The writer says, 'Thank God this "abnormal fetus" was conceived.' Is anyone in a position to make the Godlike judgment: 'It would have been better if you had not been conceived'? If we doubt our ability to make such a judgment, we have a reason for opposing policies that deliberately avoid the conception of children with severe disabilities such as spina bifida.

Degrees of Disability and the Compromise Policy

The case of the girl gives a reason in favor of intervening against disability, whereas the case of the woman gives a reason against intervening. What should we do when such strong reasons point in opposite directions?

One response is to take the view that each reason applies in its own case. The two cases are very different. The woman is glad to be alive. The girl never reached the stage where she could have understood such questions, but those closest to her thought she had little reason to be glad to be alive. One could support intervention against conditions as severe as EB, but oppose intervention against those less severe, such as the degree of spina bifida experienced by the woman.

It is worth distinguishing disastrous disability (where life is so bad that death would be a release and it would be cruel to bring someone into the world to face such a life) from moderately severe disability. The boundary between the two degrees of disability obviously is blurred, and reasonable people will often disagree about a particular case. And character and circumstances can make a difference. Some people with terrible disabilities reveal extraordinary qualities, which enrich their own lives and those of people around them. Sometimes a terrible medical condition can be transformed by a loving and supporting family. But a blurred boundary does not mean there is no difference between the cases that fall on either side. It is reasonable, therefore, to see one of the cases considered here as disastrous and the other as moderately severe. (There is also a boundary problem between moderately severe disability and less severe conditions. I am relying on an intuitive understanding that color blindness, for instance, is not even moderately severe.)

The compromise policy would recommend screening against disastrous disability, but not against moderately severe disability. It is attractive because it acknowledges each line of thought that arises out of the two cases we have looked at. But both parts of the compromise policy must be examined. Before that, however, the policy of screening against disastrous disability needs to be considered in the context of some general objections to screening.

OBJECTIONS TO SCREENING

Disabled people who oppose selective abortion or screening programs make a point that is hard to answer: supporting a screening program is in effect saying that it would have been better if every disabled person had never been born. This forceful point is critical of the arrogant assumption that anyone is qualified to play God and decide who is or is not fit to be born. Implicit in such a criticism is the negative effect that such a view has on the rights of disabled people.

Playing God

Is it objectionably Godlike to decide that it is better for one person to live than another? We want to say that all people are of equal value and that no one is in the position of being able to estimate the worth of another person's life. Who are we to make these huge decisions about who shall live?

This line of thought evokes a strong response, but it is not decisive as an objection to all screening policies. The suggestion that it is arrogant to presume to make such decisions is false in at least some cases, including those where the disability is disastrous. The parents of the girl with EB need not be the slightest degree arrogant to want no other child of theirs to have such a life.

And when couples in quite ordinary circumstances choose to have or not to have a child, they indeed are making a Godlike decision. Perhaps we are not sufficiently awed by this familiar choice. It is possible to look at one's children and be retrospectively unnerved by how their very existence depends on decisions that one participated in and that could so easily have been different. But even if those familiar choices should be more impressive than they are, they provide a context in which it is hard to argue against reproductive decisions on the grounds that by making such decisions we are presuming a Godlike power over the existence of other people.

Disabled People and Equality of Respect

Having a severe disability is not a reason for being treated in any way as a second-class citizen. Opting for the existence of normal rather than disabled people is sometimes presented as a civil rights issue. Do such decisions violate the rights of people with disabilities? This criticism arises particularly in the context of prenatal screening leading to abortion. There its main force depends on one's view about whether fetuses have rights.

Some people would argue that such screening is effectively a form of discrimination against disabled people in general. Among the worst problems that disabled people must confront are the attitudes of many other people. And screening programs aimed at preventing the birth of disabled people could reinforce those attitudes. It may be difficult to feel self-esteem when people are doing all they can to avoid having a child like you.

That it is a threat to equality of respect clearly is a possible objection to screening. But equality of respect is a complex concept. Showing respect for people has two aspects. The first requires that we respect their rights: for instance, that we do not assault them, steal their property, tap their telephones, or prevent them from expressing religious or political beliefs. (Deciding exactly what people's rights are is a problem, but that does not undermine the claim that showing people respect requires not violating their rights, whatever they are.)

The other aspect of showing respect is more difficult to pin down, but hardly less important. It is a matter of attitude. It is a matter of not treating people with contempt or condescension. It is absent, to different degrees, in a caste system, or in a snob, or in someone who never listens but always interrupts. It is what makes our attempts to teach children to be courteous and considerate more than indoctrination in a set of arbitrary rules.

Much of what is involved in equality of respect is compatible with screening. Aiming for the conception and birth of normal people, for instance, is perfectly compatible with insisting that the rights of disabled people be fully respected and with seeing them as equals. Medical treatment presupposes that health is better than sickness, but those who believe in it treat sick people as their equals.

It may be said that the case is not parallel: the screening programs aim not to cure disabled people but to replace them with normal people. But even so, treatment as equals is possible. Something similar could be said about people who are not disabled. At the time I was conceived, if there had been a choice between my conception and that of someone just like me but more athletic or more imaginative, it might have been better if the other person had been conceived instead of me. I incline to this view, and if you do as well, this need not affect your attitude toward me for the worse. (Of course, a major disability may be more central to someone's life than not being athletic is to mine, so the chances of a screening program leading to loss of esteem are greater. But it is true of all of us that someone better in some ways could have been conceived instead. Accepting this about a particular person does not mean that one feels contempt or condescension toward him or her.)

The Slide to Positive Eugenics

Many people believe that gene therapy and genetic screening of embryos is dangerous. They believe that these policies may lead to eugenic policies that are positive rather than negative; that is, designed to 'improve' people who suffer from no medical disorder.

Positive eugenic programs raise large and controversial questions. Which characteristics are to be encouraged and which discouraged? Who is to decide on a matter so fundamental to other people's futures? Is there not a risk of appalling and perhaps irreversible mistakes? Most people shudder at the thought of positive eugenics. Perhaps this reaction is too hasty. Before banning positive eugenics in principle forever, it may be a good idea to ask whether in the distant future such a ban would counteract some huge gain, and whether it is certain that the problems of positive eugenics could never be surmounted. But even if such programs should not be absolutely excluded, a strong case can be made for a ban on them at least for now. The problems they raise are so deep, and so far from being solved, that it would be wise to consider carefully their dangers and problems.

There are good reasons for resisting any current proposal that is likely to result in positive eugenics. But there is no obvious reason why gene therapy or embryo screening must slide into positive eugenics. No doubt the boundary between medical and nonmedical intervention is sometimes blurred. But conventional boundaries often exist (as in the speed limit) where there is no sharp boundary in reality. To avoid positive eugenics, it seems more rational to draw the boundary where we really want it.

Evaluating the Objections

The playing God objection is not a clear one. For it to be taken seriously would require some explanation of why deciding which kind of child to have is so much more presumptuous than deciding whether to have a child at all.

The apparently Godlike policy of 'replacing' one potential child with another is not necessarily sharply distinct from the familiar decision about having a child at all. The boundaries of replacement are blurred. Go back to a 'natural' version of replacement. Suppose the man my grandmother first loved had not been killed in the First World War. Suppose they had married and had three children: first two boys, Michael and Henry, and then their younger sister, Susan. Which of those children, if any, did my mother (who was my grandmother's only child) replace? As my grandmother's 'first' child, was she replacing Michael, or as my grandmother's daughter, was she replacing Susan? Or was she replacing Henry, who would have been born on the same day she was? And would there have been one particular grandchild whom I am replacing, and a particular great-grandchild whom each of my children counts as replacing? And must my mother have replaced one of the children my grandmother would have had in her alternative marriage, or one of the children my grandfather might have had in an alternative marriage?

In this case, the idea of one child replacing another becomes too vague to be worth discussing. It seems better just to talk of the children and grand-children of the alternative marriages who were not conceived, and of the offspring of the actual marriage who were conceived, without attempting these comparisons.

Something close to this may be true of the couple who decide not to have a child who would be disabled. Suppose that after deciding against implant-ing an embryo that would develop into a child with a disability, they wait a few months before conceiving again. Who is their next child replacing? Is she replacing the child who would have developed from that embryo, or is she replacing the child they might have conceived immediately after deciding against implantation?

Or suppose several attempts to conceive a normal child result in fertilized eggs found to have a disorder and thus not implanted. When a normal child is finally conceived, is that child a replacement for the first nonimplanted embryo, or for the most recent? Again, it seems less misleading to give up claims about replacement and to talk instead about deciding not to have one child and deciding to have another child, without bringing in the com-parison. If this is correct, in such cases the supposedly Godlike decision about replacement collapses into two decisions of a kind made all the time.[1]

Although this weakens the playing God objection by blurring the bound-ary between replacement and everyday decisions, it does not make talk of replacement wrong in all cases. When a couple have decided to have only one child and they abort a fetus with a severe disorder, the child they later do have can be seen as replacing the one who would have been born. And the same holds when there is a choice between implanting one of only two embryos. These few special cases can be described as 'clear replacement,' and the larger number of other cases as 'blurred replacement.' Cases of blurred replacement seem no more vulnerable to the charge of Godlike

---

[1] This line of thought was suggested to me by Christopher Shields.

arrogance than everyday decisions about whether to have a child. But it is hard to see why clear replacement should be either more arrogant or more morally objectionable than blurred replacement. That would require us to accept that it might be objectionable to transfer one embryo out of two, but perfectly acceptable to transfer one out of three. How the presence of a third embryo could make such a difference is difficult to explain.

To be convincing, the objection to screening that foresees a positive eugenics would need more evidence. The most serious objection is based on the interests of already disabled people.

Because attitudes to disability are among its greatest disadvantages we are reluctant to say anything that might seem to belittle disabled people. And in light of how some people triumph over disability, it is difficult to assert that a particular disability totally excludes a fulfilled life.

These responses seem appropriate. But they may distort our thinking about the problem. Our reluctance to believe that a disabled person necessarily has a less fulfilled life may lead to denying the need for screening programs that assume that the birth of a normal child is preferable to that of a disabled one. Such a preference may seem like a form of prejudice against the disabled.

But these thoughts in fact do not follow from the responses mentioned. Although a particular disability may not make a fulfilled life impossible, it is likely to make such a life more difficult. Consider the theoretical possibility of screening to ensure that only a disabled child would be conceived. This would surely be monstrous. And we think it would be monstrous because we do not believe it is just as good to be born with a disability.

If this is true, then it is not intrinsically wrong to prefer the birth of a person without disability and to base screening policies on that preference. It is desirable, however, to resist any tendency for such policies to spill over into discriminatory attitudes toward those who are disabled. If such a spillover cannot be avoided, this argument must be weighed against the case for favoring the birth of a normal person.

DISASTROUS DISABILITY

Wrongful Life

In some legal cases it has been argued, on behalf of people with severe disabilities, that they were harmed by being brought into the world. The idea of 'wrongful life' first appeared in American lawsuits in which illegitimate children claimed damages. In general, such claims were rejected. Later, wrongful life suits centered on children born with severe disabilities or diseases. Both parents and children acted as plaintiffs. The defendants were usually laboratories. Sometimes an action was brought against the parents themselves on the grounds of 'negligence,' for not having aborted the fetus.

The legal aspects of these cases are not important here. The central moral issue raised is whether parents and doctors ought to take what steps they can to prevent the birth of a child at risk of extreme disability. To put it more strongly, does a child have a right to life without severe disability, or failing that, a right to be prevented from being born?

One question about any such right is exactly on whom it imposes an obligation. Is it the duty of doctors and genetic counselors to prevent the conception or birth of such babies? This seems implausible. In general, their obligation is to provide information to enable the potential parents to make that decision. Perhaps things are different when the intervention of doctors, through IVF and so on, is required to bring the child into existence. But if there is a right not to be born with severe disability, it imposes duties mainly on the parents. This right may clash with the rights of the potential parents.

We must be cautious about assuming that there is a right not to be born with a severe handicap. Nonetheless, there are cases where it might have been better for the child not to have been born. This is related to the questions of suicide and voluntary euthanasia. Whatever the best approach to these questions, they arise because some kinds of life are perhaps worse than not to be alive at all. In one way, these questions are different, because the person is alive to make his or her own judgment about them. But if people can see death as being in their own interests, it seems equally possible that parents or doctors could think that not being born might be in the interests of a potential child. But a potential child is not like a potential immigrant, someone waiting to be admitted. Here the problem is whose interests are at issue.

Harm and the Comparison with Nonexistence

The claim under consideration is that to be brought into existence with an extremely severe disability may not be in the best interest of a child. This entails a general problem of comparing existence with nonexistence.

When medical techniques determine that some people rather than others come into existence, can those people be said to be better or worse off for the intervention? There are obvious difficulties in making comparisons between being alive and any state of being unconceived. This is a problem if we ask whether anyone is worse off when a child with a disability is born rather than a normal one. (And the idea of replacing someone else is not always clear-cut.) Yet despite these slippery conceptual problems, it does matter whether a normal or a disabled child is conceived. We need to think about these problems in a way that does not undermine this thought, but that avoids sliding into paradox or absurdity.

One approach is to find some national way of making the comparison with nonexistence, perhaps by treating it on a par with being unconscious. Just as it is better to be unconscious than to experience the pain of a major operation, so it could be better not to be conscious at all than to experience certain kinds of life. Being dead or being unconceived could be treated as equivalent to permanent unconsciousness. This provides the necessary comparison, but at the cost of a certain artificiality: a particular person is unconscious during the operation, but no particular person exists in the state of being unconceived. The claim has to be that if a child is brought into the world with a disastrous disability, that child will have a life that is worse than no life. And this is a good reason for preventing the conception of such a child.

MODERATELY SEVERE DISABILITY

The Family

Many people would take as axiomatic that it is better, when possible, to bring into the world a child without even a moderate disability. There is a problem with this view. Moderate disabilities are a substantial disadvantage, but not such that it would be better for the person not to have been born.

One approach would be to base screening policies on the interest of the parents in having a fully normal child. This is a difficult issue, because the effect on a family of having a child with a disability varies enormously. Sometimes the disabled child has qualities that enrich the family. Sometimes the other members of the family are enriched by the qualities brought out in them by the care they need to give. In other families, however, the unavoidable demands create exhaustion and strain, making the parents feel that, in Philip Larkin's words, 'something is pushing them to the side of their own lives' and contributing to depression and divorce. And sometimes the demands of care for the disabled children consume attention that otherwise would go to the other children in the family.

This is a matter where everything depends on the individual case. But there is evidence that a substantial number of parents would support screening for some conditions. A 1983 survey of parents of children with Down's syndrome in the *Journal of Medical Ethics* asked what they would do if they knew that an expected child would have a severe mental disability. A total of 78 percent said they would want the pregnancy terminated. If it is reasonable to suppose that abortion arouses greater opposition than screening, it seems likely that at least this percentage would support a screening program.

It has been suggested that parental interests do not justify preventing the conception or birth of a disabled child, and that the child should be adopted. In some cases where parents do not want to bring up a child with a disability, people may be willing to adopt. But to the extent that the interests of the parents are being considered, it is worth remembering that giving away a child is not easy. From the parents' point of view, a screening program may be the best alternative.

While acknowledging that parental interests are important, supporters of screening policies may think that more is at stake.

Who is Harmed?

Let us put to one side the interests of other people, such as family members, and consider only the handicapped person. Take a case where the rest of the family is not worse off because of the birth of a disabled child. Suppose this child has a moderate disability. Has the failure to prevent the child's existence done any harm? It would be hard to argue that the disabled person has been harmed, for he or she is leading a worthwhile life. There is no reason to think that the alternative (no life at all) would have been better for that person. Can the wrong decision have been made if no one is worse off as a result?

According to one moral principle, something is wrong only when it makes someone worse off than he or she would have been. This person-affecting principle, apart from its general plausibility, is thought to have played a useful role in reproductive ethics. One version of utilitarianism holds that a good way of increasing total happiness is to bring into the world more happy people. This conjures up two nightmares. One is a world where people are obligated to have many children in order to increase total happiness. The other, what Derek Parfit called the 'repugnant conclusion,' is a world with a huge total of happiness resulting from enormous numbers of people whose average level of happiness is low.[2] Jan Narveson once argued that the utilitarian principle should be interpreted in person-affecting terms; that is, to make people happy, not to make happy people.[3] This seems to offer a way around those unattractive alternatives.

[2] Derek Parfit, *Reasons and Persons* (Oxford: Oxford University Press, 1984), ch. 17.
[3] Narveson, 'Utilitarianism and New Generations,' *Mind*, 76/301 (1967), 62–72.

The person-affecting view also has the virtue of backing up one part of the compromise policy on screening. The child with a moderate disability has not been harmed by the absence of a screening program. Where the family and others are not harmed, the person-affecting principle gives no support to such a program.

Two Surrogate Mothers

The person-affecting principle has a platitudinous air, but reproductive ethics can make paradoxes out of apparent platitudes. The difficulty can be brought out by considering a surrogate mother variant of a case discussed by Parfit.[4]

There are two kinds of surrogate mothers. One provides the egg, and so is fully the biological mother. The other, the 'womb-leasing' surrogate mother, does not supply the egg. Agencies often screen potential womb-leasing surrogate mothers in the interest of the future child, for instance to exclude those who are likely to smoke during pregnancy. It is surely right to protect the future child in this way from risk of disability.

Should a similar screening take place for the egg-donor surrogate, for instance, to exclude carriers of genetic disorders? In this case, a different surrogate mother will result in a different child. So where the disability is a moderate one, the person-affecting principle would not require screening. The disabled child is not worse off than he or she would otherwise have been.

Some people believe that the need for screening should not depend on the type of surrogate. For those who take this view, the person-affecting principle is inadequate.

Gene therapy and other genetic engineering, if safe versions are developed, will also raise problems for the person-affecting principle. It is not clear that there is any way of drawing a boundary between genetic changes that occur in the same person and those that cause a change of person. So the boundaries of acting on the person-affecting principle may become blurred.

Impersonal Harms

There may be certain biological mechanisms that favor the conception of normal babies over those that would be abnormal. Imagine that a factory

---

[4] Parfit, *Reasons and Persons*, ch. 16.

emits a chemical that reverses one such mechanism. This mechanism now favors the conception of children who are blind. The pollution seems to have done some harm. But to whom is the harm done? It has not made those children worse off than they would have been, since otherwise they would not have existed. The case that any particular person has been harmed is hard to sustain. Yet we are surely justified in seeing the pollution as harmful and in trying to stop it.

If this is correct, reproductive ethics as a field is characterized by impersonal harms and benefits. Harm can be done even though identifiable people are no worse off than they otherwise would have been. In explaining why it is better to avert the conception of someone with a severe medical condition, we can use the idea of impersonal harms, without having to resort to metaphysical claims about benefits to a particular nonexistent person.

Many find the idea of impersonal harms counterintuitive. One reason for this is a general one underlying the appeal of person-affecting approaches to ethics. For some of us, anything put forward as a moral rule whose justification does not lead back to people (or—not to exclude other animals—at least to conscious beings) has no force. It is a natural progression to think that for an action to be right or wrong someone must be better or worse because of it. The idea of an impersonal harm then seems an evasion of this requirement. Yet the idea is necessary for a plausible account of reproductive ethics.

There is a way of retaining the intuitive spirit of the person-affecting approach while bringing in the substance of the idea of impersonal harm. This is to expand the person-affecting principle through comparisons with alternatives. The pollution that damaged the filter mechanism did not make the blind children worse off than they would have been. But their state is worse than that of the children who would have been born in the absence of the pollution.[5] This comparative version of the person-affecting principle is perhaps a more palatable version of the impersonal approach. By eliminating the impersonal flavor, this approach clearly remains rooted in people and their lives, rather than derived from mere abstract rules.

Disability and Population Size

One reason Narveson introduced the person-affecting approach was to avoid a commitment to creating as many happy people as possible. Does the move toward including impersonal harms lead back to this unattractive commitment?

[5] Hare, 'Abortion and the Golden Rule,' *Philosophy & Public Affairs*, 4 (1975), 201–22.

The creation of many happy people may be in itself a good thing. The idea of it being a duty, however, is outweighed by other considerations, such as loss in the quality of the lives people would lead. But the move to impersonal harms need not involve valuing larger numbers. When picking the best apples, there is no commitment to picking as many as possible.

This discussion has tended to undermine the part of the compromise policy that excludes screening for moderately severe disabilites. It has done so by criticizing one main argument against screening, which appeals to the claim that no one is harmed by the absence of screening. The counterclaim is that the children born because of screening will on the whole benefit more than the children born because of the absence of screening, and that this is relevant. Also relevant are the interests of other members of the family, such as the parents of children with Down's syndrome.

People are faced with different choices. (They normally must choose between different probabilities rather than between the certainty of one outcome or another, but this can be ignored here.) One choice is that between having a normal child and having a moderately disabled child. The appeal to impersonal harms gives a reason for choosing the normal child.

In another kind of choice, the condition may be so severe that the parents (like those of the girl with EB) are not prepared to risk conceiving a child who would have to endure it. Their only option may be to have no child. But the existence of a screening program, by removing the risk, could make a child possible for them. This is a strong point in favor of such a program.

Another choice is that between the risk, or even certainty, of having a child with a moderately severe disability and having no child at all. Here a widely held feeling conflicts with the results of looking in a more detached way at the two outcomes. The widely held feeling is that it surely cannot be right deliberately to produce a child who will suffer from a fairly severe disability. But the couple want the child, and the child, while regretting the disability, will not regret having been born. So no one is made worse off by the decision to have the child. And as no possibility exists of having another child without the disability, there is no impersonal harm. In such a case, the arguments support having the child.

The main arguments of this chapter support screening programs. But there is one argument that tends in the other direction: the danger of undermining respect for people with disabilities. It is important that screening programs be accompanied by social policies that protect and enlarge the civil rights of the disabled. It is even more important that equality of respect be extended to all. Individual differences of ability are quite irrelevant.

14

WRONGFUL LIFE: PARADOXES IN THE MORALITY OF CAUSING PEOPLE TO EXIST

JEFF McMAHAN

I HARM AND IDENTITY

The issue I will discuss can best be introduced by comparing two cases, both of which involve a *Negligent Physician*.

The Preconception Case
A man and a woman are considering having a child but suspect that one of them may be the carrier of a genetic defect that causes moderately severe cognitive impairment. They therefore seek to be screened for the defect. The physician who performs the screening is negligent, however, and assures the couple that there is no risk when in fact the man is a carrier of the defect. As a result, the woman conceives a child with moderately severe cognitive impairments.

Had the screening been performed properly, a single sperm from the man would have been isolated and genetically altered to correct the defect. The altered sperm would then have been combined *in vitro* with an egg drawn from the woman and the resulting zygote would have been implanted in the woman's womb, with the consequence that she would later have given birth to a normal child.

Notice, however, that the probability is vanishingly small that the sperm that would have been isolated and altered would have been the very same sperm that in fact fertilized the egg during natural conception. And let us suppose that the egg that would have been extracted for *in vitro* fertilization would also have been different from the one that was fertilized during natural conception. In that case the child who would have been conceived had the screening been done properly would have developed from a wholly different pair of gametes and would thus in fact (even if it is not a matter of metaphysical necessity) have been a *different* child from the retarded child who now exists.

Now compare the Preconception Case with:

This chapter is an abridged and slightly revised version of a paper with the same title from Jules Coleman and Christopher Morris (eds.), *Rational Commitment and Social Justice: Essays for Gregory Kavka* (Cambridge: Cambridge University Press, 1998), 208–47.

The Prenatal Case
A physician negligently prescribes a powerful drug for a woman who is in the eighth month of pregnancy. The drug causes damage to the fetus's brain and the child to whom she gives birth is, as a consequence, moderately cognitively impaired.

Assume that each of us began to exist prior to eight months after the conception of his or her organism. (I have elsewhere defended at length the claim that each of us began to exist when the brain of his or her fetal organism developed the capacity for consciousness and mental activity—which happened sometime between the 20th and the 28th week of fetal gestation.)[1] In that case, it seems clear that the retarded child who develops as a result of the brain damage is numerically the same child as the child who would have existed had the damage not been done.

There is a sense in which the outcomes of the two cases are the same: a retarded child exists rather than a cognitively normal child. The difference is that, in the Prenatal Case, the retarded child and the possible normal child are the same child in two different possible lives, whereas in the Preconception Case the retarded child and the hypothetical normal child are different children. This latter fact poses a problem, which Derek Parfit calls the *Non-Identity Problem*.[2] Assume that, in both cases, the retarded child's life, though drastically limited in the goods it can contain, is not so bad as not to be worth living. If that is so, it seems that the Negligent Physician's action in the Preconception Case was not worse for the child. For if the Negligent Physician had not acted negligently, *that* child would never have existed; and to exist with a life that is worth living cannot be *worse* than never to exist at all.

So, in the Prenatal Case, the Negligent Physician's action was worse for the retarded child (because it caused him to be retarded rather than normal), while in the Preconception Case it was not. Is this a morally significant difference? And, if the objection to the Negligent Physician's action in the Preconception Case is not that it harmed or was worse for the child, what is it? How can we explain our sense that the Negligent Physician's action was morally objectionable in that case?

It is clear that, in both cases, the Negligent Physician's negligence has harmed the couple, who have been denied many of the joys of parenthood and who instead have the often anguishing burden of caring for a relatively unresponsive and highly dependent child. In the law they would be warranted in bringing a 'wrongful birth' suit against the physician, in which they

[1] See Jeff McMahan, *The Ethics of Killing* (New York: Oxford University Press, forthcoming 2001), chs. I and IV.
[2] Derek Parfit, *Reasons and Persons* (Oxford: Oxford University Press, 1984), ch. 16.

as plaintiffs would claim damages for the harms his negligence has caused them.

But there seems to be more to it than this, even in the Preconception Case. Most of us believe that, quite independently of the impact of the physician's action on the parents, the retarded child in the Preconception Case ought not to have been caused to exist and that, given that he *has* been wrongfully caused to exist, the physician should be required to pay damages not only to compensate the parents for the injury done to them but also, insofar as possible, to enhance the life of the child. This latter conviction lingers even when we understand that, because of the Non-Identity Problem, the Negligent Physician's action was not worse for the child.

In discussing a similar pair of cases, Parfit claims that, given that the outcome is the same in each (that an individual is caused to exist with a disability), it makes no difference that in one case the outcome is worse for the individual whereas in the other case it is not. He calls this the *No-Difference View*. This view is plausible in our two cases. It implies that the objection to the Negligent Physician's action in the Preconception Case is equally strong as the objection to his action in the Prenatal Case. 'This suggests,' Parfit contends, 'that there is the same objection to each act.'[3] Since the objection to the physician's action in the Preconception case cannot be that it harmed or was worse for the retarded child, it follows, if Parfit is right, that this cannot be the objection to his action in the Prenatal Case either. Generalizing, Parfit claims that the fact that an effect is *worse for people*, or bad *for them*, is never part of the fundamental explanation of why the effect is bad. The area of morality 'concerned with beneficence and human well-being,' he writes, 'cannot be explained in person-affecting terms.'[4] It must instead be explained in *impersonal* terms.

The latter inference has broad-ranging implications for moral theory. I will explore these in some detail in Section III; for the moment I will illustrate the significance of Parfit's claim by noting one implication that is of particular interest. I cited earlier the view that each of us began to exist only when the brain of his or her physical organism developed the capacity to generate consciousness and mental activity. This understanding of personal identity, if correct, provides the basis for what seems to be a plausible argument for the permissibility of early abortion. For, according to this view, an early abortion does not kill one of us but instead merely prevents one of us from coming into existence. The organism that is killed is not numerically identical with the later person and thus is not deprived of the later life that is

---

[3] Derek Parfit, 'Comments,' *Ethics*, 96 (1986), 858.
[4] *Reasons and Persons*, 370–1.

precluded. Early abortion, then, is morally comparable to contraception: there need be no one for whom it is worse. The power of this view is illustrated by its ability to explain a common but otherwise puzzling judgment: namely, that it is less objectionable to *kill* a perfectly healthy early fetus than it is to injure or damage it in a comparatively minor way, e.g., a way that causes the subsequent person to have a minor physical disability. The explanation is that, provided that the abortion is desired by the parents, killing the fetus is not worse for anyone, while damaging the fetus harms the person to whose existence the fetus subsequently gives rise. In short, the instance of prenatal injury has a victim while early abortion does not.

According to the No-Difference View, however, that an act is bad or worse *for someone* is no part of the explanation why its effects are bad; accordingly, an act may have a bad effect, and thus be seriously morally objectionable, even if there is no one for whom it is worse or bad in any way. Hence, if Parfit is right, the fact that prenatal injury is worse for the future child does not explain why it is bad to injure a fetus; nor can one infer from the claim that an early abortion is worse for no one that it is not bad. For it might be bad impersonally. The No-Difference View thus appears to undermine both a seemingly plausible basis for distinguishing between prenatal injury and abortion and a powerful argument for the permissibility of early abortion.

II APPROACHES THAT IDENTIFY A VICTIM

Some writers have sought to address the threats that the Non-Identity Problem poses to common sense beliefs by arguing that, in such cases as the Preconception Case, a child born with a disability is adversely affected by the act that causes the disability, even if its life is worth living and it would never have existed had the act not been done. Imagine, for example, that yet another Negligent Physician gives a woman who is having trouble conceiving a child an inadequately tested fertility drug that both allows her to conceive a child and causes the child to suffer from some dreadful disease later in life. It seems reasonable to say that the Physician's act was the cause of the child's contracting the disease and that, in causing the terrible disease, the act *harmed* the child—even though it was not, on balance, worse for the child that the act was done. And, according to one proponent of this approach, 'that an agent is morally accountable for someone's suffering a harm, by virtue of having performed a certain action, seems a perfectly intelligible "person-affecting" explanation why his action is objectionable.'[5]

---

[5] Matthew Hanser, 'Harming Future People,' *Philosophy and Public Affairs*, 19 (1990), 59.

This approach has to be extended somewhat if it is to be applied to cases such as the Preconception Case. For, while contracting a disease is a discrete event that involves the worsening of a prior condition, congenital mental retardation is an inherent, constitutive aspect of a person's nature, not a contingent addition to his life. It is less easy, therefore, to regard the fact that the child in the Preconception Case is retarded as *a harm*. Still, we may invoke Joel Feinberg's notion of a 'harmed condition' in order to assimilate this case into the paradigm to which the vocabulary of harm is applicable. A harmed condition is 'a condition that has adverse effects on [an individual's] whole network of interests,' and is 'the product of a prior act of harming.'[6] Congenital retardation seems to doom many of the retarded individual's interests to frustration. And we may, if only for the sake of argument, grant that the Negligent Physician's action in the Preconception Case counts as an act of harming. The objection, then, to the Physician's action is that it causes the child to exist in a harmed condition. The child is therefore appropriately seen as the victim of this action.

It is not clear whether this approach, which may be called the *harm-based approach*, presupposes that it can be a harm to be *caused to exist* in a harmed condition. Some proponents of the harm-based approach might wish to avoid being committed to the claim that to be caused to exist can be either good or bad for a person. They will therefore want to claim that the Negligent Physician harms the retarded child not by contributing to causing his existence but instead by causing him to be cognitively disabled. It is not obvious, however, that this distinction is tenable, since *this* child can exist only if he is disabled and the actual effect of the Negligent Physician's action is simply to cause this child to exist rather than another child. But I will put this problem aside and assume for the sake of argument that the Negligent Physician's action causes the child's harmed condition—namely, its cognitive disability.

The harm-based approach raises many questions. What, for example, counts as a harmed condition? Is physical unattractiveness or low IQ a harmed condition? Presumably those who argue for this approach wish to avoid the implication that those whose genes make it likely that their offspring would be physically unattractive or have a low IQ would harm their children by causing them to exist (and therefore presumably ought not to have children). There are several options. One would be to equip the notion of a harmed condition with a threshold that would place ordinary ugliness or low intelligence below the threshold but would locate moderately severe

[6] Joel Feinberg, 'Wrongful Life and the Counterfactual Element in Harming,' in his *Freedom and Fulfillment* (Princeton: Princeton University Press, 1992), 6.

mental retardation above it. But in restricting the harm-based approach to cases involving only relatively serious conditions, this revision leaves us without a response in a wide range of cases in which the Non-Identity Problem arises. Consider, for example, a further variant of the Preconception Case in which a couple seek screening for a genetic defect that causes one's child to have an IQ that is roughly 60 points lower than it would otherwise be. As a result of the Physician's negligence, they have a child with an IQ of 90. If the defect had been detected, the man's sperm would have been altered to correct the defect and they would have conceived a different child with an IQ of 150. Surely we want to condemn the Physician's negligence in this variant on substantially the same ground on which we condemn it in the original Preconception Case. But, on the assumption that an IQ of 90 counts as only ordinary low intelligence, the Negligent Physician has not caused the child in this variant to exist in a harmed condition. So, when it incorporates the stipulated threshold, the harm-based approach lacks the resources to explain how the Physician's action has had any bad effect other than the effect on the couple.

Another option is to try to distinguish among the various cases on the basis of differences in causal responsibility. It can be argued, for example, of parents who have a child that is predictably physically unattractive or of low intelligence that, while they are responsible for the child's existence, the fact that the child is unattractive or unintelligent is not attributable to the act that caused the child to exist. There is, in fact, *no* act that causes the child to be unattractive or unintelligent; this is just the way the child is. Thus parents who have an unattractive or unintelligent child do not thereby harm the child. By contrast, consider again the Negligent Physician who administers an untested fertility drug that enables a child to be conceived but also causes the child to develop a serious disease later in life. In this case one and the same act is both a causally necessary condition of the child's existence and the cause of the disease. This act harms the child, though it is not worse for him.

The problem with this response is that it does not seem to divide the cases in the desired way. Reconsider the original Preconception Case. Here the Negligent Physician's action is a causally necessary condition of the retarded child's existence, but it does not seem to be the cause of the retardation, any more than the act of conceiving a predictably ugly child is the cause of the child's ugliness. In each case, that is just the way the child is. So any conception of causal responsibility that allows us to deny that the parents of an ugly child harm the child by causing him to exist seems also to imply that the Negligent Physician in the original Preconception Case does not harm the retarded child. Yet the desire to show that the Physician *does* harm the child is precisely what motivates people to accept the harm-based approach.

Assume, then, that the harm-based approach accepts that to cause someone to exist with a congenital genetic defect is to harm that person if the defect constitutes or inevitably causes a harmed condition. In that case, it seems that we must revert to the option of distinguishing between congenital conditions that count as harmed conditions and those that are insufficiently serious, or perhaps sufficiently widespread or normal, not to count as harmed conditions. (Otherwise the same objection to causing the retarded child to exist in the Preconception Case will apply in *all* cases of causing people to exist, since *everyone* has congenital characteristics that adversely affect their interests—e.g., I have a constellation of interests having to do with achieving great things in philosophy but am thwarted by deficiencies in native intelligence.) As I noted above, this means that the harm-based approach is at most only a partial solution to the Non-Identity Problem; but even a partial solution may constitute progress.

There remains, however, a further problem. In the Preconception Case, and the other cases with which we are concerned, the child whose existence inevitably involves a harmed condition nevertheless has a life that is worth living. The life is worth living because the goods it contains together outweigh the badness of the harmed condition and its effects within the victim's life. Why cannot we say that the act that harmed the child by causing him to have a harmed condition was not bad because the harmed condition is compensated for by the goods of life that the child would not have had if the act had not been performed? There are many instances in which it is best to harm a person for the sake of the compensating benefits that the harmful act brings to that same person—for example, painful or disfiguring medical procedures that are necessary to save a life. If it is not bad, overall, to cause these harms, why is it bad for the Negligent Physician to cause the harm he causes, which is similarly outweighed? (It might be argued that what makes medical procedures that cause harm permissible is the patient's consent; thus the relevant difference between these cases and the Preconception Case is that in the latter the retarded child cannot consent to accept his retardation as the cost of having the compensating goods of life. But it is easy to imagine cases in which it is best to perform a disfiguring or otherwise harmful operation to save a person's life even when the person cannot consent—e.g., because he is unconscious at the time that the decision to operate must be made.)

The problem here is more serious than it may initially seem. In any case in which a child is caused to exist there is a finite probability that the child will have a congenital defect that will constitute or inevitably cause a harmed condition. If, in cases of causing a person to exist, a harmed condition cannot be outweighed by the goods that the life will contain—in the sense that it remains worse, other things being equal, to cause the child to exist—then it is difficult to see how the *probability* of a congenital harmed condition can be outweighed by the probability that the life will also contain compensating goods. But, if the probability that a child will have a congenital harmed condition cannot be outweighed by the probability of compensating goods, then it seems that, at least where *expected* effects are concerned and when other things are equal, it is worse to have a child than not to have a child.

One response to this objection is to claim that, in the Preconception Case, the Negligent Physician is responsible for the harmed condition (i.e., cognitive disability) but not for any of the goods that the retarded child's life contains. The goods are attributable to other causes. On this view, there are no benefits attributable to the Negligent Physician's action that are capable of compensating the child for the harm that the action has caused. This response, however, seems untenable. If the Negligent Physician is responsible for the retardation because it is an inherent aspect of the child's nature and is therefore attributable to those causal factors that produced *that* child with *that* nature, he should be equally responsible for those inherent aspects of the child's nature that are good or beneficial for the child. If it makes sense to say that the retardation adversely affects the child's interests, it should also make sense to say that the good inherent aspects of the child's nature positively affect the child's interests.[7] Finally, if to cause the retardation is to cause a harm (or a harmed condition), then to cause the good aspects of the child's nature should be to cause benefits (or beneficial conditions). If all this is right, the Negligent Physician's action not only harms but also benefits the child—not necessarily by causing the child to exist but by causing the child's life to contain certain goods. And, since the child's life is worth living, it is reasonable to suppose that the benefits outweigh the harms.

A second response to the objection is to claim that, in the case of ordinary procreation, the risk of harming the child by causing him to have a congenital harmed condition is outweighed not by any probable compensating

---

[7] Are a congenitally retarded child's interests adversely affected by the retardation? Consider a nonhuman animal with cognitive and emotional capacities and potentials comparable to those of the retarded child. Are its interests adversely affected by the fact that its cognitive capacities are significantly lower than ours? If not, it is not obvious why one should suppose that the interests of the retarded child are adversely affected by his or her cognitive capacities. One's interests are shaped by one's cognitive capacities. See Jeff McMahan, 'Cognitive Disability, Misfortune, and Justice,' *Philosophy & Public Affairs*, 25 (1996), 3–34.

goods that the child's life might contain but instead by the expected benefits to the parents (and perhaps others in the society) of having the child. It might be thought that this response prevents us from objecting if a couple *deliberately* conceive a child with a congenital harmed condition rather than a normal child. But this worry can be dispelled by noting that parental interests may be sufficiently important to outweigh a *slight* risk of causing a harmed condition without being important enough to outweigh a *high* risk of causing a harmed condition, which there would presumably be if the parents *intended* to cause such a condition. Still, the appeal to parental interests cannot rescue the harm-based approach. For this appeal in effect grants the objection that there is always a presumption against procreation based on the risk of causing a congenital harmed condition—a risk that cannot be offset by the probability of compensating benefits within the life. But it is hard to believe that procreation is, in ordinary conditions, an activity that requires the interests of the prospective parents or of other preexisting persons to tip the balance in favor of permissibility. In ordinary circumstances, there simply is no prima facie objection to or presumption against procreation—or, rather, if there is such a presumption, it derives from current conditions of overpopulation rather from the risk of causing a congenital harmed condition.

The harm-based approach fails because it has no explanation of why an act that is assumed to cause a congenital harmed condition ought not to be done even when it also causes compensating benefits. There is, however, an alternative approach of the same sort—one that identifies a victim—that offers such an explanation. According to this approach, which we may call the *rights-based approach*, there are certain harmed conditions that are sufficiently serious that to cause them constitutes a violation of the victim's rights.[8] Assume that, according to this view, the Negligent Physician in the Preconception Case violates one of the retarded child's rights. (Again this is problematic. It is not obvious exactly what right is supposed to be violated or that the requisite causal connections obtain between the Negligent Physician's action and the relevant aspect of the child's condition.[9] But waive these difficulties.) While the Negligent Physician's action was not worse, or bad on balance, for the child, since the harm it caused is outweighed by compensating goods, that is not a sufficient justification for the action. For,

[8] For a careful exposition of an approach of this sort, see James Woodward, 'The Non-Identity Problem,' *Ethics*, 96 (1986), 804–31.

[9] One way of dealing with this difficulty is to claim not that the Negligent Physician violates the child's rights but that his action causes the child to exist with rights that cannot be fulfilled. Respect for the potential child's rights therefore required that he refrain from doing what would cause the child (and therefore the rights) to exist. Compare Jeff McMahan 'Problems of Population Theory,' *Ethics* 92 (1981): 125.

even if an act is on balance beneficial to a person, or on balance promotes the person's well-being or good, that is in general not a justification for the act if the act also violates the person's rights. Our rights protect us even from certain well-meaning forms of action aimed at our own good. Thus the central objection to the harm-based approach—that it cannot explain why the Negligent Physician's action is wrong if the harm it causes is outweighed by compensating benefits—is met by the rights-based approach.

But the rights-based approach faces other objections. Imagine a disability—*condition X*—that is not so bad as to make life not worth living but is sufficiently serious that to cause someone to exist with condition X would be, according to the rights-based approach, to violate that person's rights. One objection to the rights-based approach is that, if it is wrong to cause someone to exist with condition X, it should also be wrong to save someone's life if the only way of doing so would also cause the person to have condition X and it is not possible to obtain the person's consent to being saved in this way. Suppose, for example, that a late-term fetus (which we may assume would be numerically identical with the person into whom it would develop) contracts a disease that requires a certain treatment in order to survive but that the treatment inevitably causes condition X. Whether or not there is a strong moral reason to save the fetus for its own sake, it seems intuitively clear that it would not be *wrong* to treat the fetus, thereby saving its life. But saving it involves causing it to have condition X and thus, apparently, violates its rights. If it is not permissible to violate a right on the ground that the act that violates the right on balance benefits the right-bearer, then it seems that the rights-based approach implies that it *would* be wrong to save the fetus.

The proponent of the rights-based view may reply that this is a case involving a conflict of rights. While the fetus has a right not to be caused to have condition X, it also has a right to be saved.[10] And in this case the right to be saved, being more important, overrides the right not to be caused to have condition X. This reply assumes, however, that priority between the two rights is determined by the comparative strengths of the interests they protect. But the strength of a right does not vary proportionately with the strength of the interest it protects (assuming that it protects an interest at all). The importance of any interest it might protect is only one of a number of factors that contribute to determining the strength of a right. Among the more important determinants is whether the right is positive or negative. The right to life, or the right not to be killed, and the right to be saved both protect the same interest: namely, the interest in continuing to life or in

[10] I owe this response to Frances Kamm.

avoiding death. But the right not to be killed is a negative right and is thus held, by theorists of rights, to be considerably stronger, other things being equal, than the right to be saved. But if negative rights are in general considerably stronger than corresponding positive rights, it is at least arguable that the negative right not to be caused to be disabled is stronger, or more stringent, than the positive right to be saved.

Let us suppose, however, if only for the sake of argument, that it is true that the late-term fetus's right to be saved overrides its right not to be caused to have condition X, so that the rights-based approach does not imply that it would be wrong to save the fetus. Now consider a parallel case involving an *early-term* fetus. The fetus has a disease that will rapidly be fatal unless it is treated; but the treatment causes condition X. Assume that the claim that I noted earlier is correct—namely, that individuals such as you and I do not begin to exist until our organisms acquire the capacity to support consciousness and mental activity. If that is right, an early-term fetus does not support the existence of an individual of the sort that you and I essentially are. There is no one there to have a right to life or a right to be saved. Hence, according to the rights-based approach, there is a strong reason *not* to treat the fetus, since treating it would violate the right of the later person not to be caused to have condition X, but no countervailing rights-based reason to treat it. The rights-based approach therefore implies that it would be *wrong*, other things being equal, to treat the fetus.

This seems an implausible result. But what is even more implausible is that the rights-based approach distinguishes morally between the case of the late-term fetus and the case of the early-term fetus, claiming that one may treat the former but not the latter. As I indicated, the approach *may* imply that it is wrong to treat the late-term fetus as well. If so, the approach would avoid the embarrassment of treating the two cases asymmetrically. But the claim that it is wrong to treat the late-term fetus is itself quite implausible. There is, of course, a way around the dilemma, which is to reject the view that we do not begin to exist until the fetal organism develops the capacity to support consciousness. If we begin to exist when the human organism begins to exist, shortly after conception, it may be defensible to claim that in both cases the fetus has a right to be saved and that this makes it permissible to treat the fetus despite the fact that doing so infringes its right not to be caused to be disabled. But the supposition that even early fetuses have a right to be saved from death is quite a radical view, with implications for abortion and other issues that many will be reluctant to accept.

If I am right about the metaphysics, the case of the early-term fetus involves a choice between causing a child to exist with a disability and allowing it to be the case that the child fails to come into existence. It is *not* a feature of the case that, if the early-term fetus is untreated, a different, normal child (i.e., without either the disease or condition X) will be caused to exist instead. Cases of this sort are helpful in testing the plausibility of the harm-based and rights-based approaches. For these approaches hold that what is fundamentally objectionable about causing a person to exist with a congenital disability (i.e., one that constitutes a harmed condition or necessarily causes a right to remain unfulfilled) is found in the inherent condition of the person, not in anything extrinsic to the person's life. Thus their plausibility can best be tested by reference to cases in which the only conceivable objectionable features are intrinsic to the life of a person caused to exist with a disability. In other cases, such as the Preconception Case, in which a person is caused to exist with a disability *and* there was the alternative of causing a normal child to exist instead, these approaches may yield the intuitively correct judgment but for the wrong reason. For it may be that the comparative dimension to the case—i.e., that the Negligent Physician causes a disabled child to exist *rather than* a normal child—is an essential part of the explanation of why it is objectionable to cause the disabled child to exist.

To test the approaches that identify a victim, we should therefore consider cases that lack this comparative dimension. Imagine, then, a situation in which *any* child one might cause to exist would have a congenital harmed condition, or a right that would necessarily remain unfulfilled. It is not possible, in the circumstances, to cause a normal child to exist instead. Would it be wrong for a couple who wish to have a child to conceive a child in these circumstances? Most people believe that, provided that the child's life would be worth living and that the motives of those who would cause the child to exist would not be discreditable, it would not be worse, or bad, or wrong (other things being equal) to cause the child to exist. This is not just an intuition. The reason that it is not bad to cause the child to exist is, as I suggested in discussing the harm-based approach, that the goods that the child's life contains compensate for the presence of the harmed condition, without which the child would not exist. Thus the fact that the harm-based and rights-based approaches imply that it *would* be wrong to cause the child to exist constitutes a serious objection to them.[11]

What we need is an account that explains why it is objectionable to cause a disabled child to exist when it would be possible to cause a normal child to exist instead (as in the Preconception Case) but accepts that it is not bad, and is thus permissible if other things are equal, to cause a child to exist with

---

[11] For an intricate and detailed critique of the harm-based and rights-based approaches, see Parfit, 'Comments,' 854–62.

the same disability when any child one might cause to exist would necessarily have that disability. It is difficult to find an approach of the victim-based type that does both these things since these approaches do not locate the objection to causing a disabled child to exist in factors that are comparative or in any way extrinsic to the condition of the child. There is, however, one approach of this sort that has a certain amount of promise. This account invokes the notion of a *restricted life*—a notion introduced by Kavka in his influential and important paper on the Non-Identity Problem.[12] Kavka defines a restricted life as 'one that is significantly deficient in one or more of the major respects that generally make human lives valuable and worth living.' He goes on to note, however, that 'restricted lives typically will be worth living, on the whole, for those who live them.'[13] I will use Kavka's suggestive term in a slightly different way to refer to a life that is objectively not worth living but is subjectively tolerable, and may indeed be overall enjoyable to the individual whose life it is. Such a life is, I will say, subjectively worth living but objectively not worth living. (I put aside the question whether there could be a life that was objectively worth living but subjectively not worth living.) As an example, consider the life of Adolf Hitler. There is reason to believe that Hitler was, during most of his adulthood, abundantly satisfied with his life. Judged by the usual standards, he was a reasonably happy man. His life was therefore subjectively worth living: *he* found it well worth living. But was his life *objectively* worth living? Was this in reality a good life for him to have—better, at least, than no life at all? It is plausible, I think, to claim that Hitler's adult life was a *dreadful* life—not just in its effects on others but dreadful *for him* (even though he himself failed to recognize this). This is not the kind of life that it could be good for anyone to have. It would have been better *for Hitler* if he had died in his twenties.

How does the notion of a restricted life help with the Non-Identity Problem? Assume that the retarded child in the Preconception Case has a restricted life. This explains why it was bad that the Negligent Physician's action resulted in the child's existence: the child's life is not worth living; it is objectively bad *for the child* to exist with that sort of life. If the child's life is genuinely restricted, the goods that it contains do not, on balance, compensate for the child's harmed condition. This also supports the claim that the Negligent Physician owes the child compensation. For the Physician's negligence was culpable and had a victim: the child, for whom the Physician's action was bad.

---

[12] Gregory S. Kavka, 'The Paradox of Future Individuals,' *Philosophy & Public Affairs*, 11 (1982), 93–112.
[13] Ibid. 105.

458   JEFF McMAHAN

This explanation is, however, essentially noncomparative: it does not mention the alternative possible outcome in which a normal child would have existed. It focuses entirely on the intrinsic features of the retarded child's life. How, then, can it explain the permissibility of causing a child with a life like this to exist when it would not be possible to cause a normal child to exist instead? This approach must, it seems, claim that there is a serious prima facie reason not to have such a child—namely, that it would be objectively bad for the child. Yet, although a life that is objectively not worth living is bad, it is not nearly so bad if it is subjectively worth living as it would be if it were also subjectively not worth living. For a life that is objectively not worth living but is nevertheless subjectively worth living is not experienced as a burden by the person whose life it is. Thus the moral presumption against causing a person to exist with a restricted life may be overridden by countervailing considerations that are considerably weaker than those that would be required to override the much stronger presumption against causing a person to exist with a life that would be both subjectively and objectively not worth living. Assuming, then, that the desire to have a child has a certain normative force (e.g., that it is supported by a right of procreation), it might be that the desire of a couple to have a child could be sufficient to outweigh the harm they would do to the child by causing it to exist with a restricted life. But this same desire would be insufficient to justify causing a child to exist with a restricted life when it would be possible to have a normal child instead. For the reasonable desire to have a child could be satisfied by having the normal child. There would have to be some *other* reason to justify doing what would cause a child with a restricted life to exist rather than a normal child. And in the ordinary circumstances of life it is doubtful that there could be a reason sufficiently strong to justify the harm to a child with a restricted life.

Even when it would be permissible for a couple to cause a child to exist with a restricted life, the child would have a claim to compensation comparable in force to that which the retarded child has against the Negligent Physician in the Preconception Case. In practice this means that a couple that chose to have a child with a restricted life would be morally required to make sacrifices for the child that would not be part of the normal burden of child-rearing. This, however, seems entirely plausible. Whether such parents would owe as much as the Negligent Physician depends on whether the fact that he is at fault compounds his liability.

The appeal to the notion of a restricted life thus has a certain promise. But it nevertheless faces serious objections. It may be objected, for example, that the killing of people judged to have restricted lives could be justified as euthanasia. This, however, is not a serious concern. For the morality of killing is not governed solely by considerations of harm and benefit. Even though there is a sense in which it would be better for a person with a restricted life to die rather than continue to live, it certainly does not follow that it would be permissible to kill that person against his or her will. It has to be conceded, however, that the notion of a restricted life is an exceedingly dangerous one; for it asserts the possibility that others could know that one's life was not worth living even if one were oneself convinced that it was worth living. As a matter of principle this in fact seems to be right: it is possible to believe that one's life is worth living when in fact it is not. But surely this occurs very rarely and in most cases one's judgment about whether one's own life is worth living is, if not authoritative, then at least so nearly infallible that it would be the height of presumption for another person to dispute it.

This observation reveals the central weakness of the appeal to the notion of a restricted life—that there are scarcely any plausible instances of lives of this sort.[14] Perhaps the most plausible examples are of people whose lives, while enjoyable, are utterly morally debased. But these cases are largely irrelevant to the morality of causing people to exist because of the impossibility, at least at present, of predicting before a life begins that it will be morally degraded. Among predictable conditions, it is difficult to identify *any* that clearly make a life objectively not worth living without making it subjectively not worth living as well. Perhaps the most plausible candidate is severe congenital cognitive incapacity. Loren Lomasky contends that, 'were one condemned . . . to remain a child throughout one's existence, or to grow in bulk without simultaneously growing in the capacity to conceptualize ends and to act for their sake, it would be a personal misfortune of the utmost gravity.'[15] The idea that the severely retarded are appropriately viewed as permanently infantile suggests that a life in this condition may be objectively degraded or unworthy, even if it is subjectively tolerable. It is, however, difficult to reconcile this judgment with the commonly accepted assumption that the lives of nonhuman animals with comparable cognitive capacities may be worth living and are certainly not objectively degraded simply because they are not guided by the exercise of our higher cognitive capacities.[16]

The Non-Identity Problem arises in a large number of cases. Since it is

---

[14] The limited applicability of Kavka's notion of a restricted life to the Non-Identity Problem is noted by Derek Parfit in his reply to Kavka, 'Future Generations: Further Problems,' *Philosophy & Public Affairs*, 11 (1982), 120–1.

[15] Loren Lomasky, *Persons, Rights, and the Moral Community* (New York: Oxford University Press, 1987), 202.

[16] Cf. 'Cognitive Disability, Misfortune, and Justice.'

difficult to think of a single case in which a predictable condition causes a person to have a restricted life, it is safe to conclude that the appeal to the notion of a restricted life cannot solve this problem.[17]

III THE IMPERSONAL COMPARATIVE APPROACH

Other writers have discussed cases with the same structure as the Preconception Case under the heading of 'wrongful life.' Some have contended that the fundamental objection in these cases to causing a child to exist with a disability is that this gratuitously increases the amount of evil, or that which is bad, that the world contains. Joel Feinberg, for example, claims that the agent in a case such as the Preconception Case 'must be blamed for wantonly introducing a certain evil into the world, not for harming, or for violating the rights of, a person.' He then goes on to elucidate the nature of the evil when he observes that one could make the willful creation of a disabled child a criminal act on the ground that 'the prevention of unnecessary suffering is a legitimate reason for a criminal prohibition.'[18] These remarks are echoed by John Harris, who writes: 'What then is the wrong of wrongful life? It can be wrong to create an individual in a harmed condition even where the individual is benefited thereby. The wrong will be the wrong of bringing avoidable suffering into the world, of choosing deliberately to increase unnecessarily the amount of harm or suffering in the world.'[19]

To say that some instance of suffering is 'unnecessary' or 'avoidable' is to imply that it is wrong to cause that suffering. But what exactly does it mean to say that suffering is unnecessary or avoidable? In one sense, it means simply that the suffering could have been avoided. But that is true of *all* human suffering, since it has always been possible for people simply to stop procreating. Thus those unguarded forms of Negative Utilitarianism that call simply for the minimization of suffering have notoriously been accused of implying that it is wrong ever to cause a sentient being to exist. But this is surely not the sense of 'unnecessary' intended by Feinberg and Harris. The normal implication of the claim that some instance of suffering is unnecessary is that the suffering is not instrumental to or a necessary accompani-

[17] It may be easier to find examples in which a *part* of a life is restricted. Imagine that a person whose life has hitherto been devoted to intellectual pursuits suffers brain damage and becomes a contented idiot. Her subsequent life may be subjectively tolerable from her present point of view but objectively not worth living in the light of values that she autonomously embraced prior to the loss of her cognitive competence.

[18] Feinberg, 'Wrongful Life and the Counterfactual Element in Harming,' 27 and 28.

[19] John Harris, *Wonderwoman and Superman: The Ethics of Human Biotechnology* (Oxford: Oxford University Press, 1992), 90.

ment of some greater good for the person who experiences the suffering. Thus suffering that is *not* unnecessary is suffering that has to occur if certain compensating goods are to be had by the sufferer. In this sense, the foreseeable suffering that any life that is worth living will inevitably contain is not unnecessary. But then this applies equally to the foreseeable suffering within the lives of the congenitally disabled, provided that their lives would be worth living. Their suffering is not unnecessary in this second sense.

Feinberg and Harris must therefore be invoking a third sense in which suffering may be unnecessary. Consider again the Preconception Case. Whatever suffering the child experiences as a result of the retardation is not unnecessary for the compensating goods of *that* life. But it is unnecessary for goods of the same type—indeed a greater quantity of those goods—within a *different* life that might have been caused to occur instead. The objection urged by Feinberg and Harris therefore takes an impersonal, comparative form. For it is not concerned with effects for better or worse on any particular individual but with the comparison between the possible effects on one possible individual with those on another. The objection to causing the retarded child to exist is that it was possible to cause a *different* child to exist whose life would have contained at least as much good but less of what is bad—in particular, less overall suffering. It is in this impersonal sense that the retarded child's suffering is unnecessary.

A more precise articulation of this sort of approach has been formulated by Parfit in the following principle: 'If in either of two possible outcomes the same number of people would ever live, it would be worse if those who live are worse off, or have a lower quality of life, than those who would have lived.'[20] Call this the *Impersonal Comparative Principle*. Notice that it is explicitly restricted to what Parfit calls 'Same-Number Choices'—that is, cases in which the same number of people would exist in all the possible outcomes of a choice between acts. Note furthermore that, being impersonal, the Impersonal Comparative Principle is consistent with the No-Difference View, which asserts, in effect, that the correct principle of beneficence must take a fully impersonal form. Finally, notice that this principle presupposes that possible people count morally and must be taken into account in moral deliberation.

The Impersonal Comparative Principle has a distinct advantage. It does seem, intuitively, that the morality of causing a disabled child to exist is affected by whether or not it would be possible to cause a normal child to exist instead. The Impersonal Comparative Principle captures this. Thus it

---

[20] *Reasons and Persons*, 360. Kavka proposed a similar principle but rejected it in 'The Paradox of Future Individuals,' 99–100.

condemns the Negligent Physician's action in the Preconception Case because the normal child who might have existed would have been better off than the retarded child is. But it does not condemn a couple for having a child with the same disability provided that the child's life is worth living and that any child they might have would also have that disability. It does not condemn such a couple because it has *no* implications for their choice. Their choice is between having a disabled child and having no child. It is therefore not a Same-Number Choice but what Parfit calls a 'Different-Number Choice'—that is, a case in which different numbers of people would exist in some of the possible outcomes of a choice between acts.

Does the Impersonal Comparative Principle support the intuition that the Negligent Physician in the Preconception Case owes compensation to the retarded child? Here is an argument for the claim that it does. According to the Impersonal Comparative Principle, the Physician has a moral reason *ex ante* to ensure that a normal child exists rather than a disabled child. Indeed, his general reason to bring about the better outcome is strengthened in this case by his professional commitment. Presumably he would even have been required, if necessary, to accept certain costs in order to ensure the conception of a normal child rather than a retarded child. (The extent of the cost he should accept in order to ensure the better outcome is of course limited. If, for example, the cost to him of ensuring the conception of a normal child rather than a disabled child would be as great as the cost to a couple of being unable to have a child, then it might be permissible for him to allow the conception of a disabled child. But it is hard to imagine circumstances in which personal costs this great would be required from a physician in order to ensure the conception of a normal rather than a disabled child.) Let us stipulate that the Negligent Physician in the Preconception Case would have been required to accept costs up to amount x in order to ensure that the couple would conceive a normal rather than a disabled child. If that is true, it seems reasonable to suppose that, since his negligence has brought about the worse outcome, he should be required *ex post* to pay costs at least up to amount x in order to repair the result of his fault. In particular, he should be required to pay up to amount x, if necessary, to try to make the disabled child's life as good as the normal child's life would have been. If the compensation could succeed in benefiting the disabled child to that extent, this would cancel the bad effect of his previous action.

This argument is vulnerable to several objections. First, it is not plausible to suppose that there are grounds for liability whenever the Impersonal Comparative Principle implies that it was worse to cause some person to exist. For the Impersonal Comparative Principle implies that it is worse, other things being equal, to cause a person to exist whenever it would be possible to cause a different, better-off person to exist instead. Thus it implies that it would be worse to cause a normal person to exist if it would be possible to cause a person with an unusually high capacity for well-being to exist instead. But if, in these circumstances, one were to cause the normal person to exist, it is implausible to suppose that this would make one liable to compensate that person for being worse off than some extraordinary possible person might otherwise have been.

Second, the case for compensation depends on the availability of a better alternative. The Impersonal Comparative Principle does not imply that there is a reason not to cause a disabled child to exist when there is no possibility of causing a better-off child to exist instead. Hence there is no reason in these circumstances for an agent to accept costs *ex ante* to avoid causing a disabled child to exist and no basis for a claim to compensation *ex post*. But now imagine two equally disabled children, only one of whom was caused to exist in conditions in which a normal child could have been caused to exist instead. Although both have the same disability, only this child can claim compensation. But it may seem unfair to deny the other compensation just because there was no possibility of causing a normal child to exist in his place.

Finally, and most importantly, recall that the reason that the Impersonal Comparative Principle holds that the Negligent Physician's action was worse is not that it harmed or wronged the retarded child. His offense was instead *impersonal*. But, if the original action was objectionable for impersonal reasons, the reason to redress the situation should be impersonal as well. There is, in other words, no reason why the remedy—that is, the action aimed at canceling the bad effect—should benefit the disabled child. After all, that child is not, according to the Impersonal Comparative Principle, a victim of the Negligent Physician's action.

Despite initial appearances, therefore, the Impersonal Comparative Principle provides no basis for liability on the part of the Negligent Physician to compensate the disabled child. This may or may not constitute an objection to the principle. For it is unclear whether, in the Preconception Case, the child in fact deserves compensation. The child may deserve special compensation through relevant mechanisms of social redistribution simply for being badly off—either in absolute terms or relative to the norms of the society. In this respect the child is on a par with others who are badly off through no fault of their own. There is no reason why the Negligent Physician in particular should be required to do more than anyone else to help the child.

But, while it is not clear whether the disabled child in the Preconception Case deserves compensation, it *is* clear that the disabled child in the Prenatal Case deserves compensation and that it is the Negligent Physician who is morally (and legally) liable to pay it. Recall, however, that according to the No-Difference View, the objection in the Prenatal Case to the Negligent Physician's causing the child to be disabled rather than normal is the *same* as the objection in the Preconception Case to the Negligent Physician's causing a disabled child to exist rather than a normal child. The objection in the Preconception Case is impersonal in character; therefore the objection in the Prenatal Case must also be impersonal—which, of course, is exactly what the Impersonal Comparative Principle implies, since it treats the two cases in exactly the same way. Indeed, according to the generalized No-Difference View, the whole of the morality of beneficence is to be explained in impersonal terms. Person-affecting principles may often yield the right answers but they *never* provide the correct explanation, which is always impersonal. If it is worse to perform some act, it is not because the act is bad or worse *for somebody*; there are never any victims in the relevant sense. Notice, however, what this implies. If the objection to the Negligent Physician's action in the Prenatal Case is impersonal, then there can be no more basis for liability here than there is in the Preconception Case. Indeed, if the generalized No-Difference View is correct, then there can never be any basis for liability to compensate an individual for harm that one has done to that individual. Or at least this is true within the area of morality concerned with beneficence, or well-being. Parfit leaves it open that there may be areas of morality governed by respect for rights, or other considerations beyond the scope of beneficence. But if, as Parfit assumes, such cases as the Prenatal Case, in which one person's negligence causes another to suffer a serious disability, come within the morality of beneficence, then it seems that the areas governed by rights cannot be more than tiny provinces at the periphery.

Most of us firmly believe that, in the Prenatal Case, the Negligent Physician owes compensation to the child he has caused to be disabled rather than normal. That the Impersonal Comparative Principle seems incapable of supporting this belief is a serious objection to it, on the assumption that the No-Difference View is true. If the Prenatal Case were outside the proper scope of the Impersonal Comparative Principle, there would be no problem. But the No-Difference View holds that there is no relevant difference between the Prenatal Case and the Preconception Case, that the objection to the Negligent Physician's conduct is therefore the same in each, and that that objection is provided by the Impersonal Comparative Principle.

That the Impersonal Comparative Principle cannot account for the Negligent Physician's liability in the Prenatal Case is only one of many problems it faces. Here is another. As it is stated, the principle refers only to people. But there is no obvious reason why it should not apply to nonpersons as well. But, when extended in this way, it implies that it is worse, and therefore presumptively objectionable, to breed one's dog rather than to have a child, if one cannot do both. For to breed the dog would be to cause a worse-off rather than a better-off individual to exist.[21] And it would be worse to breed one's lizard than to breed one's dog, if one could not do both. And so on.

These implications are implausible. There are several ways that a defender of the Impersonal Comparative Principle might seek to avoid them. One would be to appeal to side-effects—for example, by arguing that, because of overpopulation, causing a person to exist has such bad side-effects that on balance it would not be worse to breed one's dog instead. But this response is inadequate. It is not because of human overpopulation that it is permissible to breed one's dog. And in any case the principle still implies that it *was* worse, before overpopulation arose, to breed one's dog rather than to have a child.

A second possible response is to note that the Impersonal Comparative Principle, as stated by Parfit, refers only to what is *worse*, not to what is *wrong*—that is, it concerns only the evaluation of outcomes, not what one ought or ought not to do. Therefore, it is only if the principle is conjoined with something like Act Consequentialism that it has implausible implications about procreation and breeding. Again, however, this response is inadequate. For the Impersonal Comparative Principle must be conjoined with *some* principle that explains how considerations of consequences should guide our action; otherwise its utility will be extremely limited when applied to cases like the Preconception Case. It is fairly obvious in that case that the Negligent Physician brings about the impersonally worse of two possible outcomes. What is important is the further claim that this is what explains why his action was morally objectionable or wrong, other things being equal. And it is reasonable to expect that any action-guiding principle that, when conjoined with the Impersonal Comparative Principle, implies that it is wrong to bring about the worse of the two outcomes in the Preconception Case will also imply that it is wrong to bring about the worse of the two outcomes when the choice is between having a child and breeding one's dog.

Perhaps the most plausible response to this challenge is to restrict the scope of the Impersonal Comparative Principle so that it applies only to cases involving lives of the same kind. Suitably restricted, it would imply that it is worse to cause the worse-off of two possible people to exist, and worse to cause the worse-off of two possible dogs to exist; but it would have

---

[21] Here I follow Robert Merrihew Adams, 'Must God Create the Best?', *Philosophical Review*, 81 (1972), 329.

nothing to say about whether it is worse to cause a dog to exist rather than a person. While I am skeptical that a principled rationale for such a restriction could be found, I cannot exclude the possibility.

The deepest problems for the impersonal conception of beneficence that is required by the No-Difference View emerge when we try to extrapolate beyond the Impersonal Comparative Principle to a principle that covers not only Same-Number Choices but also Different-Number Choices. Among those choices in which different people exist in the different possible outcomes, Different-Number Choices are significantly more common than Same-Number Choices. It is therefore essential to have a principle that covers those choices. There is, however, a formidable obstacle to extending the impersonal approach so that it applies in these cases. The extended principle must surely imply, as the Impersonal Comparative Principle does, that an outcome is worse if the people who exist in that outcome are worse off than the people who would exist in an alternative outcome. But when different numbers of people exist in the different outcomes, it becomes very difficult to determine which group is better off than the others. One has to weigh the number of lives, or perhaps the overall quantity of life, against the overall quality of life. And one has to determine how to measure the overall quality of life in a group in which individual lives may vary considerably in overall quality. Is the group with the best overall quality of life the one with the highest average quality of life, the highest maximum, or perhaps the lowest minimum? Should the measurement of overall quality of life take into account the relative levels of equality in the quality of life within the different groups? And if so, how is equality itself to be measured?

These and other problems are explored with tremendous subtlety and ingenuity in Parfit's book, *Reasons and Persons*. He assigns the label 'Theory X' to the theory that would plausibly extend the Impersonal Comparative Principle so that it would cover Different-Number Choices. While he states a variety of requirements that Theory X would have to satisfy in order to be acceptable, he confesses his own inability to discover the content of the theory. He concludes, however, with an expression of optimism: 'Though I failed to discover X, I believe that, if they tried, others could succeed.'[22]

I believe that there is reason to doubt this. Theory X must take an impersonal form: it must presuppose that the fact that an act is bad or worse *for someone* cannot be part of the fundamental explanation of why its effects are bad or why the act itself is wrong. Because of this, I suspect that any candidate for Theory X will have implications that undermine its credibility. In order to try to substantiate this suspicion, I will indicate what I think some of these implications are. I must acknowledge, however, that I cannot demonstrate that Theory X will have these implications. As yet there is no Theory X; therefore neither I nor anyone else can say what its implications might be. My claim can only be that it is difficult to see how any candidate for Theory X can avoid the implications to which I will call attention.

Let us revert to a problem mentioned earlier in Section I: the problem of abortion. On the assumption that a new individual of our kind does not begin to exist until some time during the second half of pregnancy, the choice between having and not having an early-term abortion is a Different-Number Choice: the number of people who will ever exist if one has the abortion will be different from the number who will exist if one does not. This is, however, a very simple Different-Number Choice. Consider:

The Early-Term Abortion
A woman is in the very early stages of pregnancy. If she continues the pregnancy, the child she has will have a life that is well worth living. It would be better for her and her partner, however, if she has an abortion. But, because the society in which they live is underpopulated, the abortion would also have certain bad effects on other people. Assume that these various good and bad effects on preexisting people counterbalance one another—that is, they cancel each other out. The couple decide to have the abortion. Overall this is not worse for the people who ever exist.

Suppose we want to know which of the two possible outcomes is better *impersonally*. The complications mentioned earlier that typically make it so difficult to determine which of two different-sized groups is better off simply do not arise in this case. In the actual outcome, a certain number of people exist. If the abortion had not been performed, exactly those same people would have existed and overall their collective level of well-being would have been the same. The only difference is that in the second outcome there would have been one additional person whose life would, we may assume, have been worth living. (There are instances in which, when one thing that is good when taken by itself is added to a second thing that is also good by itself, the result is a decrease in the degree of goodness of the second thing. Nothing like this would occur if, in the Early-Term Abortion, the abortion were not performed and a new person were added to the existing population.) But if, from an impersonal point of view, the two outcomes differ only in that one contains an additional life in which the good elements outweigh the bad, then it seems that the outcome with the additional good should be better impersonally.

One might arrive at the same conclusion by a slightly more circuitous route. Let us define three outcomes: having a Happy Child, having a Less Happy Child, and having No Child. According to the Impersonal Comparative Principle, having a Less Happy Child is worse than having a Happy

Child, other things being equal. This is not because having the Less Happy Child would be bad in itself; it is just that having a Happy Child contributes more to making the world better. But if having a Happy Child is better than having a Less Happy Child because it adds more good to the world, then it seems that having a Happy Child must also be better than having No Child, other things being equal, and for the same impersonal reason.

In the Preconception Case, the Negligent Physician causes the couple to have a Less Happy Child rather than a Happy Child. In the Early-Term Abortion, the couple have No Child rather than a Happy Child. From an impersonal of view, the latter should be as objectionable as the former. If we conclude that the Negligent Physician *ought not* to have caused the less good outcome rather than the better one, and for reasons that are impersonal, it may be difficult to avoid the conclusion that the woman in the Early-Term Abortion *ought not* to have had the abortion. It seems that Theory X, which will extend the claim of the Impersonal Comparative Principle so that it covers Different-Number Choices, may imply that abortion is wrong. The impersonal approach to the Non-Identity Problem thus not only threatens a powerful argument in favor of the permissibility of abortion (as I suggested in Section I) but also supports an argument against the permissibility of abortion.

Indeed the problem runs deeper than this. The objection to abortion that seems to be implied by the impersonal approach cannot, of course, be that abortion is murder, that it harms the fetus, or that it is against the fetus's interests. It is simply that abortion prevents the existence of a person whose existence would make the outcome better in impersonal terms. But this is equally true of the use of contraception and indeed of any choice that results in abstention from procreation. To the extent that abortion is objectionable from an impersonal point of view, these other forms of behavior must be objectionable as well, other things being equal, and for the same reason.

The common sense view is of course entirely different. Most of us believe that there is no moral reason to cause a person to exist just because the person's life would be worth living—that there is no reason, other things being equal, to have a Happy Child rather than No Child. But we also believe that, *if* one is going to have a child, one has reason, other things being equal, to have a Happy Child rather than a Less Happy Child. The moral reason for having a Happy Child is conditional on a prior determination to have a child. Thus we believe that it is permissible to have No Child rather than a Happy Child even though it is wrong to have a Less Happy Child rather than a Happy Child, other things being equal. I have suggested, however, that it is difficult to see how this set of beliefs could be defensible within an impersonal conception of beneficence.

Parfit has suggested an analogy that might be thought to show how these beliefs could be consistent.[23] Suppose, Parfit writes, that I have three alternatives:

A: at some great cost to myself, saving a stranger's right arm;
B: doing nothing;
C: at the same cost to myself, saving both the arms of this stranger.[24]

Most of us believe that, if these are the alternatives, it is permissible to do B—that is, to save neither arm. But, if one has decided to help the stranger, it would be wrong to do A—that is, to save one arm rather than two. If one has decided to accept a certain cost to help the stranger, and the cost will be the same whether one saves one arm or both, it would be perverse not to do what would achieve the greater good. In short, while there is no duty to do C rather than B, there is a duty to do C rather than A.

Now alter the values of the variables so that one's alternatives are:

A: having a Less Happy Child;
B: having No Child;
C: having a Happy Child.

Again the common view is that, if these are the alternatives, it is permissible to do B—that is, it is permissible not to have a child. But, if one has decided to have a child, it would be wrong to do A—that is, to have a Less Happy Child rather than a Happy Child. As in the first set of alternatives, there is no duty to do C rather than B, though there is a duty to do C rather than A. This is the common sense conception of the morality of procreation. The parallel with the first set of alternatives suggests that this conception is defensible and hence that I was mistaken to claim that, if C is better than A, it must also be better than B.

This counterargument fails, however, for the two sets of alternatives are not in fact parallel. Once parallelism is established, the comparison between them supports rather than refutes my claim. In the first set of alternatives, C is the best outcome, impersonally considered. There is also a strong moral reason to do C rather than B. It is only because there is a great cost to the agent attached to C that it is permissible to do B rather than C. If we

---

[23] Parfit is discussing his own revised version of a principle suggested but ultimately rejected by Kavka. Thus he does not himself employ his analogy the way that I do here and my critique of the analogy is not directed against his discussion. See his 'Future Generations: Further Problems,' 127–32.

[24] Ibid. 131.

subtract the stipulations about costs from the first set of alternatives, so that this set becomes analogous to the second, one would be required to do C rather than B (which is the conclusion that I assume is implied by the impersonal approach in the second set of alternatives). Alternatively, if one adds parallel stipulations about cost to the second set of alternatives, common sense intuitions may be upheld but the explanation of why it is permissible to have No Child is no longer that this outcome is not worse than having a Happy Child. The explanation instead appeals to considerations of cost, which are extraneous to the impersonal evaluation of the outcomes.[25] Indeed, to maintain parallelism with the first set of alternatives, it must be granted that there is a strong moral reason to have a Happy Child rather than No Child. This reason is overridden only by considerations of cost to the agent.

So the point still stands: it seems that Theory X will imply that it is better for a Happy Child to exist than for No Child to exist and consequently that there is a moral reason to have a Happy Child rather than No Child. While common sense resists this claim, it is not obviously wrong. But there is worse to come. For, from an impersonal point of view, there seems to be no fundamental difference between starting a life and extending a life. Provided that each would be worth living, one's reason to create a new life is the same as one's reason to extend an existing life: namely, that doing either makes the outcome better by causing there to be more of what is good, or that which makes life worth living. This suggests that, other things being equal, Theory X will imply that there is as much reason to cause a new person to exist as there is to save a person's life. Indeed, since the outcome of saving a life contains only a *part* of that life, whereas the outcome of causing a person to exist contains the *whole* of a life, it will normally be *better*, other things being equal and from an impersonal point of view, to cause a person to exist than to save a person's life.

This is very hard to believe. But there is more. Accounts of the morality of beneficence that are impersonal in character tend to treat as irrelevant certain aspects of an agent's mode of agency. They tend, for example, to deny that there is any moral significance to the distinction between doing and allowing, or to the distinction between effects that are intended and those that are foreseen but unintended. While there is no necessary incompatibility between an impersonal theory of beneficence and claims about the significance of agency that are essentially deontological in character, it is neverthe-

---

[25] Parfit's own discussion of the parallels between the first and second sets of alternatives explicitly appeals to considerations of cost to the agent in order to explain why 'most of us ... have no duty to have unwanted children.' Ibid. 128.

less natural that a theory that evaluates outcomes impersonally should also take an impersonal view of agency. If the identity of the beneficiary or victim of an act makes no difference to the morality of the act, it should not be surprising if neither the identity of the agent nor his or her mode of agency matters either. Thus many writers who accept an impersonal theory of beneficence deny that there is any fundamental or intrinsic difference between failing to save a person and killing a person. But, if this is right, and if there is also no fundamental difference between saving a person and causing a person to exist (or between not saving a person and not causing a person to exist), it follows that there is no difference, other things being equal, between killing a person and failing to cause a person to exist. From an impersonal point of view, both are bad for the same reason: the outcome is worse because it contains less good—less good than it would have contained had a person with a life worth living continued to exist or been caused to exist. Indeed, failing to cause a person to exist will, other things being equal, be *worse*, for the same reason that it is normally impersonally worse than failing to save a person.

It might be argued that, even if Theory X has these implications, this does not show that it is unacceptable. For Theory X is an account of beneficence only, and there is more to the morality of killing than considerations of beneficence. Killing may be specially objectionable, for example, because it involves a violation of rights. But, if this defense works at all, it applies only to the comparison between killing and failing to cause a person to exist. For it is implausible to suppose that the morality of saving lives lies outside the scope of beneficence.

A second response might be to argue that it is compatible with a wholly impersonal conception of beneficence to suppose that there is a moral asymmetry between harms and benefits, or between suffering losses and forgoing gains, or something of the sort. If there is such an asymmetry, then even within the morality of beneficence killing a person is worse than failing to cause a person to exist, since killing involves harm or loss while the failure to cause a person to exist involves only the absence of benefit or gain. This, however, is a mistake. The harm of death consists primarily if not exclusively in the loss of the benefits of continued life. Death and the failure of a person to come into existence involve the same sorts of loss from the impersonal point of view.

Finally, even if there are dimensions to the morality of killing beyond the evaluation of outcomes (and I believe that there are), Theory X seems to get even the evaluation of outcomes wrong. If we compare an act of killing with a failure to cause a person to exist, it seems that the *outcome* of the killing is worse. It is a worse state of affairs when someone dies (whether from being killed or from natural causes) than it is when a person fails to come into existence, assuming that in both cases the lives would have been worth living.

In sum, it is difficult to see how Theory X can avoid implying that, other things being equal, (1) it is better to have a Happy Child rather than No Child; hence (2) there are serious moral objections to abortion, contraception, and celibacy; (3) the failure of a person to come into existence is at least as bad an outcome as the death of a person; hence (4) the failure to cause a person to exist is at least as bad as the failure to save a person's life and (5) the failure to cause a person to exist is at least as bad as killing a person. These claims, or at any rate the last three, are plainly unacceptable. The only hope for Theory X is that it can avoid having them as implications. Despite my earlier remarks, those who are attracted to the impersonal approach may remain optimistic. They may point out that there are, after all, some familiar candidates for Theory X that do not necessarily have these implications. If, for example, a Happy Child would have a level of well-being at or below the average, Average Consequentialism would not imply that it is better to have the Happy Child than to have No Child; yet it would imply that, *if* it were inevitable that *some* child was going to exist, it would be better to have the Happy Child than to have a Less Happy Child. But this is just an accident of the arithmetic. If the Happy Child would be above the average, it would be better, other things being equal, to have the Happy Child. And if the existing population were quite large and the Happy Child would be well above the average and would live long, it would be better, according to Average Consequentialism, to have the Happy Child than to save a person whose life was well below the average. It is important to note these facts, since Average Consequentialism is, in effect, concerned exclusively with the quality of life (which it measures in terms of the average) and gives no weight to increasing the number of lives except insofar as this affects the overall quality of life. Among the known impersonal theories of beneficence, therefore, it is the one least likely to have the claims cited above among its implications.[26]

IV CONCLUSION

To be acceptable, Theory X must imply that failing to save a person whose life would be worth living is, other things being equal, not just worse but significantly worse than failing to cause a person to exist. And this implica-

---

[26] Average Consequentialism has been extensively criticized. See, e.g., 'Problems of Population Theory,' 111–15.

tion must not just be a contingent feature of the way the math works out. It must instead flow from the theory in a way that plausibly explains why the death of a person is a worse outcome than the failure of a person to come into existence.

I cannot prove that no impersonal theory can satisfy this condition. Yet there is good reason to believe that no impersonal theory can. For it seems essential to the explanation of why the death of a person is worse than the failure of a person to come into existence that the former is worse *for someone* while the latter is not. Person-affecting considerations seem indispensable.

In many cases involving the Non-Identity Problem, a choice seems to have a bad effect but is nevertheless not worse for anyone. Parfit asks whether, in these cases, the fact that the choice is not worse for anyone makes a moral difference. 'There are,' he writes, 'three views. It might make all the difference, or some difference, or no difference. There might be no objection to our choice, or some objection, or the objection may be just as strong.'[27] Parfit accepts the third view, the No-Difference View. According to this view, whether or not the choice is worse for anyone is morally irrelevant; impersonal considerations alone matter. I have tried to show why I think this view will prove to be unacceptable. According to the first view, impersonal considerations have no weight; person-affecting considerations alone matter. As Parfit has shown, this first view is untenable. This leaves the second view.

As I understand it, the second view holds that an effect may be bad even if it is not worse for anyone, but not as bad as it would be if it *were* worse for someone. In short, impersonal considerations matter, but person-affecting considerations matter more. According to this view, the outcome in the Prenatal Case is worse than the outcome in the Preconception Case. In each case, an individual is caused to exist with a disability. In the Prenatal Case, this effect is worse for the individual, since he could have existed without the disability. In the Preconception Case, the effect is not worse for the individual; but it is worse impersonally, since a different child without the disability could have existed instead. According to Parfit's second view, the effect is worse when it is worse for the individual.

The three options cited by Parfit are not exhaustive. There is another view, which I will call the *Encompassing Account*, that I believe is more plausible than any of the three views Parfit mentions. It is similar to, but more complex than, the second view cited by Parfit. According to the Encompassing Account, person-affecting considerations and impersonal considerations are

---

[27] *Reasons and Persons*, 363.

distinct and nonadditive. Neither type of consideration is reducible to the other. Both matter; both provide reasons for action. But it is not always worse if a bad effect is worse for someone; sometimes it is, sometimes it is not.

Consider again the relevant effect in the Preconception and Prenatal Cases: a child is caused to exist with a disability. This effect may be worse for the child. When it is, it is *also* worse impersonally (for the world would have been better if this child had not been disabled). But the effect may be worse *only* impersonally, as in the Preconception Case. The Encompassing Account holds that, when this effect is worse for the child, as in the Prenatal Case, *that* fact provides whatever reasons there are to prevent it. That the effect is also worse impersonally is irrelevant. Yet, when the effect is worse only impersonally, as in the Preconception Case, that fact provides a reason to prevent it. In short, the objections to the Negligent Physician's action in the two cases are different. Contrary to Parfit, who claims that the relevant objection is impersonal in both cases, the Encompassing Account holds that the objection in the Preconception Case is impersonal while the objection in the Prenatal Case is that the effect is worse for the child.

How do the strengths of these objections compare? When an effect is both worse for someone and worse impersonally, as in the Prenatal Case, it is *at least* as bad as it would be if it were worse only impersonally. When an effect is worse only impersonally, as in the Preconception Case, it is *at most* as bad as it would be if it were bad for someone. Accordingly, the objection to the Negligent Physician's action in the Prenatal Case is at least as strong as the objection to his action in the Preconception Case. Thus it is possible, as Parfit claims and most of us intuitively sense, that the objections are equally strong in both cases. The impersonal objection in the Preconception Case may be as strong as the person-affecting objection in the Prenatal Case. It is not possible that the impersonal objection in the Preconception Case could be stronger, though it is possible that it could be weaker. To explain how the impersonal objection might be weaker, one might reason as follows:

In the Prenatal Case, the disabled child could reasonably (though not in practice) have this thought: 'It could have been better for me.' That is a bitter reflection. In the Preconception Case, the parallel thought to which the disabled child would be entitled is: 'A better-off person might have existed instead of me.' This is not a disturbing thought; virtually all of us could reasonably believe this of ourselves. Thus, if we take up the points of view of the two children rather than surveying the possible outcomes from a distance, we have reason to think that the effect in the Prenatal Case is worse than that in the Preconception Case. This is not because the child in the Prenatal Case would actually have this thought and be made miserable by it. It is, rather, that the accessibility of this thought to the child reveals something important about the nature of the outcome.

Even if one accepts this reasoning, however, it is hard to believe that the moral difference between the two cases could be more than very slight.

As we have seen, there are other cases in which there seems to be a significant moral difference between an effect that is worse for someone and a corresponding effect that is worse only impersonally. Compare the failure to save a child who would otherwise have lived another seventy years with the failure to cause the existence of a child who would have lived for seventy years. In each case, we may suppose, there is a roughly equal loss: seventy years of life that would have been well worth living. The difference is that in the first case this loss is worse for the child—it is *his* loss—whereas in the second case the loss is worse only impersonally. The fact that, in the first case, the bad effect is worse *for someone* seems to make a significant difference. It seems that this must be part of the explanation of why the moral objection to failing to save the one child is significantly stronger than the objection to failing to cause the other child to exist.

According to the Encompassing Account, the morality of beneficence is governed by both impersonal and person-affecting considerations. In some instances, the two types of consideration may be of comparable strengths; in others, person-affecting considerations may be far stronger than corresponding impersonal considerations. This raises large questions. For any bad effect that is worse for someone, how do we determine what counts as the corresponding or 'equivalent' effect that is worse only impersonally? Why is the comparative strength of person-affecting considerations greater in some instances than in others? And how are the two types of consideration—person-affecting and impersonal—to be integrated into a unified account of our moral reasons? I cannot answer these questions. My aim here is more modest: to suggest how one can accept that the Impersonal Comparative Principle provides the correct account of the Preconception Case without committing oneself to the generalized No-Difference View—that is, the view that the whole of the morality of beneficence must be explained in impersonal terms. One can accept that there is a dimension to the Negligent Physician's conduct in the Preconception Case that can be criticized only in impersonal terms, that the Negligent Physician's conduct in this case is no less bad than his conduct in the Prenatal Case, but that his conduct in the Prenatal Case is objectionable for entirely different reasons. Thus it may be true that in the Prenatal Case the Negligent Physician owes compensation to the disabled child while this is not true in the Preconception Case.

PART VI

PROFESSIONAL ETHICS

15

PRINCIPLISM AND ITS ALLEGED COMPETITORS

TOM L. BEAUCHAMP

In the early history of modern bioethics, principles were invoked to provide frameworks of general guidelines that condensed morality to its central elements and gave people from diverse fields an easily grasped set of moral standards. Principles gave an anchor to a youthful bioethics in the 1970s and early 1980s and contributed a sense that the field rests on something firmer than disciplinary bias or subjective judgment.

After the mid-1980s, however, serious questions were raised about the adequacy and sufficiency of frameworks of general principles. Several different methods or types of moral philosophy then came into prominence in bioethics. Although often presented as rival methods or theories, I believe these approaches are compatible with principles. I will argue for this thesis after outlining the approach to biomedical ethics that James Childress and I have defended since the mid-to-late 1970s, primarily in *Principles of Biomedical Ethics*.[1] Ours is not the only principle-based approach in bioethics, as Robert Veatch points out in his defense of a version of principles in this issue of the *Kennedy Institute of Ethics Journal*,[2] but it is the only version I will discuss.

From Tom L. Beauchamp, 'Principlism and its Alleged Competitors,' *Kennedy Institute of Ethics Journal*, 5/3 (1995), 181–98. © 1995 by The Johns Hopkins University Press

[1] See Tom L. Beauchamp and James F. Childress, *Principles of Biomedical Ethics*, 4th edn. (New York: Oxford University Press, 1994) and Raanan Gillon and Ann Lloyd (eds.), *Principles of Health Care Ethics* (New York: Wiley, 1994). The latter book has a series of illuminating essays on the former, including articles by each of the authors discussed below; see especially the articles by Albert R. Jonsen, 'Clinical Ethics and the Four Principles'; K. Danner Clouser and Bernard Gert, 'Morality vs. Principlism'; and Edmund D. Pellegrino, 'The Four Principles and the Doctor–Patient Relationship: The Need for a Better Linkage.' Also relevant to the arguments below are the articles in this journal by Povl Riis, 'The Four Principles in Practice'; Howard Brody, 'The Four Principles and Narrative Ethics'; R. H. Nicholson, 'Limitations of the Four Principles'; Raanan Gillon, 'The Four Principles Revisited—a Reappraisal'; John M. Stanley, 'The Four Principles in Practice'; H. Tristram Engelhardt Jr. and Kevin William Wildes, 'The Four Principles of Health Care Ethics and Post-Modernity: Why a Libertarian Interpretation is Unavoidable'; and Henrik R. Wulff, 'Against the Four Principles: A Nordic View.'

[2] Robert M. Veatch, 'Resolving Conflicts among Principles: Ranking, Balancing, and Specifying,' *Kennedy Institute of Ethics Journal*, 5 (1995), 199–218.

THE NATURE AND ROOTS OF PRINCIPLES

Childress and I use the term 'principles' to designate the most general normative standards of conduct. Our set of principles was developed specifically for biomedical ethics and was never presented as a comprehensive ethical theory. In this respect, our account is similar to Edmund Pellegrino's and Robert Veatch's theories of medical ethics, but differs from Albert Jonsen's casuistry and K. Danner Clouser and Bernard Gert's impartial rule theory, which are general ethical theories developed independently of bioethics and then used to treat its problems. Childress and I use four principles as the basis of many more specific rules for health care and research ethics. However, neither rules nor judgments can be *deduced* directly from the principles, because additional interpretation, specification, and balancing of the principles is needed in order to formulate policies and decide about cases. Our system is therefore not an example of what has been called deductivism. We have been as interested in treating cases through the specification of principles as in the principles and rules themselves.

The principles in our framework are grouped under four general categories: (1) respect for autonomy, (2) nonmaleficence, (3) beneficence, and (4) justice. The choice of these four types of moral principle as the framework for moral decision making in health care derives in part from professional roles and traditions. Health professionals' obligations and virtues have for centuries been framed by professional commitments to provide medical care, to protect patients from the harms of disease, injury, and system failure, and to produce benefits that compensate for any harms introduced. These obligations have been expressed through rules of nonmaleficence and beneficence, and our principles build on this tradition.

But our structure of principles also reaches beyond these commitments by including parts of morality that traditionally have been neglected, especially respect for autonomy and justice. In the early days of modern bioethics, health care's traditional preoccupation with nonmaleficence-based and beneficence-based models of ethics needed correction toward an autonomy model of patient care at the same time as it needed to confront a wider set of moral and social concerns, particularly those of achieving social justice through the protection of vulnerable persons and through an appropriate social system for the distribution of benefits and burdens. All four types of principle, then, are needed to provide a comprehensive framework for biomedical ethics.

Some writers distinguish sharply between principles and rules—see, for example, the discussion of Clouser and Gert, below—but Childress and I offer distinctions based only on differences in the level of abstraction.

Principles and rules in our approach are explicated on the model of W. D. Ross's account of *prima facie* duties: Principles are always binding *unless* they conflict with other obligations.[3] When a conflict of norms occurs, some balance, harmony, or form of equilibrium between two or more norms must be found; or, alternatively, one norm overrides the other.

This way of handling conflict seems to our critics problematic, because principles seem too flexible and unable to resolve hard cases by themselves. Childress and I handle this problem through an account of balancing and specification, both of which involve the exercise of judgment in resolving conflicts. We see no reason why judgment by appeal to general principles should be condemned as 'subjective' or merely 'intuitive'—two terms of abuse at the hands of many writers in contemporary moral philosophy. From our perspective, the principles are not merely intuitive, and if an agent takes seriously the demands of the applicable set of principles and associated rules, then the judgments are neither subjective nor unprincipled.

However, this viewpoint requires amplification if principles are to be extended to policies and judgments. Many authors have pointed out that all general norms exhibit an indeterminacy that needs reduction, and principles are prime examples: They underdetermine almost all moral judgments because there is too little content in abstract principles themselves to determine concrete judgments. How is the underdetermined to become *determining*? How does one fill the gap between abstract principles and concrete judgments?

The answer is that norms must be specified to overcome their lack of content and to handle moral conflict. Specification is the progressive filling in and development of principles and rules, shedding their indeterminateness and thereby providing action-guiding content.[4] Increase of substance through specification is essential for both policy and clinical decision making, but it is, in my judgment, more useful for the formulation of policy—itself a statement of general norms—than for decision making in a particular case, which usually involves a balancing of moral considerations in a specific context.

Principles should therefore be understood less as norms that are applied, in the model of 'applied ethics,' and more as guidelines that are *interpreted and made specific* for policy and clinical decision making. A coherent development of principles and rules, not merely an application, is essential.

---

[3] W. D. Ross, *The Foundations of Ethics* (Oxford: Clarendon Press, 1939), 19–36.

[4] Henry S. Richardson, 'Specifying Norms as a Way to Resolve Concrete Ethical Problems,' *Philosophy and Public Affairs*, 19 (1990), 279–310; David DeGrazia, 'Moving Forward in Bioethical Theory: Theories, Cases, and Specified Principlism,' *Journal of Medicine and Philosophy*, 17 (1992), 511–39.

Clouser rightly insists in his article in this volume[5] that we do not invent morality, in the sense of creating its basic norms. However, when we put general norms to work in particular contexts, we do invent through specification and judgment. That is, the norms are not invented, but inventiveness and imaginativeness in their use is essential and to be encouraged.[6]

Moral progress is made through this work of specification, which often involves a balancing of considerations and interests, a stating of additional obligations, or the development of policy. Through progressive specification, bioethics becomes increasingly more practical, while maintaining fidelity to the original principles and rules. This specification is also connected, in our account, to a larger method of coherence: The best method for *justifying* a proposed specification is not determined by the model of specification, but by a coherence theory of justification.

In the current issue of this journal, Robert Veatch suggests that balancing models such as the one Childress and I adopt produce 'strongly counter-intuitive implications',[7] though he himself adopts a balancing model with constraints. He mentions problems in the history of medical research in which patients were, without their consent, exploited to the ends of science for the benefit of society. Presumably he has in mind Tuskegee-type cases or some of the more recent examples of unregulated human radiation experiments in the 1940s and 1950s. If public utility is sufficiently large in such cases, he suggests, 'balancers' must allow it to override the considerations of autonomy on which rules of consent are based.

Veatch evidently would support a model of basic moral protections that cannot be violated under any circumstances, even if there is a clear and substantial benefit for society. His deontological restrictions are analogous to constitutional rights that constrain conduct and prohibit balancing of interests in various political and social matters. Writing in the liberal individualist and contractarian traditions, he holds that a specified social space should be carved out within which the individual is absolutely protected against state or other forms of social intrusion. As he puts it in his prime example, we might 'choose a rule that flatly prohibits research without consent.'

Veatch's goal and the motivation behind it are commendable, but every attempt to carry it out in moral philosophy—through rules or other constraints that, in effect, are absolute—has failed. This approach to bioethics

---

[5] K. Danner Clouser, 'Common Morality as an Alternative to Principlism,' *Kennedy Institute of Ethics Journal*, 5/3 (1995), 219–36.

[6] J. L. Mackie, *Ethics: Inventing Right and Wrong* (Harmondsworth: Penguin, 1977), 30–49, 105–10, 122–4.

[7] Veatch, 'Resolving Conflicts among Principles,' 209.

itself produces highly counter-intuitive results, because society and individual actors are absolutely rather than contingently constrained in many cases in which balancing is justified. A good example is the current absolute prohibition of physician-assisted suicide in physician ethics and social policy, even though a significant percentage of both the physician population and the public believes that at least some cases of physician-assisted suicide are justified. The absence of an appropriate mechanism for balancing patient needs and protection of society has led to serious problems because of an inability to meet the needs of dying patients in these cases.

A model of balancing keeps options open without 'flatly prohibiting' them, as Veatch puts it. Consider, for example, how organ procurement policies might be restructured in the U.S. by balancing the interests of all who are affected by these policies. Protection of individual rights were paramount when the Uniform Anatomical Gift Act was adopted in the late 1960s and early 1970s, giving individuals the right to make decisions about the donation of their organs through a donor card. However, few individuals sign donor cards, and the signatures of those who do sign are often not available when they die. As a result, our capacity to promote the common good through more collectivist public policies has been paralyzed by a public policy entirely protective of autonomy rights. An absolutist account of individual rights leaves no opportunity to formulate more stringent policies for the procurement of tissues and organs, which I believe must be handled by balancing principles of public utility and respect for autonomy. The social ideals of beneficence are as critical to social morality as individual rights are.

With this account of principles before us, the discussion can now shift to contemporary writers in bioethics who present models that deemphasize principles, even if they do not altogether reject them. Several accounts have emerged in recent years, but I will consider only those reflected in the other articles in the present issue of this journal. These alternatives are (1) *Impartial Rule Theory* (as defended in this issue by Clouser), (2) *Casuistry* (as defended in this issue by Jonsen), and (3) *Virtue Ethics* (as defended in this issue by Pellegrino).[8] I will argue that these alternatives are consistent with and not rivals of a principle-based account.

---

[8] Clouser, 'Common Morality as an Alternative to Principlism'; Albert Jonsen, 'Casuistry: An Alternative or Complement to Principles?', *Kennedy Institute of Ethics Journal*, 5/3 (1995), 237–51; Edmund D. Pellegrino, 'Toward a Virtue-Based Normative Ethics for the Health Professions,' *Kennedy Institute of Ethics Journal*, 5/3 (1995), 253–77.

CLOUSER AND GERT'S ALTERNATIVE: IMPARTIAL RULE THEORY

Dan Clouser and Bernard Gert coined the term 'principlism' in an article that alleged certain defects or forms of incompleteness in the account of principles that Childress and I propose.[9] Paradoxically, Clouser and Gert are probably as close to us in their conception of the content of morality and philosophical method as they are to any other writers in biomedical ethics. The problem is that, although they accept general rules of obligation, they do not believe that principles provide a reliable framework. They look to more specific rules arranged in a structured system as the proper surrogate.

Clouser and Gert have brought several accusations against principles, many of which are restated in Clouser's article in this issue of the *Journal*.[10] In particular, they maintain that 'principles' function more like chapter headings in a book than as directive rules and theories. That is, principles indicate important moral themes by providing a general label for those themes, but they do not function as practical action guides. Therefore, receiving no directive guidance from the principle, a moral agent thinking through a problem is free to deal with it in his or her own way and may give the principle whatever weight he or she wishes.

Clouser is particularly fond of pointing to these deficiencies in the principle(s) of justice. There is, he says, no specific guide to action or any theory of justice in the 'principle(s).' Principlism instructs the agent to 'Be alert to matters of justice' and 'Think about justice,' nothing more. Since this injunction vastly underdetermines solutions to problems of justice, the agent is free to decide what is just and unjust, as he or she sees fit. Other moral considerations besides the principle(s) of justice, such as intuitions and theories, are certain to be beckoned to determine the solution. Although more obvious in the case of justice, Clouser thinks the same problem afflicts all general principles. Our four-principle schema allegedly fails to provide a theory of justification or any kind of moral theory that systematically unifies the principles and situates them in a tidy and integrated theory that can handle conflict among the principles.[11]

These accusations are serious and merit sustained attention. For many years before Clouser and Gert stepped forward to critique our formulations,

---

[9] K. Danner Clouser and Bernard Gert, 'A Critique of Principlism,' *Journal of Medicine and Philosophy*, 15 (1990), 219–36.

[10] Clouser, 'Common Morality as an Alternative to Principlism.'

[11] Clouser and Gert, 'A Critique of Principlism,' and 'Morality vs. Principlism,' in Gillon and Lloyd (eds.), *Principles of Health Care Ethics*; Ronald M. Green, Bernard Gert, and K. Danner Clouser, 'The Method of Public Morality versus the Method of Principlism,' *Journal of Medicine and Philosophy*, 18 (1993), 179–97.

Childress and I viewed these problems as needing a deeper resolution than we had provided. We have tried to address a number of them by developing a coherence model of justification and the aforementioned methods of specification and balancing.[12] I cannot summarize these accounts here, but I do need to consider whether the rule-based alternative presented by Clouser and Gert is itself free of the problems they direct at us. If their system is free of these defects, then it clearly is a superior system. However, I believe their theory of impartial rules fares no better than our account and inconsistently incorporates some of the very views that it explicitly claims to reject.

The first matter of importance is the specificity and directiveness of general norms. Clouser and Gert maintain that our principles lack what their rules provide: a deep and directive moral substance. This point is obviously correct for *unspecified* principles, but their unspecified rules have a near-identical problem, one level down. Their rules, being one tier less abstract than principles, reside on the first level of the specification of principles; and it is only for this reason that their rules have a more directive and specific content. Childress and I have noted this problem about general principles since the first edition of *Principles of Biomedical Ethics* (in 1979). We have insisted that many rules must be much more specific than even the rules presented by Clouser and Gert and that mere unspecified principles are insufficient for practical decision making.

Moreover, a set of rules almost identical to Clouser and Gert's is already included in our account of principles and rules. We maintain that principles lend support to more specific and directive moral rules, including those accepted by Clouser and Gert, and that more than one principle—respect for autonomy and nonmaleficence, say—may support a single rule—of, for example, medical confidentiality. Below is a comparison between a sample of the rules we defend under the heading of the principle of nonmaleficence and a directly related sample of basic moral rules defended by Gert and Clouser:

Beauchamp and Childress	Gert and Clouser
4 Rules Based on Nonmaleficence	*4 of the 10 Basic Rules*
1. Do not kill.	1. Don't kill.
2. Do not cause pain.	2. Don't cause pain.
3. Do not incapacitate.	3. Don't disable.
4. Do not deprive of goods.	4. Don't deprive of pleasure.

No substantive moral difference distinguishes these two sets of rules. The method of deriving and supporting the rules is different in our accounts, but

[12] Beauchamp and Childress, *Principles of Biomedical Ethics*, chs. 1–2.

at present I only want to show that their rules either do not or need not differ in content from ours and that their rules are no more specific and directive than ours.

Second, Gert and Clouser are critical of us for making both nonmaleficence *and* beneficence principles of obligation. They maintain that there are no moral rules of beneficence that state obligations; our only obligations in the moral life, apart from duties encountered in roles and other stations of duty, are captured by moral rules of nonmaleficence, which prohibit causing harm or evil. Their reason is that the goal of morality is the minimization of evil, not the promotion of good. Rational persons can act impartially at all times in regard to all persons with the aim of not causing evil, but they cannot impartially promote the good for all persons at all times. As Clouser puts it in his article in this journal:[13]

Each of the moral rules admonishes us to avoid causing a harm . . . Thus the moral rules are formed around these harms to be avoided . . . They are all prohibitions . . . [By contrast,] moral ideals can only be encouraged . . . [The] principle of beneficence [a moral ideal] fails to recognize the limits, constraints, and dangers of the action-guide: 'Help others.'

This thesis is neither morally correct nor supported within their own account of moral obligations. The major implication of this claim is that one is never morally required, i.e., obligated by moral rules, to *prevent* or *remove* harm or evil, but only to *avoid causing* it. There is no requirement to *do* anything, only to avoid causing harmful events. Childress and I believe this thesis misreads common morality. The following cases of what one is not obligated to do in the official Clouser–Gert account of obligations of beneficence indicate why we think their view is incorrect:

1. Mr. X's life is in great peril, but if I warn him through a phone call of the peril, he will be fine. I am not *obligated* to make the phone call.
2. A young toddler has wandered onto a busy street, having become separated from his mother. I can save his life simply by picking him up. It would be nice of me to do so, but I am not obligated to do so. After all, there are no obligations, ever, to prevent harm, apart from roles that fix obligations for us. A policeman would be obligated to lift the child from the street, but not I.
3. A blind man on the street has obviously lost his way, and he asks me for directions. I am not obligated to provide the directions.
4. I am the only witness to a serious automobile accident that has left the

---

[13] Clouser, 'Common Morality as an Alternative to Principlism,' 230–1.

drivers unconscious. I am neither obligated to stop nor to pick up my car telephone and call an ambulance as I speed on my way.

These examples suggest that there are moral obligations of beneficence and that they should be included in any system whose goal is to capture the nature and scope of morality. If Clouser and Gert believe that we are never under such obligations and that a morality of obligations does not contain at least as much beneficence as these four examples suggest, then we do indeed deeply disagree about the content of morality. However, as Gert points out in his book *Morality: A New Justification of the Moral Rules*,[14] which Clouser acknowledges to be 'the basis' of his understanding of method and content in ethics,[15] Gert *does* believe that one is morally obligated to act in circumstances precisely like those in my four examples. His reason is his acceptance of the general rule 'Do your duty,' which he gives an interpretation broad enough to incorporate the principle of beneficence. He explains his system and its commitments as follows:

Although duties, in general, go with offices, jobs, roles, etc., there are some *duties that seem more general* . . . A person has a duty . . . because of some special circumstances, for example, his job or his relationships . . . In any civilized society, if a child collapses in your arms, you have *a duty to seek help*. You cannot simply lay him out on the ground and walk away. In most civilized societies one has a *duty to help* when (1) one is in physical proximity to someone in need of help to avoid a serious evil, usually death or serious injury, (2) one is in a unique or close to unique position to provide that help and (3) it would be relatively cost-free for one to provide that help.[16]

Although Gert insists that these requirements are all supported by the moral rule, 'Do your duty,' they are effectively identical to those obligations that follow from what Childress and I call—following moral tradition in the eighteenth, nineteenth, and twentieth centuries—beneficence. It therefore *cannot* be the case that in Gert's system there are no obligations of beneficence in *our* sense of beneficence. Gert and Clouser cannot be criticizing our views about beneficence, because we are in effect in agreement on all the substantive issues about what is morally required, even if our methods differ. Often when Clouser and Gert critique our views it appears that they want to categorize all obligations of beneficence as moral ideals, but it would be inconsistent to take this line about *our* account of beneficence, given the latent commitments to beneficence in Gert's book.

To generalize, a great deal in principlism that Clouser and Gert appear to reject can be situated in their account under Gert's final rule, 'Do your job'

---

[14] (New York: Oxford University Press, 1988).
[15] Clouser, 'Common Morality as an Alternative to Principlism,' 221.
[16] Gert, *Morality*, 154–5.

(or 'Don't avoid doing your job'). If this interpretation is correct, our theories are far more compatible than they allow, though it is always worth bearing in mind that Childress and I are defending only a professional ethics, not a general moral theory like Gert's. But it is hard to see how the impartial rule theory of Clouser and Gert provides any real alternative to our substantive claims about the nature and scope of obligations. I have not here discussed methodology, but our methods are also, in many respects, compatible. Gert and Clouser therefore seem much more like good friends than hostile rivals.

I will now argue that much the same conclusion should be reached about Albert Jonsen's defense of casuistry.

JONSEN'S ALTERNATIVE: CASUISTRY

Jonsen sees ethics as rooted in the experience of deciding hard cases. Like classical rhetoricians, the casuist is concerned about the resolution of cases that are unique in their circumstances, yet similar in relevant respects to other cases. Each change in the circumstances changes the case—a fact, Jonsen claims, that has been forgotten in recent moral philosophy. The casuistic method begins with *paradigm cases* whose moral features and conclusions have already been decided; it then compares the salient features in the paradigm cases—i.e., morally determinate cases—with the features of cases that require a decision. Analogical reasoning links one case to the next and serves as the primary model of moral reasoning.[17]

As I understand him, Jonsen does not dismiss principles, but he does downgrade them in importance because he thinks moral reasoning starts at a different point. He places weight on shared maxims, which are normative statements that reflect a consensus of opinion, for example, 'the intended effect must be to alleviate pain.' These maxims inform judgment about the case by providing what Jonsen calls 'the "morals" of the story.' In difficult cases, several morals emerge because maxims give conflicting advice. The casuist's job is to determine which maxim is to rule in the case and how powerfully it is to rule.

In a very important statement in his article in this journal, Jonsen writes:

When maxims, such as 'Do no harm' or 'Informed consent is obligatory,' are invoked,

[17] Albert Jonsen and Stephen Toulmin, *The Abuse of Casuistry* (Berkeley: University of California Press, 1988), 11–19, 66–7, 251–4, 296–9; Albert Jonsen, 'Casuistry and Clinical Ethics,' *Theoretical Medicine*, 7 (1986), 67–71; 'Practice versus Theory,' *Hastings Center Report*, 20/4 (1990), 3234; 'Casuistry as Methodology in Clinical Ethics,' *Theoretical Medicine*, 12 (1991), 299–302; John Arras, 'Principles and Particularity: The Role of Cases in Bioethics,' *Indiana Law Journal*, 69 (1994), 983–1014.

they represent, as it were, cut-down versions of the major principles relevant to the topic, such as beneficence and autonomy cut down to fit the nature of the topic and the kinds of circumstances that pertain to it.[18]

This statement is no rejection of principles, and Jonsen rightly points out, in his informative segment on principles, that casuistry is 'complementary to principles' in a manner that still needs to be worked out in moral philosophy[19]. In my view, in using the language of 'cut-down versions'—one could also think of them as 'built-up,' since there is a specification of content rather than a pruning—Jonsen points in the same direction that Childress and I do in using the language of 'specification,' 'support,' and the like. Like us, Jonsen sees an intimate connection between principles and what we call progressive specification to rules (maxims, etc.) in order to meet the demands of particular contexts. His fear, which we share, is that principles will be interpreted inflexibly, without regard to the nuances of cases, generating a gridlock of conflicting principled stands.[20] While Jonsen insists that principles and rules are too indeterminate to serve as the only basis of moral judgments and that the 'application' of a principle to a case cannot be the basic model of moral reasoning, again, Childress and I quite agree.

In his early writings on casuistry, Jonsen seemed to many interpreters to say that cases lead to moral paradigms, analogies, and judgments by reference to the salient features of the case and without making any appeal to hidden evaluative assumptions.[21] However, Jonsen recognizes in his recent work that this way of portraying the case is improper. The salient moral features of cases cannot be recognized as such without assuming values already recognized as morally important. No fact or set of facts will lead to a moral conclusion unless some general *value* premises play a role in the reasoning. Jonsen's account of maxims and principles now thoroughly appreciates this point.

The best way to understand his idea of *paradigm cases* is as a combination or blend of (1) *facts* that can be generalized to other cases—for example, 'The patient refused the recommended treatment'—and (2) *settle values*—for example, 'Competent patients have a right to refuse treatment.' In a

[18] Jonsen, 'Casuistry: An Alternative or Complement to Principles?', 244.

[19] Ibid. 249.

[20] Jonsen's collaborator in casuistry Stephen Toulmin aims at 'the cult of absolute principles' ('The Tyranny of Principles,' *Hastings Center Report*, 11/6 (1981), 37). *Prima facie* principles of the sort Childress and I accept thus do not seem to fall within the scope of his critique. Of course, any type of general norms—whether principles, maxims, or rules—can be interpreted either rigidly or flexibly, just as the principles in a principle-based system can be. There is no escape from rigidity merely by emphasizing the importance of cases and maxims.

[21] Kevin William Wildes, 'The Priesthood of Bioethics and the Return of Casuistry,' *Journal of Medicine and Philosophy*, 18 (1993), 33–49.

principle-based system, these settled values are called principles, rules, rights, maxims, and the like; and they are analytically distinguished from the facts of particular cases. In casuistry, rather than *separate* values from facts, the two are bound together in the paradigm case; however, the central values are generalizable and must be preserved from one case to the next. For a casuist to reason morally, one or more settled values must connect the cases, hence the necessity of maxims. The greater the level of generality in the norms the closer the connecting norm will come to status as a rule or principle. But if the generality is at a very high level, a loss of specific guidance will occur, and the reasoning cannot handle a case.

Casuists and principlists should be able to agree that when they reflect on cases and policies, they rarely, if ever, have in hand either (1) principles that were formulated without reference to experience with cases or (2) paradigm cases that have not become paradigmatic *because* of a prior commitment to general norms. When philosophers now speak, as they often do, about 'the top' (principles, theories) and 'the bottom' (cases, individual judgments) in moral philosophy, it is doubtful that these poles can be either a starting point or a resting point without some form of cross-fertilization and mutual development. Childress and I have emphasized this point since the first edition of *Principles of Biomedical Ethics* by pointing out the dialectical character of moral reasoning, and, in the fourth edition, by developing its connection to reflective equilibrium.

I doubt that Jonsen has ever had any doubts about the need for principles to be brought into close connection with reasoning about particular cases and circumstances. It is a little known fact, but a fact nonetheless, that the final comprehensive drafting of *The Belmont Report* of the National Commission for the Protection of Human Subjects,[22] widely interpreted as a principlist document, was done by three people in a small room at NIH: Al Jonsen, Stephen Toulmin, and me. Toulmin and Jonsen made significant and commendable contributions to the polishing of the statement of *principles* in that report. I do not recall any objection that the strategy of using principles should be anything other than central to the Commission's statement of its ethical framework, especially in the attempt to justify its reasoning about cases. They did, as one would expect, mention that the Commission was engaged in casuistry, but they understood the Commission's casuistry to be consistent with and supported by its invocations of moral principles. So, despite what several commentators have made of our differences in inter-

[22] National Commission for the Protection of Human Subjects of Biomedical and Behavioral Research, *The Belmont Report: Ethical Principles and Guidelines for the Protection of Human Subjects of Research*, DHEW Publication No. (OS) 78–0012 (Washington, DC: US Government Printing Office, 1978).

preting the work of the Commission.[23] I believe those differences to be minor and insignificant.

It is hard to understand, then, how casuistry is a rival paradigm to principlism, although it has been so received in contemporary bioethics. Moreover, I believe the methodology for bioethics that Childress and I have defended—a method of coherence, specification, and balancing—need not deviate from the methods and standards proposed by Jonsen. If so, principlism and casuistry also seem more like allies than enemies.

PELLEGRINO'S ALTERNATIVE: VIRTUE THEORY

In addition to principles, obligations, rights, and cases, there are the agents who perform actions, have motives, and make judgements in cases. Proficient use of principles requires judgment, which depends on personal characteristics, such as a sense of personal responsibility and integrity. These properties of persons cannot be reduced either to principles or to behavior that conforms to principles. Sensitive and judicious decisions are not 'principled' in the sense of being straightforward applications of principles. They are simply the judgments of sensitive and judicious persons. Childress and I have therefore always considered the virtues to be central to our system, and we claim that a moral philosophy rooted in the virtues complements a framework of principles.

Writers in virtue theory today sometimes suggest that virtues are more basic than, or at least more valuable than, principles.[24] Among the most interesting recent theses tending in this direction is that of Annette Baier,[25] who has written extensively about how the virtuous and tender sentiments, as Hume called them, are more pervasive in the moral life than normative precepts such as Kantian moral laws. She finds sympathy, virtue, and various emotional capacities at least as fundamental in the moral life as the categories of rationality, obligation, justice, and rights. She argues that moral philosophy should broaden its scope to consider virtues of caring, loving,

---

[23] Jonathan D. Moreno, *Deciding Together: Bioethics and Consensus* (New York: Oxford University Press, 1995), 76–8.

[24] Alasdair MacIntyre, *After Virtue* (Notre Dame, Ind.: University of Notre Dam Press, 1981); Stanley M. Hauerwas, 'On Medicine and Virtue: A Response,' in Earl Shelp (ed.), *Virtues and Health Care* (Dordrecht: Reidel, 1984); and see commentary by Kurt Baier, 'Radical Virtue Ethics,' in Peter A. French, Theodore E. Uehling Jr., and Howard K. Wettstein (eds.), *Midwest Studies in Philosophy*, xiii: *Ethical Theory: Character and Virtue* (Notre Dame, Ind.: University of Notre Dame Press, 1988).

[25] Annette Baier, *Moral Prejudices* (Cambridge, Mass.: Harvard University Press, 1994).

trusting, gentleness, and the like, and deemphasize the reigning Kantian framework of principles of autonomy and categories of duty and law.

Edmund Pellegrino in his contribution to this issue rightly does not insist on some form of competition between virtues and principles.[26] He proposes to relate virtue-based theory to principle-based theory in order to achieve a comprehensive account adequate for the health professions. To this end, he discusses various relationships between principles, rules, and virtues, which he had treated more fully in previous works.[27] He seems to believe, as Childress and I do, that principles and virtues are mutually supportive, rather than mutually exclusive, despite the fact that he emphasizes the foundational importance of virtue theory and describes his account as a virtue-based ethic.

Pellegrino stands in the tradition of those writings in ancient, medieval, and modern medicine that conceive the health professional's obligations and virtues through professional commitments to provide care. His reconstruction of the traditional beneficence model moves without fear of loss or theoretical problem between principles and virtues. Note the following quite explicit appeal to principles in an earlier book he coauthored with David Thomasma: 'Beneficence remains the central moral principle of the ethics of medicine . . . Our aim is to redefine, and refine, the notion of beneficence in terms of the new practicalities and dimensions of the physician-patient relationship today.'[28]

The operative concept in the beneficence model embraced by Pellegrino is what he calls beneficence-in-trust, meaning that physicians and patients hold in trust 'the goal of acting in the best interests of one another in the relationship.'[29] The trust aspect is the cement of the relationship, and in this way Pellegrino can make appeals to the principle of beneficence simultaneously with appeals to the importance of the virtues of benevolence and trustworthiness in physicians.[30] This structure is similar to that which Childress and I adopt in our chapter on the virtues.[31]

[26] Pellegrino, 'Toward a Virtue-Based Normative Ethics for the Health Professions.'

[27] Edmund D. Pellegrino and David C. Thomasma, *The Virtues in Medical Practice* (New York: Oxford University Press, 1993), pp. xii, 19–27, 183–91.

[28] Edmund D. Pellegrino and David C. Thomasma, *For the Patient's Good: The Restoration of Beneficence in Health Care* (New York: Oxford University Press, 1988), 7–8.

[29] Ibid. 54–5. The philosophical basis for this view of medical morality was developed in their first book, *A Philosophical Basis of Medical Practice* (New York: Oxford University Press, 1981), esp. ch. 9; see also Edmund D. Pellegrino, 'Toward a Reconstruction of Medical Morality: The Primacy of the Act of Profession and the Fact of Illness,' *Journal of Medicine and Philosophy*, 4 (1979), 32–56.

[30] Pellegrino and Thomasma, *For the Patient's Good*, 25, 32, 46.

[31] However, the Pellegrino–Thomasma defense of the beneficence model has structural features that make it very different from our system. They maintain the absoluteness of the principle that physicians should 'act in the patient's best interest.'

Virtue theory is of the highest importance in a health-care context because a morally good person with the right motives is more likely to discern what should be done, to be motivated to do it, and to do it. The person who simply follows rules and possesses no special moral character may not be morally reliable. Often the reactions people have to those in the past who wronged patients—in research, for example—is that they lacked discernment, compassion, and trustworthiness, not that they failed to act in accordance with a rule or principle. People recommend and hold up as a moral model not the rule follower, but the person disposed by character to be attentive, generous, caring, compassionate, sympathetic, fair, and the like.

Again, however, there is no reason to suppose that we need to dispatch or minimize the importance of principles and rules in order to embrace these virtues. The two kinds of theory have different emphases, but they are compatible. A moral philosophy is simply more complete if the virtues are integrated with principles. Again, then, we have grounds to declare virtue theory and principlism partners rather than competitors.

Pellegrino observes in his essay that:

> Today's challenge is not how to demonstrate the superiority of one normative theory over the other, but rather how to relate each to the other in a matrix that does justice to each and assigns to each its proper normative force.[32]

I quite agree. In this essay I have tried to show only that principles can still provide defensible normative frameworks in bioethics despite the criticisms of principles that have emerged since the late 1980s. Impartial rule theory, casuistry, and virtue ethics are all consistent with rather than rivals of a principle-based account when it is properly conceived.

[32] Pellegrino, 'Toward a Virtue-Based Normative Ethics for the Health Professions,' 273.

16

NOT JUST AUTONOMY: THE PRINCIPLES OF AMERICAN BIOMEDICAL ETHICS

SØREN HOLM

INTRODUCTION

It is obviously an impossible project to diagnose the state of the whole of the field of bioethics in the USA in anything less than a book-length treatment. The aim of this paper is therefore somewhat more modest, and it will only look at one specific influential school of thought within American bioethics.

The paper will proceed by offering close readings and analyses of important sections in the latest edition of the most read bioethics textbook in the USA (and probably in the world) *Principles of Biomedical Ethics*, in its fourth edition (PBE4) by Tom Beauchamp and James Childress.[1]

Through this process it will become evident that the ethical system propounded by Beauchamp and Childress lacks the necessary resources satisfactorily to handle the ethically complex situations created in the interface between medicine and social justice.

Just looking at one specific approach in American bioethics could be seen as setting up a straw man, but this method is justified by the widespread use of the four principles framework in medical and nursing ethics, both academically and in practice: PBE4 is not just a small and insignificant part of American bioethics.

Another problem is that the book contains 526 pages of densely printed

From Søren Holm, 'Not just Autonomy: The Principles of American Biomedical Ethics', *Journal of Medical Ethics*, 21/6 (1995), 332–8.

This paper was written in pursuance of the project for the European Commission Biomedical and Health Research Programme: *AIDS: Ethics, Justice and European Policy*. The author gratefully acknowledges the stimulus and support provided by the commission. A preliminary version of this paper was read at a seminar at Ersta Institute of Health Care Ethics, Stockholm. I thank all the participants for their comments. I also thank the editor and two anonymous referees for their helpful comments and suggestions.

[1] T. L. Beauchamp and J. F. Childress, *Principles of Biomedical Ethics*, 4th edn. (New York: Oxford University Press, 1994).

text, and any extract of this is liable to be accused of selection bias. In the present case this is in one sense true. I only cite material which is relevant for the critique I want to put forward, but to avoid bias I have tried to provide fairly extensive quotes, and summaries of pertinent parts of the discussion which cannot be quoted at length.

In PBE4 the authors give a much longer and more in-depth account of their views on ethical theory than in the previous editions of The *Principles of Biomedical Ethics*, and this makes it possible to trace the basis of their theory in more detail than was previously possible.

The *Principles of Biomedical Ethics*, 4th edn., is a very rich book, and does reward careful study. It may well be that the widespread resistance to the four principles in the bioethics community would not have occurred if every student and end-user of the principles had been required to read the whole book. But, on the other hand, if this had been a requirement, the principles would probably never have gained the same degree of popularity among health care professionals.

KEY WORDS

Principlism; beneficence; justice; specification; balancing.

NOT JUST AUTONOMY?

The ethical system put forward in PBE4 is usually known as principlism. This specific version of principlism is often referred to as the 'Georgetown mantra' or 'The four principles', and its most vigorous European proponent is Raanan Gillon.[2] The present paper is primarily concerned with the version of the four principles found in PBE4. The version put forward by Gillon is, for instance, somewhat different from the PBE4 version, and some of the argument presented here may not affect this or other non-PBE4 versions of the four principles approach.

The PBE4 version of principlism incorporates four principles as the basis for bioethical thought: respect for autonomy; non-maleficence; beneficence; and justice.

The authors go to great lengths to emphasize that this listing of the principles does not imply a ranking, thereby trying to answer a common criticism that whereas PBE4 mentions four principles, only one or two (ie,

[2] R. Gillon, *Philosophical Medical Ethics* (Chichester: Wiley, 1986); R. Gillon (ed.), *Principles of Health Care Ethics* (Chichester: Wiley, 1994).

autonomy and non-maleficence) are really important, when it comes to analysing bioethical problems.

The authors of PBE4 reject foundationalism in bioethics, and instead develop their theory as a common-morality theory: 'A common-morality theory takes its basic premises directly from the morality shared in common by the members of *a* society—that is, unphilosophical common sense and tradition.'[3]

The fact that common-morality theory necessarily uses the shared morality in a *a specific society* as its basic premise, is often overlooked by both proponents and opponents of the four principles.

These basic premises derived from common morality are further analysed and re-arranged in order to reach a coherent moral theory, but it should come as no surprise that the content of this theory will be influenced by its basic premises, and therefore by the morality and culture of the society from which it originates.

Because the theory of PBE4 is developed from American common morality (and in reality only from a subset of that morality) it will mirror certain aspects of American society, and may, for this reason alone, be untransferable to other contexts and other societies.

Beauchamp and Childress do not explicitly limit the scope of application of their principles to the USA, or indicate that the approach should only be used by persons working in American health care institutions. It seems fair to assume that the authors must know that their book is widely read outside the USA, given that it is now in its fourth edition. If they themselves believed that the application of their principles should be restricted to the culture from which they are derived, or that transfer to other cultural contexts requires changes in form or content, then they could have written a few lines about how such a transfer might be accomplished.

One way to accomplish a relatively un-problematic transfer would be to build on the premise that the form of the ethical system is constant, ie, the four principles point to important parts of morality in all cultures, but that the exact content and strength of the individual principles may vary between cultures. This seems to be the approach advocated by Gillon,[4] but it does not seem to be available to Beauchamp and Childress. First of all, they use more than 60 pages to specify the contents of each of the four principles, without any disclaimers that this content is only valid for the USA. Secondly, they explicitly reject the criticism put forward by Clouser and Gert that the principles are 'little more than names, checklists, or headings for values worth

[3] Beauchamp and Childress, *Principles of Biomedical Ethics*, 100.
[4] Gillon (ed.), *Principles of Health Care Ethics*.

remembering, leaving principles without deep moral substance or capacity to guide actions'[5] by claiming that they agree that the principles need additional content and specificity before they are of use, and that this content is supplied in the four long chapters describing the principles.

A more general problem with an account which construes the four principles as relatively contentless pointers or labels is that it can obscure important differences in moral outlook. Let us imagine that I read a paper which states: 'Based on the principle of beneficence x, y, and z follow'. If the four principles are just pointers or labels, then I would have to know what version of the principle of beneficence the author is talking about (ie, beneficence (USA), beneficence (Denmark), or beneficence (India), etc) before I could assess the reasoning and engage in discussion. If I just assume that the author's principle of beneficence has the same content as my own, I may be seriously misled.

The American influence on the content of the principles as they are explicated in PBE4 is, for instance, exemplified in an analysis of the duties of a physician who happens to pass by the scene of an accident where people are injured. The authors wonder whether the physician has any special duty of beneficence in this situation, just because he is a physician, and reach the following conclusion: 'The physician at the scene of an accident is obligated to do more than the lawyer or student to aid the injured, in accordance with the need for the skills of the medical profession; yet a physician-stranger is not morally required to assume the same level of commitment and risk that is legally and morally required in a prior contractual relationship with a patient or hospital'.[6]

It may well be true in the context of American and British common morality and law that the physician is only obligated to a limited extent, but this analysis does not travel well to many countries in continental Europe, where Good Samaritan laws have been on the statute books for at least one hundred years, and physicians have been held answerable to the full extent of their professional duties even if no prior contract was established.

BENEFICENCE AND JUSTICE THE AMERICAN WAY!

The greatest influence of American common morality can be detected in the analysis of the principles of beneficence and justice. This is of the greatest importance in the present context. The cost of optimal (or even good)

[5] Beauchamp and Childress, *Principles of Biomedical Ethics*, 106.
[6] Ibid. 271.

treatment and care for diseases like cancer or HIV/AIDS, from the time of diagnosis to the time of death, is so large that it is outside the economic possibilities of most private persons. In the end people with these diseases will therefore have to rely on the beneficence and sense of justice of their fellow citizens.

The fourth edition of *Principles of Biomedical Ethics* defines the scope of the duty of beneficence in the following way:

Apart from special moral relationships such as contracts, a person X has a determinate obligation of beneficence toward a person Y if and only if each of the following conditions is satisfied (assuming X is aware of the relevant facts):

1. Y is at risk of significant loss of or damage to life or health or some other major interest.
2. X's action is needed (singly or in concert with others) to prevent this loss or damage.
3. X's action (singly or in concert with others) has a high probability of preventing it.
4. X's action would not present significant risks, costs, or burdens to X.
5. The benefit that Y can be expected to gain outweighs any harms, costs, or burdens that X is likely to incur.[7]

The crucial clause in this analysis, and the one which most clearly reflects American common morality, is clause 4, which states that a duty of beneficence only exists if it can be discharged without incurring significant risks, costs, or burdens. We probably all agree that there is some limit to the burdens a moral agent can be expected to incur in order to help others, but it seems strange to state that the *moral duty* of beneficence is only operative if it can be discharged without significant risk. On the previous pages of PBE4 the authors discuss the suggestion by Peter Singer that: 'If it is in our power to prevent something bad from happening, without thereby sacrificing anything of comparable moral importance, we ought, morally, to do it.'[8]

This claim is immediately rejected, and it is suggested that if we require sacrifice of people in the discharge of their duty of beneficence, we may require something which is beyond the capability of most moral agents. This seems to me to be an extremely bleak view to take of human nature. We may all agree that beneficence must be restricted both in degree and in scope, there cannot be a duty to devote all our time and resources to acting beneficently. However, if a duty of beneficence is to have any meaning, it must at

---

[7] *Principles of Biomedical Ethics*, 266.
[8] Ibid. 264; P. Singer, 'Affluence and Morality', *Philosophy & Public Affairs*, 1 (1972), 229–43.

least contain the notion of the possibility of sacrifice of personal interests in the discharge of the duty.

The authors then continue with a discussion of Singer's later proposal that 10 per cent of one's income given to good causes is the minimum that any reasonable ethical standard requires, and they seem to accept this, but as a maximum instead of a minimum.

In light of this, clause 4 above must therefore be interpreted as stating that a duty of beneficence only exists if it can be discharged within the yearly allocation of 10 per cent of one's income, where risks and non-monetary burdens are represented by their comparable money value. An interpretation taking this limit at face value must therefore lead to the conclusion that a society can only legitimately collect taxes amounting to 10 per cent of the income of individual citizens in order to pay for those parts of the public social and health care programmes that cannot be legitimated by reference to their prudential value for the individual (for example, by reference to their function as an insurance substitute). And even this 10 per cent tax must be reduced if citizens are simultaneously obligated to perform other acts of beneficence.

It is also interesting to note that a strict interpretation of clause 5 would entail that it would never be morally required to put one's life at risk to save *one* other person, except within the special moral relationships mentioned in the initial *ceteris paribus* clause.

Even earlier in their exposition the authors of PBE4 distinguish rules of beneficence from rules of non-maleficence, and present two strong claims: 'But, with rare exceptions, obligations of non-maleficence must be discharged impartially and obligations of beneficence need not be discharged impartially.[9]

'Advocates of a principle of general beneficence, however, argue the far more demanding thesis that we are obligated to act impartially to promote the interests of persons beyond our limited sphere of relationships and influence.'[10]

The reason for these assertions/conclusions is given in the following way: 'It is possible to act non-maleficently toward all persons, but it would be impossible to act beneficently toward all persons.'[11]

[9] Beauchamp and Childress, *Principles of Biomedical Ethics*, 263.
[10] Ibid.
[11] Ibid. 262.

SIMPLY WRONG

But this is simply wrong. It is possible to act beneficently toward all persons (for example, if I made a will dividing my property into six billion equal shares, given that my property was of a sufficient size, and I had no natural heirs); and, as marxist and feminist analyses have shown, it may very well be impossible to act non-maleficently towards all because of necessarily oppressive societal structures. It may simply be impossible to live as a citizen in a modern, first-world country without harming somebody through one's action. On one, not totally ludicrous, interpretation it is, for instance, the case that every time I buy coffee in my local supermarket I act maleficently towards a large number of people in the third world. I may not be aware that that is what I am doing, but I am inflicting harm. I might claim that this harmdoing is not intentional, but this seems a rather disingenuous excuse, given that it would only require minimal effort to make myself aware of the consequences of my act.

It could be argued that I cannot in reality act beneficently towards all, because I cannot act beneficently towards future persons. If we accept that future persons fall within the scope of the principle of beneficence that may well be true. Even if I benefit every living person, I cannot be certain that this will also benefit future persons, and I cannot benefit future persons directly; but the same argument goes for non-maleficence. The future consequences of my present acts of non-maleficence are equally uncertain, and acting non-maleficently may in the long run create more harm than is prevented.

If future persons fall within the scope of the principle of beneficence, then they must also fall within the scope of the principle of non-maleficence, since both principles are of the same person-affecting kind. But, in that case the impossibility of acting beneficently towards all, caused by the problem of future persons, implies a similar impossibility of acting non-maleficently towards all.

The content of the principle of beneficence which emerges in PBE4 is, as we have seen, very limited, and it is not strange that critics of the PBE4 framework have claimed that beneficence disappears when compared to respect for autonomy and non-maleficence.

The principle of justice fares equally badly. Very early on in the book we read: 'For example, if the theory proposed such high requirements for personal autonomy ... or such lofty standards of social justice ... that, realistically, no person could be autonomous and no society be just, the proposed theory would be deeply defective.'[12]

---

[12] *Principles of Biomedical Ethics*, 47.

A JUST SOCIETY

It is interesting to note in this context that on most accounts of justice it is actually the case that it will be very difficult or realistically impossible to create and maintain a just society. It seems impossible to claim that any presently existing society is just in a strict sense, and no realistic plans have been put forward to rectify this lamentable state of affairs. But on the PBE4 account we can probably instead simply choose to abandon our ideas about justice, since they are obviously too strict and stringent.

Whether this conclusion follows in a way which is damaging to the PBE4 account of justice depends on the meaning of the clause 'realistically could'. The fourth edition of the *Principles of Biomedical Ethics* uses a notion of 'realistic possibility' or 'practicality' to distinguish between obligatory and supererogatory acts, and in the assessment of ethical theories. The exact meaning of this notion is never made explicit, but it is, for instance, used to cast doubt on utilitarianism as a viable moral theory because of its stringent moral demands, and it is claimed that utilitarians cannot maintain the crucial distinction between the obligatory and the supererogatory. This is a fairly commonplace objection, and could be made even if the PBE4 notion of practicality put the dividing line between the obligatory and the supererogatory so that the area of obligation became very large. The PBE4 discussion of supererogation at the end of the book does, however, support a reading which points towards the area of obligation as being rather restricted. The closest possible approximation to the PBE4 idea of 'realistically could' one can get to is therefore something like 'within the reach of the average person.'

According to this conception of realistic possibility, it seems that the authors of PBE4 must place the quest for a just society within the realm of the supererogatory, and outside of the obligatory, because the chance of reaching a just society is small (or non-existent), and the effort required great. But it is difficult to see how the fulfilment of a putative obligation to work towards a just society could ever be supererogatory. If I know that the society in which I live is unjust, then I must have an obligation to try to rectify this state of affairs, even though that obligation might well be unfulfillable.

In their chapter on the principle of justice the authors discuss Michael Walzer's contention that within the sphere of health care there is a distinctive logic that 'Care should be proportionate to illness and not to wealth'[13]

---

[13] Ibid. 339; M. Walzer, *Spheres of Justice: A Defense of Pluralism and Equality* (New York: Basic Books, 1983).

and that this distinctive logic forms part of common morality. The fourth edition of the *Principles of Biomedical Ethics* rejects this contention: 'It is doubtful that equal access to health care finds stronger support throughout the American tradition than free-market principles or beliefs in the right to a decent basic minimum of health care.'[14]

From this, probably correct, interpretation of the American moral tradition PBE4 can only draw the conclusion that an egalitarian health care system is not morally mandated, but only some form of two-tier or multi-tier system with a decent minimum of health care for everybody: 'The first tier would *presumably* cover *at least* public health measures and preventive care, primary care, acute care, and special social services for those with disabilities.'[15]

' . . . the decent-minimum proposal has proved difficult to explicate and implement. It raises problems of whether society can fairly, consistently, and unambiguously devise a public policy that recognizes a right to care for primary needs without creating a right to exotic and expensive forms of treatment, such as liver transplants costing over $200,000 for what many deem to be marginal benefits in quality-adjusted life-years.'[16]

It is only with great hesitancy that I invite the reader to ponder how many people would evaluate the costs and benefits in using $50,000 each year for a number of years on the care and treatment of a drug-addict with HIV-infection and multi-resistant tuberculosis.

If the content of common morality is to any extent dependent on the number of members of the community who hold a certain point of view, I will safely predict that this treatment scenario falls outside what American (and European) common morality countenances.

And even if we reject clearly prejudicial components in common morality, it seems that the present cost-benefit ratio of AIDS care or care for persons with untreatable cancers may put it beyond the decent-minimum commitment in the communal first tier.

A common theme which emerges in the treatment of beneficence and justice in PBE4 is a reluctance to endow these principles with much substantive content. There are many rejections of other authors who put forward too demanding and stringent conceptions of either principle, and through the gradual grinding down by removing the demanding components of the duty of beneficence and the principle of justice we end up with a totally watered-down conception without any substance or moral bite.

[14] Beauchamp and Childress, *Principles of Biomedical Ethics*, 339.
[15] Ibid. 356; my emphasis.
[16] Ibid. 357.

SPECIFICATION AND BALANCING

Another serious problem with the moral framework put forward in PBE4 is its lack of explicit decision rules. According to PBE4 good moral theories and principles should have 'output power', they should give 'creative and practical solutions', and be 'adaptive to novelty'.[17] The principlism in PBE4 fulfils all these criteria, but unfortunately at the expense of any clear guidance as to how we are to reach answers to moral questions. The theory may have a lot of output power, but what is produced is produced via, but not by, the theory.

What do I mean by this?

According to PBE4 moral judgment can be aided by reflecting on the four principles, and by applying them to the case at hand through the processes of specification and balancing. Specification and balancing are not parts of the generic four principles approach (which would then be a six principles approach), but they are integral parts of the model for justification in morality which is developed in PBE4, and the total PBE4 model cannot be assessed just by looking at the four principles. Without specification and balancing the four principles are morally inert.

Specification takes place when we explicate the exact content of a given principle, norm, or rule. When we, for instance, specify the rule, 'Doctors should put their patients' interests first' we see that it does not imply that they should falsify information on insurance forms.[18] Specification involves one principle and can resolve some moral conflicts, whereas moral problems involving more than one principle also requires balancing between these principles (see below). Unfortunately no procedural rules are put forward to guide the process of specification, apart from the rules of justification and coherence regulative for all rational discourse.

When it comes to balancing we get some more specific guidance. The fourth edition of the *Principles of Biomedical Ethics* accepts the distinction between *prima facie* and actual obligations as proposed by W. D. Ross, but the authors further argue for a set of conditions that must be met to justify infringing one *prima facie* norm in order to adhere to another:

1. Better reasons can be offered to act on the overriding norm than on the infringed norm . . .
2. The moral objective justifying the infringement has a realistic prospect of achievement.
3. No morally preferable alternative actions can be substituted.

---

[17] Ibid. 26.   [18] Ibid. 29.

4. The form of infringement selected is the least possible, commensurate with achieving the primary goal of the action.
5. The agent seeks to minimize the negative effects of the infringement.[19]

The authors note that some of these conditions appear to be tautological, and it is difficult not to agree with them. If one applies the 'not test' by trying to assert the opposite of the five conditions it is obvious that they are not only nearly tautological but also totally uncontroversial. It would indeed be strange to override a *prima facie* obligation if 'Only worse reasons can be offered to act on the overriding norm than on the infringed norm'!

But can the five conditions help us, if we don't have any further conditions delimiting the field of considerations that can validly be introduced in the balancing?

Not very much, because they are almost purely formal. We are given no criteria with which we can decide whether something is a relevant *moral* consideration.

Strangely enough the authors of PBE4 seem to see this as a strength in their theory: 'As with specification, the process of balancing cannot be rigidly dictated by some formulaic "method" in ethical theory. The model of balancing will satisfy neither those who seek clear-cut, specific guidance about what one ought to do in particular cases nor those who believe in a lexical or serial ranking of principles with automatic overriding conditions'.[20]

I will leave aside the question of lexical ranking, but a balancing model, which is a central component in a moral theory put forward for use in the health care context, must be able to give 'clear-cut, specific guidance about what one ought to do in particular cases' in a reasonably large number of cases, otherwise it is at greater risk of becoming at rhetorical justification of intuitions or prejudices.

It is evident that a lack of definitive moral decidability will greatly expand the output power of a moral theory, at least in terms of the number of answers produced, and that this lack will also enhance the ability to give 'creative and practical solutions' (although they will not be definitive), and the ability to be 'adaptive to novelty'. Unfortunately the answers produced will be underdetermined by the content of the theory, and the final choice between available answers will have to be made on the basis of considerations outside of the PBE4 framework. We can only hope that these decisive considerations will be moral considerations.

---

[19] *Principles of Biomedical Ethics*, 34.   [20] Ibid. 36.

   The theory in PBE4 therefore, not surprisingly, fulfils all the PBE4 criteria
for a good moral theory, but the cost which has been paid is very high.

CONCLUSION

The problem with the principlism of PBE4 is thus not only the explicitly
American nature of the model, with its subsequent underdevelopment of the
positive obligations incorporated in beneficence and justice, but also that we
are presented with a structure for moral reasoning which cannot give any
definite answers to moral problems, or perhaps more accurately can produce
almost any answer we want.
   This problem is freely acknowledged by the authors, but they fail to see
that it shifts the ground beneath their elaborate theoretical structure. They
write: 'The attempt to work out the implications of general theories for
specific forms of conduct and moral judgment will be called *practical ethics*
here . . . The term *practical* refers to the use of ethical theory and methods of
analysis to examine moral problems, practices, and policies in several areas,
including the professions and public policy. Often no straightforward
movement from theory or principles to particular principles is possible in
these contexts, although general reasons, principles, and even ideals can play
some role in evaluating conduct and establishing policies'.[21]
   'We have not attempted a general ethical theory and do not claim that our
principles mimic, are analogous to, or substitute for the foundational principles in leading classical theories such as utilitarianism (with its principle of
utility) and Kantianism (with its categorical imperative) . . . As we have
acknowledged, even the core principles of our account are so scant that
they cannot provide an adequate basis for deducing most of what we can
justifiably claim to know in the moral life.'[22]
   But what use do we have in the practical health care setting for an account
where even the proponents claim that ' . . . even the core principles of our
account are so scant that they cannot provide an adequate basis for
deducing most of what we can *justifiably claim to know in the moral life*'.[23]
   One answer could be, that even if the four principles approach cannot
provide definitive answers it can provide an initial mapping of the moral
domain in individual problem cases, it can facilitate the identification of the
morally relevant facts, and it can thereby create the basis for an adequate
discussion of such cases.
   This suggestion raises two questions: a. does the PBE4 framework map the

---

[21] Ibid. 4; italics in original.   [22] Ibid. 106–7.   [23] Ibid.; my emphasis.

whole moral domain, and b. does the PBE4 framework contain sufficient guidance about the moral relevance of specific considerations?

There is no doubt that large parts of the moral domain can be accommodated within the four principles approach, but the inclusion in PBE4 of a chapter on 'Virtues and ideals in professional life' enumerating four(!) focal virtues, suggests that even the inventors of the four principles approach believe that there is more to morality than principles. Using only the four principles as an analytic tool, may therefore leave out other important moral considerations.

Within the PBE4 framework, the only guidance about the moral relevance of specific considerations is found in the chapters explicating the content of the four principles. I have argued above that much of this content is only applicable within an American context, and that it cannot be transferred in any straightforward manner to other cultural contexts. Even if this is only partly true it leaves the non-American user of the PBE4 approach with limited or no guidance as to the moral relevance of specific considerations falling within one of the four broad principles. Any use of the PBE4 approach as an analytic tool outside America can therefore only proceed, if the content of the four principles is worked out for the specific cultural context in which the framework is applied.

The two considerations mentioned here indicate that although the PBE4 approach may have value as a tool for elucidating specific moral problems, this value is predicated on a re-working of the content of the four principles for each new cultural context, and on an explicit recognition that the four principles must be supplemented by further moral considerations.

17

TELLING THE TRUTH, CONFIDENTIALITY, CONSENT, AND RESPECT FOR AUTONOMY

RAANAN GILLON

TELLING THE TRUTH AND MEDICAL ETHICS

In this book I have discussed four principles for guiding action that seem to be required by any adequate philosophical theory of medical ethics: a principle of respect for persons, notably for their autonomy; a principle of beneficence; a principle of non-maleficence; and a principle of justice. Much moral debate stems either from disagreement about scope (about what sorts of entity are owed what sorts of moral concern) or from disagreement about the relative importance of these four principles. In the next four chapters I shall look at examples of conflicts in the context of medical ethics that are primarily between the principle of respect for autonomy on one hand and the principles of beneficence and non-maleficence on the other. I shall start with the issue of telling the truth.

Telling the Truth

'In much wisdom is much grief: and he that increaseth knowledge increaseth sorrow' (Ecclesiastes 1: 18). Thus Dr Maurice Davidson began his chapter on truth telling in his 1957 book on medical ethics.[1] Davidson, however, argued against the tendency of 'so many medical practitioners to withhold the facts from their patients, especially in cases of grave illness, and to insist that the truth must at all costs be kept from them.' Rejecting this as a 'fetich,' which was wholly unjustifiable, he argued that real harm rarely resulted from honesty in response to patients who wanted reliable information about their

From Raanan Gillon, 'Telling the Truth and Medical Ethics,' 'Confidentiality,' 'Consent,' and 'Where Respect for Autonomy is not the Answer,' chapters 16–19 in his *Philosophical Medical Ethics* (Chichester: Wiley, 1985).

[1] M. Davidson, 'What to Tell the Gravely Ill Patient, or One who has to Undergo a Serious Operation,' in Davidson (ed.), *Medical Ethics: A Guide to Students and Practitioners* (London: Lloyd-Luke, 1957).

condition. They might have 'vitally important duties' that they could carry out only if they were given such information, and failure to divulge the plain facts was in the long run 'a frequent cause of the greatest distress.' As Davidson freely admitted, he was unusual among doctors in holding these views, but he remained unconvinced that the arguments of his colleagues against such frankness were 'anything but an excuse for evading what is admittedly an extremely unpleasant duty.'

Sympathetic as I am to Davidson's position, I think the opposing position needs more consideration. The case for deception in medical practice, whether in the context of fatal or grave disease or in informing patients of the risks of treatment or research, is usually based on three major arguments (elegantly dissected, among many others, by the philosopher Sissela Bok in her book *Lying*[2]).

The Case for Deception

The first argument in favour of deception is, as indicated above, that doctors' Hippocratic obligations to benefit and not harm their patients override any requirement of not deceiving people. For example, by definition patients with serious illness already have severe problems; the doctor adds to these problems by giving patients distressing news; moreover, patients' prospects of recovery often depend crucially on their morale and perhaps on some element of placebo effect or, in Balint's memorable phrase, 'the drug doctor,' or both. Passing on unpleasant medical information will probably undermine these and thus impair patients' prospects of recovery.

The second argument in favour of not telling the truth is that it cannot be communicated, both because a doctor is rarely, or never, in a position to know the truth (he can never be sure of the diagnosis or prognosis) and because even if he were the patient would rarely, if ever, be in a position to understand it. Even common words such as 'cancer' are likely to be radically misunderstood by patients unless they have had a medical training. The wide range of conditions and prognoses and all other technical nuances implied by the word are probably not taken into consideration and are often replaced by a single dark understanding that cancer is simply another word for a peculiarly horrible death. As an American doctor emphatically summarised this argument, 'It is meaningless to speak of telling the truth, the whole truth and nothing but the truth to a patient. It is meaningless because it is

---

[2] S. Bok, *Lying: Moral Choice in Public and Private Life* (Hassocks: Harvester Press, 1978).

impossible' (he went on to recommend the 'far older' medico-moral guide, 'So far as possible do no harm').[3]

The third common medical argument against telling the truth is that patients do not wish to be told the truth when it is dire, particularly when they have a dangerous or fatal condition.

Precedence of Beneficence and Non-Maleficence

With regard to the first argument—that the principles of beneficence and non-maleficence must take precedence over any requirement of not deceiving people—I showed in the chapter on autonomy how even for utilitarians (for whom the overriding moral principle is to maximise welfare and minimise harm) the principle of respect for autonomy is a crucial moral principle, while for Kantians respect for people and their autonomy is itself the overriding moral principle.

As deceiving people in medical contexts usually means failing to respect their autonomy (usually in each of the categories I outlined: thought, intention, and action) by denying them adequate information for rational deliberation, even from a utilitarian viewpoint it is probably morally unacceptable unless there is strong reason to believe that in a particular case overall welfare would be maximised by deception. Furthermore, the various arguments adduced in my discussion of medical paternalism apply to this specific example: not only can welfare be expected to be increased by honesty and frankness but also there is no reason to assume that doctors are particularly skilled judges of what course of action maximises welfare. Generally, so far as the welfare of individual patients is concerned they themselves are probably the best judges of whether knowing the truth about unpleasant facts will or will not improve their welfare.

There is, of course, an important practical difficulty here: how is the doctor to find out a patient's views without disclosing any unpleasant facts to those patients who would rather not know such information? There is no simple answer to this, but by sensitive questioning or by simply (but genuinely and at different times) offering to answer any questions, and giving adequate time for this, skilful doctors can often master this difficult medical art. In this context the remarkable psychological defence mechanism of denial may be reassuring; even after being told of their impending demise many patients seem to eliminate this information from their minds and deny

[3] L. Henderson, 'Physician and Patient as a Social System,' *New England Journal of Medicine*, 212 (1935), 819–23.

that they have been given it, and, according to Kubler Ross, most people who know they are fatally ill tend to move in and out of such denial, more so to start with than later on.[4] Perhaps denial is a natural defence against being overburdened with such difficult thoughts when people are unable to cope with them. In addition to skilful and sympathetic discussion with patients after unpleasant information has been discovered, pilot studies could be run to find out the pros and cons of asking patients in advance their views on being deceived about unpleasant news, and indeed on a whole range of other medicomoral issues—an upgraded version of asking them what religion they espouse. For example, when they first registered with a doctor or attended a hospital patients could be offered an opportunity to answer a questionnaire about such matters, including how much they would like to participate in decision making or how much they would prefer to leave it to medical people; how much they would want to be told any bad news or how much they would wish to be shielded from it; whether or not they would wish to donate their organs if they died; whom they would allow to be told about their medical condition and whom not; which matters, if any, they considered to be particularly sensitive; and so on?

It astonishes me how, with a few exceptions, whenever I suggest this idea to medical colleagues there is widespread scorn—for example, 'You'll terrify them,' 'What they say when they are fairly well couldn't be relied on when they are ill,' 'They might have changed their minds,' 'Suppose they have not understood the questions,'—yet when I suggest it to non-medical people the idea is usually embraced enthusiastically and the counterarguments rejected—'It might be worrying but at least the doctors would know what you wanted,' 'One wouldn't say something important unless one felt fairly sure about it,' 'Why shouldn't they design the questionnaire so that you did understand it?'

At the very least, it seems worth investigating such a scheme on a pilot basis to see if it offers any advantages in patient care and to find out what the problems are. Such an investigation would surely be as worthwhile for an MD thesis as many a more technical topic.

Impossibility of Communicating the Truth

The second argument against telling the truth concerns a fundamental confusion between the moral issue of truth telling and truthfulness on one hand and the epistemological, logical, and semantic problems that beset the

---

[4] E. Kubler-Ross, *On Death and Dying* (London: Tavistock, 1970), 34–43.

concept of truth itself. Although these last three issues are of central importance in philosophy, they have little to do with the question of what it is right to do with such knowledge of the truth as a person believes himself to have. Here, the crucial moral issue concerns the doctor's intentions—in particular, does he intend to discover what the patient would wish to know and does he intend to try to meet such wishes when they concern the transmission of information that the doctor believes to be both true and likely to distress the patient, or does he intend to deceive the patient? Of course, most medical information is typically probabilistic, of course, patients will vary in their ability to understand complex medical information, of course, 'the whole truth' is usually a mirage, and, of course, even philosophers disagree about what is meant by 'truth.' In the ordinary case none of these difficulties are relevant to the moral dilemmas of truthfulness and deceit. Those with residual doubts should, as Sissela Bok suggests,[2] imagine what their response would be to a used car dealer who used such arguments to justify his deceit.

Patients' Wish not to Know

Finally, there is the argument that patients do not want to be told the truth about their fatal condition. This is an important argument as it implicitly acknowledges that doctors ought to respect their patients' wishes. Several papers have, however, indicated that most people surveyed (usually over 80%) would like to be told the truth.[5] On the other hand, until fairly recently most American doctors surveyed generally withheld the truth about diagnoses of cancer from their patients,[6] though recently this has changed radically, with up to 97% of responding doctors preferring to tell patients with cancer their diagnosis.[7] Again this is an empirical question, but if the premise on which it is based is accepted—notably the desirability of doing what the patient wants—then the important issue is not what most patients or doctors think but what the particular patient in the particular circumstances

---

[5] N. H. Cassem and R. S. Stewart, 'Management and Care of the Dying Patient,' *International Journal of Psychiatry and Medicine*, 6 (1975), 2–304; R. Veatch, *Death, Dying and the Biological Revolution* (New Haven: Yale University Press, 1976), 229–35; J. Aitken-Swan and E. C. Easson, 'Reactions of Cancer Patients on Being Told their Diagnoses,' *British Medical Journal*, 1 (1959), 779–83; J. McIntosh, 'Patients' Awareness and Desire for Information about Diagnosed but Undisclosed Malignant Disease,' *Lancet*, 7 (1976), 300–3; W. D. Kelly and S. R. Friesen, 'Do Cancer Patients Want to be Told?', *Surgery*, 27 (1950), 822–6.

[6] D. Oken, 'What to Tell Cancer Patients,' *Journal of the American Medical Association*, 175 (1961), 1120–8.

[7] D. H. Novack, R. Plumer, R. L. Smith, H. Ochtill, G. R. Morrow, and J. M. Bennett, 'Changes in Physicians' Attitudes toward Telling the Cancer Patient,' *Journal of the American Medical Association*, 241 (1979), 897–900.

wants. There seems to be no real doubt that the third argument is false and that at least some, possibly many, patients would wish to be dealt with honestly.

It should be emphasised that the forgoing counterarguments do not support indiscriminate, casual, curt, or unsupportive truth telling to all patients, approaches that are alas not unknown in medical practice, as Goldie disconcertingly recounts.[8] Nor do they deny the considerable difficulties concerned. They do reiterate that avoiding deceit is a basic moral norm, defensible from several moral perspectives, including those primarily concerned with maximising welfare, provided that welfare is not assessed simplistically on the basis of mere consideration of a patient's immediate distress on being told dire news.

CONFIDENTIALITY

The principle of medical confidentiality—that doctors must keep their patients' secrets—is one of the most venerable moral obligations of medical ethics. The Hippocratic Oath enjoins: 'Whatever, in connection with my professional practice, or not in connection with it, I see or hear, in the life of men, which ought not to be spoken of abroad, I will not divulge, as reckoning that all such should be kept secret.'[9] The obligation is widely regarded as being exceedingly strict. Indeed, according to the World Medical Association's International Code of Medical Ethics it is an absolute requirement, even after the patient's death:[10] an absolutist claim echoed in a leading article in the *BMJ*.[11] (Ironically, two years later the General Medical Council (GMC) officially indicated to the editor of the *BMJ* that an obituary he had published of a famous soldier had transgressed medical confidentiality.)[12] In France so strict is the obligation of medical confidentiality that it is apparently enshrined in law as an absolute medical privilege which no one, including the patient, is allowed to override, even when to do so would be in the patient's interest.[13]

In practice, on the other hand, doctors do not seem to regard confidentiality as an absolute requirement, as many relatives of seriously ill patients could testify. The BMA handbook of medical ethics lists five types of

---

[8] L. Goldie, 'The Ethics of Telling the Patient,' *Journal of Medical Ethics*, 8 (1982), 128–33.
[9] British Medical Association, *The Handbook of Medical Ethics* (London: BMA, 1984), 69–70.
[10] Ibid. 70–2.
[11] R. Parkes, 'The Duty of Confidence,' *British Medical Journal*, 285 (1982), 1442–3.
[12] S. Lock, 'A Question of Confidence,' *British Medical Journal*, 288 (1984), 123–5.
[13] J. Havard, 'Medical Confidence,' *Journal of Medical Ethics*, 22 (1985), 8–11.

exception to the need to maintain medical confidentiality[14] and the GMC
lists eight.[15] Recent British governments certainly do not regard medical
confidentiality as absolute: one of Mrs Thatcher's governments tried
(unsuccessfully, largely as a result of opposition from the BMA) to give
statutory licence to the police to search medical files,[16] and the BMA is still
unhappy about the inadequate protection afforded to health records by the
Data Protection Act 1984 and has cosponsored an interprofessional working
group partly to tighten up the Act's provisions for medical confidentiality.[17]
The campaign led by Mrs Gillick—accepted by the Court of Appeal but
then rejected by the House of Lords—clearly believed that doctors are
excessively concerned with confidentiality when it comes to prescribing oral
contraceptives to girls under 16;[18] its members would presumably approve of
the famous (or infamous) action of Dr Browne, who broke medical confidentiality and told his 16 year old patient's parents that she was taking the
pill[19] (he was not censured by the GMC). Doctors express concern about
both the threats to[20] and the relaxing standards of[21] the medical profession's
principle of confidentiality, and one doctor has advocated that patients
ought to keep their own records to preserve their confidentiality.[22] So was the
American doctor right who called medical confidentiality 'a decrepit concept'?[23] How can any sense be made of what may appear to be a chaotic
jumble of attitudes?

What is 'Medical Confidentiality'?

Some preliminary (and sketchy) analysis of the issues may be useful. What is
meant by 'medical confidentiality'? Is it morally valuable in itself or, if not,

[14] British Medical Association, *Handbook of Medical Ethics*, 12.
[15] General Medical Council, *Professional Conduct and Disciplines: Fitness to Practise* (London:
GMC, 1985), 19–21.
[16] J. Havard, 'Doctors and the Police,' *British Medical Journal*, 286 (1983), 742–3.
[17] A. W. Macara, 'Confidentiality: A Decrepit Concept?', *Journal of the Royal Society of Medicine*, 77 (1984), 577–84.
[18] 'Teenage Confidence and Consent,' Editorial, *British Medical Journal*, 290 (1985), 144–5.
[19] J. K. Mason and R. A. McCall-Smith, *Law and Medical Ethics* (London: Butterworth, 1983),
103.
[20] J. Barnes, S. Biggs, R. Boyd, *et al.*, 'Threats to Medical Confidentiality,' *The Lancet*, 2 (1983),
1422.
[21] D. Black and F. Subotsky, 'Medical Ethics and Child Psychiatry,' *Journal of Medical Ethics*, 8
(1982), 5–8; D. F. H. Pheby, 'Changing Practice of Confidentiality: A Cause for Concern,' ibid.
12–24.
[22] V. Coleman, 'Why Patients should Keep their Records,' *Journal of Medical Ethics*, 1 (1984),
27–8.
[23] M. Siegler, 'Confidentiality in Medicine: A Decrepit Concept,' *New England Journal of Medicine*, 307 (1982), 1518–21.

why is it morally important? Is it an absolute requirement? How does it relate to other obligations?

Essentially medical confidentiality is the respecting of other people's secrets (in the sense of information they do not wish to have further disclosed without their permission). There is obviously no general moral duty to respect other people's secrets (imagine a thief whom one had surprised saying 'Shh, don't tell the police, it's a secret'), yet equally obviously doctors (and, of course, other groups) voluntarily undertake some general commitment to keep their patients' or clients' secrets (imagine the same thief talking about his activities in the course of a medical consultation). It seems clear that two conditions are necessary to create a moral duty of confidentiality: one person must undertake—that is, explicitly or implicitly promise—not to disclose another's secrets and that other person must disclose to the first person information that he considers to be secret. Thus there can be no transgression of confidentiality if the information is not regarded as secret by the person giving it; equally it is only because doctors have undertaken not to disclose patients' secrets that they have acquired a duty of confidentiality.

Why should doctors from the time of Hippocrates to the present have promised to keep their patients' secrets? If confidentiality is not a moral good in itself what moral good does it serve? The commonest justification for the duty of medical confidentiality is undoubtedly consequentialist: people's better health, welfare, the general good, and overall happiness are more likely to be attained if doctors are fully informed by their patients, and this is more likely if doctors undertake not to disclose their patients' secrets. Conversely, if patients did not believe that doctors would keep their secrets then either they would not divulge embarrassing but potentially medically important information, thus reducing their chances of getting the best medical care, or they would disclose such information and feel anxious and unhappy at the prospect of their secrets being made known.

Such consequentialist reasoning might well be accepted not only by utilitarians but also by many deontological pluralists. Deontologists, however, are unlikely to accept it as being adequate. They are likely to base their arguments for confidentiality not just (if at all) on welfare considerations but also on the moral principle of respect for autonomy,[24] or sometimes on a putatively independent principle of respect for privacy,[25] which is seen as a

[24] S. Benn, 'Privacy, Freedom and Respect for Persons,' in R. Wassterstrom (ed.), *Today's Moral Problems* (New York: Macmillan, 1975).

[25] H. W. S. Francis, 'Gossips, Eavesdroppers and Peeping Toms: A Defence of the Right of Privacy,' *Journal of Medical Ethics*, 8 (1982), 134–43.

fundamental moral requirement in itself.[26] Thus, while the principle of medical confidentiality is not defended as a moral end—in itself, it is defended by utilitarians and deontologists alike as a means to some morally desirable end the general welfare, respect for people's autonomy, or respect for their privacy.

Medical Confidentiality an 'Absolute' Principle . . .

I have given reasons in previous chapters why both utilitarians and pluralist deontologists would not be able, and would not try, to make a principle such as medical confidentiality into an absolute principle, whereby a patient's confidences invariably had to be respected whatever the consequences (though the duty of confidentiality of the Roman Catholic confessor appears to be regarded as absolute). I have also argued previously that although the Kantian categorical imperative is regarded as an absolute principle, it necessarily requires the interests of all affected rational agents to be taken into account in its application; Kantians too would thus have no place for a maxim that demanded absolute medical confidentiality in all circumstances. Nor, incidentally, would there be any philosophical justification within these systems for the requirement of confidentiality to be absolute after a patient's death.

Such philosophical reluctance to see medical confidentiality as an absolute requirement is matched not only by various modern codes of medical ethics (though not by the World Medical Association's international code) but also, I suspect, by the Hippocratic Oath itself. The qualifier, 'which ought not to be spoken of abroad,' though ambiguous, can plausibly be taken to imply that the oath envisaged circumstances where it was permissible for information obtained in the course of a doctor's professional activities to be 'spoken of abroad.' In general the medical profession in Britain today probably sees confidentiality as a strong but by no means absolute moral obligation. The GMC's 'blue book' lists the following eight legitimate exceptions: (a) when the patient 'or his legal adviser' gives written and valid consent; (b) when other doctors or other health care professionals are participating in the patient's care; (c) when the doctor believes that a close relative or friend should know about the patient's health but it is medically undesirable to seek the patient's consent; (d) exceptionally when the doctor believes that disclosure to a third party other than a relative would be in the

[26] A. Caplan, 'On Privacy and Confidentiality in Social Science Research,' in T. L. Beauchamp (ed.), *Ethical Issues in Social Science Research* (Baltimore: Johns Hopkins University Press, 1982); C. Fried, *An Anatomy of Values* (Cambridge, Mass.: Harvard University Press, 1970), 137–52.

'best interests of the patient' and when the patient has rejected 'every reasonable effort to persuade'; (e) when there are statutory requirements to disclose information; (f) when a judge or equivalent legal authority directs a doctor to disclose confidential medical information; (g) (rarely) when the public interest overrides the duty of confidentiality 'such as for example investigation by the police of a grave or very serious crime'; and (h) for the purposes of medical research approved by a 'recognised ethical committee.'[27]

. . . or a 'Decrepit Concept'?

Small wonder, the sceptic may be thinking, that Siegler called medical confidentiality a 'decrepit concept.' He had looked into the matter after a patient complained that all sorts of people whom he (the patient) had not authorised were looking at his notes. On investigation Dr Siegler was 'astonished to learn that at least 25 and possibly as many as 100 health professionals and administrative personnel at our university hospital had access to the patient's record and that all of them had a legitimate need, indeed a professional responsibility, to open and use that chart.'[28]

It is too harsh to call the principle of medical confidentiality 'decrepit' but it does seem to have lost its way. The problem seems to be that the moral unacceptability of an absolute requirement of medical confidentiality has been recognised by the profession, which has both officially and in practice specified—without explicitly justifying—a set of ad hoc exceptions. On the other hand, doctors in practice (including myself I must confess) are reluctant to give up thinking and talking about confidentiality as though it were an absolute requirement. This reluctance may result partly from a lingering belief that it ought to be absolute and partly from the belief that if patients find out that it is not they will feel aggrieved, even betrayed, and also will stop being honest with their doctors, thus impairing their medical care. If my personal inquiries are representative few non-doctors are aware of how many official and de facto exceptions there are to medical confidentiality. On the other hand, many believe that the supposedly absolute requirement of confidentiality is actually honoured by doctors only in so far as it suits them. If these are typical attitudes doctors' current ambivalence about confidentiality is producing an understandable but undesirable cynicism about their attitudes.

Such cynicism could be reduced—without much if any harm to patient care—by admitting openly that medical confidentiality is not absolute and

---

[27] General Medical Council, *Professional Conduct and Disciplines*, 19–21.
[28] Siegler, 'Confidentiality in Medicine.'

then justifying,[29] rather than simply stating, the sorts of exception approved by the profession, with a view to achieving a sort of 'social contract' between the profession and society about the categories of exception that would and would not be acceptable. If such justification were attempted for each of the GMC's exceptions some would probably be more easily justifiable and more widely acceptable than others. Few people would expect doctors to undertake to disobey (just) laws or facilitate substantial and probable harm to others, yet those possibilities would be entailed by an absolute commitment to medical confidentiality, and it is presumably to combat such an unacceptable commitment that the GMC specified exceptions (e), (f), and (g).

Justification of Exceptions

The other exceptions accepted by the GMC seem, however, less easily justifiable and less likely to obtain widespread social approval. Exception (h) justifies breaking confidentiality in order to carry out medical research—but ought not patients to be asked before their personal files are used for research? (This could be done routinely on admission or acceptance to a general practitioner's list and the files flagged appropriately.)

Exceptions (b, (c), and (d) are more problematical for they all depend on breaking a patient's confidence on the paternalistic assumption that to do so without consulting the patient will be in the patient's best interests. I have rehearsed the arguments against medical paternalism previously and they seem to be powerful (though I shall consider in a subsequent article certain exceptions such as emergencies, unobtainability of information about the patient's wishes, and mental incompetence or other causes of sufficiently impaired autonomy). In the normal case, however, I am persuaded that medical paternalism is an unjustifiable anachronism that would receive little if any support in any medicomoral 'social contract' and which should be avoided. (Let me reiterate, however, that to object to paternalism is not to object to doctors making decisions if that is what the patient wants—the important thing is to find out what he or she does want.) Nor does there seem much reason to believe that obtaining a patient's consent to disclosure would be excessively difficult 'at the sharp' end. ('Good morning Mrs Jones, I've been asked to give you physiotherapy, do you mind if I consult your notes to see what would be best for you?') Few patients are going to refuse what is in their own interests (especially if it is made clear that, as the GMC

[29] P. Sieghart, 'Medical Confidence, the Law and Computers,' *Journal of the Royal Society of Medicine*, 77 (1984), 656–62.

recommends, any health professional given access to the notes will be bound by the same strong though not absolute standards of confidentiality as are doctors.) If patients do refuse certain others access to medical information about themselves, whether it is in the context of (b), (c), or (d), should not their refusal be honoured just as refusal to consult some other doctor or health professional would be honoured? Why not?

An Important Principle

In summary, medical confidentiality is an important medico-moral principle that can be justified by its contribution to improving people's medical treatment and respecting their autonomy and privacy. It is not, however, an absolute obligation, and this should be made clear. On the other hand, exceptions to medical confidentiality need to be not merely specified, as they are at present, but also justified. Exceptions based on the principles of non-maleficence and justice may well be justified in particular cases, but I have argued against accepting exceptions that are justified by appeals to medical paternalism or the benefits of medical research (both variants of the principle of beneficence which ignore its integral requirement also to respect people's autonomy). In both these sorts of cases patients' permission should generally be obtained if medical information concerning them is to be disclosed to others.

CONSENT

Vets do not bother with their patients' consent: why should doctors? To address this question it is important to state which meaning of 'consent' is being used for the term is ambiguous. Under one definition it simply means agreement, acceptance, or assent. It is fairly obvious (though here unargued) that this meaning of consent is not relevant to medical interventions, whether these are investigations, treatments, or research. For medical interventions it is widely accepted that consent means a voluntary, uncoerced decision, made by a sufficiently competent or autonomous person on the basis of adequate information and deliberation, to accept rather than reject some proposed course of action that will affect him or her.[30] Consent in this

---

[30] A. W. Wilkinson, 'Consent,' in A. S. Duncan, G. R. Dunstan, and R. B. Welbourn (eds.), *Dictionary of Medical Ethics* (London: Darton, Longman & Todd, 1981); P. Taylor, 'Consent, Competency and ECT: A Psychiatrist's View,' *Journal of Medical Ethics*, 9 (1983), 146–51; P. D. G. Skegg, 'Informed Consent to Medical Procedures,' *Medical Science Law*, 15 (1975), 124–8;

sense requires action by an autonomous agent based on adequate information and is by definition informed consent.

Autonomy and Informed Consent

This analysis explains why vets do not bother with consent from their patients: their patients are not autonomous agents (or at least most of them are not—I remain agnostic about certain higher primates and dolphins), and they simply could not give consent. Given that most adult patients could give consent in this sense, why should doctors bother to ensure that they do? The most obvious answer is that generally we have a moral obligation to respect each other's autonomy, at least in so far as to do so is compatible with respect for the autonomy of others—a moral principle that I have previously shown to be supported from various moral perspectives. Doing things to other autonomous agents without their consent generally means overriding their autonomy. It is respect for people's autonomy, or self determination as Mason and McCall Smith[31] and Kirby[32] call it, that morally underpins the requirement of consent. Justice Kirby, then president of the Australian Law Reform Commission, in an excellent article on consent, wrote: '[T]he fundamental principle underlying consent is said to be a right of self determination: the principle or value choice of autonomy of the person . . . The principle is not just a legal rule devised by one profession to harass another. It is an ethical principle which is simply reflected in legal rules because our law has been developed by judges sensitive to the practical application of generally held community ethical principles.'[32]

According to the above definition, to consent to medical intervention a person requires sufficient information to be able to make an informed and

---

V. Herbert, 'Informed Consent: A Legal Evaluation,' *Cancer*, 46 (1980), 1042–3; G. R. Dunstan and M. J. Seller (eds.), *Consent in Medicine* (London: King's Fund Publishing Office and Oxford University Press, 1983); T. L. Beauchamp and J. F. Childress, *Principles of Biomedical Ethics*, 2nd edn. (Oxford: Oxford University Press, 1983), 69–93; C. W. Lidz, A. Meisel, E. Zerubavel, M. Carter, R. M. Sestak, and L. H. Roth, *Informed Consent* (London: Guilford Press, 1984); C. M. Culver and B. Gert, *Philosophy in Medicine* (Oxford: Oxford University Press, 1982), 42–63; S. Gorovitz, *Doctors' Dilemmas* (London: Collier Macmillan, 1982), 34–54; S. Gorovitz (ed.), *Moral Problems in Medicine*, 2nd edn. (Englewood Cliffs, NJ: Prentice-Hall, 1983), 153–91; W. T. Reich (ed.), *Encyclopedia of Bioethics* (London: Collier Macmillan, 1978), 751–8; R. J. Levine, *Ethics and Regulation of Clinical Research* (Baltimore: Urban & Schwarzenberg, 1981), 69–115; Z. Bankowski and N. Howard-Jones (eds.), *Human Experimentation and Medical Ethics* (Geneva: Council for International Organisations of Medical Sciences, 1982), 16–121; R. M. Veatch, *Case Studies in Medical Ethics* (Cambridge, Mass.: Harvard University Press, 1977), 290–316.

[31] J. K. Mason and R. A. M. Smith, *Law and Medical Ethics* (London: Butterworth, 1983), 120.

[32] M. D. Kirby, 'Informed Consent: What does it Mean?', *Journal of Medical Ethics*, 9 (1983), 69–75.

deliberated choice, and it is in this context that doctors often object to the requirement for such consent. Patients, they say, are unnecessarily alarmed and their medical state unnecessarily impaired if they have to be given information about their diagnosis or prognosis or risks associated with their proposed management and treatment. The alarm is compounded with confusion, the argument continues, if differential diagnoses and risks have to be mentioned and made intolerable if the patient is expected to choose between the options. As Dr Ingelfinger exclaimed, he as a patient would not want 'to be in the position of a shopper at the casbah who negotiates and haggles with the physician about what is best.' Indeed, the doctor 'who merely spreads an array of vendibles in front of the patient and then says "go ahead and choose, it's your life" is guilty of shirking his duty, if not of malpractice.'[33]

Three Counterarguments

There are least three problems with such arguments. The first is that it is dangerous for a doctor to extrapolate from his own case to generalisations about his patients (or about anybody else). The fact that the good doctor would feel like that does not ensure or even make probable that any particular patient feels like that; and, as Dr Ingelfinger's argument implicitly acknowledges, the doctor should be trying to meet his patient's wishes rather than his own. As a wise philosopher once wrote, it is not putting yourself into another's shoes that is morally relevant, it is understanding what it is like for that other person to be in his or her own shoes that is morally important.

The second problem is empirical. Is it true that patients are generally made more alarmed by open minded and sympathetic provision of information and an invitation from the doctor to express their own preferences in so far as they have any? I doubt it. In this regard Dr Ingelfinger offers a parody of respect for the patient's autonomy when he suggests that the doctor would 'haggle' with the patient or alternatively merely tell the patient the available options and then say 'Go ahead and choose, it's your life.' The doctor who really respected his patient's autonomy would discover in a sensitive way, which did not demand a particular answer, what and how much each patient really wanted to know and how much he wished to participate in the decision making. Some patients are, like Dr Ingelfinger, undoubtedly keen not to be given unpleasant information and to leave all

---

[33] F. J. Ingelfinger, 'Arrogance,' *New England Journal of Medicine*, 303 (1980), 1507–11.

the decision making to the doctor; if the doctor acts accordingly, thus respecting their autonomy, such patients will probably be happier. Other patients, however, do want to know about their medical condition and its implications and about alternative options; they also wish to be active in decision making when it affects them. Such patients will probably feel more at ease, trusting, and happy if the doctor has respected their wishes and if they have deliberately, comprehendingly, and willingly consented to their doctor's plan of management and have been 'incorporated' as key figures in the medical management team. Of course, this second counterargument is no more than an empirical claim based on clinical impressions and common sense, but then so purports to be the claim it opposes—namely, that patients will be more miserable if they are given information they want and genuine opportunities to make their own decisions about their management.

The third problem is that even if it were true that in some circumstances a patient would be made more miserable by being given information about his condition and the risks of alternative methods of management, if that is what the patient truly wishes to know, is the doctor not morally obliged to tell him? In the chapters on autonomy and paternalism I outlined what seem to me to be cogent arguments from utilitarian as well as deontological perspectives for respecting people's autonomy in so far as to do so is compatible with respecting the autonomy of others. These arguments have as much weight against witholding of relevant information required for consent as they do against lying or otherwise deceiving the patient (indeed the deliberate witholding of information relevant to decision making is a form of deceit) and against breaking confidentiality in the patients' own interests.

Doctor's Licence under English Law

A further set of common medical counterarguments to such emphasis on respect for patients' autonomy in the context of consent is that English law, at least with regard to consent to medical treatment, leaves doctors to decide, in the context of their therapeutic (as distinct from research) relationships, how much information they ought to give patients when obtaining their consent to treatment.

Accounts of what the law stipulates in any particular jurisdiction, however, do not in themselves provide moral justification for a moral claim. At most they can be used as part of a moral claim that there is a general presumption that it is a good thing to obey just laws. As I have argued previously, the possibility that there might be unjust laws (never mind the fact that there are) shows that it is not necessarily a good thing to obey all laws. Similarly, the possibility that there might be morally bad laws shows that what is legal is not necessarily morally justifiable.

The second point is that even if English law did leave it to doctors to decide how much information ought to be given to patients in the course of obtaining their consent to treatment, doctors would still be obliged to try to resolve the moral problem: to be given the legal responsibility of making a moral decision is precisely not to be absolved from doing so.

It may, however, be worth noting that English law has recently been changed considerably by the House of Lords' appeal judgment in the Sidaway case.[34] Until that case the law seemed to leave decision making to doctors, although there is no legal unanimity about this.[35] Thus according to Lord Scarman's account of the relevant leading case, in which a Mr Bolam claimed, inter alia, that he had not been adequately informed about the risks of his (then unanaesthetised) electroconvulsive therapy, doctors would not be held negligent in law provided they acted 'in accordance with the practice accepted by a responsible body of medical men,' even if there existed a different practice advocated by another responsible body of doctors.[36] In the Sidaway judgment, however, only one of the five law lords (Lord Diplock) accepted the so called Bolam doctrine in its unmodified form. Each of the four others judged that the 'professional standard' position of the Bolam doctrine required modification towards allowing patients to make their own decisions based on adequate information about treatments that included 'material' (Scarman) or substantial (Bridge and Keith) risks, or 'which might have disadvantages or dangers' (Templeman). Lords Bridge and Keith added that 'When questioned by a patient of apparently sound mind about risks involved in a particular treatment proposed the doctor's duty was to answer both truthfully and as fully as the questioner required.'[37]

Consent in Therapeutic Research

Occasionally the argument is heard that although properly informed consent is required in the context of non-therapeutic research on patients, it is not needed in the context of treatment or therapeutic research. The manifold medico-moral issues associated with medical research are complex but in this context suffice it to assert that doctors are no less morally obliged to respect

[34] *Sidaway v. Bethlem Royal Hospital and the Maudsley Hospital Health Authority and Others* (law report), *The Times*, 22 Feb. 1985, 28.

[35] K. McK. Norrie, 'Medical Negligence: Who Sets the Standard?', *Journal of Medical Ethics*, 11 (1985), 135–7.

[36] *Sidaway v. Bethlem Royal Hospital and the Maudsley Hospital Health Authority and Others.*

[37] Ibid.

the autonomy of their patients than that of their research subjects. The moral differences between the two categories relate not to respect for autonomy but to two quite different issues. The first is that there is a substantial danger that research subjects will assume that doctors' normal beneficent Hippocratic concern to do their best for their particular patients will also apply to their research subjects. In the case of non-therapeutic research this cannot be the case (by definition), and doctors therefore have a particularly strong moral obligation to make this clear to such subjects. The second, though related, point is that in the normal therapeutic relationship patients can properly assume that any risks to which the doctor proposes to subject them will be proposed only in the light of an analysis of risk and benefit that is favourable for the particular patient. Such an assumption would again be quite mistaken in the case of non-therapeutic research (in which the benefits, if any, will accrue to future patients, while the risks are taken by the research subjects). But while both these points indicate that doctors should make it crystal clear to patients when they are not acting in a therapeutic role, neither supports the claim that when doctors are acting therapeutically they need not obtain properly informed consent.

In the last three chapters I have argued that in normal cases respect for patients' autonomy takes moral priority over medical beneficence and generally precludes lying to or otherwise deceiving patients even in their own interests, breaking their confidences even in their own interests, and failing to obtain their adequately informed consent to medical intervention even in their own interests. In the next chapter I shall look at circumstances in which the principle of respect for autonomy does not seem to have priority over beneficence.

WHERE RESPECT FOR AUTONOMY IS NOT THE ANSWER

In several of the chapters in this book I have emphasised the centrality of the principle of respect for autonomy to many areas of medical ethics, as indeed to ethics in general, and I have shown how this centrality is a feature of both utilitarian and deontological theories of ethics. Undoubtedly, doctors will have thought of counterexample after counterexample deriving from their clinical practice when respect for autonomy does not seem to be the most important or relevant moral principle. In this chapter I shall outline several categories of clinical circumstances in which, so I shall argue, respect for autonomy is not the central moral issue. They include examples in which patients have given prior consent for their doctors to make decisions on their

behalf; in which respect for the autonomy of a particular patient conflicts
with respect for the autonomy of others or causes harm to others or conflicts
with considerations of justice; in which the patient has either no autonomy
or too little autonomy for the principle of respect for autonomy to apply;
and of emergencies in which it is not possible to find out what the patient
himself would wish to happen.

I have already discussed the fact that often patients positively and deliberately delegate doctors to make decisions and manage their case. Provided
the patients have made an autonomous choice then the doctor who accedes
to their request and makes the decisions is indeed respecting their autonomy.
In these circumstances the Hippocratic principles of medical beneficence
and non-maleficence to the patient are the main moral determinants,
though, as I have argued, they may have to be constrained by considerations
of justice. Let me recall that the principle of respect for autonomy—whether
in the utilitarian model of Mill or in the deontological model of Kant—has
built into it the need to consider the autonomy of others: a point too often
forgotten by overenthusiastic libertarians. I have also argued against any
moral principle being taken as absolute—the principle of respect for autonomy may conflict with the principles of beneficence, non-maleficence, and
justice (though I have also argued from both deontological and utilitarian
standpoints that where others will not be harmed such conflicts usually
require respect for the patient's autonomy).

Impaired Autonomy

The most obvious counterexamples to the primacy of respect for autonomy
arise either when the patient has no autonomy—for example, a baby has no
autonomy—or, more difficult still, when patients have considerably impaired
or otherwise inadequate autonomy—for example, when they are young and
immature or severely mentally handicapped or disordered, from whatever
cause. One of the complicating features of medical practice is that disease
and disability tend precisely to impair people's autonomy to a greater or
lesser extent.[38] The crucial question then arises, How much autonomy does a
person need to have for his autonomy to require respect?

[38] E. D. Pellegrino, 'Toward a Reconstruction of Medical Morality: The Primacy of the Act of
Profession and the Fact of Illness,' *Journal of Medical Philosophy*, 4 (1979), 32–56; A. Freud, 'The
Doctor–Patient Relationship,' in S. Gorovitz (ed.), *Moral Problems in Medicine*, 2nd edn. (Engle-
wood Cliffs, NJ: Prentice-Hall, 1983), 108–10; C. Perry, 'Paternalism as a Supererogatory Act,'
cited by G. E. Jones, 'The Doctor–Patient Relationship and Euthanasia,' *Journal of Medical
Ethics*, 8 (1082), 195–8.

   It is perhaps worth distinguishing between impairments of the three types of autonomy I discussed in my chapter on autonomy: of action, of will (or intention), and of thought. Impairment of autonomy of action, however gross, does not in itself justify overriding the principle of respect for autonomy. This becomes immediately obvious if severely physically handicapped people are considered; their impaired autonomy of action in no way reduces our moral obligation to respect their autonomy of thought and of will, though respect for their autonomy must as usual be balanced against respect for the autonomy of others. Physically handicapped people, especially those needing wheelchairs, often complain, however, that they are treated as though their autonomy is generally impaired and typically as though they are children ('Does he take sugar?').

   When autonomy of thought or will, or both, are sufficiently impaired medical intervention without consent that will benefit the person concerned—that is, paternalistic intervention—often seems to be justified, and indeed morally imperative, even when the person concerned rejects such help. A child with meningitis should surely be given her antibiotic injections even if she hates injections and volubly refuses them; a severely mentally handicapped adult should surely be operated on for appendicitis even if he does not want an operation. The most plausible justification for overriding such decisions is that (a) it is in the patient's best interests to do so and (b) such patients do not have sufficient autonomy of thought for their self damaging decisions to require the respect due to autonomous agents (though, as the American president's commission on medical ethics concluded in a useful report, this should in no way stop doctors from consulting such people and, as far as is consistent with their best interests, acceding to their opinions and preferences[39]).

   Impaired autonomy of thought is not necessarily a matter of impaired reasoning; reasoning may be fairly unimpaired but based on an information substrate that is grossly distorted by, for example, delusions, false perceptions, hallucinations, or a mixture. Even that apostle of non-paternalism, J. S. Mill, argued that paternalistic interference was justified to benefit the mad or delirious, children, and the immature and that in general 'those who are still in a state to require being taken care of by others must be protected against their own actions as well as against external injury.'[40]

---

[39] President's Commission for the Study of Ethical Problems in Medicine and Biomedical and Behavioral Research, *Making Health Care Decisions* (Washington, DC: US Government Printing Office, 1982), 181.

[40] J. S. Mill, 'On Liberty,' in M. Warnock (ed.), *Utilitarianism*, 11th edn. (Glasgow: Collins/Fontana, 1974), 135–6, 229.

Impaired Volitional Autonomy

Not only may autonomy of thought, including reasoning and cognition, be grossly impaired but so too can volitional autonomy—that is, impaired autonomy of will or intention (a point approached from a different perspective in an excellent analysis of these issues by Professors C. M. Culver and B. Gert, one a psychiatrist, the other a philosopher[41]). Such impairment of volition may be intrinsic or extrinsic. The case of extrinsic impairment raises the interesting issue of duress. Clearly, an agreement to participate in some clinical trial would hardly be voluntary if the 'volunteer' and his family were threatened with death if he refused. But what about an offer of payment? Most of our decisions are subject to some degree of external pressure. At one end of the spectrum such pressures are clearly powerful enough grossly to impair our autonomy of will or intention; at the other end they are equally clearly within the normal range of 'pros and cons,' consideration of which necessarily plays a part in voluntary choice.

Similarly, the mere presence of intrinsic pressures such as stress, neurosis, and grief, although they may diminish a person's autonomy, does not justify overriding what is left. On the other hand, gross intrinsic impairment of volitional autonomy may also occur and is especially obvious in certain psychiatric conditions, including severe depression and certain phobias. Dr Pamela Taylor, in a symposium on putatively 'irrational' yet 'competently made' decisions to refuse electroconvulsive therapy, graphically recalls that some psychiatric patients are simply not able to make voluntary decisions of any kind.[42] As well as psychiatric illnesses various severe 'physical' illnesses and toxic agents can cause grossly impaired autonomy of will (alcohol and barbiturates are used by seducers and interrogators for precisely this purpose). When people's autonomy of volition is sufficiently diminished by such impediments, though not when it is merely diminished,[43] then the autonomy that remains may justifiably be overridden not only if it threatens others but also if it threatens them.

Such examples from psychiatric practice are entirely consistent with the obvious claims that: (a) autonomy is not an all or nothing affair and (b) a basic minimum of autonomy is required for the principle of respect for autonomy to be applicable. They do not alas give answers to the

---

[41] C. M. Culver and B. Gert, *Philosophy in Medicine* (Oxford: Oxford University Press, 1982), 109–25. (See also Gillon, *Philosophical Medical Ethics*, chs. 3, 7, 8.)

[42] P. J. Taylor, 'Consent, Competency and ECT: A Psychiatrist's View,' *Journal of Medical Ethics*, 9 (1983), 146–51.

[43] 'Impaired Autonomy and Rejection of Treatment,' Editorial, *Journal of Medical Ethics*, 9 (1983), 131–2.

major question that I started with, How much autonomy is 'sufficient' for a person to be respected as an autonomous agent? Nor do they answer the questions, Who is to decide how much autonomy a particular person possesses and on what basis, and Who is to make decisions (such as giving or withholding consent by proxy to medical intervention) on behalf of those judged non-autonomous or 'incompetent,' and according to what criteria?

I can do no more than outline a few points here in the context of these important questions. Although there are no clear cut answers to the question of how much autonomy a person must have to have it respected, it appears reasonable to argue that at least in democratic, and hence in principle autonomy respecting, societies there seems no good reason for doctors to establish any higher (or lower) standards of requisite autonomy than those set democratically. In our society these standards are not high, and little autonomy is required to be allowed by law to make legally valid contracts, marry, consent to sexual intercourse, vote, make a will, go motor racing, hang gliding, horse riding, and mountaineering, join the army, drive and motor cycle, smoke, drink alcohol, and generally participate in risk taking and risk inflicting occupations and in general take responsibility for one's own decisions. It seems reasonable for doctors, unless they are required by the democratic process to do otherwise, to accept that people possessing similarly minimal standards of autonomy should none the less have that autonomy respected in the context of medical care (in so far as such respect is compatible with respect for the autonomy of others).

DIALOGUE BETWEEN THE PROFESSION AND SOCIETY

This seems pre-eminently an area in which far more dialogue is needed between the profession and society. It may be that were non-professionals to have a better awareness of the depredations of severe disease, both physical and mental, on a person's autonomy of thought or will, or both, they would wish to raise the threshold required for autonomy to be respected. People in our society might agree with those like Professor J. F. Drane who proposes that required standards of 'competence' to make decisions on medical care for oneself should vary with the seriousness of those decisions. Thus to be respected as competent to make decisions that are 'very dangerous and run counter to both professional and public rationality'—for example, a decision to refuse lifesaving treatment—would require a far higher standard of manifest competence to make informed, voluntary, deliberated, and thus autonomous decisions than would less dangerous decisions, including a decision to accept the same treatment.[44]

Dialogue between the profession and society seems necessary to decide on the two other problems mentioned: who should decide how much autonomy a person possesses, and on what criteria, and who should make decisions by proxy, and by what criteria, for those patients classified as inadequately autonomous or incompetent? Reasonable arguments could be offered for those with special training, such as forensic psychiatrists and psychologists, to make the assessments of patients' autonomy, and doing so in relation to the particular decisions that need to be made; reports on methodology abound.[45]

Similarly, reasonable arguments can be offered in favour of people previously designated by the patient, or their next of kin or other loved ones being proxies for inadequately autonomous patients (except in emergencies where delay would be dangerous), these proxies having an option to delegate part or all of their proxy decision making to doctors if they believe this to be in the patient's interests. I would, however, agree with Professor Kennedy that such proposals are not the prerogative of doctors to implement without social agreement.[46] After all, it is fairly uncontroversial to assert that the source of any authority or rights that we as a profession have to make decisions about other people's medical care, notably the source of our right to be beneficent to any patient, is either that person's own autonomous desire that we do so or something simplistically but most easily summarised as 'the will of society.' In cases where the patient does not have such an autonomous desire, including a previously expressed prospective desire,[47] it follows that the source of our authority to behave paternalistically towards him must be society. Hence our obligation to lay the ground rules for such beneficent medical paternalism in consultation with that society of which we form a part.

[44] J. F. Drane, 'The Many Faces of Competency,' *Hastings Center Report*, 15 (1985), 17–21; S. Eth, 'Competency and Consent to Treatment,' *Journal of the American Medical Association*, 253 (1985), 778–9.

[45] See n. 41. S. Bloch and P. Chodoff (eds.), *Psychiatric Ethics* (Oxford: Oxford University Press, 1981), 203–94; R. B. Edwards (ed.), *Psychiatry and Ethics* (Buffalo, NY: Prometheus Books, 1982), 68–82, 189–346, 496–605; L. H. Roth, A. Meisel, and C. W. Lidz, 'Tests of Competency to Consent to Treatment,' *American Journal of Psychiatry*, 134 (1977), 279–84; L. H. Roth, C. W. Lidz, A. Meisel, *et al.*, 'Competency to Decide about Treatment or Research: An Overview of Some Empirical Data,' *International Journal of Law Psychiatry*, 5 (1982), 29–50; R. Bluglass, *A Guide to the Mental Health Act 1983* (Edinburgh: Churchill Livingstone, 1983), 75–88.

[46] I. Kennedy, *The Unmasking of Medicine* (London: George Allen & Unwin, 1981), 76–98.

[47] G. S. Robertson, 'Dealing with the Brain Damaged Old: Dignity before Sanctity,' *Journal of Medical Ethics*, 8 (1982), 173–9.

NOTES ON CONTRIBUTORS

TOM L. BEAUCHAMP is Professor of Philosophy, Senior Research Scholar at the Kennedy Institute, Georgetown University. He took graduate degrees in theology from Yale University and in philosophy from The Johns Hopkins University where he received his Ph.D. in 1970. He then joined the Philosophy Department at Georgetown University and in 1970 accepted a joint appointment at Kennedy Institute of Ethics. In 1976 he joined the staff of the National Commission for the Protection of Human Subjects of Biomedical and Behavioural Research, where he wrote the bulk of the *Belmont Report*. He is co-author of *Principles of Biomedical Ethics* (1979) and *A History and Theory of Informed Consent* (1986). He is also one of three editors of the Clarendon Hume, a critical edition of the works of David Hume.

DAN W. BROCK is Charles C. Tillinghast, Jr. University Professor, Professor of Philosophy and Biomedical Ethics, and Director of the Center for Biomedical Ethics at Brown University. He is the author of over 130 published papers and his most recent book is *From Chance to Choice: Genetics and Justice* (with Allen Buchanan, Norman Daniels, and Daniel Wikler, 2000).

ALLEN BUCHANAN is Professor of Philosophy at the University of Arizona. He lectures and publishes mainly in Bioethics and Political Philosophy. He is the author of over one hundred articles and the following books: *Marx and Justice: Radical Critique of Liberalism* (1982), *Ethics, Efficiency, and the Market* (1985), *Deciding For Others: The Ethics of Surrogate Decision Making* (with Dan W. Brock, 1989), *Secession: The Morality of Political Divorce From Fort Sumter to Lithuania and Quebec* (1991). He served as Staff Philosopher for the Presidents commission on Medical Ethics, where he was a principal author of the Commission's two book-length reports on ethical issues in genetics (1983). As Staff-Consultant for the U.S. Advisory Committee on Human Radiation Experiments, Buchanan authored the ethical framework chapter for the Committee's final report (1995). He is also the first author (with Dan W. Brock, Norman Daniels, and Daniel Wikler) of a book on ethical issues in genetic intervention (2000).

DANIEL CALLAHAN is Director, International Program, The Hastings Center. He received his BA from Yale and a Ph.D. in philosophy from Harvard. He is an elected member of the Institute of Medicine, National Academy of Sciences and a Senior Fellow at the Harvard Medical School. He is the chairman of the ethics sub-committee of the Centers for Disease Control and Prevention. He is the author of 27 books, and is completing a book on *The Research Imperative: What Price Health?*.

NORMAN DANIELS is Goldthwaite Professor and former Chair of the Tufts Philosophy Department and Professor of Medical Ethics at Tufts Medical School. He has taught at Tufts University since 1969. He has published over 100 articles. His most recent books include *Just Health Care* (1985), *Am I My Parents' Keeper? An Essay on Justice Between the Young and the Old* (1988), *Seeking Fair Treatment: From the AIDS Epidemic to National Health Care Reform* (1995), *Justice and Justification: Reflective Equilibrium in Theory and Practice* (1996), (with Donald Light and Ronald Caplan) *Benchmarks of Fairness for Health Care Reform* (1996), (with Allen Buchanan, Dan Brock, and Dan Wikler) *From Chance to Choice: Genetics and Justice* (2000), and (with Bruce Kennedy and Ichiro Kawachi) *Is Inequality Bad for Our Health?* (2000).

RONALD DWORKIN is Quain Professor of Jurisprudence at University College London and Frank. H. Sommer Professor of Law at New York University. Ronald Dworkin is a Fellow of the British Academy and the American Academy of Arts and Sciences. He has made important contributions to questions relating to senile dementia, abortion, and health care although he has more recently been turning his attention to issues of quality and constitutional interpretation. He is a strong advocate of a bill of rights for Britain. His publications include: *Sovereign Virtue: The Theory and Practice of Equality*, (2000), *Freedom's Law: The Moral Reading of the American Constitution* (1997), *Life's Dominion: An Argument about Abortion, Euthanasia, and Individual Freedom* (1994), *A Matter of Principle* (1986), *Taking Rights Seriously* (1978).

RAANAN GILLON trained in philosophy as well as in medicine. He is part-time senior partner in a UK National Health Service general medical practice and Emeritus Professor of Medical Ethics at Imperial College, London University. Until April 2001 he was editor for 20 years of the Journal of Medical Ethics.

JONATHAN GLOVER is Director of the Centre of Medical Law and Ethics at King's College London. Previously he taught philosophy at New College, Oxford. Among his books are *Causing Death and Saving Lives* (1977), *What Sort of People Should There Be?* (1984), and *Humanity, A Moral History of the Twentieth Century* (2000).

JOHN HARRIS, BA, D.Phil., is Sir David Alliance Professor of Bioethics at the Institute of Medicine, Law and Bioethics, University of Manchester. He is a member of The United Kingdom *Human Genetics Commission* and of the *Ethics Committee of the British Medical Association*. He is General Editor of a major new series of books for Oxford University Press entitled *Issues in Biomedical Ethics*. John Harris is the author or editor of fourteen books and over one hundred and fifty papers. Publications include: *Violence & Responsibility* (1980), *The Value Of Life* (1985), *Clones Genes and Immortality* (1998), and (edited with Søren Holm) *The Future of Human Reproduction* (1998).

SØREN HOLM is Professor of Clinical Bioethics at the University of Manchester and Professor of Medical ethics at the University of Oslo. He holds degrees in medicine, philosophy, and health care ethics. He has written extensively about the problems in transferring American bioethics to a European context.

HELGA KUHSE is an Honorary Senior Research Fellow at the Centre for Human Bioethics at Monash University, and a Senior Research Associate at the University of Melbourn, Australia. She has written widely in the field of bioethics, and takes a special interest in ethical issues at the end of life.

JEFF MCMAHAN is Associate Professor of Philosophy at the University of Illinois at Urbana-Champaign. His book, *Killing at the Margins of Life*, which is the first volume of a two-part work called *The Ethics of Killing*, will be published in 2001.

RUTH MACKLIN is Professor of Bioethics at Albert Einstein College of Medicine in the Bronx, New York. She has just completed a term as President of the International Association of Bioethics, and has numerous publications in academic and professional journals. Her latest book is *Against Relativism* (1999).

DEREK PARFIT is a Senior Research Fellow at All Souls College, Oxford. He is also a Fellow of the British Academy and of the American Academy of Arts and Sciences. He has published many articles on personal identity, philosophy of mind, and ethics. His book, *Reasons and Persons*, is widely regarded as one of the most important contributions to moral philosophy in the last 100 years.

WARREN QUINN, who died in 1991, was Professor of Philosophy at U.C.L.A. Quinn laid out the foundations for an anti-utilitarian moral philosophy that was critical of much contemporary work in ethics. Quinn's own distinctive moral theory is developed in the discussion of substantial, practical moral issues. His publications include: 'Abortion: Identity and Loss.' *Philosophy & Public Affairs* (Winter 1984), 'Egoism as an Ethical System.' *Journal of Philosophy* (August 15, 1974, 'Pleasure—Disposition or Episode?' *Philosophy and Phenomenological Research* (June 1968), 'The Right to Threaten and the Right to Punish.' *Philosophy & Public Affairs* (Fall 1985), 'Theories of Intrinsic Value.' *American Philosophical Quarterly* (April 1974), and 'Truth and Explanation in Ethics.' *Ethics* (April 1986).

ERIC RAKOWSKI, A.B., Harvard University, J.D., Harvard Law School, B.Phil., D.Phil., Oxford University, is Professor of Law at the University of California, Berkeley. A former Rotary and Marshall scholar, Eric Rakowski clerked for Judge Harry T. Edwards of the U.S. Court of Appeals for the District of Columbia Circuit and for Justice William J. Brennan Jr. of the U.S. Supreme Court. He worked as a tax attorney at Davis Polk & Wardwell before joining the Boalt faculty in 1990. Rakowski is the author of *Equal Justice* (1991). He writes mainly on issues relating to taxation, distributive justice, health care, and moral philosophy. He was a visiting professor at Harvard Law School during the 1998–99 academic year and was named a UC Berkeley Chancellor's Professor for 1998–2001.

PETER SINGER is Ira W. DeCamp Professor of Bioethics in the University Center for Human Values at Princeton University. He was the founding President of the International Association of Bioethics, and with Helga Kuhse, founding co-editor of the journal *Bioethics*. He first became well-known internationally after the publication of *Animal Liberation* (1975). His other books include: *Democracy and Disobedience* (1973), *Practical Ethics* (1979), *Marx* (1980), *Animal Factories* (with Jim Mason, 1980), *The Expanding Circle* (1981), *Hegel* (1982), *The Reproduction Revolution* (with Deane Wells, 1984), *Should the Baby Live?* (with Helga Kuhse, 1985), *How Are We to Live?* (1993), *Rethinking Life and Death* (1994), and *Ethics into Action: Henry Spira and the Animal Rights Movement* (1998).

JUDITH JARVIS THOMSON works in ethics and metaphysics. Her book, *The Realm of Rights* (1990) is a study of the questions what it is to have a right, and which ones we have. An article entitled 'Self-Defense' appeared in *Philosophy and Public Affairs* (Fall 1991); a recent article entitled 'On some ways in which a thing can be good' appeared in *Social Philosophy and Policy* (Spring 1992). Her work in metaphysics has largely been on the ontology of events, and the identity across time of people and other physical objects. An article entitled 'People and their bodies,' which takes issue with views expressed by Derek Parfit in Part III of his Reasons and Persons, will appear in a collection of essays (edited by Jonathan Dancy) written on topics dealt with in that book. She is currently working on the question what it is for one event to cause another.

SELECT BIBLIOGRAPHY

The Select Bibliography begins with a fairly comprehensive list of works that are generally relevant to bioethics if not self-consciously written as works within the genre. They include law and political philosophy as well as ethics and meta-ethics.

The next section highlights (with some repetition) some of the best and most accessible texts of bioethics.

Finally there is a topical bibliography, which provides highly selected reading on particular topics.

GENERAL BIBLIOGRAPHY OF TEXTS RELEVANT TO BIOETHICS

ACKERMAN, TERRENCE F., and STRONG, CARSON, *A Casebook of Medical Ethics* (New York: Oxford University Press, 1989).

ALMOND, BRENDA (ed.), *Introducing Applied Ethics* (Oxford: Blackwell, 1995).

—— and HILL, DONALD (eds.), *Applied Philosophy*: Morals and Metaphysics In Contemporary Debate (London: Routledge, 1991).

ANNAS, GEORGE J., *Standard of Care*: *The Law of American Bioethics* (New York: Oxford University Press, 1993).

ASHTON, JOHN, and SEYMOUR, HOWARD, *The New Public Health*: *The Liverpool Experience* (Buckingham: Open University Press, 1988).

BAIER, ANNETTE, *Moral Prejudices: Essays on Ethics* (Cambridge, Mass.: Harvard University Press, 1995).

BARRY, BRIAN, *The Liberal Theory of Justice* (Oxford: Clarendon Press, 1973).

—— *Theories of Justice: A Treatise on Social Justice*, 1 (London: Harvester Wheatsheaf, 1989).

BATTIN, MARGARET PABST, *The Least Worst Death: Essays in Bioethics on the End of Life* (New York: Oxford University Press, 1994).

BEAUCHAMP, T. L., and CHILDRESS, J. F., *Principles of Biomedical Ethics*, 4th edn. (New York: Oxford University Press, 1994).

DE BEAUFORT, INEZ, and HILHORST, M. T. (eds.), *Individual Responsibility for Health: Moral Issues regarding Life Styles* (Luxembourg: Office for Official Publications of the European Communities, 1996).

BENNETT, REBECCA, and ERIN, CHARLES A. (eds.), *HIV and AIDS: Testing, Screening, and Confidentiality, Ethics, Law and Social Policy* (Oxford: Oxford University Press, 1999).

BENTHAM, JEREMY, *The Collected Works of Jeremy Bentham: An Introduction to the Principles of Morals and Legislation. An Authorative Edition with a New Introduction by F. Rosen and an Interpretive Essay by H. L. A. Hart*, ed. J. H. BURNS and H. L. A. HART (Oxford: Clarendon Press, 1996).

BEROFSKY, BERNARD, *Liberation from Self: A Theory of Personal Autonomy* (Cambridge: Cambridge University Press, 1995).

BLACK, NICK, BOSWELL, DAVID, GRAY, ALASTAIR, MURPHY, SÉAN, and POPAY, JENNIE

My colleague Charles Erin helped greatly with this bibliography.

(eds.), *Health and Disease: A Reader* (Milton Keynes: Open University Press, 1984).

BLOCH, SYDNEY, CHODOFF, PAUL, and GREEN, STEPHEN (eds.), *Psychiatric Ethics*, 3rd edn. (Oxford: Oxford University Press, 1998).

BOK, SISSELA, *Secrets: Concealment and Revelation* (Oxford: Oxford University Press, 1982).

—— *Common Values* (Columbia, MO.: University of Missouri Press, 1996).

BOUCHER, DAVID, and KELLY, PAUL, (eds.), *The Social Contract from Hobbes to Rawls* (London: Routledge, 1994).

BOYD, K. M. (ed.), *The Ethics of Resource Allocation in Health Care* (Edinburgh: Edinburgh University Press, 1978).

BRANDT, RICHARD, B. (ed.), *Social Justice* (Oxford: Clarendon Press, 1976).

—— *A Theory of the Good and the Right* (Oxford: Clarendon Press, 1979).

—— *Facts, Values and Morality* (Cambridge: Cambridge University Press, 1996).

BRATMAN, MICHAEL, *Intention, Plans and Practical Reason* (Cambridge, Mass.: Harvard University Press, 1987).

BRAYBROOKE, DAVID, *Meeting Needs* (Princeton: Princeton University Press, 1987).

BRAZIER, MARGARET, *Medicine, Patients and the Law,* 2nd edn. (Harmondsworth: Penguin, 1992).

BRITISH MEDICAL ASSOCIATION (Professional Division), *Rights and Responsibilities of Doctors*, 2nd edn. (London: BMJ Publishing, 1992).

BRITISH MEDICAL ASSOCIATION (Ethics, Science, and Information Division), *Medical Ethics Today: Its Practice and Philosophy* (London: BMJ Publishing, 1993).

BRITISH MEDICAL ASSOCIATION and the LAW SOCIETY, *Assessment of Mental Capacity: Guidance for Doctors and Lawyers* (London: BMA, 1995).

BROCK, DAN W., *Life and Death: Philosophical Essays in Biomedical Ethics* (Cambridge: Cambridge University Press, 1993).

BUCHANAN, ALLEN E., and BROCK, DAN W., *Deciding for Others: The Ethics of Surrogate Decision Making* (Cambridge: Cambridge University Press, 1990).

BYRNE, P. (ed.), *Rights and Wrongs in Medicine* (London: King Edward's Hospital Fund for London, 1986).

CAMPBELL, A. V., *Moral Dilemmas in Medicine* (Edinburgh: Churchill Livingstone, 1975).

—— and HIGGS, R., *In that case: Medical Ethics in Everyday Practice* (London: Darton, Longman & Todd, 1982).

CAPLAN, ARTHUR L., *If I were a Rich Man could I Buy a Pancreas? And Other Essays on the Ethics of Health Care* (Bloomington: Indiana University Press, 1992).

CHADWICK, RUTH, *The Right to Know and the Right not to Know* (London: Avebury, 1997).

CLARKE, PAUL A. B., and LINZEY, ANDREW, *Research on Embryos: Politics, Theology and Law* (London: Lester Crook Academic, 1988).

COHEN, M. (ed.), *Rights and Wrongs of Abortion: A Philosophy & Public Affairs Reader* (Princeton: Princeton University Press, 1960).

COOPER, DAVID E., *World Philosophies: An Historical Introduction* (Oxford: Blackwell, 1996).

COREA, GENA, *The Mother Machine: Reproductive Technologies from Artificial Insemination to Artificial Wombs* (London: Women's Press, 1988).

COUGHLIN, STEVEN S., and BEAUCHAMP, TOM L. (eds.), *Ethics and Epidemiology* (New York: Oxford University Press, 1996).

DANIELS, NORMAN, *Just Health Care* (Cambridge: Cambridge University Press, 1985).

536 SELECT BIBLIOGRAPHY

536 SELECT BIBLIOGRAPHY

—— (ed.), *Reading Rawls* (Oxford: Blackwell, 1975; repr. Stanford, Calif.: Stanford University Press, 1989).

—— *Justice and Justification: Reflective Equilibrium in Theory and Practice* (Cambridge: Cambridge University Press, 1996).

DARWALL, STEPHEN, GIBBARD, ALLAN, and RAILTON, PETER (eds.), *Moral Discourse and Practice: Some Philosophical Approaches* (New York: Oxford University Press, 1996).

DE GRAZIA, DAVID, *Taking Animals Seriously: Mental Life and Moral Status* (Cambridge: Cambridge University Press, 1996).

DOWNIE, R. S., and CALMAN, K. C., *Healthy Respect: Ethics in Health Care* (London: Faber & Faber, 1987).

—— FYFE, CAROL, and TANNAHILL, ANDREW, *Health Promotion: Models and Values* (Oxford: Oxford University Press, 1990).

DUNSTAN, G. R., and SELLER, M. J. (eds.), *Consent in Medicine: Convergence and Divergence in Tradition* (Oxford: Oxford University Press, King Edward's Hospital Fund for London, 1983).

DWORKIN, GERALD, *The Theory and Practice of Autonomy* (Cambridge: Cambridge University Press, 1988).

DWORKIN, RONALD, *Life's Dominion: An Argument about Abortion and Euthanasia* (London: HarperCollins, 1993).

DYSON, ANTHONY, *The Ethics of IVF* (New York: Mowbray, 1995).

—— and HARRIS, JOHN (eds.), *Experiments on Embryos* (London: Routledge, 1990).

—— (eds.), *Ethics and Biotechnology* (London: Routledge, 1994).

EDWARDS, STEVEN D., *Nursing Ethics: A Principle-Based Approach* (London: Macmillan, 1996).

ELLOS, WILLIAM J., *Ethical Practice in Clinical Medicine* (London: Routledge, 1990).

EMANUEL, LINDA L. (ed.), *Regulating how we Die: The Ethical, Medical, and Legal Issues Surrounding Physician-Assisted Suicide* (Cambridge, Mass.: Harvard University Press, 1998).

ENGELHARDT, H. TRISTRAM, Jr., *The Foundations of Bioethics*, 2nd edn. (New York: Oxford University Press, 1996).

EVANS, DONALD, and EVANS, MARTYN, *A Decent Proposal: Ethical Review of Clinical Research* (Chichester: Wiley, 1996).

FEINBERG, JOEL (ed.), *Moral Concepts* (Oxford: Oxford University Press, 1969).

—— *Doing and Deserving* (Princeton: Princeton University Press, 1970).

—— *Social Philosophy* (Englewood Cliffs, NJ: Prentice-Hall, 1973).

—— *Rights, Justice and the Bounds of Liberty: Essays in Social Philosophy* (Princeton: Princeton University Press, 1980).

—— *Harm to Others* (Oxford: Oxford University Press, 1984).

—— *Offense to Others* (Oxford: Oxford University Press, 1985).

—— *Harm to Self* (Oxford: Oxford University Press, 1986).

—— *Harmless Wrongdoing* (Oxford: Oxford University Press, 1990)

—— *Freedom and Fulfillment: Philosophical Essays* (Princeton: Princeton University Press, 1992).

FINNIS, JOHN, *Natural Law and Natural Rights* (Oxford: Oxford University Press, 1980).

FISCHER, JOHN MARTIN, and RAVIZZA, MARK (eds.), *Perspectives on Moral Responsibility* (Ithaca, NY: Cornell University Press, 1993).

FLANAGAN, O., *Varieties of Moral Personality: Ethics and Psychological Realism* (Cambridge, Mass.: Harvard University Press, 1991).

FLETCHER, NINA, HOLT, JANET, BRAZIER, MARGARET, and HARRIS, JOHN, *Ethics, Law and Nursing* (Manchester: Manchester University Press, 1995).

FOOT, PHILIPPA, *Virtues and Vices* (Oxford: Blackwell, 1978).

FRAZER, ELIZABETH, HORNSBY, JENNIFER, and LOVIBOND, SABINA (eds.), *Ethics: A Feminist Reader* (Oxford: Blackwell, 1992).

FULLER, LON L., *The Morality of Law*, rev. edn. (New Haven: Yale University Press, 1969).

GAYLIN, WILLARD, and JENNINGS, BRUCE, *The Perversion of Autonomy: The Proper Uses of Coercion and Constraints in a Liberal Society* (New York: Free Press, 1996).

GENSLER, HARRY J., *Formal Ethics* (London: Routledge, 1996).

GILLON, RAANAN, *Philosophical Medical Ethics* (London: Wiley on behalf of the *British Medical Journal*, 1986).

—— (ed.), *Principles of Health Care Ethics* (Chichester: Wiley, 1994).

GLOVER, JONATHAN, *Causing Death and Saving Lives* (Harmondsworth: Penguin, 1977; repr. 1988).

—— *What Sort of People should there Be? Genetic Engineering, Brain Control and their Impact on our Future World* (Harmondsworth: Penguin, 1984).

—— *I: The Philosophy and Psychology of Personal Identity* (London: Penguin, 1988).

—— *et al.*, *Fertility and the Family: The Glover Report on Reproductive Technologies to the European Commission* (London: Fourth Estate, 1989).

—— (ed.), *Utilitarianism and its Critics* (New York: Macmillan, 1990).

GOODIN, ROBERT E., *Utilitarianism as a Public Philosophy* (Cambridge: Cambridge University Press, 1995).

GORECKI, JAN, *Justifying Ethics: Human Rights and Human Nature* (New Brunswick, NJ: Transaction, 1996).

GORMALLY, LUKE (ed.), *Euthanasia, Clinical Practice and the Law* (London: Linacre Centre, 1994).

GRIFFIN, JAMES, *Well-Being: Its Meaning, Measurement and Moral Importance* (Oxford: Clarendon Press, 1986).

—— *Value Judgement: Improving our Ethical Beliefs* (Oxford: Clarendon Press, 1986).

GRIFFITHS, A. PHILLIPS (ed.), *Of Liberty*, Royal Institute of Philosophy Lecture Series, 15, suppl. to *Philosophy*, 1983 (Cambridge: Cambridge University Press, 1983).

—— (ed.), *Ethics*, Royal Institute of Philosophy Lecture Series, 35 (Cambridge: Cambridge University Press, 1994).

—— (ed.), *Philosophy, Psychology and Psychiatry*, Royal Institute of Philosophy Lecture Series, 37 (Cambridge: Cambridge University Press, 1995).

HACKER, P. M. S., and RAZ, J. (eds.), *Law, Morality and Society: Essays in Honour of H. L. A. Hart* (Oxford: Clarendon Press, 1977).

HAMPSHIRE, STUART (ed.), *Public and Private Morality* (Cambridge: Cambridge University Press, 1978).

HANRATTY, JAMES F., and HIGGINSON, IRENE, *Palliative Care in Terminal Illness*, 2nd edn. (Oxford: Oxford University Press, 1994).

HARE, R. M., *The Language of Morals* (Oxford: Clarendon Press, 1952).

—— *Freedom and Reason* (Oxford: Clarendon Press, 1963).

—— *Moral Thinking: Its Level, Method and Point* (Oxford: Clarendon Press, 1981).

—— *Essays in Ethical Theory* (Oxford: Clarendon Press, 1989).

HARRIS, JOHN, *Violence and Responsibility* (London: Routledge & Kegan Paul, 1980).

—— *The Value of Life: An Introduction to Medical Ethics* (London: Routledge & Kegan Paul, 1985).

—— *Clones, Genes and Immortality: Ethics and the Genetic Revolution* (Oxford: Oxford University Press, 1998).

—— and HOLM, SØREN (eds.), *The Future of Human Reproduction: Ethics, Choice and Regulation* (Oxford: Clarendon Press, 1998).

HART, H. L. A., *The Concept of Law* (Oxford: Clarendon Press, 1961).

—— *Essays on Bentham: Jurisprudence and Political Theory* (Oxford: Clarendon Press, 1982).

—— *Essays in Jurisprudence and Philosophy* (Oxford: Clarendon Press, 1983).

HÄYRY, HETA, *The Limits of Medical Paternalism* (London: Routledge, 1991).

HÄYRY, MATTI, *Liberal Utilitarianism and Applied Ethics* (London: Routledge, 1994).

HERMAN, BARBARA, *The Practice of Moral Judgement* (Cambridge, Mass.: Harvard University Press, 1993).

HERZOG, DON, *Happy Slaves: A Critique of Consent Theory* (Chicago: University of Chicago Press, 1989).

HEYD, DAVID (ed.), *Toleration: An Elusive Virtue* (Princeton: Princeton University Press, 1996).

HILL, THOMAS E., Jr., *Autonomy and Self-Respect* (Cambridge: Cambridge University Press, 1991).

HIRSCH, STEVEN R., and HARRIS, JOHN (eds.), *Consent and the Incompetent Patient: Ethics, Law, and Medicine* (London: Gaskell, 1988).

HOGGETT, BRENDA, *Mental Health Law*, 4th edn. (London: Sweet & Maxwell, 1996)

HOLLIDAY, IAN, *The NHS Transformed*, 2nd edn. (Manchester: Baseline Books, 1995).

HOLM, SØREN, *Ethical Problems in Clinical Practice: The Ethical Reasoning of Health Care Professionals* (Manchester: Manchester University Press, 1997).

HORAN, DENNIS J., and MALL, DAVID (eds.), *Death, Dying, and Euthanasia* (Frederick, Md.: University Publications of America, 1980).

HUNTER, KATHRYN MONTGOMERY, *Doctor's Stories: The Narrative Structure of Medical Knowledge* (Princeton: Princeton University Press, 1991).

HURSTHOUSE, ROSALIND, *Beginning Lives* (Oxford: Blackwell, 1987).

ILLICH, I., *Limits to Medicine* (Harmondsworth: Penguin, 1977).

KAMM, FRANCES MYRNA, *Creation and Abortion: A Study in Moral and Legal Philosophy* (Oxford: Oxford University Press, 1992).

—— *Morality, Mortality*, i: *Death and Whom to Save from It* (New York: Oxford University Press, 1993).

—— *Morality, Mortality*, ii: *Rights, Duties and Status* (New York: Oxford University Press, 1996).

KENNEDY, IAN, *Unmasking Medicine* (London: Paladin, 1983).

KEOWN, J. (ed.), *Euthanasia Examined* (Cambridge: Cambridge University Press, 1995).

KLEIN, RENATE D. (ed.), *Infertility: Women Speak out about their Experiences of Reproductive Medicine* (London: Pandora Press, 1989).

KLEIN, RUDOLF, DAY, PATRICIA, and REDMAYNE, SHARON, *Managing Scarcity: Priority Setting and Rationing in the National Health Service* (Buckingham: Open University Press, 1996).

KORSGAARD, CHRISTINE M., with COHEN, G. A., GEUSS, RAYMOND, NAGEL, THOMAS, and WILLIAMS, BERNARD, *The Sources of Normativity*, ed. Onora O'Neill (Cambridge: Cambridge University Press, 1996).

KUHSE, H. & SINGER, P., *Should the Baby Live? The Problem of Handicapped Infants* (Oxford: Oxford University Press, 1985).

LaFollette, Hugh, *Personal Relationships: Love, Identity and Morality* (Oxford: Blackwell, 1996).
—— *Ethics in Practice: An Anthology* (Oxford: Blackwell, 1997).
Leahy, Michael P. T., *Against Liberation: Putting Animals in Perspective* (London: Routledge, 1991).
—— and Cohn-Sherbok, Dan (eds.), *The Liberation Debate: Rights at Issue* (London: Routledge, 1996).
Lehrer, Keith, *Self-Trust: A Study of Reason, Knowledge, and Autonomy* (Oxford: Clarendon Press, 1997).
Lindley, Richard, *Autonomy* (Basingstoke: Macmillan, 1986).
Lockett, Tony, *Health Economics for the Uninitiated* (Oxford: Radcliffe Medical Press, 1996).
Lockwood, M. (ed.), *Moral Dilemmas in Medicine* (Oxford: Oxford University Press, 1985).
Lomasky, Loren E., *Persons, Rights and the Moral Community* (Oxford: Oxford University Press, 1987).
Lucas, John Randolph, *Responsibility* (Oxford: Oxford University Press, 1995).
Ludvigsen, Carol, and Roberts, Kathleen, *Health Care Policies and Europe: The Implications for Practice* (Oxford: Butterworth-Heinemann, 1996).
Lyons, David, *Moral Aspects of Legal Theory: Essays on Law, Justice, and Political Responsibility* (Cambridge: Cambridge University Press, 1993).
—— *Right, Welfare and Mill's Moral Theory* (Oxford: Oxford University Press, 1994).
McHale, Jean, and Fox, Marie, with Murphy, John, *Health Care Law: Text and Materials* (London: Sweet & Maxwell, 1997).
MacIntyre, Alasdair, *A Short History of Ethics: A History of Moral Philosophy from the Homeric Age to the Twentieth Century* (London: Routledge & Kegan Paul, 1967).
—— *After Virtue: A Study in Moral Theory*, 2nd edn. (London: Duckworth, 1985).
Mackie, J. L., *The Cement of the Universe: A Study of Causation* (Oxford: Clarendon Press, 1974; reissued 1980).
—— *Problems from Locke* (Oxford: Oxford University Press, 1976).
—— *Ethics: Inventing Right and Wrong* (London: Penguin, 1977).
—— *Hume's Moral Theory* (London: Routledge & Kegan Paul, 1980).
McLean, Sheila A. M., *A Patient's Right to Know: Information, Disclosure, the Doctor and the Law* (Aldershot: Dartmouth, 1989).
—— (ed.), *Legal Issues in Human Reproduction* (Aldershot: Dartmouth, 1989).
—— *Old Law, New Medicine* (London: Pandora, 1999).
—— and Maher, G., *Medicine, Morals and the Law* (Aldershot: Gower, 1983).
MacMurray, John, *Reason and Emotion* (London: Faber & Faber, 1935; reissued 1995).
Mason, J. K., *Medico-Legal Aspects of Reproduction and Parenthood* (Dartmouth: 1990).
—— and McCall Smith, R. A., *Law and Medical Ethics*, 5th edn. (London: Butterworth, 1998).
May, Larry, *Sharing Responsibility* (Chicago: University of Chicago Press, 1996).
Mele, Alfred R., *Autonomous Agents: From Self-Control to Autonomy* (New York: Oxford University Press, 1995).
Messerly, John G., *An Introduction to Ethical Theories* (Lanham, Md.: University of America Press, 1995).

MEYERS, DAVID W., *The Human Body and the Law*, 2nd edn. (Edinburgh: Edinburgh University Press, 1990).

MIDGLEY, MARY, *Beast and Man: The Roots of Human Nature* (Brighton: Harvester Press, 1979; repr. London: Methuen, 1980).

—— *Heart and Mind: The Varieties of Moral Experience* (Brighton: Harvester Press, 1981; repr. London: Methuen, 1983).

—— *The Ethical Primate: Humans, Freedom and Morality* (London: Routledge, 1994).

MILLER, DAVID (ed.), *Liberty* (Oxford: Oxford University Press, 1991).

—— *Casuistry and Modern Ethics* (Chicago: University of Chicago Press, 1996).

MONROE, K. R., *The Heart of Altruism: Perceptions of a Common Humanity* (Princeton: Princeton University Press, 1996).

MONTEFIORE, A. (ed.), *Philosophy and Personal Relations* (London: Routledge & Kegan Paul, 1973).

MONTGOMERY, JONATHAN, *Health Care Law* (Oxford: Oxford University Press, 1997).

MORAN, MICHAEL, and WOOD, BRUCE, *States, Regulation and the Medical Profession* (Milton Keynes: Open University Press, 1992).

MORENO, JONATHAN D., *Deciding Together: Bioethics and Moral Consensus* (New York: Oxford University Press, 1995).

MORGAN, DEREK, and LEE, ROBERT, G., *Blackstone's Guide to the Human Fertilisation and Embryology Act 1990: Abortion and Embryo Research, the New Law* (London: Blackstone, 1991).

NAGEL, THOMAS, *The Possibility of Altruism* (Princeton: Princeton University Press, 1970).

—— *Mortal Questions* (Cambridge: Cambridge University Press, 1979).

—— *The View from Nowhere* (Oxford: Oxford University Thames, 1986).

—— *What does it all Mean? A Very Short Introduction to Philosophy* (Oxford: Oxford University Press, 1987).

—— *Equality and Partiality* (New York: Oxford University Press, 1991).

—— *The Last Word* (New York: Oxford University Press, 1997).

NOZICK, ROBERT, *Anarchy, State and Utopia* (Oxford: Blackwell, 1974).

NIELSEN, KAI, *Ethics without God*, rev. edn. (Amherst, NY: Prometheus, 1990).

NUSSBAUM, MARTHA, and SEN, AMARTYA (eds.), *The Quality of Life* (Oxford: Clarendon Press, 1993).

O'NEILL, ONORA, *Constructions of Reason: Explorations of Kant's Practical Philosophy* (Cambridge: Cambridge University Press, 1989).

—— *Towards Justice and Virtue: A Constructive Account of Practical Reasoning* (Cambridge: Cambridge University Press, 1996).

PARFIT, DEREK, *Reasons and Persons* (Oxford: Oxford University Press, 1984).

PENSLAR, R., *Research Ethics: Cases and Materials* (Bloomington, Indiana University Press, 1994).

PFEFFER, NAOMI, *The Stork and the Syringe: A Political History of Reproductive Medicine* (Cambridge: Polity Press, 1993).

QUINN, WARREN, *Morality and Action* (Cambridge: Cambridge Universty Press, 1993).

QUINTON, ANTHONY, *Utilitarian Ethics*, 2nd edn. (London: Duckworth, 1989).

RACHELS, JAMES, (ed.), *Moral Problems: A Collection of Philosophical Essays*, 3rd edn. (New York: Harper & Row, 1979).

—— *The End of Life: Euthanasia and Morality* (Oxford: Oxford University Press, 1986).

SELECT BIBLIOGRAPHY 541

RACHELS, JAMES, *The Right Thing to Do: Basic Readings in Moral Theory* (New York: McGraw-Hill, 1989).
—— *The Elements of Moral Philosophy* 2nd edn. (New York: McGraw-Hill, 1993).
—— (ed.), *Ethical Theory* (Oxford: Oxford University Press, 1998).
RADCLIFFE RICHARDS, JANET, *The Sceptical Feminist* (Harmondsworth: Penguin, 1982).
RAKOWSKI, ERIC, *Equal Justice* (Oxford: Clarendon Press, 1991).
RANDALL, FIONA, and DOWNIE, R. S., *Palliative Care Ethics: A Good Companion* (Oxford: Oxford University Press, 1996).
RAPHAEL, D. D., *Moral Philosophy* (Oxford: Oxford University Press, 1981).
RAWLS, JOHN, *A Theory of Justice* (Cambridge, Mass.: Belknap Press of Harvard University Press, 1971).
—— *Political Liberalism*, The John Dewey Essays in Philosophy, 4 (New York: Columbia University Press, 1993).
REICH, WARREN THOMAS (ed.), *Encyclopedia of Bioethics*, rev. edn., 5 vols. (New York: Macmillan, 1995).
ROBERTSON, JOHN, *Children of Choice: Freedom and the New Reproductive Technologies* (Princeton: Princeton University Press, 1994).
ROBINSON, IAN (ed.), *Life and Death under High Technology Medicine* (University of Manchester Press in association with the Fulbright Commission, 1994).
ROEMER, JOHN E., *Theories of Distributive Justice* (Cambridge, Mass.: Harvard University Press, 1996).
ROLLIN, BERNARD E., *The Frankenstein Syndrome: Ethical and Social Issues in the Genetic Engineering of Animals* (Cambridge: Cambridge University Press, 1995).
RYAN, ALAN, *Justice* (Oxford: Oxford University Press, 1993).
SAMPSON, CHRIS, *The Neglected Ethic: Religious and Cultural Factors in the Care of Patients* (Maidenhead: McGraw-Hill, 1982).
SCARRE, GEOFFREY, *Utilitarianism* (London: Routledge, 1996).
SCHEFFLER, SAMUEL, *The Rejection of Consequentialism* (Oxford: Clarendon Press, 1982).
—— (ed.), *Consequentialism and its Critics* (Oxford: Oxford University Press, 1988).
—— *Human Morality* (Oxford: Clarendon Press, 1994).
SCHMIDTZ, DAVID, *Rational Choice and Moral Agency* (Princeton: Princeton University Press, 1996).
SHAPIRO, IAN (ed.), *Abortion: The Supreme Court Decisions* (Indianapolis: Hackett, 1995).
SHORTER, EDWARD, *A History of Psychiatry: From the Era of the Asylum to the Age of Prozac* (New York: Wiley, 1997).
SINGER, PETER, *Practical Ethics* (Cambridge: Cambridge University Press, 1979).
—— (ed.), *Applied Ethics* (Oxford University Press, 1986).
—— (ed.), *A Companion to Ethics* (Oxford: Blackwell, 1991).
—— (ed.), *Ethics* (Oxford: Oxford University Press, 1994).
—— *Rethinking Life and Death: The Collapse of our Traditional Ethics* (Oxford: Oxford University Press, 1995).
SKEGG, P. D. G., *Law, Ethics and Medicine: Studies in Medical Law*, rev. edn. (Oxford: Clarendon Press, 1988).
SKRABANEK, PETR, *The Death of Humane Medicine and the Rise of Coercive Healthism* (Bury St Edmunds: Social Affairs Unit, 1994).
—— and MCCORMICK, JAMES, *Follies and Fallacies in Medicine*, 2nd edn. (Chippenham: Tarragon Press, 1992).

SMART, J. J. C., and WILLIAMS, BERNARD, *Utilitarianism: For and Against* (Cambridge: Cambridge University Press, 1973).

STANWORTH, MICHELLE (ed.), *Reproductive Technologies: Gender, Motherhood and Medicine* (Cambridge: Polity Press, 1987).

STEINBOCK, BONNIE, *Life before Birth: The Moral and Legal Status of Embryos and Fetuses* (New York: Oxford University Press, 1992).

—— and NORCROSS, ALASTAIR (eds.), *Killing and Letting Die*, 2nd edn. (Bronx, NY: Fordham University Press, 1994).

STOCKER, MICHAEL, *Plural and Conflicting Values* (Oxford: Clarendon Press, 1990).

STRONG, CARSON, *Ethics in Reproductive and Perinatal Medicine: A New Framework* (New Haven: Yale University Press, 1997).

STRUMPEL, BURKHARD (ed.), *Subjective Elements of Well-Being* (Paris: OECD, 1974).

SULLIVAN, R. J., *An Introduction to Kant's Ethics* (Cambridge: Cambridge University Press, 1994).

SUMNER, L. W., *Abortion and Moral Theory* (Princeton: Princeton University Press, 1981).

—— *Welfare, Happiness, and Ethics* (Oxford: Oxford University Press, 1996).

TEICHMAN, JENNY, *Social Ethics: A Student's Guide* (Oxford: Blackwell, 1996).

THOMPSON, I. (ed.), *Dilemmas of Dying: A Study in the Ethics of Terminal Care* (Edinburgh: Edinburgh University Press, 1979).

TOOLEY, MICHAEL, *Abortion and Infanticide* (Oxford: Oxford University Press, 1983).

VEATCH, ROBERT M., *Medical Ethics*, 2nd edn. (Sudbury, Mass.: Jones & Bartlett, 1997).

WALTERS, LEROY, and PALMER, JULIE GAGE, *The Ethics of Human Gene Therapy* (Oxford: Oxford University Press, 1997).

WALTON, DOUGLAS N., *Informal Logic: A Handbook for Critical Argumentation* (Cambridge: Cambridge University Press, 1989; repr. 1994).

WARNOCK, MARY, *A Question of Life: The Warnock Report on Human Fertilisation and Embryology* (Oxford: Blackwell, 1985).

WESTON, ANTHONY, *A Rulebook for Arguments*, 2nd edn. (Indianapolis: Hackett, 1992).

—— *A Practical Companion to Ethics* (Oxford: Oxford University Press, 1996).

WILLIAMS, BERNARD, *Morality: An Introduction to Ethics* (Cambridge: Cambridge University Press, 1972).

—— *Problems of the Self: Philosophical Papers 1956–1972* (Cambridge: Cambridge University Press, 1973).

—— *Moral Luck* (Cambridge: Cambridge University Press, 1981).

—— *Ethics and the Limits of Philosophy* (London: Fontana, 1985).

—— *Shame and Necessity* (Berkeley: University of California Press, 1993).

—— *Making Sense of Humanity and Other Philosophical Papers* (Cambridge: Cambridge University Press, 1995).

WOLFF, R., *Understanding Rawls* (Princeton: Princeton University Press, 1977).

YOUNG, ROBERT, *Personal Autonomy: Beyond Negative and Positive Liberty* (New York: St Martin's Press, 1986).

GOOD AND ACCESSIBLE GENERAL INTRODUCTIONS TO MORAL PHILOSOPHY

FINNIS, JOHN, *Natural Law and Natural Rights* (Oxford: Oxford University Press, 1980).

Foot, Philippa, *Virtues and Vices* (Oxford: Blackwell, 1978).

Fried, Charles, *Right and Wrong* (Cambridge, Mass.: Harvard University Press, 1978).

Glover, Jonathan, *Causing Death and Saving Lives* (Harmondsworth: Pelican, 1977).

—— *What Sort of People Should There Be?* (Harmondsworth: Pelican, 1984).

Häyry, Matti, *Liberal Utilitarianism and Applied Ethics* (London: Routledge, 1994).

Jones, Peter, *Rights* (London: Macmillan, 1994).

Leaman, Oliver, *Death and Loss: Compassionate Approaches in the Classroom* (London: Cassell, 1995).

Lindley, Richard, *Autonomy* (London: Macmillan, 1986).

Mackie, J. L. *Ethics* (Harmondsworth: Pelican, 1977).

Midgley, Mary, *Heart and Mind* (London: Methuen, 1983).

Mill, J. S., *Utilitarianism and On Liberty*, in Mary Warnock (ed.), *Utilitarianism* (London: Fontana, 1972).

Nagel, Tom, *Mortal Questions* (Cambridge: Cambridge University Press, 1979).

Oderburg, David, *Moral Theory* (Oxford: Blackwell, 2000).

—— *Applied Ethics* (Oxford, Blackwell, 2000).

Rachels, James (ed.), *Ethical Theory* (Oxford: Oxford University Press, 1998).

Radcliffe Richards, Janet, *The Sceptical Feminist* (Harmondsworth: Penguin, 1982).

Raz, Joseph, *The Morality of Freedom* (Oxford: Oxford University Press, 1968).

Singer, Peter, *Practical Ethics* (Cambridge: Cambridge University Press, 1979).

Sorell, Tom, and Hendry, John, *Business Ethics* (Oxford: Butterworth-Heinemann, 1994).

Tooley, Michael, *Abortion and Infanticide* (Oxford: Oxford University Press, 1983).

Williams, Bernard, *Moral Luck* (Cambridge: Cambridge University Press, 1981).

—— *Ethics and the Limits of Philosophy* (London: Fontana, 1986).

TOPICAL BIBLIOGRAPHY (HIGHLY SELECTED)

The Value of Life

Dworkin, Ronald, *Life's Dominion* (London: HarperCollins, 1993).

Harris, J., *The Value of Life* (London: Routledge, 1985), esp. chs. 1, 7, and 8.

Kleinig, John, *Valuing Life* (Princeton: Princeton University Press, 1991).

Parfit, Derek *Reasons and Persons* (Oxford: Clarendon Press, 1984).

Embryo Experimentation and Use

Austyn, J. M. (ed.), *New Prospects for Medicine* (Oxford: Oxford University Press, 1988).

Caplan, Arthur L., 'Should Fetuses or Infants be Utilized as Organ Donors?', *Bioethics*, 1/2 (Apr. 1987).

Clarke, P. A. B., and Linzey, A., *Research on Embryos* (London: Lester Crook Academic, 1988).

Dawson, Karen, 'Segmentation and Moral Status *in Vivo* and *in Vitro*: A Scientific Perspective', *Bioethics*, 2/1 (Jan. 1988).

Dunstan, G. R., and Seller, M. J., *The Status of the Human Embryo* (Oxford: King Edward's Hospital Fund for London and Oxford University Press, 1988).

FLEMING, LORETTE, 'The Moral Status of the Foetus: A Reappraisal', *Bioethics*, 1/1 (1987).

HARRIS, JOHN, '*In Vitro* Fertilization: The Ethical Issues', *Philosophical Quarterly*, 33/ 132 (July 1983).

—— 'Full Humans and Empty Morality', *Philosophical Quarterly*, 35/138 (Jan. 1985).

—— and HOLM, SØREN, *The Future of Human Reproduction*, (Oxford: Oxford University Press, 1998).

LEE, BOB, and MORGAN, DERECK, *Birthrights: Law and Ethics at the Beginnings of Life* (London: Croom Helm, 1988).

MCCULLAGH, PETER, *The Foetus as Transplant Donor* (Chichester: Wiley, 1987).

ROWLAND, ROBYN, 'Making Women Visible in the Embryo Experimentation Debate', *Bioethics*, 1/2 (Apr. 1987).

WALTERS, WILLIAM, and SINGER, PETER, *Test-Tube Babies* (Melbourne: Oxford University Press, 1982).

WARNOCK, MARY, '*In Vitro* Fertilization: The Ethical Issues, II', *Philosophical Quarterly*, 33/132 (July 1983).

WEIL, WILLIAMS B., and BENJAMIN, MARTIN (eds.), *Ethical Issues at the Outset of Life* (Oxford: Blackwell Scientific Publications, 1987).

YOXEN, EDWARD, *Unnatural Selection?* (London: Heinemann, 1986).

Abortion and Infanticide

DWORKIN, RONALD, *Life's Dominion* (London: HarperCollins, 1993).

HARE, R. M., 'Abortion and the Golden Rule', in his *Essays in Biomedical Ethics* (Oxford: Clarendon Press, 1993), ch. 7.

THOMSON, J. J., 'A Defense of Abortion', in Peter Singer (ed.), *Applied Ethics* (Oxford: Oxford University Press, 1986), ch. IV.

—— 'Abortion: Whose Right?', *Boston Review*, 20/3 (Summer 1995).

TOOLEY, M., *Abortion and Infanticide* (Oxford: Clarendon Press, 1983).

—— 'Abortion and Infanticide', in Peter Singer (ed.), *Applied Ethics* (Oxford: Oxford University Press, 1986), ch. V.

Acts and Omissions

FOOT, P., 'Morality, Action and Outcome', in T. Honderich (ed.), *Morality and Objectivity* (London: Routledge, 1985), esp. 23–9.

KAMM, F., 'Harming, Not Aiding and Positive Rights', *Philosophy and Public Affairs*, 15 (1986).

KAMM, J., and HARRIS, J., 'The Doctrine of Triple Effect', *Proceedings of the Aristotelian Society*, suppl. 74 (2000).

RACHELS, J., 'Killing and Starving to Death', *Philosophy*, 54 (1979).

SEARLE, J., 'The Intentionality of Intention and Action', *Cognitive Science*, 4 (1980).

THOMSON, J. J., 'Killing, Letting Die and the Trolley Problem', *Monist* (1976).

Euthanasia

DWORKIN, R., 'Do we have a Right to Die?', in his *Freedom's Law* (Oxford: Oxford University Press, 1996), ch. 5.

FOOT, P., 'Euthanasia', *Philosophy & Public Affairs*, 6 (1977).

KEOWN, J. (ed.), *Euthanasia Examined* (Cambridge: Cambridge University Press, 1995), chs. 1–6 (exchange between Finnis and Harris).

Harm to Future People

FISHKIN, J., 'The Limits of Intergenerational Justice', in P. Laslett and J. Fishkin (eds.), *Justice between Age Groups and Generations* (New Haven: Yale University Press, 1992).
GLOVER, J., *Causing Death and Saving Lives* (London: Penguin, 1977), ch. 4.
HEYD, DAVID, *Genethics* (Berkeley: University of California Press, 1992).
KITCHER, P., *The Lives to Come* (London: Penguin, 1996), chs. 8, 9, and 10.
PARFIT, D., *Reasons and Persons* (Oxford: Oxford University Press, 1984), chs. 16 and 17.

Preventing Disability: Gene Testing, Gene Therapy, and Selective Terminations

DYSON, A. O., and HARRIS, J. (eds.), *Ethics and Biotechnology* (London: Routledge, 1994), chs. 7 and 8.
GLOVER, J., 'Future People, Disability and Screening', in P. Laslett and J. Fishkin (eds.), *Justice between Age Groups and Generations* (New Haven: Yale University Press, 1992).
HARRIS, J., 'Should we Attempt to Eradicate Disability?', *Public Understanding of Science*, 4 (1995).

Self-Ownership

JONES, P., 'Review Article: Two Conceptions of Justice', *British Journal of Political Science*, 25 (1995).
STEINER, H., *An Essay on Rights* (Oxford: Blackwell, 1994), ch. 3, sects. 3.1, 3.2, 3.3.

Markets in Organs and Blood

ARNESON, R., 'Commodification and Commercial Surrogacy', *Philosophy & Public Affairs*, 21 (1992).
ERIN, CHARLES, A., and HARRIS, JOHN, 'A Monopsonistic Market', in I. Robinson (ed.), *The Social Consequences of Life and Death under High Technology Medicine* (Manchester: Manchester University Press, 1994).
SATZ, D., 'Markets in Women's Reproductive Labor', *Philosophy & Public Affairs*, 21 (1992).

Rights

DWORKIN, R., *Taking Rights Seriously* (Cambridge, Mass.: Harvard University Press, 1977), chs. 7 and 12.
RAZ, J., 'Professor Dworkin's Theory of Rights', *Political Studies*, 26 (1978).
WALDRON, J. (ed.), *Theories of Rights* (Oxford: Oxford University Press, 1984), essays by Dworkin, Mackie, and Raz.
—— 'Liberal Rights: Two Sides of the Coin', in his *Liberal Rights: Collected Papers 1981–1991* (Cambridge: Cambridge University Press, 1993).

Consequentialism and Deontology

MACKIE, J., *Ethics: Inventing Right and Wrong* (London: Penguin, 1977), ch. 7.

NAGEL, T., 'The Limits of Objectivity', in S. McMurrin (ed.), *The Tanner Lectures on Human Values* (Cambridge: Cambridge University Press, 1980).

PARFIT, D., *Reasons and Persons* (Oxford: Oxford University Press, 1984), sects. 10–18, 21–4, 36–44.

RAZ, J., *The Morality of Freedom* (Oxford: Clarendon Press, 1984), ch. 11.

WILLIAMS, B., and SEN, A. (eds.), *Utilitarianism and Beyond* (Cambridge: Cambridge University Press, 1982), introd.

The Survival Lottery

DUXBURY, NEIL, *Random Justice* (Oxford: Clarendon Press, 1999).

GOODWIN, BARBARA, *Justice by Lottery* (New York: Harvester Wheatsheaf, 1992).

HARRIS, J., 'The Survival Lottery', in Peter Singer (ed.), *Applied Ethics* (Oxford: Oxford University Press, 1986).

NAGEL, T., *Mortal Questions* (Cambridge: Cambridge University Press, 1979).

Autonomy and Informed Consent

FEINBERG, J., *Harm to Self* (Oxford: Oxford University Press, 1986), chs. 25 and 26.

RAZ, J., *The Morality of Freedom* (Oxford: Clarendon Press, 1984), pt. 5.

——— 'Autonomy, Toleration and the Harm Principle', in S. Mendus (ed.), *Justifying Toleration: Conceptual and Historical Perspectives* (Cambridge: Cambridge University Press, 1988).

Experimentation on Humans and Animals

HARRIS, JOHN, 'Research on Human Subjects: Exploitation and Global Principles of Ethics', in Andrew D. E. Lewis and Michael Freeman (eds.), *Current Legal Issue, iii: Law and Medicine* (Oxford: Oxford University Press, 2000).

——— 'Ethical Issues in Geriatric Medicine', in R. Tallis *et al.* (eds.), *Textbook of Geriatric Medicine*, 5th edn. (Edinburgh: Churchill Livingstone, 1998).

SINGER, P., 'All Animals are Equal', in P. Singer (ed.), *Applied Ethics* (Oxford: Oxford University Press, 1986), ch. XIII.

——— *Practical Ethics* (Cambridge: Cambridge University Press, 1993), chs. 4 and 5.

Quality of Life Measures

BROCK, D., 'Quality of Life Measures in Health Care', in M. Nussbaum and A. Sen (eds.), *The Quality of Life* (Oxford: Oxford University Press, 1993).

DWORKIN, R., 'What is Equality? Part I: Equality of Welfare', *Philosophy and Public Affairs*, 10 (1981).

SINGER, P., *Rethinking Life and Death* (Oxford: Oxford University Press, 1996). chs. 7 and 8.

Macro and Micro Allocation of Health Care Resources

CUBBON, J., 'The Principle of QALY Maximization as the Basis for Allocating Health Care Resources', *Journal of Medical Ethics*, 17 (1991).

DANIELS, N., *Just Health Care* (Cambridge: Cambridge University Press, 1985), chs. 2, 3, 4, 7.

—— *Justice and Justification* (Cambridge: Cambridge University Press, 1996), chs. 9 and 11.

DWORKIN, R., 'What is Equality? Part II: Equality of Resources', *Philosophy & Public Affairs*, 10 (1981).

—— 'Justice in the Distribution of Health Care', *McGill Law Review*, 38 (1993).

GOSTIN, LAWRENCE O., *Public Health Law* (Berkeley: University of California Press, 2000).

HARRIS, J., 'Unprincipled QALYs: A Response to Cubbon', *Journal of Medical Ethics*, 17 (1991).

—— 'Double Jeopardy and the Veil of Ignorance: A Reply', *Journal of Medical Ethics*, 21 (1995).

MCKIE, J., 'Double Jeopardy, the Equal Value of Lives and the Veil of Ignorance: A Rejoinder to Harris', *Journal of Medical Ethics*, 22 (1996).

SAVVLESCU, JULIAN, 'Consequentialism, Reasons, Value and Justice', *Bioethics*, vol. 12, No. 3 (July 1998).

SINGER, P., MCKIE, J., KUHSE, H., and RICHARDSON, J., 'Double Jeopardy and the Use of QALYs in Health Care Allocation', *Journal of Medical Ethics*, 21 (1995).

WIGGINS, D., 'Claims of Need', in his *Needs, Values and Truth* (Oxford: Blackwell, 1987), ch. 1.

Paternalism, Perfectionism, and Neutrality

DWORKIN, R., 'Liberalism', in his *A Matter of Principle* (Cambridge, Mass.: Harvard University Press, 1985), ch. 8.

FEINBERG, J., *Harm to Self* (Oxford: Oxford University Press, 1986), chs. 17 and 18.

RAZ, J., *The Morality of Freedom* (Oxford: Clarendon Press, 1986), chs. 5 and 6.

Health Promotion and Lifestyles

BRAZIER, MARGARET, and HARRIS, JOHN, 'Public Health and Private Lives', *Medical Law Review*, 4 (Summer 1996).

ROEMER, J. 'Equality and Responsibility', *Democracy Project* (Apr.–May 1995) (and replies to Roemer).

WIKLER, D., 'Persuasion and Coercion for Health: Issues in Government Efforts to Change Life Style', *Milbank Memorial Fund Quarterly: Health and Society*, 56/3 (1978).

ACKNOWLEDGEMENTS

We are grateful to the following for permission to use copyright material.

BMJ PUBLISHING GROUP, for Søren Holm, 'Not Just Autonomy: The Principles of American Biomedical Ethics', *Journal of Medical Ethics*, 21/6 (1995).

COLUMBIA UNIVERSITY PRESS, for Eric Rakowski, 'Taking and Saving Lives' in 93 Colum. L. Rev. 1063, 1993. Reprinted by permission of the publisher and the author.

HARPER COLLINS PUBLISHERS, for Ronald Dworkin, *Life's Dominion*. Published by Harper Collins, 1993.

THE HASTINGS CENTER, for Daniel Callahan, 'Terminating Life Sustaining Treatment of the Demented' in *Hastings Center Report* (Nov.–Dec. 1995).

JOHNS HOPKINS UNIVERSITY PRESS, for T. L. Beauchamp, 'Principlism and its Alleged Competitors' in *Kennedy Institute of Ethics Journal* 5:3, 1995 181–92; Norman Daniels, 'Health Care Needs and Distributive Justice' in *Philosophy and Public Affairs* 10:2, 1981; Allen Buchanan, 'Advance Directives and the Personal Identity Problem' in *Philosophy and Public Affairs,* 1988; Judith Jarvis Thomson, 'A Defense of Abortion' in *Philosophy and Public Affairs* 1:1, 1971, 47–66; Warren Quinn, 'Abortion: Identity and Loss' in *Philosophy and Public Affairs* 13:1, 1984, 2454. All Copyright © The Johns Hopkins University Press. Reprinted with the permission of The Johns Hopkins University Press.

TAYLOR AND FRANCIS, for John Harris, 'The Survival Lottery' in *Violence and Responsibility*. Published by Routledge, 1980

UNIVERSITY OF KANSAS, for Derek Parfit, 'Equality or Priority' in *The Lindley Lecture,* University of Kansas, 21 Nov. 1991. Published by the Department of Philosophy, University of Kansas, 1995.

JOHN WILEY AND SONS, LTD., for Raanan Gillon, 'Telling the Truth, Confidentiality, Consent and Respect for Autonomy' in *Philosophy and Medical Ethics.* Published by John Wiley & Sons, Ltd., 1985. Reprinted by permission of the publisher.

YALE UNIVERSITY PRESS, for Jonathan Glover, 'Future People, Disability and Screening' in J. Fishkin and P. Laslett (eds.), *Justice Between Age Groups and Generations.* Published by Yale University Press, 1992.

INDEX OF NAMES